P9-CEG-132

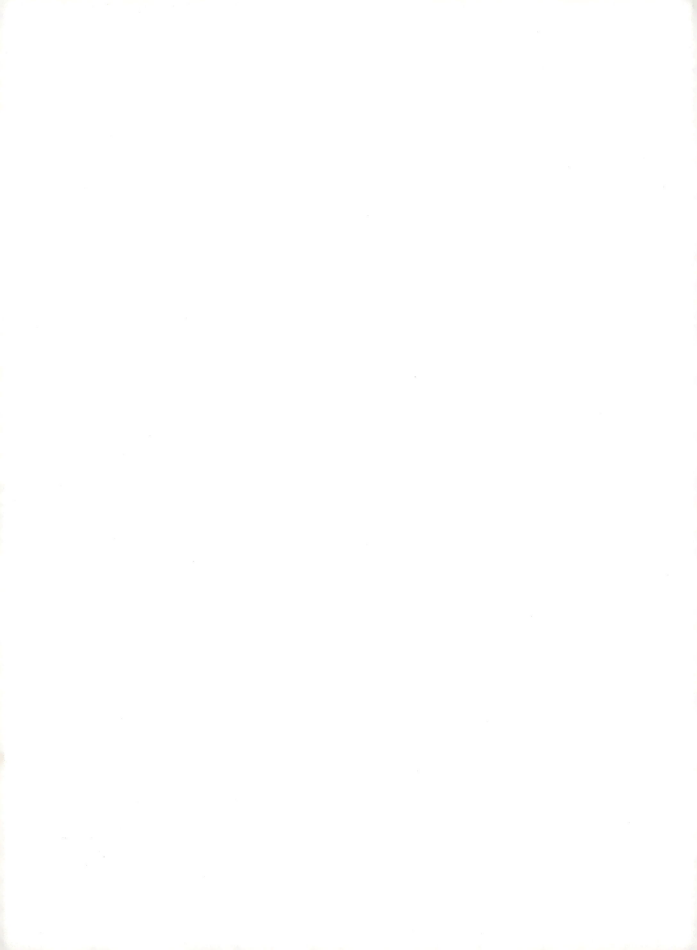

THE ULTIMATE 2015
Women's Guide to Beating Disease
AND LIVING A HAPPY, ACTIVE LIFE

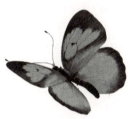

FROM THE EDITORS OF BOTTOM LINE PUBLICATIONS

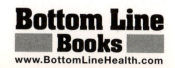

Bottom Line Books

www.BottomLineHealth.com

**The Ultimate Women's Guide to Beating Disease
and Living a Happy, Active Life**

Copyright © 2015 by Boardroom® Inc.

10 9 8 7 6 5 4 3 2 1

All rights reserved. No part of this book may be reproduced, scanned, distributed
or transmitted in any form, by any means, electronic or mechanical, without
written permission from the publisher.

ISBN 0-88723-723-1

Bottom Line Books® publishes the advice of expert authorities in many fields. These opinions
may at times conflict as there are often different approaches to solving problems. The use
of a book is not a substitute for legal, accounting, investment, health or any other professional
services. Consult competent professionals for answers to your specific questions.

Offers, prices, rates, addresses, telephone numbers and Web sites
listed in this book are accurate at the time of publication,
but they are subject to frequent change.

Bottom Line Books® is a registered trademark of
Boardroom® Inc.
281 Tresser Boulevard, Stamford, CT 06901

www.BottomLineHealth.com

Bottom Line Books® is an imprint of Boardroom® Inc., publisher of print periodicals,
e-letters and books. We are dedicated to bringing you the best information from the most
knowledgeable sources in the world. Our goal is to help you gain greater wealth,
better health, more wisdom, extra time and increased happiness.

Printed in the United States of America

CONTENTS

4 • CHOLESTEROL: A STICKY PROBLEM FOR WOMEN

5 • EVERYDAY HEART-HEALTH SECRETS

6 • LIFESAVING TREATMENTS

PART 2: CANCER

7 • WHAT WOMEN NEED TO KNOW ABOUT LUNG CANCER

8 • BREAST CANCER BREAKTHROUGHS

9 • LOWER YOUR RISK OF COLORECTAL CANCER

PART 4: CHRONIC LOWER RESPIRATORY DISEASES

14 • KEEP YOUR LUNGS HEALTHY FOR LIFE

15 • STOP SMOKING NOW

PART 5: ALZHEIMERS

16 • ALZHEIMER'S RISKS AND WARNINGS

17 • STOP MEMORY LOSS

PART 6: PHYSICAL INJURY

18 • SECRETS TO STAYING STEADY ON YOUR FEET

PART 7: DIABETES

19 • BEST WAYS TO CONTROL— EVEN CURE—DIABETES

PART 8: PNEUMONIA AND INFLUENZA

20 • EVERYTHING YOU NEED TO KNOW ABOUT PNEUMONIA

PREFACE

We are proud to bring to you *The Ultimate Women's Guide to Beating Disease and Living a Happy, Active Life*. This essential volume features trustworthy and actionable life-saving information from the best health experts in the world—information that will help women beat the conditions that are most deadly to them.* In the following chapters you'll find the latest discoveries, best treatments and scientifically proven remedies to keep you living a long, happy and active life.

Whether it's heart care, the latest on lung cancer, breast cancer prevention, breakthrough osteoporosis treatments or cutting-edge nutritional advice, the editors of Bottom Line Publications talk to the experts—from top women's health doctors to research scientists to leading alternative care practitioners—who are creating the true innovations in health care.

How do we find all these top-notch medical professionals? Over the past four decades, we have built a network of literally thousands of leading physicians in both alternative and conventional medicine. They are affiliated with the premier medical institutions and the best universities throughout the world.

We read the important medical journals and follow the latest research that is reported at medical conferences. And we regularly talk to our advisors in major teaching hospitals, private practices and government health agencies for their insider perspective.

The Ultimate Women's Guide to Beating Disease and Living a Happy, Active Life is a result of our ongoing research and connection with these experts, and is a distillation of their latest findings and advice. We trust that you will glean new, helpful and affordable information about the health topics that concern you and your family.

As a reader of a Bottom Line book, please be assured that you are receiving well-researched information from a trusted source.

But, please use prudence in health matters. Always speak to your physician before taking vitamins, supplements or over-the-counter medication…changing your diet…or beginning an exercise program. If you experience side effects from any regimen, contact your doctor immediately.

Be well,
The Editors, Bottom Line Publications
Stamford, Connecticut

*"Leading Causes of Death in Females," Centers for Disease Control and Prevention (*http://www.cdc.gov/women/lcod/2010/index.htm*).

HEART DISEASE

Cardiovascular disease remains the leading cause of death among women, surpassing all cancers. In fact, one in every four women dies from heart disease.

Knowing the signs and symptoms of a heart attack are crucial, but equally, or perhaps even more important, is understanding how to keep your heart healthy. In the following section, you'll discover the most accurate heart tests for women, how your mammogram might reveal if you're at risk for heart disease, how to tell if your heartbeat is healthy, and how you can predict a heart attack—even if you don't have symptoms. Read on to find out what puts women at risk for blood clots, and the best ways to prevent them.

Did you know that as a woman, you should probably talk to your doctor about controlling your blood pressure even if it is just 125/80? Or that after menopause, women need to take extra care with cholesterol? Before menopause, estrogen helps protect women from high cholesterol by raising levels of HDL (good) cholesterol. However, after menopause, harmful triglyceride levels increase. Although postmenopausal hormone therapy (PHT) may help women fight some conditions, the American Heart Association does not recommend it for cardiovascular protection.*

Fortunately the news is not all bad: Even if heart disease runs in your family, there are little things you can do every day that can practically erase your genetic risk of cardiovascular disease. If you do have a heart attack, or have coronary artery disease, the type of treatment you receive will often determine how you live the rest of your life. That's why it is critical that you know the best options and the latest procedures reviewed here.

*http://www.heart.org/HEARTORG/Conditions/Cholesterol/UnderstandYourRiskforHighCholesterol/Women-and-Cholesterol_UCM_305565_Article.jsp

Chapter 1

HEART HELP FOR WOMEN

Heart Attack—The Red Flags That Too Often Get Overlooked

Comedienne and former talk-show host Rosie O'Donnell recently became one of the 195,000 Americans each year who experiences a heart attack and does not even know it. O'Donnell, then age 50, reportedly did not realize what was happening to her when she became nauseated and started to feel clammy, two of the subtle, often-missed heart attack symptoms that are frequently experienced by women. (Other "atypical" heart attack symptoms in women include back or jaw pain, extreme fatigue, dizziness and light-headedness.)

An even more insidious risk: It's common for women to fail to tell their doctors about elusive heart disease symptoms that often precede a heart attack. If recognized, these symptoms often can be effectively treated to stop a heart attack before it occurs.

What Gets Missed

Most people do not realize just how important it is to report new symptoms during a doctor visit. With heart disease, in particular, there can be such a wide range of mild and/or fleeting changes in the heart, that the way you describe any possible abnormality to your doctor can mean the difference between an accurate diagnosis and a missed one. That's why you always should be sure to include details whenever you tell your physician about a symptom.

Examples: Don't just say that you're short of breath—do you feel this way all the time or just when you're climbing stairs? And don't just say that you've noticed changes in your heartbeat—is it too fast, too slow, fluttery, irregular, etc.?

Other important symptoms that should be discussed…

• **Intermittent chest pain.** The majority of heart attacks are preceded by the development of atherosclerosis, accumulations of fatty deposits in the arteries that inhibit the normal flow of blood and oxygen. When these deposits restrict blood flow to the heart, the result can be myocardial ischemia, a condition that typically causes chest pain due to a lack of oxygen.

Antonio M. Gotto, Jr., MD, DPhil, dean emeritus, Lewis Thomas University Professor and cochairman of the board of overseers for Weill Cornell Medical College in New York City. He is also coauthor of *The Living Heart in the 21st Century* (Prometheus).

Main symptom: Sharp chest pains or pressure that can last anywhere from a few seconds to about five minutes. This type of chest pain, known as angina, usually occurs during physical exertion, such as climbing stairs or working in the yard. It also can occur during cold weather, which causes blood vessels to constrict, or during stressful situations, which can increase demands on the heart and cause it to beat faster.

Exceptions: Angina isn't always painful, and you won't necessarily feel it in your chest. Patients with myocardial ischemia affecting the base of the heart might have abdominal discomfort instead of chest pain. (Some people mistake it for heartburn.) People with diabetes who have nerve damage, or those with a high pain threshold, might have no pain at all.

My advice: Suspect angina when you have chest and/or abdominal pain that occurs only during physical exertion. Rest if you experience pain in these areas. The pain should go away within five minutes if angina is the cause. In this case, call your doctor promptly to make an appointment. Call 911 if the pain isn't gone after five minutes.

• **Shortness of breath (dyspnea).** It is one of the main symptoms of heart disease, yet patients don't always mention it because they attribute it to other factors, such as smoking, advancing age and/or a lack of exercise.

Important: Shortness of breath can be caused by atypical angina. These angina patients do not experience pain as the main symptom. They are more likely to have episodes of breathlessness, weakness, fatigue and/or sweating. This is particularly common in older adults and those with diabetes.

My advice: To distinguish "normal" shortness of breath from a heart-related condition, ask yourself whether the dyspnea is out of proportion to what you're doing.

For example, people do not normally get winded from unloading the dishwasher or walking to the mailbox. If you do—and you haven't been diagnosed with a condition to explain it, such as lung disease—see your doctor. Also, any change in your tolerance for exercise could indicate a heart problem. If you experience unexplained shortness of breath or a significant change in your tolerance for exercise, see your doctor as soon as possible.

Call 911 if you have severe shortness of breath that comes on suddenly, especially if it's accompanied by chest pain, fainting or nausea—these could be signs of heart attack or pulmonary embolism.

• **Palpitations.** Everyone has occasional changes in the heart's pumping rhythm. You might notice that your heartbeat is rapid, pounding or fluttering, particularly during exercise or when you're stressed. The heart is probably still pumping blood effectively, but you'll want to talk to your doctor anyway.

The risk: Heart palpitations can indicate that you have arrhythmias, problems with the heart's electrical systems. A heartbeat that's too rapid (tachycardia), too slow (bradycardia) or irregular (atrial fibrillation, among others) can be life-threatening.

Example: Atrial fibrillation is common in older adults. The heart usually regains its normal rhythm within a few seconds, but not always. There's an increased risk for stroke if the irregular heartbeat continues for more than 24 hours.

My advice: Call 911 immediately if palpitations are accompanied by other symptoms, such as fainting, heavy sweating or extreme anxiety—all of which can signal a heart attack or an impending one. If you have palpitations without other symptoms, make an appointment to see your doctor as soon as possible.

• **Leg pain.** It's normal to experience occasional "charley horses," cramps in the muscles in your legs. It's not normal to have frequent pain in a foot, calf, thigh or buttock when you're walking or doing other activities. Leg pain that develops during exertion is often a sign of peripheral artery disease, a form of atherosclerosis that occurs in arteries in the leg. Patients with peripheral artery disease have a high risk of having (or developing) cardiovascular disease.

My advice: If you notice aching, cramping or pain in one or both legs during physical activity, see your doctor. Peripheral artery disease also can cause a sensation of "burning," tingling or numbness in the legs and/or feet. These symptoms indicate that the leg isn't getting enough oxygen-rich blood—and there's a good chance that your heart arteries are also at risk. With advanced peripheral artery disease, the symptoms occur even when the body is at rest.

•**Hair loss on the legs/feet.** Sedentary patients with peripheral artery disease might not notice leg pain or cramps. However, they might have other "silent" symptoms that indicate impaired circulation, including hair loss on the legs and/or feet.

My advice: See your physician as soon as possible if you notice hair loss on the legs or feet or one of the other possible signs of peripheral artery disease—one leg/foot that is colder than the other…sores that are slow to heal…a "shine" to the skin…or thick, slow-growing toenails. The symptoms may occur in both legs, but patients often report that only one leg is affected.

When to Call 911…

Severe chest pain (often described as "crushing" pain) is the heart attack symptom that everyone knows about—and fears. You most likely are having a heart attack if you have severe, unexplained chest pain that lasts longer than 20 minutes. But do not wait that long before getting help.

Call 911 even if your chest pain has lasted just a few minutes—or if you do not have chest pain but are experiencing other symptoms that could indicate a heart attack, such as unexplained nausea, breaking out in a cold sweat, dizziness, shortness of breath or extreme anxiety accompanied by a feeling of impending doom.

Emergency personnel may advise you to chew aspirin while you wait for help to arrive, so always keep a bottle of aspirin handy.

Heart Attack Can Be Predicted—Even Without Symptoms

Scientists gave EKGs to 2,192 healthy adults (age 70 and older) and followed their health outcomes for eight years.

Result: Those whose EKGs showed abnormalities—but no chest pain or other symptoms—were at increased risk for heart attacks and coronary heart disease.

If you have an EKG that shows any abnormalities: Talk to your doctor about what you can do to decrease your risk for heart disease, such as being screened for high blood pressure, high cholesterol and diabetes.

Reto Auer, MD, research fellow, department of epidemiology and biostatistics, University of California, San Francisco.

What Your Age at Menopause Means for Your Heart

Dhananjay Vaidya, PhD, MPH, assistant professor in the division of general internal medicine at the Johns Hopkins University School of Medicine in Baltimore and coauthor of a study on heart risk published in *Menopause.*

What's not to love about menopause? No more period pimples, belly bloat, monthly messes or birth control hassles—hurrah! But one aspect of menopause that's not so cheer-worthy is the increased risk for heart problems that it brings. The connection? When periods stop, production of heart-protecting estrogen decreases dramatically.

Now a recent study adds to that concern by highlighting the fact that women who reach menopause at a relatively young age are particularly likely to develop heart problems. Given that cardiovascular disease is the number-one killer of US women, we

5

can't afford to ignore these findings. *Here's the scoop…*

Previous research linked early menopause to heart disease in Caucasian women, but there has been little such info about risk among other ethnicities. So for the more recent study, researchers analyzed data on 2,509 women (ages 45 to 84) who were either non-Hispanic white…black…Chinese… or Hispanic. All were free of cardiovascular disease at the start of the study and were followed for an average of nearly five years.

Findings: 28% of the women reached menopause before age 46, either naturally or due to oophorectomy (surgical removal of the ovaries, often done in conjunction with hysterectomy). These women were more than twice as likely to suffer a fatal or nonfatal heart attack or stroke during the study as women who entered menopause later. This held true across all ethnicities and regardless of any other heart-related risk factors the women may have had.

If you're premenopausal: To help guard against early menopause, don't smoke—research shows that smokers reach menopause two years earlier, on average, than nonsmokers. Also, if your doctor suggests a hysterectomy, get a second opinion…and if surgical removal of your uterus truly is necessary, discuss whether you can keep your ovaries. This is particularly important for Hispanic and black women, who tend to hit menopause somewhat earlier than women of other ethnicities.

If you did reach menopause early: Though it's wise for everyone to follow a heart-healthy lifestyle, you should be especially careful about eating right, exercising regularly, maintaining an appropriate weight and not smoking. What about using hormone therapy (HT) to replace some of the estrogen lost at menopause? Whether HT helps or harms heart health is a subject of intense debate, though in this study, HT users did not have any cardiovascular advantage—and HT does increase the risk for breast cancer.

HPV May Raise Women's Cardiovascular Risks

Several types of the human papillomavirus cause cervical cancer—and new evidence suggests that women with certain strains of HPV are more than twice as likely to have a heart attack or stroke as women not infected with the strains. The HPV vaccines, which protect against certain cancers, have not yet been proven to have cardiovascular benefits.

Hsu-Ko Kuo, MD, MPH, medical resident, University of Texas Medical Branch, Galveston, and leader of a study of 2,450 women, ages 20 to 59, published in *Journal of the American College of Cardiology.*

Better bet: Be sure that your current doctor is aware of the age at which you reached menopause…and work with your physician to keep any other cardiovascular risk factors, such as blood pressure and cholesterol levels, well under control.

According to naturopathic physician Andrew L. Rubman, ND, medical director of the Southbury Clinic for Traditional Medicines in Southbury, Connecticut, certain nutritional supplements also have been shown to protect cardiovascular health. Ask your doctor about taking 200 mg to 300 mg of magnesium daily (as long as you don't have kidney problems)…and 3,000 mg a day of fish oil (as long as you are not on a blood thinner).

Yes, this all adds up to a bit of effort, but look at it this way—it's for a very good cause. Working at getting and staying healthy will result in a longer, healthier and happier life, which gives you all the more time to enjoy doing other things that make you happy!

Cardiac Screening Tests That Do More Harm Than Good

C. Noel Bairey Merz, MD, director of the Women's Heart Center and the Preventive and Rehabilitative Cardiac Center at Cedars-Sinai Heart Institute and professor of medicine at Cedars-Sinai Medical Center, all in Los Angeles.

Today, more American women die from heart disease than from all cancers combined—so it's tempting to try to protect yourself by getting cardiac screening tests during your annual checkup.

However: For women who have no signs or symptoms of heart problems and who are not at high risk for heart disease, certain screening tests are a waste of time and money.

Reasons: They are unlikely to provide information that is useful—and they even may be dangerous because they involve radiation.

In addition, false positive test results can lead to expensive and possibly dangerous follow-up tests.

Concern for women: The more radiation you receive over a lifetime, the higher your risk for cancer. Women are advised to get regular mammograms to screen for breast cancer. Because mammography uses X-rays, women's radiation exposure already tends to be higher than men's. That is why women must be especially wary of increasing their radiation exposure and consequent cancer risk with unnecessary cardiac testing.

Here's what women need to know about heart disease screening tests…

Tests to Avoid

In certain circumstances, cardiac diagnostic tests are potentially lifesaving and well worth the risks involved. The four tests described below may indeed be necessary if you have any signs or symptoms of heart problems, such as chest pain, irregular heartbeat, short-ness of breath, dizziness, fainting, or pain or swelling in the limbs.

These tests also may be appropriate if you have one or more factors that place you at high risk for heart disease—such as high blood pressure, high cholesterol, high triglycerides (a type of blood fat), diabetes, obesity, high-fat diet, sedentary lifestyle, smoking habit or family history of heart disease.

However: If you do not have any signs, symptoms or risk factors, there's no reason to get the four tests below. They can cost hundreds or thousands of dollars—and health insurance typically does not pay for them for screening purposes. So if your doctor recommends testing, ask for a clear and detailed explanation of why each test is being ordered in your particular case.

• **Coronary artery calcium (CAC) scan.** This checks for deposits of calcium that are associated with plaque in the coronary arteries. You lie on a table while a computed tomography (CT) scanner takes multiple X-rays from various angles and uses these to create a three-dimensional image. White spots suggest calcium deposits.

Problem: The National Cancer Institute reports that the average radiation exposure from having this test every five years would cause 62 additional cases of cancer per 100,000 women (and 42 additional cases per 100,000 men).

Also: CAC scans have not been shown to be effective at saving lives in people with no heart disease symptoms or significant risk factors.

• **CT angiogram.** The goal is to detect blockages of fatty plaque in the blood vessels or chambers of the heart. A tiny tube is inserted into your arm, then dye is injected to make blood vessels visible by X-ray. You may be given beta-blocker medication to slow your heart during the procedure.

Problem: This test is less accurate in women than in men because women's plaque tends to be more evenly distributed throughout the arteries.

Risks: There is radiation...the dye may cause an allergic reaction...or the beta-blocker may trigger asthma or slow the heart too much, leading to low blood pressure, fainting or (rarely) death.

•**Exercise electrocardiogram (ECG).** This provides a graphic record of the heart's electrical activity. Wires taped to your skin connect you to an ECG machine while you walk on a treadmill.

Problem: Because women's heart vessels differ somewhat from men's, an exercise ECG is less accurate at detecting large artery blockages in women. Though there is no radiation, the test is not worth the effort or expense for a patient without signs or symptoms of heart disease.

•**Cardiac ultrasound.** Also called an echocardiogram, or echo, this uses sound waves to generate a picture of the heart. A conductive gel is spread over your chest, then a handheld transducer is moved over the area to produce sound waves.

Problem: Though this test is safe and it helps diagnose the cause of existing heart disease, it does not reliably identify heart problems before symptoms develop. For this reason, the cardiac ultrasound is not a good general screening tool.

Tests Worth Doing

Every adult woman should be assessed annually for heart health.

How: During your routine physical, your doctor should record your height, weight, waist circumference and blood pressure...order fasting blood tests for glucose, cholesterol and triglyceride levels...and discuss your diet, exercise habits, alcohol consumption, cigarette use and family history. Based on these factors, your doctor calculates your risk for heart disease, heart attack and stroke.

If this annual evaluation indicates that your risk for heart disease may be elevated, your doctor may consider doing the following safe, radiation-free tests to get a clearer picture of your heart health...

•**Resting ECG.** This is an electrocardiogram taken while you lie quietly. It is able to identify atrial fibrillation, an irregular quivering of the heart muscle that increases stroke risk.

Insurance does pay if a physician orders this test for an approved indication. Unfortunately, many insurance companies now refuse to cover the test as part of a routine physical—so ask your doctor if you should consider getting it anyway and paying out-of-pocket.

Cost: $75 to $400, depending on your location and provider.

•**Carotid intima-media thickness (C-IMT) measurement.** The test uses ultrasound to measure the thickness of the arterial wall in the carotid artery in the neck, which is an indicator of plaque buildup. Repeating this test as directed by your physician may help detect changes in your cardiovascular health.

The test works as well for women as for men and can help your doctor determine whether you would benefit from taking a daily aspirin or statin drug.

Cost: $250 to $500, usually not covered by insurance. If you are at intermediate risk, your doctor may advise you to pay for this test if the results could help determine the best course of action.

•**High-sensitivity C-reactive protein test (hs-CRP).** The regular CRP blood test measures levels of a protein linked to inflammation, which in turn is linked to heart disease. The high-sensitivity version more accurately reveals when the protein concentrations are only slightly elevated, so it is more useful in predicting a healthy person's heart disease risk.

Among people whose hs-CRP levels are in the high end of the normal range, heart attack risk is one-and-a-half to four times higher than in people whose CRP is at the low end.

Cost: About $50, often covered by insurance.

Free self-assessment tool: To get an idea of your chances of developing heart disease within 10 years, check the online calculator from the National Heart, Lung and Blood Institute at *http://cvdrisk.nhlbi.nih.gov*.

Can Mammograms Screen for Heart Disease, Too?

Peter F. Schnatz, DO, associate chairman and residency program director in the department of obstetrics and gynecology at The Reading Hospital and Medical Center in Pennsylvania, and lead author of a study on 1,454 women.

Today we go for routine mammograms expecting to learn whether our breasts are healthy—but soon that test also may reveal whether we're at risk for heart disease, recent research suggests.

Background: Breast arterial calcification (BAC), or calcium buildup in breast arteries, is visible on 3% to 29% of regular mammograms but is not routinely included in mammography reports.

In the recent study, published in *Obstetrics & Gynecology*, women underwent mammograms and then were followed for five years. Coronary heart disease developed in 21% of women whose mammograms had revealed BAC, compared with only 5% of those without BAC. Women with BAC also were significantly more likely to suffer a stroke.

Surprising: The heart disease risk associated with BAC was even greater than that associated with better-known risk factors, such as high cholesterol, hypertension or family history of coronary heart disease!

Best: Ask your radiologist to include BAC status in your mammography report. Since no extra testing is needed, there should be no additional cost. While the ultimate meaning of BAC is not yet definitively known, the information may prove helpful, researchers say…and if you do have BAC, it is even more important to have your other heart disease

risk factors assessed. As usual, be sure to follow your doctor's recommendations on exercising, not smoking, and controlling diabetes, cholesterol and/or blood pressure. While these measures are unlikely to make BAC go away (since BAC probably is a marker for other factors), they will help reduce your overall heart risk.

How Antidepressants May Hurt Your Arteries

Amit J. Shah, MD, cardiology fellow, Emory University School of Medicine, Atlanta.

There's a little-known way that antidepressants may hurt your cardiovascular system—they may thicken your artery walls. Few studies to date have examined this phenomenon, yet it poses a serious health risk. Narrowed arteries raise your risk for heart attack and stroke. According to the National Institute of Mental Health, more women than men are likely to be diagnosed with depression in any given year.

At Emory University School of Medicine in Atlanta, cardiologist Amit J. Shah, MD, and his colleagues decided to study this topic because the potential connection between antidepressant use and heart disease has been poorly understood.

One Thickening, Sickening Problem

To rule out genetics as a factor, Dr. Shah and his colleagues analyzed people from one of the largest twin databases in the country—513 pairs of identical and fraternal male twins (average age 55). At the time of the research, about 16% of the men were taking antidepressants—all different kinds, though 60% of the antidepressants were selective serotonin reuptake inhibitors (SSRIs), such as *fluoxetine* (Prozac), *duloxetine* (Cymbalta) and *sertraline* (Zoloft). The researchers didn't record how long the men had been taking the medications or the exact dosages. They used ultrasound to take one measurement of the thickness of the linings of the mens' carotid arteries (the main arteries in the neck that supply blood to the brain).

What the study found: As we grow older, our arteries naturally thicken at the rate of about 10 microns (one millionth of a meter) per year, but Dr. Shah discovered that participants who had been taking any type of antidepressant had experienced substantially greater artery thickening. When the researchers looked at the 59 twin pairs in which one twin was taking an antidepressant and the other wasn't, the carotid artery lining was, on average, about 40 microns (about 5%) thicker in the twin taking the drug.

The men were not followed to see who developed cardiovascular disease and who didn't, but previous research has revealed that each 10-micron increase in carotid artery thickness is associated with a 1.8% increase in risk for cardiovascular disease, so that 40-micron increase in thickness could correlate to about a 7.2% increased risk for cardiovascular disease in the men who were on antidepressants. *Another way to look at it:* Their arteries were, in effect, four years older than their brothers' arteries, noted Dr. Shah.

This finding took into consideration other factors that can affect artery thickness, including alcohol and coffee intake, previous history of heart disease, history of post-traumatic stress disorder and depression. "A higher level of depressive symptoms was associated with higher artery thickness only in those taking antidepressants," said Dr. Shah. "Therefore, antidepressants may act synergistically with depressive symptoms to increase risk for artery thickness."

Why the Disheartening Effect?

Dr. Shah theorized why the antidepressants might have been associated with having thicker arteries. Antidepressants, of course, work by increasing levels of neurotransmitters. Yet while these chemicals act in your brain to relieve symptoms of depression, Dr. Shah said that they also may cause blood vessels elsewhere in the body to constrict or tighten, which can lead to thicker arteries.

Dr. Shah cautioned that this is an observational study—not a test of cause-and-effect—so we can't definitively conclude from it that antidepressants cause artery thickening. Further research is needed to confirm these results.

Weigh the Pros and Cons

So if you're on an antidepressant, what should you do? "No one taking antidepressants should stop taking them based solely on the results of this study," said Dr. Shah. That is undoubtedly true. But keep in mind that, like all drugs, antidepressants have side effects—some that we can see and feel (e.g., agitation, insomnia, sexual dysfunction) and perhaps others that we cannot. And if you're considering taking an antidepressant, consider natural treatment first, such as exercise, healthy eating and talk therapy. Sit down with your doctor and carefully discuss the pros and cons for your particular situation.

Is Your Heartbeat Healthy…or Not? What Women Must Know About Arrhythmia

Jennifer Cummings, MD, associate professor of medicine at Northeastern Ohio Universities College of Medicine in Rootstown, Ohio, and a cardiologist with City Cardiology Associates in Akron. She serves on the American College of Cardiology's Committee for Clinical Electrophysiology and is an ad hoc peer reviewer for *Journal of Cardiac Electrophysiology, Annals of Internal Medicine* and *Circulation*.

A 70-year-old woman recently woke feeling so dizzy that she couldn't walk or even sit up in bed. She phoned her son, a doctor, who told her to get to the ER stat. There she was diagnosed with a dangerously slow heartbeat, a condition called bradycardia.

A pacemaker fixed the problem, and she recovered—but her scare shows how truly vital a steady heartbeat is…and how much can go wrong with the heart's rhythm. And even though some people think of heart problems as mostly affecting men, the fact remains that heart disease is a leading cause of disability and the number-one killer of women in the US.

Has your heart ever "skipped" a beat? Or have you noticed that your heart was racing or fluttering? Occasional irregularities in the heart's rhythm, known as arrhythmias, generally are harmless for people without underlying heart problems. But some arrhythmias indicate a serious disruption in the heart's electrical pathways.

Example: More than 325,000 Americans die from sudden cardiac arrest each year. The impulses that regulate the heartbeat become too rapid, too chaotic or both—and the heart simply stops.

What you need to know now about arrhythmia…

Transmission Errors

The heart beats in an on-off rhythm, a cycle that allows the heart to fill with blood and then pump the blood through the body.

How it works: Each heartbeat originates in the sinoatrial node, a cluster of cells in the atria, the top chambers of the heart. Signals from the sinoatrial node cause the atria to contract and pump blood into the ventricles beneath. When the ventricles are full, that electrical signal crosses over a "bridge" to the bottom chambers, causing them to contract and push blood outward into the body.

When you feel as though your heart has "skipped" a beat, what most likely has happened is that either the atria or the ventricles pulsed prematurely. These are premature atrial contractions (PACs) or premature ventricular contractions (PVCs). This type of arrhythmia may not cause symptoms and doesn't need treatment—although anyone who gets it frequently should undergo testing to make sure that his/her heart is healthy.

Other common arrhythmias that can be more serious.…

Atrial Fibrillation (AF)

This is the most common serious arrhythmia in adults. It is suspected that nearly 50% of patients either have no symptoms or aren't bothered by the symptoms that they do experience.

What happens: Rather than producing a single, forceful beat, the atria "quiver" for a few minutes to more than an hour and can beat faster than 300 times a minute.

During these episodes, eddies of blood can cause a clot—the trigger of most strokes. Depending on other risk factors, the risk for a stroke in people with AF can be from 5% to 25% higher than in people without this condition.

Symptoms: Sensation of irregular or racing heartbeats…sometimes fatigue and shortness of breath.

Treatment: Anticoagulant therapy to lower the risk for stroke. A daily low-dose aspirin—81 milligrams (mg)—is enough for many patients. Those with a higher risk for stroke will need stronger anticlotting agents, such as *warfarin* (Coumadin) or *dabigatran* (Pradaxa). *Other treatments…*

•**Medications that slow the heart rate,** including beta-blockers, such as *propranolol* (Inderal), or calcium-channel blockers, such as *verapamil* (Isoptin). Some patients may need stronger antiarrhythmics.

•**Cardioversion,** an outpatient procedure in which surface electrodes shock the heart back into normal rhythm. This can restore a normal heartbeat for months or even years, especially if combined with antiarrhythmic medication.

•**Ablation therapy,** in which one or more catheters are threaded through blood vessels into the heart. The tips of the catheters are positioned near the areas of the heart that are causing arrhythmias. Heat from the catheter tips destroys (ablates) small patches of heart tissue and blocks irregular electrical signals. Ablation therapy can reduce or eliminate arrhythmias in 70% to 80% of cases. The procedure, usually done under general anesthesia in a hospital, can take four to six hours.

Bradycardia

This is an umbrella term that refers to a slow heartbeat. Anyone whose heart beats less than 60 times a minute has bradycardia, but this doesn't always mean that he/she has a dangerous condition.

Example: Many healthy adults have a normal heart rhythm of 40 to 60 beats a minute—in athletes, the heart can beat as slowly as 30 times a minute. Bradycardia is a problem only when the heart beats so slowly that it causes symptoms.

Symptoms: Low blood pressure, dizziness, light-headedness, fatigue.

Drug side effects are the main cause of symptomatic bradycardia. This often happens when medications used to lower blood pressure, such as calcium-channel blockers or beta-blockers, slow the heart too much. Bradycardia also can be caused by a number of conditions, including inadequate levels of thyroid hormone, an electrolyte imbalance (such as low levels of calcium or magnesium) or kidney disease.

Treatment: A medication review. In some cases, patients need to stop taking certain medications, or take a lower dose, to see if the heart rate increases—this should be done only under a doctor's supervision. Or patients may be prescribed medications that don't have this effect (such as diuretics for hypertension).

Another option: A pacemaker, a device surgically implanted under the skin near the collarbone with electrodes that run to the heart. The pacemaker detects when the heart is beating too slowly and delivers a series of electrical signals that speed up the heart.

In cases where a medical condition is causing bradycardia, treating the underlying problem will correct the heart rate.

Calcium Supplements May Cause Heart Attacks

According to a recent study, people who took calcium supplements were more than twice as likely to have heart attacks as people who did not take the supplements. (Foods with added calcium were not studied.)

Best: Get calcium naturally from foods such as dairy products, sardines and kale.

Sabine Rohrmann, PhD, MPH, head of cancer epidemiology and prevention at Institute of Social and Preventive Medicine, University of Zurich, Switzerland, and coauthor of a study of 23,980 people, published in *Heart*.

Ventricular Tachycardia/ Fibrillation

These are among the most serious arrhythmias. When you hear that someone "dropped dead" from a heart attack, a ventricular tachycardia/fibrillation most often is the cause.

What happens: Electrical signals in the ventricles are so rapid and chaotic that the heart is unable to pump blood.

Result: A rapid drop in blood pressure cuts off circulation to the brain and other organs. Patients will collapse within seconds—most will die without emergency treatment.

Many patients who experience these arrhythmias have underlying heart disease, damage from a previous heart attack or electrical and/or valve abnormalities that have a genetic origin.

Symptoms: Racing heartbeat, loss of consciousness.

Treatment: Call 911 immediately. If an automated external defibrillator (AED) is available, it should be used. This portable device analyzes the heart's rhythm. If arrhythmias are present, the machine will instruct the operator to press a "shock" button. The heart rhythm will again be analyzed to determine if additional shocks are needed. The machine won't deliver a shock if the heart rhythm is normal.

Patients with cardiac risk factors, including a previous heart attack, should ask their doctors if they should buy an AED.

If an AED is not available and the heart has stopped, cardiopulmonary resuscitation (CPR) should be done until an ambulance arrives. To learn how to do CPR, go to the American Heart Association Web site, *www. Heart.org* (put "CPR" in the search box).

Other treatment options: Patients who have survived a heart attack but have a weakened heart muscle may be advised to get an implantable cardioverter defibrillator (ICD), a device that continuously analyzes the heart and administers electrical shocks, as needed, to treat ventricular fibrillation. The procedure takes about an hour and often can be done on an outpatient basis.

In some cases, radiofrequency ablation can be helpful. Your doctor can decide what is right for you.

Supraventricular Tachycardia (SVT)

These originate in the area above the ventricles, causing a burst of rapid beats that begin suddenly and can last up to an hour. SVTs usually occur in young adults. They're uncomfortable but rarely dangerous in people without other heart disorders.

Symptoms: Rapid heartbeat that starts and stops suddenly. It may be associated with dizziness, chest pressure and/or shortness of breath. Some people have no symptoms.

Treatment: Patients may be taught how to do a vagal maneuver, such as coughing or holding their breath while bearing down. This stimulates the vagus nerve and slows the electrical impulses that cause rapid beats. If that doesn't work, radiofrequency ablation can eliminate the problem in most patients. Or patients may be advised to take a beta-blocker or other antiarrhythmic medications that will reduce the frequency of these episodes.

Light-Headedness Upon Standing Up? It's More Dangerous Than You Think

Christine DeLong Jones, MD, preventive medicine resident, University of North Carolina at Chapel Hill.

You stand up, and suddenly your head is spinning—you freeze for a moment or grab onto something to hold yourself steady.

After a few seconds or minutes, the feeling passes and you get on with your business. Everything seems OK.

But everything is not necessarily OK. Those moments of light-headedness signal that your blood pressure suddenly dropped when you stood up. You might have what's called orthostatic hypotension (OH). If you have OH often and/or severely (bouts during which you almost pass out or do pass out), it can lead to some major consequences.

According to a new study, those with OH are at higher risk for something very serious—heart failure.

Not So Benign

OH is defined by a blood pressure drop upon standing of at least 20 mmHg systolic (the top number in a blood pressure reading) or 10 mmHg diastolic (the bottom number). OH may come and go—or may last forever—depending on what's causing it, which could be dehydration...standing up quickly after eating...blood loss...certain medications (such as those for high blood pressure, anxiety, depression and erectile dysfunction)...certain diseases (such as atherosclerosis, diabetes, Parkinson's and thyroid problems)...prolonged bed rest...crossing your legs while sitting...and other factors. The chance of experiencing OH rises as you age.

So how is this related to something as dangerous as heart failure, where the heart can't pump enough blood?

Low-Carb/High-Protein Diet Increases Heart Disease Risk in Women

According to a recent study, eating a diet similar to the Atkins diet—with low carbohydrate intake and more protein intake—was linked to a greater risk for cardiovascular disease in women ages 30 to 49.

Study of data from the Swedish Women's Lifestyle and Health Cohort (43,396 women ages 30 to 49) by researchers at University of Athens, Greece, published in *BMJ*.

The Heart of the Matter

The new study, from the University of North Carolina at Chapel Hill, found that people between the ages of 45 and 64 with OH had a 54% greater risk of developing heart failure. This finding held true even after controlling for cardiac risk factors such as diabetes, high blood pressure, coronary heart disease and medications that can cause blood pressure drops.

Dealing With Dizziness

So how do you know whether you have OH and, if you do, what you should do about it? When we spoke with study coauthor Christine DeLong Jones, MD, a preventive medicine resident at the university, her first piece of advice was to drink plenty of water, because dehydration is one of the most common (and reversible) causes of OH. If you're hydrated and light-headedness continues, she said, then it's reasonable to ask your doctor about having a series of blood pressure measurements to test for OH.

If you have OH, work with your doctor to figure out the cause, said Dr. Jones. For example, you may be taking a medication that's causing the problem and your doctor may be able to prescribe a different drug or an alternative treatment.

But if the cause is something that you can't change (such as a disease) and OH persists, Dr. Jones said to consider it a red flag that you must act to prevent or treat other conditions that can contribute to heart failure—including coronary heart disease, diabetes and hypertension. In that case, think of your episodes of light-headedness as a friendly warning—much friendlier, at least, than heart failure!

Heartwarming News... Sort of

Peter Briss, MD, MPH, medical director of the National Center for Chronic Disease Prevention and Health Promotion at the Centers for Disease Control and Prevention in Atlanta.

Any good news about heart health is welcome, given that cardiovascular disease causes one in three deaths among Americans each year. So, you'll be happy to hear that the data for 2007 to 2008 (the latest period for which figures are available) show an 8.1 percentage point decrease since 1999 to 2000 in the percentage of US adults ages 20 and older who have at least one of three major preventable risk factors for cardiovascular disease.

The not-so-good news: 47% of us still have one or more of those risk factors—uncontrolled high blood pressure, uncontrolled high cholesterol levels and/or a current smoking habit. While that represents progress over the previous rate of 57.8%, it remains alarmingly high.

Fun source of inspiration: Check out *http://MillionHearts.hhs.gov*, a national initiative designed to prevent one million heart attacks and strokes over the next five years.

Hidden Causes of Heart Disease: Little-Known Risk Factors

Stephen Sinatra, MD, board-certified cardiologist and assistant clinical professor of medicine at University of Connecticut School of Medicine in Farmington and a fellow in the American College of Cardiology and the American College of Nutrition. Dr. Sinatra is author or coauthor of numerous books, including *The Healing Kitchen* (Bottom Line Books). *www.Bottom LinePublications.com/HealingKitchen*

There are well-known risk factors for heart disease, such as high blood pressure, diabetes, being overweight and a family history of early heart attacks. But some little-known risk factors are as threatening to your heart as those you're familiar with—in some cases, doubling your risk for disease.

Here are five of these "secret" risk factors, revealed by recent scientific studies—*and how to reduce your risk…*

• **Bisphenol A (BPA).** BPA is a chemical frequently found in food and beverage containers, such as plastic bottles and the lining of metal cans. It can harm your arteries.

Recent research: In a study of 591 people published in *PLOS One*, those with the highest urinary levels of BPA were the most likely to have advanced coronary artery disease—severely narrowed arteries ripe for the blockage that triggers a heart attack.

What happens: BPA sparks the chronic inflammation that drives arterial damage and heart disease.

My recommendation: Reduce your exposure to BPA. Avoid canned foods as much as possible because cans may have an epoxy liner that leaches BPA into food. Or look for cans labeled BPA-free. Drink water out of glass or stainless steel bottles that don't have a plastic liner. Don't microwave food in plastic or use plastic containers for hot foods or liquids—the heat can cause BPA to leach out.

Exception: Soft or cloudy-colored plastics typically do not contain BPA—they usually are marked on the bottom with the recycling labels #1, #2 or #4.

• **Shift work.** Dozens of studies have linked shift work—an ongoing pattern of work that is not roughly 9 am to 5 pm—to higher heart disease risk, but the link has always been speculative. The latest study—a so-called "meta-analysis" of previous research—changes the shift work/heart disease hypothesis into scientific fact.

Recent research: The study, published in *BMJ*, analyzed data from 34 studies involving more than two million people and found that shift work was linked to a 23% increased risk for heart attack. The researchers concluded that 7% of all heart attacks—about one out of every 14—are directly attributable to shift work.

What happens: Shift work disrupts the normal sleep-wake cycle, throwing every system in your body out of balance, including the autonomic nervous system, which regulates heartbeat. An irregular heartbeat (arrhythmia) can cause a type of heart attack.

My recommendation: A key way to balance your autonomic nervous system is to increase your intake of foods rich in omega-3 fatty acids, such as wild-caught fatty fish (salmon, sardines, mackerel, tuna), grass-fed red meats, free-range poultry, walnuts and flaxseed oil. Also, take a daily fish oil supplement that delivers one to two grams of the essential fatty acids EPA and DHA.

If your work schedule includes shift work, pay attention to other heart disease risk factors and go for regular screenings.

• **Diabetes drugs.** A generic, low-cost class of antidiabetes drugs called *sulfonylureas* (*glipizide, glyburide* and *glimepiride*) help control type 2 diabetes by stimulating the pancreas to produce insulin, a hormone that regulates blood sugar levels, but these drugs can be dangerous to your heart.

Recent research: Researchers at the Cleveland Clinic analyzed data from nearly 24,000 patients who had taken either a sulfonylurea drug or *metformin*, another generic, low-cost drug used to control diabetes. Compared with metformin, the sulfonylureas were linked to a 50% greater risk for death.

What happens: It's likely that sulfonylurea drugs are toxic to the body's mitochondria, the energy-generating structures in every cell that are crucial to health and longevity.

My recommendation: If you're taking a sulfonylurea drug, ask your doctor to switch you to metformin.

Even better: In a major, multiyear study, losing weight and exercising outperformed metformin in regulating blood sugar.

•**Early menopause.** Menopause, and its accompanying drop in heart-protecting estrogen, increases the risk for heart disease. So it's no surprise that early menopause (starting at age 46 or younger) is a risk factor.

Recent research: In an eight-year study published in *Menopause,* researchers found that women who enter menopause early are twice as likely to suffer from heart disease and stroke.

My recommendation: There are several ways menopausal women can lower their risk for heart disease…

•Eat more noninflammatory foods, such as fresh, organic vegetables and fruits and wild-caught fatty fish.

•Minimize your intake of inflammatory simple sugars (white bread, pastries, cookies, pastas, candies, etc.).

•Exercise regularly, such as a daily 30-to-60-minute walk.

•In addition to a multivitamin, take daily supplements that strengthen the heart and circulatory system, including CoQ10 (60 mg to 100 mg)…fish oil (one to two grams)…vitamin C (1,000 mg)…and magnesium (400 mg to 800 mg).

•Reduce stress with meditation, yoga and/or tai chi. Other ways to reduce stress include socializing with friends and doing hobbies you enjoy.

•**Psoriasis.** The chronic inflammatory disease of psoriasis causes patches of dry, itchy skin. A recent study shows that it also damages arteries.

Recent research: In a study in *Journal of Investigative Dermatology,* researchers found that chronic inflammation of the skin is accompanied by chronic inflammation in blood vessels. And in a study published in *Circulation: Cardiovascular Imaging,* researchers found that treating psoriasis patients with the anti-inflammatory drug *adalimumab* decreased inflammation in the arteries (carotid and ascending aorta) often involved in heart attack and stroke.

My recommendation: All psoriasis patients should go on a gluten-free diet, eliminating inflammation-sparking grains such as wheat, rye and barley. They also should take inflammation-reducing omega-3 fatty acids (three to four grams daily). In addition, people with psoriasis should be screened regularly for heart disease.

More Risk Factors for Heart Attack from Top Heart Expert

Michael Ozner, MD, medical director of the Center for Wellness & Prevention at Baptist Health South Florida in Miami and a past chairman of the American Heart Association of Miami. He is author of four books, including *Heart Attack Proof: A Six-Week Cardiac Makeover for a Lifetime of Optimal Health* (BenBella). *www.DrOzner.com*

When determining one's odds of having a heart attack, two factors often are overlooked…

•**Periodontal disease.** Many doctors have been slow to recognize how poor dental hygiene can increase a person's heart attack risk.

Here's what happens: If you don't brush and floss regularly, small particles of food get trapped between your teeth and gums, which promotes the buildup of plaque as well as inflammation and infection. Periodontal disease, in turn, causes a generalized inflammatory response that can increase heart attack risk.

In fact, a recent seven-year study of more than 100,000 people with no history of heart attack or stroke showed that those who had their teeth cleaned by a dentist or hygienist at least twice a year over a two-year period had a 24% lower risk for heart attack compared with people who did not go to the dentist or went only once in a two-year period. *My approach:* Brush and floss regularly…and see your dentist at least every six months.

• **Sleep apnea.** Recent research shows that this nighttime breathing disorder increases a person's risk for heart attack and stroke.

What's the connection? With sleep apnea, the upper airway narrows or collapses during sleep, often disrupting sleep hundreds of times each night. This sleep disturbance decreases oxygen saturation in the bloodstream. Sleep apnea also raises adrenaline and inflammation—both of which increase risk for heart attack.

My approach: Patients who have signs or symptoms of sleep apnea—such as snoring, periods of breathing cessation during sleep, daytime fatigue and/or morning headaches—should see a doctor. There is some evidence that treating sleep apnea can lower heart attack risk.

Why a Creased Earlobe May Kill You

Anne Tybjaerg-Hansen, MD, DMSc, professor of clinical biochemistry, University of Copenhagen, and chief physician in the department of clinical biochemistry at Copenhagen University Hospital, Denmark.

When it comes to your cardiovascular health, you might think that if you don't have any typical risk factors for heart attack or coronary artery disease, such as obesity, high blood pressure or high cholesterol, then your heart is in good shape.

But a recent study may make you think twice.

A Happy Heart Is a Healthy Heart

When researchers surveyed 5,654 adults, those who were secure in their romantic relationships (that is, able to get close to others and willing to let others depend on them) had lower rates of high blood pressure, heart attack and stroke than those who were anxious in their relationships (for example, needy and worried about rejection).

Theory: Anxiety in relationships can negatively affect your cardiovascular system.

Self-defense: If you are having problems in your relationships, consider seeking advice from a therapist, who may help you learn more about your relationship style.

Lachlan McWilliams, PhD, associate professor of psychology, Acadia University, Nova Scotia, Canada.

It may sound crazy, but how you look—as in, whether you look young or old for your age—can actually affect your risk for certain cardiovascular problems.

In fact, researchers have pinpointed four specific physical traits.

So check out what the four traits are and then take a look in the mirror…

The Heart of the Matter

After studying 35 years of data from nearly 11,000 male and female volunteers, Danish researchers found that two of the traits are fairly common and easy to recognize—a receding hairline and a bald spot on the head. (If a participant was mostly or completely bald, that person was put into the "bald spot" group.) The association of baldness and cardiovascular risk was seen among both men and women, though baldness was much less common in women.

The third trait is a little more obscure—a crease in one or both earlobes. And the fourth is having small, lumpy, yellow deposits on, above, below or next to the eyelids, a condition called *xanthelasma* that's caused by excess cholesterol under the skin.

The study showed that the more of these traits a person had, the higher his or her chance of having a heart attack or developing coronary artery disease. For example, the researchers discovered that for people with three or four of these traits, the chances of suffering a heart attack are 57% greater and the chances of developing coronary artery disease are 39% greater, on average, than for people who have none of these traits.

What's remarkable is that these elevated risks held true even when researchers controlled for other common risk factors for cardiovascular problems, such as age, high blood pressure, high cholesterol, excess weight, poor nutrition, smoking, not exercising, gender and a family history of heart disease.

Why are these traits associated with these serious cardiovascular problems—and what might your doctor be able to do to help treat each trait? *We asked the lead author of the study, Anne Tybjaerg-Hansen, MD, DMSc, and here's what she said…*

• **Xanthelasma.** This condition remains a mystery to medical science. One potential cause of these fatty eyelid deposits is a diet that includes too much saturated fat—because saturated fat can raise your cholesterol levels. A doctor may advise you to eat a healthier diet and get more exercise, which may help lower your cholesterol numbers, and, in turn, prevent more fatty deposits from appearing. But it's possible to have a normal cholesterol level and still have xanthelasma. Other potential causes of xanthelasma are diabetes, certain cancers and cirrhosis of the liver. You can have the deposits surgically removed, but unless the underlying cause is treated, the deposits may return and your cardiovascular risk would not be reduced.

• **Hair loss.** There are a wide variety of potential causes for hair loss. It could be due to genetics (male pattern baldness)…a hormone imbalance…a drug (for instance, some medications that treat cancer, arthritis, depression and high blood pressure are associated with hair loss)…a thyroid prob-

Alcohol Is More Dangerous for Women Than Men

Women who drink to excess are at much greater risk for liver, brain and heart damage than men who drink to excess. Women have more body fat than men, less water in their systems and lower levels of an enzyme that breaks down alcohol, so the effects of alcohol are more acutely concentrated in women. Excessive drinking is an average of four or more drinks within two hours for women and five or more drinks within two hours for men.

Deidra Roach, MD, program director, division of treatment and recovery research, National Institute on Alcohol Abuse and Alcoholism, Bethesda, Maryland. www.niaaa.nih.gov

lem…the disease alopecia, in which the immune system destroys hair follicles…a scalp infection…a skin disorder (such as lichen planus or lupus)…emotional or physical shock (due to, say, a death in the family or sudden weight loss)…anxiety (certain mental disorders make people want to pull hair from their heads)…a certain hairstyle (pulling hair too tightly can cause it to break and fall out)…overusing hair products (when hair gets too brittle, it can break and fall out)…or improper nutrition (a lack of iron and protein can cause hair to thin). If you have a treatable condition that's causing your hair loss, treating the condition may or may not have a positive effect on your cardiovascular risk factors—we don't know.

• **Earlobe crease.** This is a tricky trait. You might have an earlobe crease if the trait is passed down genetically through your family. As far as what else may cause this, that's up for debate. One theory suggests that it could be due to impaired circulation leading to a collapsed blood vessel near the earlobe. Another theory, which comes from a dermatologist, is that it may develop from a combination of aging and sleeping on one particular side of your body. But the cause is hard to pin down and there aren't any current treatments for it.

So all in all, it's not entirely clear why these traits are associated with certain increased cardiovascular risks and it's not yet known how to counteract these increased risks. But if you have at least one of these traits, Dr. Tybjaerg-Hansen said it probably wouldn't hurt to talk to your doctor about making more aggressive lifestyle changes, even if you're already eating some healthy foods and exercising a little. Your test results may lead you to believe that you're in the clear, but these findings show that you're not! It's possible that you'll need to make more of an effort than most people to protect your heart health.

Don't Let Unemployment Hurt Your Heart

People who were jobless because they had been fired, laid off or quit a job earlier in life had a 35% higher risk for heart attack after age 50 than people who remained employed. Multiple job losses posed as much of a threat to heart health as smoking, high blood pressure and diabetes. Talk to your doctor about heart-health strategies, such as reducing stress.

Matthew Dupre, PhD, assistant professor of community and family medicine, Duke University, Durham, North Carolina, and leader of a study of 13,451 people, ages 51 to 75, published online in *Archives of Internal Medicine*.

Restless Legs May Indicate Heart Problems

Restless legs may be a sign of hidden heart problems, warns Arshad A. Jahangir, MD. People whose legs move very frequently during sleep (more than 35 times per hour) are almost twice as likely to have a thickened heart muscle as people whose legs move less frequently. Thickening of the heart muscle can increase the risk for arrhythmias, heart attack or heart failure.

Self-defense: If you have been diagnosed with restless legs, ask your physician about cardiac testing.

Arshad A. Jahangir, MD, a heart rhythm specialist at Mayo Clinic Arizona, Scottsdale, and leader of a study of 584 people with restless legs syndrome, presented at a recent American College of Cardiology conference.

Insomnia Raises Heart Disease Risk

Insomnia raises heart disease risk, warns Lars Erik Laugsand, MD.

Recent finding: People who have trouble falling asleep most nights have a 45% higher risk for heart disease than people who don't have trouble falling asleep. Those who have trouble staying asleep have a 30% higher risk.

Possible connection: Insomnia may be linked to increased stress hormones, blood pressure and inflammation, all of which increase the risk for heart disease.

Lars Erik Laugsand, MD, a public health researcher and internist at Norwegian University of Science and Technology, Trondheim, and lead author of a study of 52,610 people, published online in *Circulation*.

Your Job Can Hurt Your Heart

Job stress hurts women's hearts, we hear from Michelle Albert, MD, MPH. Over 10 years, researchers studied the link between work stress and cardiovascular health in 22,000 women (average age 57).

Result: Women with the most stressful jobs, including those with high demands and little opportunity to make decisions or use creativity, were 38% more likely to suffer heart-related events such as stroke or death than those with less stressful jobs. Risk for heart attack was 70% higher.

If you have a stressful job: Talk to your doctor about ways to protect your heart health, including effective strategies to cope with stress.

Michelle Albert, MD, MPH, associate professor of medicine, Harvard Medical School, Boston.

Can a Broken Heart Really Kill Someone?

Amir Lerman, MD, cardiologist, Mayo Clinic, Rochester, Minnesota.

Recent research has identified that some people have a vascular abnormality that may make them vulnerable to a heart attack as a result of suffering intense emotional anguish. It turns out that these patients have blood vessels that react very differently to stress than those of other people, triggering physiological changes that may increase vulnerability to heart attack—and, in extreme cases, actually bring one on.

Extra-Sensitive People

The medical name for broken heart syndrome is *apical ballooning syndrome (ABS)*. Seen in men and young women only very occasionally, the problem mainly affects postmenopausal women, probably because menopause brings hormonal shifts that change the way their blood vessels respond to stress.

Amir Lerman, MD, a Mayo Clinic cardiologist and coauthor of a recent study on the topic (published in the *Journal of the American College of Cardiology*), explained that awareness of this problem has grown in recent years. He and others are now working to take the knowledge further and develop a way to identify these very sensitive people in advance so that they can take steps to avoid the problem.

The Challenge

The study: To learn more about the cause of this condition, researchers examined 28 postmenopausal women—12 with ABS, 12 without ABS and four who had suffered classic heart attacks. The participants were asked to complete a series of mental stress tests, including complex memory and mathematical tasks. As they did this, researchers used a finger cuff (called an EndoPAT) to monitor changes in their blood volume as a way to determine how their blood vessels reacted when they were experiencing mental stress.

Normal blood vessels dilate during stress, allowing more blood to flow to the heart, but the opposite occurs in people with ABS. Researchers found that, compared with both other groups, these patients had "decreased endothelial function," causing their blood vessels to constrict under stress. The endothelium or inner layer of the vessels regulates the activity of the vessels, allowing blood flow to increase when we're in demanding situations, such as exercising or under mental stress. Endothelial dysfunction also can contribute to decreased blood flow to the heart, which—if dramatic enough—can lead to a heart attack and also to weakening of the left ventricle, the heart's main pumping chamber.

What Can You Do?

"If you're under stress and your blood vessels narrow rather than dilate, there's a discrepancy between how much blood flow you need and how much you get," explains Dr. Lerman, noting that this is what causes the chest pains or shortness of breath that ABS patients often experience. The good news is this isn't usually as dangerous as it feels. There's no actual blockage involved with ABS and it usually doesn't cause permanent damage, he said.

Might you have ABS? Well, if you have noticed that when you're really stressed your chest hurts and you're short of breath, then Dr. Lerman advises that you discuss the condition with your doctor. He suggests asking to have your endothelial function tested with noninvasive devices, such as the EndoPAT used in the study, and adds that it's a good idea for anyone who has experienced heart attack-like symptoms but hasn't actually had a heart attack to be tested as well.

Dr. Lerman explained that people with ABS usually respond quite well to treatment, which may involve medication, such as beta-blockers and other drugs to lower blood pressure, and/or relaxation techniques, such as meditation or yoga, to help them learn better ways to handle stressful situations. The goal, said Dr. Lerman, is for people to learn coping skills that bring greater resilience so that they can learn to tolerate sadness and loss without allowing it to, literally, "break their hearts." It's a simple and healthful fix—for all of us, in fact, not just people who have ABS!

Grief and Your Heart

In one recent study, physicians tested the blood of 80 newly bereaved adults (average age 66), comparing their cardiovascular risk factors with those of 80 adults who were not bereaved.

Result: Within two weeks of the loss of a spouse or child, three measures of inflammatory and clotting risk increased significantly. Six months later, the overall risk dropped but still tended to be higher than the non-bereaved. The higher clotting levels may be related to increased stress hormones, as well as behavioral changes, such as reduced sleep.

Anyone who has recently lost a loved one should take care of his/her heart by getting regular sleep, eating well and avoiding smoking and other cardiovascular strains.

Geoffrey Tofler, MD, professor of medicine, University of Sydney, Australia.

New (and Serious) Risk for Arthritis Sufferers

Jesper Lindhardsen, MD, research fellow and physician in the department of cardiology at Copenhagen University Hospital in Gentofte, Denmark. His study was published in *BMJ*.

If you have rheumatoid arthritis (RA), you're probably most concerned about managing joint pain. But the disease can have more serious, life-threatening adverse effects that don't always have symptoms, so it's an insidious killer.

Prior studies have shown a link between RA and stroke, and a recent study out of Denmark says that those with RA are at risk for yet another serious heart condition—a heart rhythm disorder called atrial fibrillation.

An Out-of-Control Heartbeat

The study looked at the health records of the entire Danish population (about four million people), including Danes who had been diagnosed with RA and were taking RA drugs.

Researchers wanted to compare that group to the general population to see who had atrial fibrillation or a stroke during the five-year study period.

Here is what they found: The RA patients were, on average, 40% more likely to have atrial fibrillation than the general population. Futhermore, all RA patients (whether they had atrial fibrillation or not) were, on average, 30% more likely to have a stroke than the general population.

Stroke can, of course, sometimes cause death, paralysis and other serious complications, and atrial fibrillation can also have severe consequences, including stroke and heart failure.

One limitation of the study is that it did not consider whether the medications that these patients were on might be somewhat or fully responsible for the increased incidence of atrial fibrillation or stroke. But when we spoke with the study's lead author, Jesper Lindhardsen, MD, research fellow and physician in the department of cardiology at Copenhagen University Hospital, he pointed out that RA is a disease that causes inflammation of all of the body's systems—not just the joints—and that inflammation is what's thought to lead to atrial fibrillation and stroke.

Speak Up, Get Monitored

Stroke, of course, usually has symptoms—and they're often quite obvious (including sudden loss of balance, inability to speak or slurred speech, paralysis or numbness on one side of the body, blurred vision or severe headache).

Atrial fibrillation, on the other hand, sometimes has symptoms and sometimes does not. And when it does, the symptoms can be subtle. So if you have RA, said Dr. Lindhardsen, it's important that you be on the lookout for the following red flags that may indicate atrial fibrillation…

• **Palpitations or a sudden pounding,** fluttering or racing sensation in the chest—often described as "butterflies."

• **Irregular pulse.**

• **Intermittent lightheadedness or dizziness.**

Since atrial fibrillation can be symptomless, if you have RA it's also wise to ask your doctor to check your heart for atrial fibrillation at your annual checkup. This check would include an assessment of your heartbeat and—if deemed necessary—an electrocardiogram or ECG.

If atrial fibrillation is detected, your treatment will depend on the severity of the problem. Some fibrillation is constant, while some is intermittent. Your doctor will help you decide whether you should be treated with an antiarrhythmic, a drug intended to make the heartbeat even, or with other medicine designed to slow the heart rate. Your doctor might also prescribe an anticoagulant to prevent the blood clots that often result from atrial fibrillation. A naturopathic physician might also try to solve the underlying problem of atrial fibrillation by administering L-carnitine (an amino acid), by ensuring that adequate calcium and magnesium are delivered to the heart and/or by providing omega-3 oils and polyphenolic plant extract.

Brittle Bones— "Brittle" Heart

Susan Steinbaum, DO, preventive cardiologist, director of Women and Heart Disease at Lenox Hill Hospital in New York City and a spokesperson for the American Heart Association.

You might think of brittle bones and heart disease as two entirely different, unrelated health problems. The heart is a muscle, after all, while bones are the tough stuff of the body. But recent scientific findings from Norway suggest that a person with an ailing heart muscle may also be prone to weak bones…and vice versa.

The implications of this are frightening, given that an estimated 44 million Americans have either full-fledged osteoporosis or low bone density (and are at risk for osteoporosis), while 17.6 million Americans have heart disease.

The study: Examining the medical records of some 6,000 men and women over a three-year period, researchers found that those with low bone density were also likely to have arterial damage, indicating that they are at risk for heart disease and stroke. And, in a previous study from the same Norwegian researchers, those women who had suffered from a stroke were found to have a much lower bone density, on average, than other women of the same age.

To see what we might be able to learn about this connection, we called preventive cardiologist Susan Steinbaum, DO, director of Women and Heart Disease at Lenox Hill Hospital in New York City and a spokesperson for the American Heart Association. She said that this latest study is just one of several pointing to an association between brittle bones and heart disease, and she said that while the reason for the link is not fully understood yet, one theory points to inflammation as the culprit. "We know that inflammation inside the lining of the arteries leads to heart disease," Dr. Steinbaum said, adding that some researchers theorize that weak bones may be the result of cell wasting caused by that same inflammation. She noted that the good news is that "a lot of the lifestyle recommendations for heart disease are the same as for osteoporosis, so what works to prevent one can also help prevent the other."

To Keep Both Heart and Bones Healthy

What to do? Most of the advice on how to keep your heart and bones healthy will sound very familiar, but it is nonetheless worthy of review...

• **Get regular exercise.** You need 150 minutes per week of moderate intensity cardiovascular exercise—walking fast, pushing a lawnmower, playing doubles tennis—to protect your heart. For your bones, you should also do weight-bearing exercises—yes, as in lifting weights—two to three times per week.

• **Watch your diet.** "In some people, a high-fat, high-meat diet is associated with heart disease," Dr. Steinbaum said, adding that evidence suggests that a diet high in saturated fats such as those found in red meat is the type of diet that also is linked with osteoporosis. Choose lean proteins and eat plenty of fruits and vegetables to protect against both.

• **Stop smoking.** The many reasons to give up cigarettes include preventing heart disease, but cigarette smoke has also been linked to low bone density, the precursor to osteoporosis.

Cautionary Notes

There are a few bits of advice that aren't the same for heart and bones. Heart medications don't seem to harm the bones, but medications known as bisphosphonates prescribed for osteoporosis have been associated with the heart disorder atrial fibrillation in some patients who took them. There's also evidence that long-term use of these drugs can lead to fracture in the spine, hip and leg bones along with, in some people, deterioration of the jawbone. If you need these drugs, they should be used for only a limited period of time and under the close supervision of a doctor.

Ask for This Test!— Finally, You Can Know for Sure If You're Getting Enough Omega-3s

Christopher D. Abel, MD, an internist and a preventive medicine specialist at Cooper Clinic in Dallas, where he is executive vice president, medical director and director of laboratory services. The Cooper Clinic, which specializes in comprehensive preventive medical exams, was founded in 1970 by Kenneth H. Cooper, MD, who coined the term "aerobics." *www.CooperAerobics.com*

T he positive research just keeps on coming. First, scientists told us that omega-3 fatty acids help guard against heart disease. (Although a large study recently disputed fish oil and heart health, some heart experts disagree.) Then research showed that these healthful fats also may help prevent other serious conditions, such as Alzheimer's disease, depression, rheumatoid arthritis, macular degeneration and polyps that can lead to colon cancer.

What we're not being told: A little-known report from the US Dietary Guidelines Advisory Committee has estimated that about 70% of Americans are deficient in omega-3s.

So how do you know whether you're getting enough of them?

Recent development: A simple test that measures total omega-3s in the blood can tell you whether your levels are adequate. With this information, you don't have to guess any longer whether you need to eat more omega-3–rich foods or take a dietary supplement.

A Test for All Adults

To gain the wide-ranging health benefits of omega-3s, we have all been encouraged to eat oily fish, such as salmon and sardines, at least twice a week…and/or increase our intake of plant foods, such as flaxseed or walnuts, that contain alpha-linolenic acid, which helps the body manufacture the omega-3 fatty acids eicosapentaenoic acid (EPA) and docosahexaenoic acid (DHA). In many cases, people also take fish oil supplements to boost their omega-3 levels.

But even by boosting your intake of omega-3–rich foods and/or taking a supplement, you might not have enough of the fatty acids in your body—everyone absorbs varying amounts of omega-3s and needs different amounts to optimize health.

That is why I recommend an omega-3 blood test for all adults. Not all doctors offer this test, but it's the best way to determine exactly what levels of omega-3s are in your body. *What you need to know about omega-3 testing…*

• **How it is done.** The omega-3 index is a simple blood test. Your doctor will take a blood sample, which is analyzed in a laboratory. Home tests are also available in which you do a "blood stick" and mail the sample to a testing laboratory. However, I prefer the test that is performed in a doctor's office.

• **What it does.** The test measures the two omega-3 fatty acids, EPA and DHA, that are present in the membranes of red blood cells.

Omega-3s are deposited in these membranes whenever you consume food or supplements that contain the fatty acids or alpha-linolenic acid, which is converted into the healthful fats. Red blood cells live for about four months in the body, so the test shows what level of omega-3s you've absorbed over that period.

• **What to look for.** The test lists your level of omega-3 fatty acids as a percentage of total fatty acids in cell membranes.

The optimal level of omega-3s (EPA and DHA combined) is 8% or higher—this means that you have the lowest risk of developing heart disease (not including risks from other factors, such as smoking, elevated blood fats, hypertension and diabetes). Below 4% indicates an elevated risk of developing heart disease. A level between 4% and 8% is considered suboptimal.

Typical cost: $100 to $200. The test is not covered by insurance, but this might change in the future as more doctors recognize its clinical value. Labs that offer the test include Health Diagnostic Laboratory, 877-443-5227, *www.HDLabInc.com*…and OmegaQuant, 800-949-0632, *www.OmegaQuant.com.*

Now What?

The most important question to ask after any medical test is, "What do I do with the results?" The omega-3 index can be a strong motivator. People already know if they are eating a little or a lot of fish…they also know if they are taking omega-3 supplements.

What people don't know—without testing—is whether they have enough omega-3s in the bloodstream. When they see that they have a low percentage of omega-3s, they're more likely to make the necessary changes. *My advice…*

• **Get tested annually.** First, get an initial baseline test. If a patient's levels are low, I typically advise that he/she eat more oily fish. Since many people don't like the taste of fish, it's fine to take a daily fish oil supplement instead. The test can then be repeated in a year.

• **Eat much more fish.** If you do eat fish, the American Heart Association's advice to consume it twice a week probably represents the minimum that you need to derive health benefits from omega-3s. More is better, particularly if you already have heart disease (or risk factors for it) and/or your omega-3 levels are low.

My advice: Eat fatty fish at least four times a week (avoid fish that is high in mercury, such as king mackerel). Keep in mind that some people can eat fish every day and still have suboptimal omega-3 levels due to variations in absorption and metabolism. These people will need to also take supplements to raise their omega-3 levels.

• **Take fish oil supplements.** They are an effective way to increase blood levels of omega-3s. Ask your doctor what dosage is most appropriate for you.

Also important: Be sure to check with your doctor if you take a blood thinner. Because fish oil has a blood-thinning effect, there is the possibility of excessive bleeding in people taking *warfarin* (Coumadin) or another blood thinner.

• **Reduce side effects.** Fish oil supplements are among the safest dietary supplements. Some patients might complain about minor stomach upset or the occasional fishy burp. However, the majority of people taking fish oil have no side effects at all.

Helpful: Divide the dose by taking half in the morning after a meal and the second half later in the day after a meal. This helps prevent an upset stomach and other possible side effects.

• **"Burp-free" fish oil supplements are another option.** They do not cause a fishy aftertaste. Look for products that state "odorless" or "burp-free" on the label.

Migraine With Aura: A Big Risk Factor for Heart Disease

Tobias Kurth, MD, ScD, director of research, French National Institute of Health and Medical Research, Bordeaux, France, and adjunct associate professor of epidemiology, Harvard School of Public Health, Boston. His study was presented at a recent meeting of the American Academy of Neurology in San Diego.

You know that high blood pressure, diabetes and obesity increase your risk for cardiovascular disease—but you may not know that your heart risk also rises if you suffer from migraine with aura (aura means visual or other sensory disturbances that precede the headache). Yet that's the startling news from a recent study.

The researchers analyzed data on nearly 28,000 women age 45 and older. The participants, none of whom had cardiovascular disease at the start of the study, answered various questions about their health, including whether they had a history of migraine with aura. The participants were then followed for 15 years, with researchers scouring medical records to see who ended up having or dying from a cardiovascular "event" (heart attack or stroke).

Troubling finding: After analyzing the data, the researchers found that migraine with aura was the second biggest individual risk factor for cardiovascular disease, with an incidence of 7.9 events per 1,000 women. The only risk factor that surpassed it was having very high blood pressure (180 or higher for the top number of a blood pressure reading), with an incidence of 9.8 events per 1,000 women.

To put these numbers into perspective, consider that the incidence associated with diabetes was 7.1 cardiovascular events per 1,000 women…for smoking, it was 5.4 events per 1,000 women…for severe obesity (a body mass index of 35 or higher), it was 5.3 events per 1,000 women.

This study does not prove that migraine with aura causes cardiovascular disease, only that the two are associated. And questions remain, of course. For instance, since the recent study included only women, we don't know whether men who experience migraines with aura are similarly at risk. Also, it is not known whether controlling migraines with medication would reduce heart risk…or whether migraine medications themselves (such as those that work by constricting the blood vessels) might contribute to heart risk—though the researchers said that this was unlikely, given that patients who experience migraine without aura also take these drugs yet the study found no link between cardiovascular disease risk and migraine without aura.

Still, until more information is available, women (and men) who have a history of migraines with aura would be wise to mention this study to their doctors and ask for a careful assessment of their individual risk factors for cardiovascular disease—including physical condition, lifestyle and family history—and then follow up if changes are needed to lower their risk.

Are Swollen Ankles a Serious Problem? It May Mean Heart Disease

Leo Galland, MD, director of the Foundation for Integrated Medicine in New York City...founder of Pilladvised.com, an online resource for learning about medications, supplements and food...and author of *Power Healing: Use the New Integrated Medicine to Cure Yourself* (Random House). *www.mdheal.org*

Dismissing ankle swelling as inconsequential can sometimes be a big mistake, according to Leo Galland, MD, a practicing physician, author and director of the Foundation for Integrated Medicine in New York City. He explained, "In some cases, ankle swelling is a warning sign of a serious underlying medical condition that requires a doctor's attention or even emergency care." It could indicate congestive heart failure...

This condition develops when the heart is unable to pump as efficiently as it should, so blood backs up in the veins and fluid accumulates in the lungs.

Watch for swelling that...
- **Affects both ankles.**
- **Gradually worsens.**
- **Causes little or no discomfort.**
- **Leaves indentations** when the skin is pressed (called "pitting edema").

Accompanied by...
- **Chronic cough.**
- **Increased heart rate.**
- **Fatigue.**
- **Shortness of breath** that worsens with physical exertion or when lying down.

What to do: See your doctor. This is a serious condition that needs monitoring and may require treatment to avoid permanent damage to the heart.

Reassuring: Most cases of ankle swelling are not caused by any hidden dire condition, but instead have a harmless or obvious cause, such as...

- **Fluid retention**—brought on by an impending menstrual period, a recent high-salt meal or too many hours spent sitting still. In this case, swelling affects both ankles, causes no discomfort and goes away within a day or two.

Helpful: Sit down and elevate your legs, ideally higher than the level of your heart, for 30 minutes.

- **Varicose veins**—which develop when tiny, one-way valves inside veins don't work well enough to keep blood circulating efficiently through the legs. One or both legs may be affected. Ask your doctor if you could benefit from wearing support stockings, which create a pressure gradient that helps prevent fluid from pooling in the legs.

See pages 30, 421 and 446 for more information on swollen ankles.

Chapter 2

BLOOD CLOTS: THE INSIDE STORY

Millions of Americans Die of Blood Clots

It can happen to anyone at any age. Clots form in the deep veins, usually in the legs. Patients with this deep vein thrombosis might experience leg pain, redness or swelling…or they might have no symptoms at all.

These clots can break free and travel to the lungs, blocking blood flow. This condition, a pulmonary embolism, can easily be fatal.

Who's at Risk

The risk is elevated in people who…

•**Are immobile for extended periods.** The veins require muscle movements to push blood back to the heart. If you can't move your legs freely—because of an injury, a hospitalization or a long car or plane trip—blood tends to pool in the veins and gets "sludgy."

•**Have cancer or are receiving chemotherapy.** Some cancers and cancer treatments increase levels of procoagulants, clot-promoting substances in the blood.

•**Have an inherited blood-clotting disorder** that causes blood to clot more easily.

•**Have a personal history or family history of deep vein thrombosis or pulmonary embolism.**

Medications

Patients with deep vein thrombosis always are treated with an anticlotting medication, such as *heparin* or *warfarin*. (Heparin is given as an injection and acts quickly. Warfarin is a pill that takes two to three days to start working.) The drugs prevent a clot from getting larger while the body's anticlotting mechanisms slowly break it down.

Anticlotting medication also may be given as a preventive measure. Patients undergoing an orthopedic procedure, such as knee or hip replacement, are routinely given anticlotting medication prior to surgery. (In the past, before anticlotting drugs, between 50% and 70% of patients would develop clots after surgery.)

Patients taking anticlotting medications should limit their consumption of foods high in vitamin K, which can affect how drugs

Geno J. Merli, MD, FACP, FHM, FSVM, an internist and a leading specialist in vascular medicine. He is a professor of medicine and codirector of Jefferson Vascular Center, part of Thomas Jefferson University Hospitals in Philadelphia. He specializes in the treatment and prevention of deep vein thrombosis and pulmonary embolism.

such as warfarin work. Foods high in vitamin K include leafy green vegetables and canola and soybean oils.

Other medications your doctor might prescribe…

•**Low-dose aspirin.** Two recent studies in *The New England Journal of Medicine* found that patients with deep vein thrombosis who were treated for three to six months with anticlotting medication could be started on 100 milligrams of aspirin after these medications were stopped. This prevented recurrent clots.

•*Rivaroxaban* **(Xarelto).** This is an oral blood thinner approved by the Food and Drug Administration for the treatment of blood clots. It also reduces the recurrence of clots.

Your doctor may recommend compression stockings, which usually are worn from your foot to about knee level. These exert pressure on the legs and cause less pooling of blood. They are recommended for patients who have had a blood clot in the legs.

Different patients require different amounts of leg pressure. I usually recommend stockings with a pressure of 20 to 30 mmHg (millimeters of mercury). These are available at pharmacies for about $20 a pair—much less than prescription stockings.

Prevention

Even if you have never had a blood clot, you still need to take measures to prevent one…

•**Flex and extend feet and knees.** It's among the best ways to prevent clots from forming in the leg veins. When you're sitting or lying down for more than two hours—in the hospital, on an airplane—rotate your ankles and flex your toes at least three times an hour. If you're able to stand, flex the calf muscles by rising up and down on your toes. It pushes blood out of the veins.

•**Drink more water.** Dehydration is a common cause of clots because it decreases blood volume and makes blood "sticky." It's particularly important to drink more water during airplane flights because the dry air increases dehydration. Drink a large glass of water before getting on a plane, and have several glasses during your flight.

•**Lose weight.** Patients with a body mass index (BMI) of 40 or higher have an elevated risk for clots when they are immobile or have surgery. Those who lose weight and lower their BMI can reduce their blood clot risk. In addition, quit smoking and control your blood pressure—these measures also can lower your risk.

Symptoms of Pulmonary Embolism

A pulmonary embolism can be fatal. It's important to seek medical attention if you…

•**Have sudden, unexplained shortness of breath.**

•**Experience chest pain or discomfort** that worsens when you take a deep breath or cough.

•**Feel dizzy, faint.**

•**Have a rapid pulse.**

•**Cough up blood.**

The Most Dangerous Birth Control Pills

Margaret Polaneczky, MD, an associate professor of clinical obstetrics and gynecology at Weill Cornell Medical College in New York City.

You might use an oral contraceptive for birth control…or for another reason, such as heavy periods, acne or premenstrual dysphoric disorder (PMDD), which involves having symptoms of depression, irritability and tension before menstruation. Whatever the reason, it's important to know—many birth control medications may slightly raise your risk for blood clots.

These clots can occur in any artery or vein in the body. Sometimes they dissolve and cause no problems, but other times—

depending on where they occur—they can cause life-threatening problems, such as pulmonary embolism (blocked blood flow to the lungs), ischemic stroke (blocked blood flow to the brain) or angina (blocked blood flow to the heart).

Recently, the FDA announced that certain birth control pills may raise that risk more than other types of birth control pills—and will require new labels. So which pills are the culprits? And what should you do if you're taking one of them? We posed these questions, as well as others, to Margaret Polaneczky, MD, associate professor of clinical obstetrics and gynecology at Weill Cornell Medical College in New York City.

Some Pills Are Riskier Than Others

Dr. Polaneczky explained that the FDA based its recent decision on large studies that were released in 2011. These studies revealed that birth control pills containing a synthetic form of progesterone known as *drospirenone* may create up to three times as much risk for blood clots as birth control pills containing other types of progesterone. Brands that contain drospirenone include the popular Yaz and Yasmin, as well as Beyaz, Gianvi, Loryna, Ocella, Safyral, Syeda and Zarah.

It's important to note that these are not the only types of birth control that have been linked to higher risks for clots. Dr. Polaneczky noted that in the late 1990s, the FDA found a similarly increased risk for clots from birth control pills containing *desogestrel* (the brands Desogen, Mircette and their generics), and that in 2011 the FDA announced that the Ortho Evra patch could create higher clot risks than low-dose oral contraceptive pills. And though the FDA hasn't formally addressed this yet, recent research suggests that the NuvaRing (a vaginal insert) may also raise the risk for clots more than other types of birth control. (Editor's note: As of February 2014, Merck, the manufacturer of NuvaRing agreed to a $100 million settlement with claimants.)

When you look at all the findings, she said, they suggest that the lowest clot risk might be found in older birth control pills containing *levonorgestrel* or *norethindrone* and newer birth control pills containing *norgestimate*.

Why the Difference in Risk?

It's maddening when drugs are approved by the FDA and then later discovered to be riskier than previously thought. Why didn't we know about this danger sooner? "Before drugs are approved by the FDA, they are tested in clinical trials. And clinical trials may be too small to detect a statistically significant increase in clots. It's often only when a drug makes it out into the general population of millions of women that an increased clot risk becomes evident," Dr. Polaneczky said.

Right now, she added, we don't know why this particular form of progesterone increases clot risk even more. So what should you do if you're on one of these drospirenone-containing pills?

Put the Risk in Perspective

The first thing to remember, said Dr. Polaneczky, is that there's a difference between relative risk and absolute risk. The relative risk of these brands may be higher when compared with that of other pills. But the risk for blood clot is very low to start with, so even when that risk is raised, the absolute risk is still very low.

If 10,000 women took birth control pills that didn't contain drospirenone for one year, three would be likely to develop clots caused by the pills…and if 10,000 women took pills that did contain drospirenone for a year, nine would be likely to develop clots caused by the pills.

But keep in mind, Dr. Polaneczky said, that if you've been taking one of the brands listed above for more than one year, you're already at a lower risk for clotting, since most pill-caused clots occur in the first year of use.

If you took a pill that contains drospirenone and then stopped and are now taking it again, there's a chance that your risk might be as elevated as it would be during your first year taking it, said Dr. Polaneczky, so talk to your doctor about your specific risks.

What You Can Do About It

If you use any of the brands mentioned earlier, talk to your doctor, said Dr. Polaneczky, who added that the decision may be different for each woman. For example, if you're taking the pill for only birth control and you tolerate other types of birth control pills that don't contain drospirenone, then it might make sense to switch, she said. But beyond clot risk, each type of birth control pill has its own set of risks and side effects. If you use the pill to treat PMDD and it's the only one that provides relief for you and/or it's the only one that doesn't trigger side effects, then perhaps it's worth accepting the increased blood clot risk.

We asked Dr. Polaneczky what all women—especially those taking the brands mentioned earlier—can do to lower their clot risk.

Answer: On long car trips or flights (or when you're at a desk for many hours), avoid crossing your legs...do calf raises (lift your heels as high as you can, hold for two seconds and then repeat 10 times)...walk around periodically...and stay hydrated.

Are Swollen Ankles a Serious Problem? It May Mean Blood Clots

Leo Galland, MD, director of the Foundation for Integrated Medicine in New York City...founder of Pilladvised.com, an online resource for learning about medications, supplements and food...and author of *Power Healing: Use the New Integrated Medicine to Cure Yourself* (Random House). *www.mdheal.org*

Dismissing ankle swelling as inconsequential can sometimes be a big mistake, according to Leo Galland, MD, a practicing physician, author and director of the Foundation for Integrated Medicine in

New York City. He explained, "In some cases, ankle swelling is a warning sign of a serious underlying medical condition that requires a doctor's attention or even emergency care." It could be a sign of blood clots in the leg, which could ultimately affect your heart...

The primary concern is that if a clot in a deep vein breaks off and travels to the lungs, it can be fatal.

Watch for swelling that...
- **Affects one ankle.**
- **Appears suddenly.**

Accompanied by...
- **Pain or tenderness in the calf.**
- **Unusual warmth in the skin of the affected area.**
- **A hardened spot beneath the skin.**
- **Red or bluish skin discoloration.**

What to do: If you have possible symptoms of a blood clot in the leg, alert your doctor immediately. For more information about swollen ankles, see pages 26, 421 and 446.

Safer Clotbuster Saves Lives

Tod Engelhardt, MD, chair of the cardiovascular and thoracic surgery division at East Jefferson General Hospital, Metairie, Louisiana.

Blood clots are bad anywhere...but terribly frightening when they travel through your heart and then to your lungs, cutting off your body's oxygen supply and keeping your heart from working properly.

A clot that reaches the lungs is called a pulmonary embolism (PE). Unless the clot is treated quickly after it reaches the lungs, the patient may die of heart failure. In fact, the National Heart Lung and Blood Institute says that at least 100,000 people a year experience PEs in the US and about 30% of them die.

PE patients typically are given anticoagulants such as *heparin* and *warfarin* (Coumadin). These don't dissolve the clot—they just help prevent the clot from growing and new clots from forming. However, for "massive" PEs, doctors can administer a risky drug called a *tissue plasminogen activator* (tPA) to dissolve the clot. The problem is that high doses of tPA often result in catastrophic bleeding.

A High-Tech Approach

That's where ultrasound comes in. With the use of an ultrasonic drug-delivery catheter, tPA can be delivered directly into the clot. The ultrasonic energy makes the clot more permeable to the drug, and much less drug is used—resulting in fewer side effects (i.e., bleeding). "The way that it works is that you have a catheter with small ultrasound transducers attached. There also are holes in the catheter, so it works as a tiny drug-delivery hose as well as a source of ultrasonic energy," Tod Engelhardt, MD, chair of the cardiovascular and thoracic surgery division at East Jefferson General Hospital, Metairie, Louisiana, explained. "That means that I can give a much lower dose of tPA. The traditional systemic dose is 100 milligrams given over two hours, versus 20 milligrams over 12 hours with the ultrasonic-enhanced catheter."

"My first case was an extreme emergency—a patient who was dying. So I decided to use the device, and it worked very well," Dr. Engelhardt said. That was about two and a half years ago. Since then, he has treated 36 PE patients with this new ultrasonic-enhanced catheter, and he's gotten "great results" each time.

The catheter was approved in 2011 in Europe for treating PEs. In the US, the Food and Drug Administration has okayed ultrasound for treating clots in the arms and legs but has not yet specifically approved it for use in the lungs. Dr. Engelhardt, who has made it a personal mission to campaign for the ultrasound technique, said East Jefferson and several other hospitals are conducting clinical trials for FDA approval.

Until ultrasonic-enhanced catheter use becomes more widespread in treating PEs, Dr. Engelhardt urges anyone diagnosed with a PE to ask his/her doctor if he is aware of the technology.

Prevention

To reduce the chance of developing a blood clot that can travel to the lungs, the National Heart Lung and Blood Institute advises people to exercise their calf muscles whenever they sit for a long time. The Institute also advises people to get out of bed and move around as soon as possible after surgery or an illness…drink plenty of fluids to keep the blood thin…and follow the doctor's advice on anticlot medication after certain types of surgery.

See a doctor immediately if you have any symptoms of a PE—chest pain…unexplained shortness of breath, problems breathing or persistent coughing…an irregular heartbeat…coughing up blood…light-headedness…an unexplained sudden feeling of dread or anxiety.

The Deadly Clot-Buster Filter

Peter L. Faries, MD, Franz W. Sichel Professor of Surgery, chief of the division of vascular surgery and a professor of radiology at Mount Sinai School of Medicine in New York City. Winner of numerous professional awards, he is listed among *Castle Connolly's Top Doctors* and *New York* magazine's *Best Doctors.*

Frances feels like a ticking time bomb. Six years ago, during cancer surgery, her surgeon implanted a special metal filter in her inferior vena cava (IVC), the large vein in the abdomen that returns blood from the lower body to the heart in order to guard against postoperative blood clots. Frances was told that if a clot formed, it could become a pulmonary embolism, a potentially deadly condition in which a clot travels to the lungs.

But ironically, the filter that was supposed to protect Frances has itself become a grave concern—because it is breaking apart. Bits of the device have snapped off, moved through her circulatory system and lodged in her lungs…and the rest of the filter has embedded itself so firmly in the blood vessel wall that her surgeon failed in his attempt to remove it.

Frances is far from alone. The FDA has received more than 900 reports of problems, including filter fractures…migration of filters or detached pieces to other parts of the body, such as the heart, lungs and intestines…perforation of the inferior vena cava…and, ironically, increased risk for the formation of the very clots that the device is meant to guard against. Those cases may represent just the tip of the iceberg, given that about 167,000 patients received IVC filters in 2007 and 259,000 were expected to get them in 2012. Meanwhile, reports of complications continue to emerge.

You may have one of these filters now—or your doctor may someday recommend one. Either way, you need to know about the risks and how to protect yourself. For information, we contacted Peter L. Faries, MD, chief of the division of vascular surgery at Mount Sinai School of Medicine. *What we learned…*

What's Going On?

Many different types of surgery (including orthopedic surgeries, cancer operations, even outpatient procedures) increase a person's odds of developing a blood clot. An IVC filter may be implanted when a patient is deemed to be at particular risk for postsurgical clotting.

The filter, a metal device several inches long with multiple spidery legs, resembles the metal ribs of an umbrella. It is inserted into the patient's IVC via a catheter threaded through a vein in the groin or neck. Once in place, the filter opens like an umbrella. If a clot forms, breaks off and gets carried into the IVC, the filter's job is to catch it and hang on to it (while the body's own clot-dissolving mechanisms and/or blood-thinning medications encourage it to dissolve) so it never reaches the lungs. Retrievable IVC filters gen-

erally are intended to be removed after a few months, when the risk for postsurgical clotting subsides…permanent filters are specifically designed to be left in place.

Concerns about IVC filters came to light when a study by cardiologist William Nicholson, MD, was published in *Archives of Internal Medicine*. After a patient complained of chest pains, Dr. Nicholson discovered that a leg of his IVC filter had migrated to his heart, necessitating open-heart surgery. Then the doctor contacted all patients at his institution who had received this particular type of device (the Bard Recovery filter) and discovered that 25% had broken filters! Among patients who had a newer version, the Bard G2, 12% had broken filters.

If retrievable filters are left in long after the risk for postsurgical clotting has passed, breakage can occur when metal fatigue sets in. Some doctors may be lax about recommending follow-up care, as Frances said that her doctor was. In other cases, patients neglect to return to the doctor as scheduled to have the filter removed. Dr. Faries explained, "Often a person has a removable filter inserted before a big surgery, then afterward, there's recovery and rehab. The patient thinks, 'I've been through a lot already, I don't want to go back to the doctor just now'—and then never gets around to the follow-up."

If Your Doctor Recommends an IVC Filter

Some patients truly are at increased risk for a postsurgical pulmonary embolism—for instance, because they have a history of clots or cannot take blood-thinning medication. In such cases, an IVC filter can be lifesaving, Dr. Faries said—and so its benefits far outweigh its risks.

But in other cases, doctors seem to be too quick to jump on the IVC filter bandwagon.

Evidence: In a recent study in *Archives of Internal Medicine*, 26% of filter placements were deemed inappropriate and another 23% were considered debatable. Clearly, when a patient doesn't really need the filter, getting one "just in case" creates unnecessary risks.

Blood Clots Could Mean DVT

Recent research: In a study of 46 men and women with superficial vein thrombosis (clotting in blood vessels close to the skin), 24% of the patients were found to also have deep vein thrombosis (DVT), a condition in which blood clots form—usually in the leg—and can break away and travel to the lungs or brain, causing stroke or death.

If you have been diagnosed with superficial vein thrombosis: Ask your doctor to evaluate you for DVT.

Barbara Binder, MD, associate professor, department of dermatology, Medical University of Graz, Austria.

Suppose that your doctor someday suggests that you need an IVC filter. *Here's what to discuss before you say OK…*

• **Why is a filter advisable for you personally?** The doctor should explain which factors in your individual health history tip the balance of benefits versus risks.

• **Are there other options?** Many at-risk patients can be treated with blood-thinning medication, such as *warfarin* (Coumadin), rather than a filter.

• **What information is there on the long-term safety of the particular product to be used?** Your doctor should be able to discuss the specific brand.

• **Will the filter be implanted temporarily or permanently?** Though the best answer depends on your individual needs, the doctor ought to explain his or her recommendation to you.

• **If the filter is to be permanent, will you receive a product specifically designed for permanent placement?** The answer must be yes—these filters have had fewer reports of breakages, Dr. Faries noted.

• **If the filter is temporary, when will it be removed?** Again, the answer varies from patient to patient—but the FDA recommends that physicians consider removing retriev-able IVC filters as soon as protection from pulmonary embolism is no longer needed. Remember, what's important is to follow up in a timely manner. You can't just leave the thing in and forget about it! As Dr. Faries emphasized, care of the filter must remain a priority.

If You Already Have An IVC Filter

Did you receive an IVC filter in the past? *What to do…*

If you are overdue for a filter follow-up visit, contact your doctor without delay. An X-ray can check for breakage…additional testing can determine where broken pieces have gone and whether they can be surgically removed.

Ask your doctor whether the filter itself—intact or not—should and could be removed. In many cases, removal is a relatively simple procedure similar to the insertion method, Dr. Faries said.

If your doctor says that your filter is not retrievable, get a second or even a third opinion. If it turns out that you must live with the filter, follow your doctor's recommendations regarding ongoing follow-up and surveillance.

Be on the lookout for possible warning signs—unexplained shortness of breath, chest pain, abdominal pain—that could signal filter breakage, migration or clotting. If you experience any such symptoms, call your doctor immediately.

Tall People Have a Higher Risk for Blood Clots

In taller people, blood must be pumped a longer distance, so there may be reduced blood flow in the legs—raising clot risk. Clot risk is greatest in men who are tall and heavy. Obese men who are five feet, 11 inches tall have five times the risk of normal-weight men who are about five feet, seven inches tall or less. In obese, tall women—more than five feet, six inches—the risk is 2.9 times greater than in normal-weight women, who are five feet, 2.6 inches tall or less.

Sigrid Braekkan, PhD, researcher, Hematological Research Group, University of Tromsø, Norway, and investigator of a study of 26,714 Norwegian people, published by the American Heart Association in *Arteriosclerosis, Thrombosis and Vascular Biology.*

Breaks Can Stop Blood Clots

Blood clots in the legs can occur in office workers as well as long-distance travelers. A potentially deadly clot, called deep vein thrombosis, can occur when a person is seated in one position for prolonged periods.

Reality: There are more people seated for long periods every day in offices than there are airline travelers.

Self-defense: Take regular breaks while working or flying. Get up, stretch your legs and walk around—to prevent clots from forming.

Richard Beasley, DSc, director, Medical Research Institute of New Zealand, Wellington, and leader of a study of 61 patients, published in *Internal Medicine Journal.*

Blood Thinners: Too Risky?

Emile Mohler, MD, associate professor of medicine, Hospital of the University of Pennsylvania, Presbyterian Medical Center of Philadelphia, and director of vascular medicine, Penn Heart and Vascular Center, Penn Medical, Philadelphia.

A study from Vanderbilt University Medical Center in Nashville, published recently in the *Archives of Surgery,* underscored the dangers blood thinners carry, when it found that people on the popular anticoagulant *warfarin* (Coumadin) who sustained a traumatic injury (and this can be

Post Surgery Blood Clot Prevention

Dangerous blood clots are likely up to 12 weeks after surgery. Patients who have recently undergone surgery are up to 110 times more likely to be admitted to a hospital because of potentially fatal thromboses (blood clots) than people who have not had surgery.

Self-defense: Anticlotting drugs and physical measures, such as compression stockings, can reduce risk.

Jane Green, MD, PhD, group head and principal investigator, Cancer Epidemiology Unit, University of Oxford, England, and coauthor of a study of thromboses in 947,454 women, published in *BMJ Online First.*

something as simple as falling in your bathtub and hitting your head) were twice as likely to die as those not on the drug.

Different Meds, Different Risks

What can you do to best protect yourself? According to Emile Mohler, MD, director of vascular medicine at the Penn Heart and Vascular Center in Philadelphia, even people who take these drugs can get confused about the exact nature of the medicine they are on. In fact, calling the drugs "blood thinners" is technically incorrect—the drugs do not thin blood but rather act on clots that can form in the blood. And, while the group of drugs overall is referred to as "anticoagulants," this too is actually not quite correct since different drugs act in different ways. *Here is an explanation of the drug categories and how they differ…*

•**Anticoagulants**—e.g., *warfarin* (Coumadin). These do not dissolve clots but inhibit clot production and prevent clots from enlarging. They are used for atrial fibrillation, an erratic heartbeat that can create clots that travel to the brain, triggering stroke, as well as for other situations in which clots may form in the heart, such as during heart-valve replacement. These drugs treat blood clots in a deep vein, usually in the legs. This condition is known as deep vein thrombosis (DVT). Anticoagulants also help prevent second strokes or heart attacks.

• **Antiplatelets**—e.g., aspirin, *clopidogrel* (Plavix). Platelets are cells in the blood that form clots to repair damaged blood vessels. Unfortunately platelets also can create harmful clots—and so antiplatelet drugs are used to prevent the kind of platelet "clumping" that starts a clot. Antiplatelets are used for heart attacks caused by a clot (myocardial infarction), for angioplasty/stent patients and to prevent future heart attacks in patients who have already suffered one.

• **Thrombin inhibitors**—e.g., *heparin*. These are fast-acting drugs that are used, usually on a short-term basis, right after many types of surgery to prevent clot formation or to treat patients with vein clots.

Your Safety on Anticoagulants

Dr. Mohler describes these drugs as "incredibly lifesaving," noting that most of the time the drugs' benefits outweigh their risks. Nevertheless, he says it is indeed a tough balance between clot protection and bleeding. "There is always going to be a risk of bleeding whatever the specific drug, because otherwise it would mean the drug isn't effective," he explains. *To maximize your safety, Dr. Mohler offered the following information and advice…*

• **Although Coumadin is the most widely used anticoagulant,** it is a difficult drug for both patients and doctors, says Dr. Mohler, because "however carefully blood levels are monitored, they can change quickly, and the foods you eat impact your blood levels as well."

For your safety: Strictly adhere to a schedule of monitoring with International Normalized Ratio (INR) blood tests (through a Coumadin clinic) to be sure that your blood levels remain in the proper range. Diet is critical—Coumadin blocks the clotting action of vitamin K, but if you eat foods that are high in K (leafy greens, especially spinach and kale), it can negate the effect of the Couma-

din. Limit yourself to the number of servings per week that your doctor advises.

• **Patients on low-dose aspirin therapy** must be careful when taking additional aspirin for painkilling purposes, as it can jeopardize the antiplatelet effect.

For your safety: Never take additional aspirin. If you need a painkiller, take acetaminophen instead—or if you take ibuprofen, which is more similar to aspirin, always take the additional painkiller at least 30 minutes after taking the daily aspirin to be sure that the other drug will not interfere with the antiplatelet action of the aspirin.

• **Surgery patients need to clot in order to heal,** but when taking blood thinners it is tricky, Dr. Mohler says. Depending on the level of clot risk, there are a variety of ways for doctors to handle this problem, including using heparin in place of warfarin for a few days.

For your safety: Before surgery, discuss with your doctor how this will be handled to best protect you.

• **Accidents that healthy people are likely to recover from quickly** can cause deep bruises and bleeding when a patient is on these drugs.

For your safety: Avoid situations with a high risk for injury—even minor injury—such as rough sports, difficult hiking, etc. Always carry a card or wear a medical ID bracelet that lets emergency medical professionals know you are on an anticoagulant or antiplatelet…be sure to inform all of your health-care professionals, including pharmacists, about your drug.

Brighter Days Ahead

There are hopeful developments in the world of anticoagulants with new drugs in development. One called *dabigatran* (Pradaxa) is already available and may one day replace Coumadin. It is easier to monitor, and diet does not interfere with it. However, you need to take it twice a day, and the drug is very expensive. Another group of anticoagulants called factor Xa inhibitors are available, and

Dr. Mohler says these too may replace Coumadin in some instances, especially for DVT. Perhaps most intriguing of all, there is a study under way at The University of Pennsylvania that should make treatment easier and safer. Researchers are investigating patients' DNA for mutations that affect blood clotting. The hope is that with information specific to individuals, doctors will be able to adjust drug dosages to create optimal levels in each person's blood.

Fight Killer Blood Clots—Reduce Your Risk for Heart Attack and Stroke with These Nondrug Approaches

Decker Weiss, NMD, a naturopathic medical doctor who specializes in integrative cardiology. He is the founder and owner of Weiss Natural Medicine, in Scottsdale, Arizona, *www.weissnaturalmedicine.com*, and author of *The Weiss Method: A Natural Program for Reversing Heart Disease and Preventing Heart Attacks* (Shannake).

Millions of Americans take anticlotting medications, or "blood thinners," including aspirin and *warfarin* (Coumadin), to prevent clots and reduce the risk for such conditions as heart attack and stroke.

These drugs are extremely effective. Daily aspirin, for example, can reduce the risk for a first heart attack by 44%, according to data from the *Physicians' Health Study*.

The downside: Even at low doses, every anticlotting agent can cause bleeding—often from the stomach, gums or intestines—as a side effect. Sometimes, gastrointestinal bleeding can occur even without causing noticeable symptoms.

In addition, warfarin, one of the leading blood thinners, doubles the risk for intracerebral hemorrhage (bleeding in the brain).

Natural Blood Thinners

The good news is that certain herbs and other supplements can be used for their anti-clotting properties—and may have a reduced risk for side effects, such as bleeding.

This approach is not intended to replace medications—patients with a high risk for clotting need to take such drugs. Under a doctor's supervision, these supplements can be combined with blood-thinning medications to boost the drugs' effectiveness and potentially allow you to take a lower dose, thus reducing the risk for bleeding.

Those with only a slight risk for clots (due to family history, for example) may want to consider using natural anticoagulants alone, under a doctor's supervision, to promote better circulation.

Bonus: Natural blood thinners usually have anti-inflammatory properties. This is important because most chronic diseases, including heart disease, rheumatoid arthritis and stroke, are caused in part by inflammation.

The supplements below can be taken alone or in combination, depending on the degree of protection that's required.

Some of these supplements may interact with prescription medications, so consult a doctor who is knowledgeable about supplement use.* *Best choices*…

•**Fish oil.** Studies of large populations show that people who eat a lot of cold-water fish, such as salmon and mackerel, tend to have lower heart attack death rates than people who don't eat fish.

The omega-3 fatty acids in cold-water fish are strong anticlotting agents. Fish oil is thought to inhibit platelet aggregation (clumping), part of the clotting process. One report, published in *The Annals of Pharmacotherapy*, found that taking fish oil along with warfarin caused an increase in anticlotting activity.

Typical dose: Depending on other risk factors, such as elevated cholesterol and high blood pressure, one tablet twice daily

*To find a doctor who has experience treating patients with supplements, consult the American Association of Naturopathic Physicians, 866-538-2267, *www.naturopathic.org*.

of Vectomega's Whole Food Omega-3 DHA/ EPA Complex—it provides 292 mg of omega-3s (DHA and EPA balanced) in a phospholipid peptide complex, in which the fish oil is bound to peptides to increase absorbability. Or one teaspoon twice daily of Nordic Naturals' Ultimate Omega Liquid, which provides 1,626 mg of EPA and 1,126 mg of DHA.

• **Ginger and curcumin.** Ginger reduces levels of fibrinogen, a precursor to fibrin, a protein that is a major component of blood clots. Curcumin has only modest effects on coagulation but is a stronger anti-inflammatory agent. That's why I advise patients to take these herbs together. Studies have shown that both ginger and curcumin can reduce inflammation in the body. An Australian study found that substances in ginger inhibited the activity of arachidonic acid, part of the chemical sequence involved in clotting. In the study, ginger compounds were more effective than aspirin at blocking platelet activity.

Typical dose: Twice daily, 50 mg to 100 mg of ginger and one or two 375-mg capsules of curcumin.

Good products: Gaia Herbs' Ginger Supreme Phyto-Caps and EuroPharma's Cura Med curcumin complex.

• **Nattokinase.** Extracted from soybeans, nattokinase is an enzyme that helps prevent clot formation—it also makes platelets less likely to clump together. Unlike warfarin, which only prevents clots, nattokinase appears to break down clots that already have formed.

Typical dose: Depending on other risk factors, one to two capsules or tablets (2,000 fibrin units per 100 mg) twice daily.

Important: I recommend taking nattokinase between meals. The anticlotting properties are strongest when it is taken without food.

• **Vinpocetine.** This supplement is extracted from periwinkle. It's extremely important to take vinpocetine under a doctor's supervision. Vinpocetine is the most potent natural substance for preventing clots—and, like

prescription anticlotting agents, it can cause internal bleeding in some patients. For this reason, I recommend it mainly for high-risk patients who are unable to take warfarin because of side effects and/or complications.

Typical dose: 2 mg total—in divided doses twice daily. Higher doses (5 mg total in divided doses) might be needed, but don't increase from the starting dose without talking with your doctor. Should be taken without food.

• **Ginkgo.** The extract from the dried leaves of the ginkgo biloba tree has traditionally been used to treat intermittent claudication, leg pain caused by insufficient blood flow, as well as cognitive impairments (such as memory problems) due to poor blood circulation in the brain.

Ginkgo is effective at reducing clots and also acts as a vasodilator that helps improve blood flow to the brain, heart and other parts of the body. I don't recommend it as often as other anticoagulants because it has little effect on inflammation. If you use ginkgo, ask your doctor about combining it with curcumin or other anti-inflammatory herbs/supplements.

Typical dose: About 40 mg, three times daily.

• **Garlic.** Studies have shown that patients who take garlic supplements have a lower risk for clots. Use only those products that list a high allicin content—the main active ingredient in garlic. This can be found frequently in fresh garlic supplements.

Typical dose: The optimal dose for garlic hasn't been definitively established. However, some studies indicate that you need at least 180 mg of allicin twice daily.

Good brand: Allimax.

Important: In general, natural therapies should be started at low doses that are slowly increased, under a doctor's supervision, over time. I recommend that the supplements described in this article be used at least twice daily to ensure that adequate levels of the therapeutic compounds are maintained in the body.

Chapter 3

BEST WAYS TO CONTROL YOUR BLOOD PRESSURE

Blood Pressure Medications May Increase Breast Cancer Risk

What is the most common chronic medical condition among US adults? High blood pressure. And what is one of the most common cancers among women? Breast cancer.

Now, no one is suggesting that the high blood pressure causes breast cancer...but because they're both so common, it just makes sense to look for any possible links. And researchers have found one.

It turns out that a certain type of drug used to treat high blood pressure is associated with more than double the risk for breast cancer...while a different type of blood pressure drug is associated with a reduced risk for breast cancer.

If you or a woman you love takes blood pressure medication, you should know which is which.

In-Home Interviews For Accuracy

Previous studies that looked for a connection between blood pressure drugs and breast cancer had only small numbers of patients... did not factor in how long the drugs were used...and/or relied on patients' own recall about medication use, which can be inaccurate. So epidemiologists at Fred Hutchinson Cancer Research Center in Seattle tackled the subject in a unique way.

The study participants included nearly 2,000 Seattle-area postmenopausal women who had been diagnosed between 2000 and 2008 with either invasive ductal breast cancer (the most common form, which arises in the milk ducts) or invasive lobular breast cancer (which arises in the milk glands)...plus nearly 900 cancer-free postmenopausal women who served as controls.

To ensure that participants' reports about medication use were as accurate as possible, the women were interviewed in their own homes and asked to show the researchers the actual bottles of all medications that they were currently using. To aid participants' memories of past medication use, the researchers also showed the women photographs of commonly used blood pressure drugs, along with cards listing their brand

Christopher I. Li, MD, PhD, epidemiologist specializing in breast cancer, division of public health sciences, Fred Hutchinson Cancer Research Center, Seattle. His study was published in *JAMA Internal Medicine*.

and generic names. In addition, the women answered detailed questions about medication dosages and dates of usage…and about other risk factors for breast cancer, including their reproductive, medical and family health histories.

Breast Cancer/Blood Pressure Connection

The rate of high blood pressure was the same—44%—among the women with breast cancer and the women without breast cancer. Researchers analyzed the data several different ways, cross-comparing women with and without breast cancer…women with and without high blood pressure…women who did and did not take the various types of blood pressure drugs…and short-term versus long-term use of the drugs. The researchers also adjusted for age and other breast cancer risk factors, such as smoking, alcohol use and family history of breast cancer.

Here's what they found…

Using a type of blood pressure drug called a calcium-channel blocker for 10 years or more was associated with 2.4 times higher risk for ductal breast cancer and 2.6 times higher risk for lobular breast cancer. There was some indication that risks were even greater—3.7 times higher for ductal breast cancer and 3.6 times higher for lobular breast cancer—among current users of the so-called short-acting calcium-channel blockers. However, because short-acting formulations are prescribed less often, the effect of duration of use could not be assessed.

Using drugs known as ACE inhibitors for 10 years or longer was associated with a 30% reduced risk for ductal breast cancer and a 40% reduced risk for lobular breast cancer. Using an ACE inhibitor for less than 10 years did not significantly decrease or increase breast cancer risk.

There was no increase or decrease in breast cancer risk among women taking other types of blood pressure drugs—diuretics, beta-blockers or angiotensin receptor blockers (ARBs).

Women's Blood Pressure Should Be Lower Than Men's

Researchers analyzed data on 3,344 hypertension patients (average age 52.6) for more than five years.

Result: Women were at greater risk for cardiovascular events, such as heart attack and stroke, than men when their daytime blood pressure readings were 125/80 mmHg or above and nighttime readings were 110/65 or above—far below the current threshold for hypertension for both sexes of 140/90.

Theory: Women's blood pressure is typically lower than men's, so it should be monitored differently.

If you're a woman with blood pressure of 125/80 or above: Talk to your doctor.

Ramon Hermida, PhD, director, bioengineering and chronobiology laboratory, University of Vigo, Spain.

Help for the Hypertensive Woman

The different blood pressure drugs work in different ways. Calcium-channel blockers work by preventing calcium from entering the cells of the heart and blood vessels, which allows the muscle cells to relax and thus reduces blood pressure. Nearly 15% of blood pressure drug prescriptions are for calcium-channel blockers such as *amlodipine* (Norvasc)…*diltiazem* (Cardizem)…*felodipine* (Plendil)…*isradipine* (Dynacirc)…*nicardipine* (Cardene)…*nifedipine* (Procardia)…and *verapamil* (Calan).

Why are calcium-channel blockers associated with increased risk for breast cancer? That's not known, and this study wasn't designed to answer that question. Researchers also could not say why ACE inhibitors were associated with lower breast cancer risk, and they noted that this finding needs to be replicated in future studies that include a greater number of long-term users of ACE inhibitors. The current study results must be interpreted with caution and should not yet affect clinical practice, the researchers said—so clearly, more research is needed.

What can you do in the meantime? Reduce your blood pressure naturally—which may reduce your need for any sort of blood pressure drug—by eating right. See "Foods That Help Control Blood Pressure" on page 48.

High Blood Pressure in Pregnancy May Predict Later Ills, Study Says

Circulation, news release

Women who have high blood pressure during pregnancy are at increased risk for heart disease, kidney disease and diabetes later in life, according to a recent study.

The increased risk was seen even in women who had only one or two high blood pressure readings during their pregnancy, the researchers said.

"All of the later-life risks were similar in pregnant women who could otherwise be considered low-risk—those who were young, normal weight, nonsmokers, with no diabetes during pregnancy," said study lead author Tuija Mannisto, MD, PhD, a postdoctoral fellow at the US National Institute of Child Health and Human Development.

"According to our findings, women who have had high blood pressure during pregnancy or who are diagnosed with high blood pressure in pregnancy for the first time might benefit from comprehensive heart disease risk factor checks by their physicians, to decrease their long-term risk of heart diseases," Dr. Mannisto added.

It's known that women with preeclampsia—a serious pregnancy-related disease marked by high blood pressure and protein in the urine—are at increased risk for heart and kidney disease.

Even Slightly High Blood Pressure May Raise Stroke Risk

People who have prehypertension—defined by systolic blood pressure (top number) of 120 mmHg to 139 mmHg or diastolic pressure (bottom number) of 80 mmHg to 89 mmHg—are 55% more likely to have strokes than people with normal blood pressure.

Self-defense: If your blood pressure is even slightly high, ask your doctor about ways to bring it down, such as losing weight and reducing salt intake.

Bruce Ovbiagele, MD, MSc, professor, department of neurosciences, University of California, San Diego, and leader of a review of 12 studies involving 518,520 adults, published online in *Neurology*.

Study Details

This study looked at less serious forms of high blood pressure that are much more common in pregnant women. The study included Finnish women who had babies in 1966 and were followed for 40 years.

One-third of the women had at least one high blood pressure reading during pregnancy. These women were 14% to 100% more likely to develop heart disease later in life than those with normal blood pressure throughout their pregnancy, according to the study in the journal *Circulation*.

Women with any high blood pressure during pregnancy also had a two to five times increased risk of dying from a heart attack and a 1.4 to 2.2 times higher risk of developing diabetes. Women who had any high blood pressure, with and without measurable protein in the urine, during pregnancy had a 1.9 to 2.8 times greater risk of developing kidney disease later in life.

The study also found that women with high blood pressure during pregnancy but normal blood pressure after pregnancy still had a 1.6 to 2.5 times greater risk of having high blood pressure requiring medication or hospitalization later in life.

Dr. Mannisto said future research should explore whether lifestyle changes and post-pregnancy follow-up could change these women's long-term health.

For more information about high blood pressure during pregnancy, visit the US National Heart, Lung, and Blood Institute Web site at *www.nhlbi.nih.gov/health/public/heart/hbp/hbp_preg.htm.*

What Your Doctor May Not Tell You About High Blood Pressure

Mark C. Houston, MD, associate clinical professor of medicine at Vanderbilt University School of Medicine and director of the Hypertension Institute at Saint Thomas Medical Group, both in Nashville. He is author of four books, including *What Your Doctor May Not Tell You About Hypertension* and the upcoming *What Your Doctor May Not Tell You About Heart Disease* (both from Grand Central). *www.hypertension institute.com*

A woman—let's call her Naomi—was diagnosed with high blood pressure and went on medication prescribed by her doctor. Within a few months, she was back at the doctor's office, her blood pressure heading up instead of down. It turned out that she was not taking her medication properly—and that the drug she had been given was not the most appropriate one for her.

Naomi is hardly alone. Nearly one-third of US adults have hypertension (blood pressure higher than 140/90), a symptomless disease that, if not appropriately managed, can result in a heart attack or stroke.

Mark C. Houston, MD, is director of the Hypertension Institute at Saint Thomas Medical Group in Nashville and author of *What Your Doctor May Not Tell You About Hypertension*. He explained that failure to take medication properly is one primary reason why high blood pressure is often so hard to get under control.

Another problem is that finding the right medication or combination of medications can be tricky, and often doctors have resorted to a "try this, try that" approach.

Good news: Recent research has helped clarify which types of drugs are likely to work best for certain patients. (See the following article "Are You Taking the Right Blood Pressure Medication?" for more information.) So if you have recently been diagnosed with hypertension or if your medication is not working, it's time to talk to your doctor about…

•**Your levels of the blood pressure-modulating enzyme renin.** A recent study showed that people with different blood levels of renin responded differently to various hypertension drugs—and that taking the wrong kind of medication actually made blood pressure go up.

Patients with high-renin hypertension responded best to…

•Angiotensin-converting enzyme (ACE) inhibitors, which reduce blood pressure by blocking an enzyme that produces angiotensin II (a hormone that causes blood vessels to narrow)…dilating arteries…and reducing inflammation and oxidative stress. They also decrease clotting, further protecting against heart attack and stroke.

•Angiotensin receptor blockers (ARBs), which work by blocking receptors for angiotensin I (the precursor to angiotensin II). They also dilate blood vessels and ease inflammation and oxidative stress.

•Direct renin inhibitors, which reduce angiotensin I and relax blood vessels.

•Beta-blockers, which reduce blood pressure by reducing nerve signals to the heart and blood vessels and slowing the heart rate.

People with low-renin hypertension responded best to…

•Calcium channel blockers, which combat high blood pressure by preventing calcium from moving into arteries and heart muscle cells and allowing arteries to dilate.

•Diuretics, which cause kidneys to remove excess sodium and water from the body and dilate blood vessel walls.

•**How your blood pressure is being measured.** The blood pressure cuff in your doctor's office may not be reliable if you are prone to "white-coat hypertension" (blood pressure that rises from the anxiety of being in the doctor's office) or "masked hypertension" (lower blood pressure numbers in the doctor's office but consistently higher numbers at other times).

Ask your doctor if you might benefit from using a high-quality home blood pressure monitor (sold over the counter in pharmacies and online for $50 to $150) to keep track of your readings every day. Also discuss the option of using a 24-hour ambulatory blood pressure monitor. A cuff worn on your arm and a small device clipped to your belt record your pressure every 15 to 30 minutes for 24 hours…then your doctor analyzes that data.

•**How consistently you take your medicine.** The different types of hypertension drugs can cause a variety of side effects, such as fatigue, memory problems and sexual dysfunction. If you experience these or other problems, do not suffer in silence—and certainly do not keep silent if you sometimes skip doses to avoid side effects. Tell your doctor and discuss alternative drugs.

But if you are conscientious about taking your meds, be sure your doctor knows that, too. Otherwise he or she may wrongly assume that any lack of effectiveness is due to your noncompliance rather than to a need for a different medication.

•**When to take your medication.** Since blood pressure medications are effective for only 24 hours, it is important to take them at the same time every day. Don't drive yourself crazy if you are an hour early or an hour late, but do not be off by several hours.

Very important: Most heart attacks and strokes happen between 3 am and 10 am, which is when blood pressure typically is highest. That's why the new recommendation generally is to take your medicine at night, Dr. Houston said—to block that early morning blood pressure spike.

Are You Taking the Right Blood Pressure Medication?

Samuel J. Mann, MD, professor of clinical medicine at Weill Medical College of Cornell University and a hypertension specialist at New York-Presbyterian Hospital, both in New York City. Dr. Mann has written more than 50 scientific articles and book chapters about hypertension. He is also author of *Hypertension and You: Old Drugs, New Drugs and the Right Drugs for Your High Blood Pressure* (Rowman & Littlefield).

If you're one of the roughly 75 million Americans with high blood pressure (hypertension), you might like to believe that lifestyle changes, such as losing weight, exercising and cutting back on salt, can control it. In some cases, it can. But like it or not, most people who have hypertension end up on medication.

The problem is that more than one-third of patients on medication still have elevated blood pressure readings. In many instances, they are not on medication or a dosage that is right for them. Millions also are suffering from avoidable side effects.

There are more than 60 drugs for hypertension—too many for most physicians (even specialists) to know about in detail. What's more, your drug treatment needs to be targeted to match the cause of your hypertension.

What's Your Hypertension?

Of the millions of Americans with inadequately controlled hypertension, nearly all could have blood pressure in the normal range simply by adjusting their medication. What most patients don't realize is that hypertension is driven by different mechanisms that respond to different treatments.

The three mechanisms underlying hypertension in most cases—and the best treatments for each…

#1: Hypertension driven by sodium/volume. This is the most common form of high blood pressure, affecting at least half of hypertensive patients.

The kidneys do not excrete sodium efficiently and, as a result, the body starts to accumulate sodium and fluid. This increase in fluid volume raises blood pressure. In addition, elevated sodium can trigger arterial constriction in some patients, which further raises blood pressure.

Telltale signs: Fluid retention in the legs (edema) and low levels of the hormone renin (as measured with a widely available blood test). African-Americans, people over age 65 and those who are "salt-sensitive" are more likely to have sodium/volume hypertension.

Main treatment: A diuretic (water pill) that increases sodium excretion or a calcium-channel blocker, such as amlodipine (Norvasc), that dilates arteries.

#2: Hypertension driven by the renin-angiotensin system (RAS).

The kidneys have sensors that monitor blood pressure and blood volume. When either is low, the kidneys secrete the hormone renin, which triggers the formation of angiotensin II, constricting arteries and raising blood pressure.

Telltale signs: High renin levels in the blood, the absence of edema and lack of response to diuretics prescribed to reduce blood pressure. It's more common in Caucasians under age 50.

Four classes of drugs that block RAS activation…

•**Angiotensin-converting enzyme (ACE) inhibitors,** such as *enalapril* (Vasotec) and *captopril* (Capoten).

•**Angiotensin-receptor blockers (ARBs),** such as *losartan* (Cozaar) and *valsartan* (Diovan).

•**Direct renin inhibitor (DRI).** *Aliskiren* (Tekturna)—the only drug within this class.

•**Beta-blockers,** an older drug class, which includes *metoprolol* (Toprol). In most patients with RAS-mediated hypertension, ACE inhibitors and ARBs are preferred over beta-blockers—outcomes are better, and they cause fewer side effects, such as fatigue.

Approximately 80% of hypertension patients will respond to drugs that target sodium/volume or the RAS, or to a combination of drugs that targets both.

#3: Hypertension driven by the sympathetic nervous system (SNS). The SNS is responsible for hypertension in about 15% of cases and frequently is overlooked by physicians. Stimulation of the SNS, which is the primary link between our brain and our blood pressure, results in adrenaline-induced increases in heart rate and cardiac output (the amount of blood pumped by the heart) and arterial constriction. Emotions stimulate the SNS and may be the source of SNS hypertension.

Effective drugs include beta-blockers, which slow down the heart, often in combination with an alpha-blocker, such as *doxazosin* (Cardura), which dilates arteries. Drugs like *clonidine* (Catapres), a central alpha-receptor stimulator, reduce SNS outflow from the brain but cause fatigue in most patients.

Telltale signs: Conditions such as alcohol abuse and sleep apnea can trigger SNS-driven hypertension. Other indicators are episodic hypertension and hypertension that is not controlled by drugs that target sodium/volume and the RAS.

Prescription Pitfalls

There are many effective drugs on the market, but unless they are correctly prescribed, hypertension won't be controlled and avoidable side effects may occur. *Common errors you should watch out for…*

•**Widespread overtreatment.** Millions of Americans are on more medication than they need, including many people who might not need any at all.

The most common reasons doctors overprescribe: Anxiety that raises blood pressure when visiting the doctor, incorrect measurement of blood pressure at the doctor's office and/or at home, and the addition of medication in patients with

Better Blood Pressure Drug

33,000 adults with high blood pressure took the generic diuretic *chlorthalidone* or one of two newer, brand-name drugs—the calcium channel blocker Norvasc or the ACE inhibitor *lisinopril*—for nine years, on average.

Result: Compared with those taking a diuretic, those taking Norvasc were 12% more likely to have died from or been hospitalized for heart failure, and those taking Lisinopril were 20% more likely to have died from stroke.

When exercise and diet changes don't lower blood pressure: Ask your doctor about diuretics.

Paul Whelton, MD, former president and CEO, Loyola University Health System, Chicago.

well-controlled hypertension who have an occasional elevated reading.

• **Not enough diuretics.** In many people, a low dose of a diuretic, such as 25 mg of *hydrochlorothiazide*, is sufficient—a higher dose is not needed and even can be harmful. But in some, a higher dose or a combination of two diuretics is essential. Studies show that in half of people with uncontrolled hypertension, blood pressure can be brought under control by strengthening the diuretic regimen.

• **Underuse of some highly effective older drugs.** New drugs are promoted, while some older drugs are nearly forgotten. Older diuretics such as *amiloride* (Midamor) and *torsemide* (Demadex), and beta-blockers such as *betaxolol* (Kerlone) and *bisoprolol* (Zebeta) are examples of excellent older drugs that are not commonly prescribed but should be.

• **Overuse of beta-blockers.** Beta-blockers can cause fatigue and, in older patients, can affect cognitive function. Modifying or eliminating use of the beta-blocker can improve cognitive function in some patients and should not be overlooked as a consideration

in the evaluation of cognitive decline. Many patients taking a beta-blocker for hypertension don't need to be on one!

• **Lack of appreciation for emotional factors.** Decades of studies have failed to prove that such factors as stress, anger and anxiety lead to hypertension. However, some studies suggest that repressed emotions, the emotions we are unaware of, might contribute. If your hypertension is driven by emotional factors, you will respond better to drugs that target the SNS.

Summing up, nearly all patients with hypertension can be treated successfully with available drugs. The goal is a normal blood pressure without drug side effects. You should not settle for less.

Should you see a hypertension specialist? If your hypertension is under control with one or two drugs, and you have no side effects, you don't need to see a specialist.

Otherwise, consider seeking the opinion of a physician specializing in hypertension. To find one, go to *www.ASH-US.org*, the Web site of the American Society of Hypertension (under "Patients," click on "HTN Specialists Directory").

Are You Taking Blood Pressure Medications That You Don't Need?

Steven Burgess, MD, chief resident in family medicine at Texas Tech University Health Sciences Center, School of Medicine, Amarillo.

Here's a disturbing bit of news: A recent study reports that 81% of blood pressure measurements taken by doctors and nurses are done improperly, resulting in numerous misdiagnoses. This means that many people are taking medications that they really don't need!

The American Heart Association has published guidelines recommending a particular methodology to follow when taking blood pressure measurements in a clinical setting, such as a doctor's office. In an earlier study, researchers evaluated pressure-taking techniques of 172 doctors and nurses and reported that none were following guidelines set by the American Heart Association—this inspired Steven Burgess, MD, chief resident in family medicine at Texas Tech University Health Sciences Center School of Medicine in Amarillo, to undertake a study to evaluate how these potentially erroneous measurements impact patient care.

What he learned is disconcerting, to say the least—he said that the mistakes made when taking blood pressure readings were significant enough to change treatment recommendations for more than half the patients in the study! "My study showed that if someone initially has elevated blood pressure and we redo the reading in accordance with the guidelines, over 50% of the time the new 'correct' pressure puts the patient into a different category, which would cause treatment to be different," he said, noting that the pressure is virtually always lower when taken "correctly."

Mistakes Are Made

The most common blood pressure measurement mistake being made by health-care practitioners is to take a blood pressure reading immediately after a patient sits down. The guidelines say that patients should rest quietly for five minutes first. Why? Because physical activity raises blood pressure, often by 10 mmHg or more.

In his 18-month study of 56 patients, Dr. Burgess found that when blood pressure is measured properly, the average patient's systolic (top number) reading is 15.7 mmHg lower than when the guidelines aren't being followed. For more than half (56.4%) of the patients, using the correct technique—compared with doing it the wrong way—meant that patients were fine without medication or changes to their current therapy.

Measure by Measure...

Here are the American Heart Association's guidelines regarding the proper technique for measuring blood pressure...

• **Patients should not exercise, drink caffeine or smoke** for 30 minutes prior to measurement and should sit quietly for five minutes immediately before.

• **While the measurement is being taken, the patient should be comfortably seated with his/her back supported** (not perched on a stool or a table) and with feet flat on the floor. The patient's bare arm (the sleeve can be rolled up or, if it is too constricting, the shirt can be removed) should be supported at the level of his heart. In other words, the patient should lean his arm on an armrest or table or the doctor or nurse taking the reading should hold the patient's arm, not let it hang at the patient's side.

• **The cuff must fit properly according to specific guidelines.** For most people, a standard cuff will satisfy these guidelines, but large or obese patients or those who are unusually small require special-sized equipment.

• **For professional equipment (what's used by a health-care professional), the cuff should be placed one inch above the elbow.** For digital monitors designed to be used at home, the cuff should be centered over the inside of the elbow.

• **No talking—by either the patient or the practitioner.** Speaking not only raises blood pressure, it also interferes with the practitioner's ability to focus on your pulse while taking a reading.

• **At an initial visit, two readings should be taken and the results should be averaged.** If the readings differ by more than 5 mm Hg, a third reading should be taken and averaged with the other two. (*Note*: At subsequent visits, a single reading may be sufficient.)

Homework

Lots of people now monitor their blood pressure at home—so it's important that everyone recognizes that these readings must be done in the proper way. Be sure you are using the right type of equipment and following instructions. Also check to see whether your equipment gives you readings that match those taken in your doctor's office.

Is Your Doctor Checking Your Blood Pressure Wrong?

Christopher E. Clark, MBChB, MSc, FRCP, FRCGP, clinical academic fellow, Primary Care Research Group at the Peninsula College of Medicine & Dentistry, University of Exeter and Plymouth, England.

At your annual physical, after your doctor wraps that blood pressure cuff around one of your arms, does he/she then wrap it around your other arm?

It's most likely that he or his assistant does not.

So what? Well, a recent British study adds to the growing body of research showing that blood pressure measurements in both arms are critical, because each arm may have a different measure—and the size of that difference can play a large role in your risk for cardiovascular problems.

The Heart of the Matter

Researchers at the Peninsula College of Medicine & Dentistry in England analyzed data from more than 20 studies on blood pressure monitoring.

What they found: After five to 16 years of follow-up, researchers found that a difference of 15 mmHg of systolic pressure (the top blood pressure reading) between the two arms indicated 2.5 times the risk for peripheral artery disease...a 60% higher risk for stroke...and a 70% higher risk of dying of heart disease, compared with those whose left- and right-arm systolic pressure differed by less than 15 mmHg. And the risk for these

events increased as the difference in systolic blood pressure increased over 15 mmHg.

Those particular increased risks were the same whether a patient's two systolic numbers were, say, 115 and 100 or 170 and 155. But hypertensive patients, those with blood pressure readings over 140/90, are still at more overall risk, the researchers noted.

Double Checking

If so many studies keep showing that the difference in blood pressure between the two arms matters, then why aren't more doctors measuring both arms? *Lead study author Christopher E. Clark, MD, clinical academic fellow at the college, explains...*

If your systolic pressure varies between arms, what's likely going on? Dr. Clark said that, just like with past research, he and his coauthors suspect that there is a narrowing of the arteries (or a full-on blockage) on one side of the body compared to the other—the result of arterial disease—and that this narrowing can cause the systolic blood pressure to drop on that side.

Dr. Clark said that doctors in Europe and in the US are taught that taking blood pressure on both sides is a good idea, but it's not mandatory in either place. In fact, fewer than half of doctors in Britain say that they regularly measure blood pressure in both arms, said Dr. Clark. He doesn't have statistics for the US, but he speculates that the data is probably similar here. "Most doctors probably perceive taking a second measurement in the other arm as needlessly time-consuming. And, until now, the importance of doing so hasn't been well-publicized," he said. Hopefully, since his findings were published in January 2012 in *The Lancet*, the practice will become more widespread.

Speak Up

You could be at higher risk for cardiovascular problems than you realize. So on your next trip to the doctor, ask that your blood pressure be measured in both arms, said Dr.

Clark. And in case the nurse or your doctor asks why, bring this article with you.

If you do have a dangerous difference in the measurements between arms, knowing early matters, because the sooner you are aware of your risk, the sooner you can start discussing lifestyle changes with your doctor, such as quitting smoking, exercising more and eating healthier foods—and possibly, pursuing cardiovascular medical treatment.

So don't be shy—be a proactive patient!

Pinching Back on Salt Restrictions

Martin J. O'Donnell, MB, PhD, associate clinical professor of medicine, McMaster University, Hamilton, Ontario, Canada.

It's a mantra that we've heard for years—cut back on salt! But a recent study dashes that advice, demonstrating that it's not just too much salt that's bad for our hearts but apparently also too little.

Not all of this is surprising because many practitioners of natural medicine have long held the view that advice on salt intake should be individualized—and not simply be "less is best" for everyone. So we spoke with the study's lead author, Martin J. O'Donnell, MB, PhD, an associate clinical professor of medicine at McMaster University in Canada, to learn more about the research.

Shaking Up Conventional Wisdom

Dr. O'Donnell said that his study—published in the *Journal of the American Medical Association*—is the first large study to report potential heart health risks for both low and high salt intake in a single study.

Dr. O'Donnell and his colleagues examined data from nearly 29,000 men and women (all age 55 or over) from 40 countries who either had heart disease or were at increased risk for it because of prior history and co-morbidity factors such as diabetes. They looked at how much sodium was excreted in their morning fasting urine (so it wasn't self-reported salt intake) at the start of the study. The participants were not aware that their salt consumption was being measured, nor were they asked to raise or lower their intake—they just ate the amount that they normally ate.

What the researchers found was that, over four years, those who consumed higher-than-average amounts of salt and those who consumed lower-than-average amounts of salt experienced more heart problems (including deaths) than those with an average intake.

What's "Average"?

It's worth noting that the "average" salt consumption among participants in this study—estimated between 4,000 mg and 6,000 mg per day—is much higher than the recommended upper limits of 1,500 mg per day (the advice of the American Heart Association) or 2,300 mg per day (the recommended dietary guideline from the US Department of Agriculture). And yet in this study it was the people who consumed this much salt who had the least number of heart problems.

The study showed that those with the highest and lowest amounts of sodium excretion had the highest risk. For example, those who consumed more than 8,000 mg daily were at a 50%-to-70% higher risk of suffering a cardiovascular event over the four-year period, compared with the "average" salt group. And, not quite as alarming but still of concern, among those whose daily salt intake was between 2,000 mg and 3,000 mg, the likelihood of dying from a cardiac event related to congestive heart failure rose by 20%, compared with the "average" salt group.

Now, it's important to note that patients who ate the least amount of salt might have been doing so because they were at very high risk for disease and their doctors had insisted that they cut back severely on salt.

In other words, their risk uptick might not be due to their salt intake (or their salt intake alone), but also due to poor health. "We did some analysis to address this issue, but we can't exclude this possibility—larger clinical trials will be the only way to truly answer this question," said Dr. O'Donnell.

The mystery is—how could consuming a low amount of salt increase cardiovascular risk? There may be several potential reasons for this, Dr. O'Donnell said, but the most prominent hypothesis is that lower salt intake activates the body's renin-angiotensin system, which results in narrowed blood vessels, which of course makes it harder for blood to flow to and from the heart.

What's the Salt Solution?

This study—and others that have recently shown that similarly negative health effects may be associated with a low-salt diet—caught the attention of the government. Congress has already put on hold its plans to legislate lower sodium levels for school lunches, requesting more information from the US Department of Agriculture before putting it to vote. Dr. O'Donnell said that there is "an urgent need to establish a safe range for sodium intake."

In terms of how much salt you should eat, talk to your doctor about your particular risk factors—and remember that the jury is still out.

Foods That Help Control Blood Pressure

Janet Bond Brill, PhD, RD, a registered dietitian and a nationally recognized expert in nutrition and cardiovascular disease prevention. She is author of *Blood Pressure Down: The 10-Step Plan to Lower Your Blood Pressure in 4 Weeks Without Prescription Drugs* (Three Rivers). *www.DrJanet.com*

Considering all the dangers of high blood pressure (including increased risk for heart attack, stroke and de-mentia), we definitely want to do everything we can to keep our blood pressure levels under control. But are we? Unfortunately, one surprisingly simple step—eating the right foods—consistently gets ignored as an effective technique for controlling blood pressure.* Of course everyone knows that a low-sodium diet helps some people maintain healthy blood pressure levels. But there's a lot more to blood pressure control than avoiding that bag of potato chips, extra dash of soy sauce or a crunchy dill pickle (just one dill pickle contains about 875 mg of sodium, or nearly 40% of recommended daily sodium intake).

What most people are missing out on: With the right combination of blood pressure–controlling nutrients, you often can avoid high blood pressure altogether…or if you already have the condition and are being treated with medication, you may be able to reduce your dosage and curb your risk for troubling side effects, such as fatigue, depression and erectile dysfunction.

The best foods for blood pressure control…

Eat More Bananas

Bananas are among the best sources of potassium, a mineral that's crucial for blood pressure control. A typical banana contains about 450 mg of potassium, or about 10% of the amount of potassium most people should aim for each day.

Potassium works like a "water pill." It's a natural diuretic that enables the kidneys to excrete more sodium while also relaxing blood vessels—both functions help control blood pressure.

Scientific evidence: In a large study of nearly 250,000 adults published in the *Journal of the American College of Cardiology*, people who increased their intake of potassium by 1,600 mg daily were 21% less likely to suffer a stroke than those who ate less. Kiwifruit also is a concentrated source of potassium with more than 200 mg in each small fruit.

*In addition to smart eating habits, a blood pressure–controlling action plan includes regular exercise (ideally, 30 minutes of aerobic activity, such as brisk walking or swimming, at least five times a week) and a stress-reducing regimen.

Recommended daily amount of potassium: 4,700 mg. A good potassium-rich breakfast is oatmeal made with soy milk (300 mg), one cup of cantaloupe (430 mg), one cup of fresh-squeezed orange juice (496 mg) and one cup of coffee (116 mg).

Other good potassium sources: Potatoes (purple potatoes have the most), avocados, pistachios and Swiss chard.

Good rule of thumb: To control blood pressure, try to consume three times more potassium than sodium.

Pile On the Spinach

Even if you eat plenty of bananas, all of that potassium won't lower your blood pressure unless you also get enough magnesium. It is estimated that about two-thirds of Americans are deficient in magnesium—and while magnesium supplements might help in some ways, they do not reduce blood pressure. Only magnesium from food—such as spinach, nuts, legumes and oatmeal—offers this benefit due to the nutrients' synergistic effect.

Recommended daily amount of magnesium: 500 mg. One cup of cooked spinach provides 157 mg of magnesium.

Also good: Two ounces of dry-roasted almonds (160 mg).

Dip into Yogurt

Calcium helps the body maintain mineral balance that regulates blood pressure. Dairy products, such as yogurt, contain a milk-derived protein that works like a natural ACE inhibitor (one of the most common types of blood pressure medications) and prevents the constriction of blood vessels that raises blood pressure.

Important: Stick to low-fat or no-fat yogurt, milk and cheese—the saturated fat in whole-fat dairy products appears to cancel the blood pressure–lowering effects. In addition, opt for "plain" yogurt to avoid the added sugar that's found in many brands of yogurt. If you don't like the taste of plain yogurt, add

a little granola, honey, nuts, seeds, fresh berries or banana.

For a tasty "pumpkin pie" snack: Add plain canned pumpkin, walnuts, pumpkin pie spice and Splenda to plain yogurt and top it with fat-free whipped cream.

Other high-calcium foods: Leafy greens and sardines (with the bones). Calcium supplements also can help keep blood pressure down, but recent research has linked them to increased cardiovascular risk. Talk to your doctor about these supplements.

Recommended daily amount of calcium: Women age 51 and older need 1,200 mg (1,000 mg for men age 51 to 70…1,200 mg for men age 71 and older). Eating two fat-free yogurts (830 mg), one cup of cooked spinach (245 mg) and three kiwifruits (150 mg) will easily get you to your daily calcium goal.

Enjoy Soy

Soy foods, including tofu, soy nuts and soy milk, may be the most underrated blood pressure–lowering foods. Research shows that people who regularly eat soy can reduce their blood pressure as much as they would by taking some medications. Soy increases nitric oxide, a naturally occurring gas that lowers blood pressure.

Helpful: If you can't get used to the taste (or texture) of tofu, drink chocolate soy milk. An eight-ounce glass has 8 g of soy protein. Unsalted, dry-roasted soy nuts are an even richer source with about 10 g in a quarter cup.

Recommended daily amount of soy: 20 g to 25 g of soy protein. This translates to two to four servings of soy nuts or soy milk. Women at high risk or who are being treated for breast, ovarian or uterine cancer should discuss their soy intake with their doctors—it can affect hormone levels that can fuel these cancers.

Sip Red Wine

Too much alcohol increases risk for high blood pressure—as well as heart disease and stroke. In moderation, however, red wine relaxes arteries and reduces risk for diabetes, a condition that often increases blood pressure. White wine and other forms of alcohol also reduce blood pressure, but red wine is a better choice because it contains more heart-protecting antioxidants known as flavonoids.

You'll get significant flavonoids from wines with a deep red color, such as cabernets. Specifically, grapevines that face harsher sun exposure and nutrient deprivation produce more flavonoids—cabernet sauvignon tops the list.

Red wine also is high in resveratrol, another antioxidant. One glass of red wine contains enough resveratrol to stimulate the body's production of nitric oxide. Pinot noir wine has more resveratrol than other types.

Recommended daily limit for red wine: No more than two glasses for men or one glass for women.

For people who can't drink alcohol, purple grape juice has some flavonoids and resveratrol but doesn't contain the full benefit provided by red wine.

More from Dr. Bond Brill...

Slow Breathing Lowers Blood Pressure

You've probably heard that yoga, meditation and other forms of relaxation can reduce blood pressure.

An even simpler solution: Merely breathing more slowly, for just a few minutes a day, can do the same thing—and research shows that for some people, combining slow breathing with relaxation techniques can be as effective as drug therapy.

What to do: Once a day, take a little time to slow your breathing. Breathe in deeply for 10 seconds, then breathe out at the same rate. Repeat the cycle for 15 minutes. Or try Resperate, an electronic breathing device that helps you synchronize your breathing (from $120, *www.Resperate.com*).

The Sweet Snack That Does Wonders for Blood Pressure

Harold Bays, MD, medical director and president of the Louisville Metabolic and Atherosclerosis Research Center in Louisville, Kentucky, and principal investigator of a study on the effects of raisins on blood pressure, presented at the American College of Cardiology's 61st Annual Scientific Session.

It's always good news when a study produces scientific evidence in support of advice that seems sensible but previously lacked proof. And it's particularly nice when that advice deals with something sweet and yummy. In this case, the good news is that raisins can reduce blood pressure.

Why is this important? Blood pressure that is even slightly elevated—a condition called prehypertension—increases the risk for heart attack, stroke and kidney disease. Prehypertension is defined as a systolic pressure (the top number in a blood pressure reading, as measured in "millimeters of mercury" or mmHg) of 120 to 139...or a diastolic pressure (the bottom number) of 80 to 89.

For the recent study, researchers randomly assigned 46 prehypertension patients, average age 61, to eat a snack three times a day for 12 weeks. For one group, each snack consisted of a one-ounce package of raisins. The other group ate prepackaged processed commercial snack foods, such as crackers or cookies, that did not contain raisins, other fruit or vegetables. The raisins and the other snacks each contained about 90 to 100 calories per serving. Participants' blood pressure was measured at the start of the study and after four, eight and 12 weeks.

Results: Blood pressure did not change significantly among participants in the commercial snacks group. In comparison, in the raisin group, systolic pressure decreased significantly, with reductions ranging from 5 mmHg to 7 mmHg—an amount that has cardiovascular benefits, clinical trial evidence suggests. Raisin eaters' diastolic pressure also dropped, though not as much.

Explanation: Raisins are high in potassium, a mineral that reduces blood pressure by promoting the proper balance of electrolytes and fluids in the body...helping offset the adverse effects of dietary sodium...and increasing the amount of sodium excreted via the urine. Raisins also have antioxidants and other components that may make blood vessels less stiff.

Best: If your blood pressure is elevated—or if your blood pressure is fine and you want to keep it that way—consider forgoing processed snack foods in favor of a handful of natural raisins. Not fond of raisins or crave more variety? Other potassium-rich snack options include bananas, cantaloupe, carrots, honeydew melon, papayas and yogurt.

The Mysterious Link Between Popcorn and Blood Pressure

In a recent study, researchers who reviewed health and nutrition data for 31,684 men found that those who consumed the most whole grains (about 52 g daily) were 19% less likely to develop high blood pressure than those who consumed the least whole grains (about 3 g daily).

Best sources: Oatmeal (instant or cooked)—one cup, 30 g to 35 g...popcorn —one cup, 10 g to 12 g...whole-wheat bread—one slice, about 15 g...and bran cereal—one cup, 5 g to 10 g.

Alan Flint, MD, DrPH, research scientist, department of nutrition, Harvard School of Public Health, Boston.

Hibiscus Tea Lowers Blood Pressure

Hibiscus tea lowers blood pressure, reports Diane L. McKay, PhD, FACN. Herbal tea containing hibiscus seems to relax the blood vessels, having an effect similar to that of the hypertension medicines called ACE inhibitors. Hibiscus also is thought to be a diuretic—and removing water from the body can reduce blood pressure. Talk to your doctor about drinking hibiscus tea for high blood pressure.

Diane L. McKay, PhD, FACN, a scientist at the Antioxidants Research Laboratory of the Jean Mayer USDA Human Nutrition Research Center on Aging at Tufts University, Boston, and leader, a study of 65 people, published in *Journal of Nutrition*.

Sesame Oil Blend Lowers Blood Pressure

In a study of 300 people (average age 57) with mild to moderately high blood pressure, those who added about one ounce of a blend of sesame oil and rice oil to their meals daily had average blood pressure drops of 14 points systolic (top number) and 11 points diastolic (bottom number). This was almost as much as blood pressure dropped in those taking the blood pressure drug *nifedipine* (Procardia).

Theory: The antioxidants and fatty acids found in these oils may have a blood pressure–lowering effect. The blend of oils used in the study is not commercially available, but you can make your own 50/50 mix.

Devarajan Sankar, MD, PhD, researcher, Fukuoka University Chikushi Hospital, Chikushino, Japan.

Nighttime Aspirin Lowers Blood Pressure

Previous studies have linked nighttime aspirin use with lower blood pressure, but there was no explanation for the drug's effect.

Recent research: Bedtime aspirin use was found to lower blood and urine levels of naturally occurring chemicals associated with high blood pressure in a study of 16 adults with untreated, mildly elevated blood pressure.

If your doctor has prescribed daily aspirin: Ask about taking the pill at night.

Jaapjan Snoep, MSc, researcher, department of clinical epidemiology, Leiden University Medical Center, the Netherlands.

Cola, Not Coffee, Raises Blood Pressure in Women

The association between hypertension and caffeine had been attributed to coffee, but a recent study shows that caffeinated colas increase women's risk of hypertension. Researchers speculate that some other compound in soda is responsible for increased risk.

Wolfgang Winkelmayer, MD, department of pharmacoepidemiology and pharmacoeconomics, Brigham and Women's Hospital, Boston, and leader of an analysis of 12 years of data from 155,594 women, published in *The Journal of the American Medical Association.*

A Top Doctor's Natural Cure for Blood Pressure

C. Norman Shealy, MD, PhD, founding president of the American Holistic Medical Association, a leading advocate for the use of holistic and integrative medicine by health-care providers. He has done extensive research on nontraditional therapies and has written many books, including *The Healing Remedies Sourcebook* (Da Capo). *www.NormShealy.com*

Most patients do significantly better when they use natural therapies that restore physical as well as emotional balance. Of course, always check with your doctor before trying any new remedy.

Problem: High blood pressure.

Remedy: L-arginine.

L-arginine is an amino acid found in meats, grains, fish and other foods. When you take higher, supplemental doses, it increases blood levels of nitric oxide, which dilates arteries and reduces blood pressure. Studies have shown that patients who take L-arginine can reduce their blood pressure by 20 points or more. Also, L-arginine appears to reduce atherosclerosis, buildups in the arteries that lead to most heart attacks.

How to use it: Take 1,000 milligrams (mg) twice a day. Use a time-release form—it will stay active in the body throughout the day.

Caution: L-arginine can interact with some medications, including high blood pressure medications and *nitroglycerin.*

Stress Busters for Women That Help Beat High Blood Pressure

C. Tissa Kappagoda, MBBS, PhD, a professor of medicine in the Preventive Cardiology Program at the University of California, Davis. Dr. Kappagoda has published more than 200 medical journal articles on matters relating to cardiology and cardiovascular health.

High blood pressure is becoming an increasingly significant problem for women. *Consider…*

A recent study in the journal *Circulation* found an alarming trend—that rates of uncontrolled hypertension are increasing among women even as rates among men are decreasing.

The Centers for Disease Control and Prevention reports that more than one-third of women age 45 to 54 now have high blood pressure…while among women age 75 and older, 80% do!

A more recent report from the National Center for Health Statistics states that, in the past decade, there has been a 62% increase in the number of visits to the doctor due to high blood pressure.

C. Tissa Kappagoda, MBBS, PhD, a professor in the preventive cardiology program at the University of California, Davis, explained, "Chronic stress raises blood pressure by increasing levels of adrenaline and cortisol, hormones that promote artery spasm and salt retention. It also increases vascular resistance, the resistance to flow that must be overcome to move blood through the blood vessels, which is a primary cause of hypertension." Stress also can impede basic self-care, such as eating healthfully and exercising—which probably explains why stress is such a "massive multiplier of the effects of conventional risk factors," Dr. Kappagoda added.

Though high blood pressure doesn't cause pain or other obvious symptoms, it does damage arteries—increasing the risk for heart attack, diabetes, stroke and kidney problems. How high is too high? Hypertension is diagnosed when blood pressure hits 140/90 mmHg or higher...but doctors now realize that prehypertension (blood pressure between 120/80 and 139/89) also is risky.

Of course, it's important to follow your doctor's advice regarding blood pressure-lowering lifestyle changes, such as limiting salt and alcohol and losing excess weight. But stress reduction should be a priority, too, Dr. Kappagoda said—and may reduce the need for hypertension medication. That's good, because these drugs can have side effects, such as dizziness, chronic cough and muscle cramps, and often are taken for the rest of a person's life.

Research shows that the following stress-lowering techniques help reduce blood pressure. *If you have hypertension or prehypertension, consider...*

•**Breathing control.** When you're relaxed, your breathing naturally slows...and if you slow down your breathing, your body naturally relaxes. This encourages constricted blood vessels to dilate, improving blood flow.

Target: Practice slow breathing for 15 minutes twice daily, aiming to take six breaths per minute.

If you find it difficult (or even stressful!) to count and time your breaths, consider using a biofeedback device instead. One example designed for home use is Resperate (877-988-9388, *www.Resperate.com*, from $300), which looks like a portable CD player with headphones and uses musical tones to guide you to an optimal breathing pattern. Typically, Resperate is used for 15 minutes three or four times per week, and results are seen within several weeks. In studies, users experienced significant reductions in systolic pressure (the top number of a blood pressure reading) and diastolic pressure (bottom number). There are many similar and effective devices, said Dr. Kappagoda, so ask your doctor about the options. Biofeedback devices are safe and have no side effects.

•**Meditation.** A recent analysis of nine clinical trials, published in *American Journal of Hypertension,* found that regular practice of transcendental meditation reduced blood pressure, on average, by 4.7 mmHg systolic and 3.2 mmHg diastolic. Though these results are for transcendental meditation specifically, many experts believe that any type of meditation works.

Goal: Meditate for 20 minutes daily.

•**Exercise.** Regular physical activity reduces blood pressure not only by alleviating stress, but also by promoting weight loss and improving heart and blood vessel health. Research shows that becoming more active can reduce systolic pressure by 5 mmHg to 10 mmHg, on average. An excellent all-around exercise is walking, Dr. Kappagoda said—so with your doctor's OK, take a 30-minute walk at least three times weekly.

Caution: Weight training can trigger a temporary increase in blood pressure during the exercise, especially when heavy weights are used. To minimize this blood pressure spike, use lighter weights to do more repetitions...and don't hold your breath during the exertion.

Reduce High Blood Pressure By Tapping Your Toes

Ann Marie Chiasson, MD, family practitioner and clinical assistant professor of medicine, Arizona Center for Integrative Medicine, University of Tucson. She is author of *Energy Healing: The Essentials of Self-Care* (Sounds True). *www.AnnMarieChiassonMD.com*.

There's a killer running rampant amongst us—and its name is high blood pressure.

Overly dramatic? Not really.

High blood pressure increases your risk not only for heart attack, heart failure and stroke, but also for grave maladies that you may never have considered, such as kidney failure, dementia, aneurysm, blindness and osteoporosis.

Yeah, medications help reduce blood pressure…but their nasty side effects can include joint pain, headache, weakness, dizziness, heart palpitations, coughing, asthma, constipation, diarrhea, insomnia, depression and sexual dysfunction!

But there's a promising alternative therapy that's completely risk-free—and costs nothing!

We're talking about tapping, which is based on the principles of Chinese medicine. *Here's how it works…*

Vitamin C Can Reduce Blood Pressure

In a recent study, about 500 milligrams (mg) of vitamin C taken daily for eight weeks reduced systolic pressure—the more important top number—by 3.84 Hg…and by 4.85 Hg in patients with hypertension. The dose is well below the daily limit of 2,000 mg.

Edgar Miller III, MD, PhD, associate professor of medicine and epidemiology at Johns Hopkins University School of Medicine, Baltimore, and senior author of an analysis of 29 studies, published in *American Journal of Clinical Nutrition*.

Something Old, Something New

Ann Marie Chiasson, MD, of the Arizona Center for Integrative Medicine, described the tapping method for us. For her own patients with high blood pressure, Dr. Chiasson has adapted a tapping technique that is part of the ancient Chinese practice called qigong.

Qigong involves simple movements, including tapping on the body's meridians, or "highways" of energy movement. These meridians are the same as those used during acupuncture and acupressure treatments. According to a review of nine studies published in *The Journal of Alternative and Complementary Medicine*, qigong reduced systolic blood pressure (the top number) by an average of 17 points and diastolic blood pressure (the bottom number) by an average of 10 points. Those are big reductions! In fact, they are comparable to the reductions achieved with drugs—but the qigong had no unwanted side effects.

Though Dr. Chiasson has not conducted a clinical trial on her tapping protocol, she has observed reductions in blood pressure among her patients who practice tapping. The technique she recommends also could conceivably benefit people who do not have high blood pressure if it reduces stress and thus helps lower the risk of developing high blood pressure.

Tap Away

Some tapping routines are complicated, involving tapping the top of the head, around the eyes, side of the hand and under the nose, chin and/or arms. But Dr. Chiasson's technique is a simpler toe-and-torso method that is quite easy to learn. It is safe and can be done in the privacy of your own home—so if it might help you, why not give it a try?

First, you may want to get a blood pressure reading so you can do a comparison later on. If the tapping technique is helpful, you eventually may be able to reduce or even discontinue your high blood pressure drugs (of course, for safety's sake, you should not stop taking any drugs without first talking to your doctor about it).

Dr. Chiasson's plan: Each day, do five minutes of toe tapping (instructions below)…five minutes of belly tapping…and five minutes of chest tapping. You may experience tingling or a sensation of warmth in the part of the body being tapped and/or in your hands, which is normal. You can listen to rhythmic music during your tapping if you like. As you tap, try to think as little as possible, Dr. Chiasson said—just focus on your body, tapping and breath.

Rate: For each tapping location, aim for a rate of about one to two taps per second.

• **Toe tapping.** Lie flat on your back on the bed or floor. Keeping your whole body relaxed, quickly rotate your legs inward and outward from the hips (like windshield wipers), tapping the sides of your big toes together with each inward rotation. Tap as softly or as vigorously as you like.

• **Belly tapping.** Stand with your feet a little wider than shoulder-width apart. Staying relaxed, gently bounce up and down by slightly bending your knees. At the same time, tap softly with gently closed fists on the area below your belly button and above your

pubic bone. Try to synchronize your movements to give one tap per knee bend.

• **Chest tapping.** Sit or stand comfortably. Using your fingertips, open hands or gently closed fists, tap all over your chest area, including the armpits. Tap as softly or as vigorously as you like without pushing past your comfort level.

Cautions: If you are recovering from hip or knee surgery, skip the toe tapping (which might strain your joint) and do only the belly tapping and chest tapping. If you are pregnant, stick with just the chest tapping—lying on your back during toe tapping could reduce blood flow to the fetus…and tapping on your belly may not feel comfortable and could stimulate the acupressure points used to induce labor, Dr. Chiasson said.

Follow-up: Continue your tapping routine for eight weeks, then get another blood pressure reading to see whether your numbers have improved. If they have—or if you simply enjoy the relaxing effects of the tapping—you might want to continue indefinitely. To see a video in which Dr. Chiasson explains more about energy healing and tapping, visit *http://www.youtube.com/watch?v=KF4ELjSBioU.*

Chapter 4

CHOLESTEROL: A STICKY PROBLEM FOR WOMEN

Cholesterol Myths

For years, we have been told that high cholesterol causes heart attacks. But that is a dangerous over-simplification.

What most people don't know: Nearly 50% of heart attack patients who are tested for cholesterol turn out to have normal levels, according to data from the large Framingham Heart study.

What's true—and what's not—about cholesterol and heart attack risk…

Myth 1: **LDL cholesterol is always bad.** This type of cholesterol is often referred to simply as "bad" cholesterol. But we now know that LDL cholesterol isn't a single entity. Scientists have identified seven different subtypes, and there are probably more. Some forms of LDL do contribute much more to atherosclerosis and heart attacks—others are not as harmful.

Yet the standard cholesterol tests don't make this distinction. A patient with high LDL is assumed to have an elevated risk for heart disease and probably will be treated with a cholesterol-lowering statin drug, even though his/her LDL might consist primarily of one of the less harmful forms.

Fact: Some LDL subtypes are large and buoyant—and less likely to cause heart disease than others that are small and dense. Small forms are most likely to settle into artery walls and cause inflammation and atherosclerosis, increasing risk for a heart attack.

Example: A person with high levels of Lp(a), an extremely dense form of LDL, is up to three times more likely to develop heart disease or have a heart attack than someone with lower levels, even when the total LDL is the same in both people.

Implication: Newer, expanded cholesterol tests that measure individual types of LDL particles may prove to be more useful than standard cholesterol tests. Lp(a) screening is not yet widely used—ask your doctor whether you should have it. Some insurers cover the cost of this test.

Ronald M. Krauss, MD, senior scientist and director of atherosclerosis research at Children's Hospital Oakland Research Institute. He is an adjunct professor in the department of medicine at the University of California, San Francisco, and in the department of nutritional sciences at the University of California, Berkeley. He is a member of one of the US National Cholesterol Education Program's expert panels, and founder and past chair of the American Heart Association's Council on Nutrition, Physical Activity and Metabolism.

Myth 2: **High cholesterol numbers mean high risk.** Depending on an individual's risks and other factors, optimal cholesterol is roughly defined as having a total number below 200 mg/dL...LDL below 100 mg/dL... and HDL, the so-called "good" cholesterol, greater than 40 mg/dL for men and 50 mg/dL for women.

Fact: The standard test numbers may matter less than experts once thought.

More important: The ratio of small-to-large LDL particles, known as the size pattern.

Patients with Pattern A have a higher concentration of large, buoyant particles. Those with Pattern B have a higher concentration of small, dense particles. A patient with Pattern A is at least three times less likely to develop heart disease than someone with Pattern B.

Implication: Don't assume that you need a statin drug just because your LDL is high.

Example: Suppose that your LDL is 160. If you happen to have Pattern A, taking a statin may provide only a modest benefit. If you happen to have the more dangerous Pattern B, taking a statin may not provide maximal benefit either, so other treatment may be necessary to reduce heart disease risk. Taking high doses of a statin may result in side effects such as muscle pain or weakness. Advanced lipid testing determines one's LDL size pattern.

Myth 3: **Saturated fat is the enemy.** We've all been told that reducing dietary fat, particularly saturated fat, is among the most important ways to lower cholesterol and protect the heart.

Fact: A diet high in saturated fat clearly increases LDL. However, much of this increase is due to a corresponding increase in large, buoyant particles. In other words, saturated fat seems to trigger the less harmful Pattern A composition. Also, saturated fat increases the beneficial HDL cholesterol.

Implication: For years, Americans have been advised to keep their intake of dietary fat under 30% of total calories, with less than 7% of the fat calories coming from saturated fat. This now seems overly cautious. Americans who slightly exceed 10% saturated fat in their diets probably experience no increase in cardiovascular risks. However, people should avoid harmful trans fats in partially hydrogenated vegetable oils, found in packaged baked goods and fast foods.

Myth 4: **It's OK to replace fat with carbohydrates.** Doctors have routinely advised patients to eat more carbs and less fat to help manage their cholesterol levels.

Fact: A high-carbohydrate diet may be more likely than a diet high in fat to increase cardiovascular risks.

Reason: Replacing fat with carbohydrates seems to shift LDL to the more dangerous Pattern B.

Important: Researchers suspect that it's mainly refined carbohydrates, such as soft drinks, white rice, white pasta, sugary desserts, etc., that cause this shift. Unprocessed carbohydrates that are high in fiber, such as whole grains, legumes, fruits and vegetables, are less likely to increase risk.

Implication: It's more important to cut back on refined carbohydrates than to cut back on fat. Danish researchers who followed 53,644 adults for an average of 12 years found that those who replaced saturated fat with refined carbohydrates were 33% more likely to have a heart attack. Those who ate healthier carbohydrates, on the other hand, had a slightly lower risk.

Myth 5: **Statins are the best way to prevent a heart attack.** Estimates show that 20 million Americans take statin drugs, such as *atorvastatin* (Lipitor), *pravastatin* (Pravachol) and *simvastatin* (Zocor).

Fact: Even though statins do lower LDL, these drugs appear to have a limited ability to change LDL size pattern.

Implications: If you have high LDL, first control your diet and get more exercise. If your LDL level is still high, ask your doctor about advanced lipid testing to determine your LDL size pattern. Especially if you have Pattern B, discuss taking a statin with your doctor.

If necessary, also talk to your doctor about adding niacin. In high doses, niacin lowers Lp(a) by about 30% in some patients.

If you use niacin, you should be supervised by a physician and receive periodic blood tests to ensure that your liver is functioning properly. If too much niacin is taken, it can damage the liver.

Become Heart Attack Proof—Here Are the Tests and Other Strategies You Really Need...

Michael Ozner, MD, medical director of the Center for Wellness & Prevention at Baptist Health South Florida in Miami and a past chairman of the American Heart Association of Miami. He is author of several books, including *Heart Attack Proof: A Six-Week Cardiac Makeover for a Lifetime of Optimal Health* (BenBella). *www.DrOzner.com*

There are few things as reassuring as hearing your doctor say that your cholesterol levels are "normal." But don't assume that these test results mean you have dodged the heart attack "bullet."

Surprising fact: About half of all heart attacks occur in people with normal LDL "bad" cholesterol levels. Other important facts you should know about testing to increase your odds of being heart attack proof...

Don't Settle for Normal

Most doctors rely heavily upon the results of their patients' basic cholesterol tests to determine their heart attack risk. Total and LDL cholesterol—both measured by routine blood tests—are useful indicators of heart attack risk.

The problem is that the desirable levels recommended by the National Cholesterol Education Program are not the optimal levels that can protect you from having a heart attack.

For example, the optimal total cholesterol level is less than 150 mg/dL (rather than the standard recommendation of less than 200 mg/dL).

Dr. William Castelli of the landmark Framingham Heart Study noted that none of the participants with a total cholesterol level of less than 150 mg/dL had suffered a heart attack.

In addition, the desirable LDL cholesterol is listed as less than 100 mg/dL, yet clinical studies have demonstrated that the optimal level should be less than 70 mg/dL.

Why wait until you have already suffered a heart attack to strive for the optimal cholesterol levels?

My approach: All adults should aim for optimal levels of total cholesterol and LDL cholesterol by following a healthy lifestyle. If you are not able to achieve optimal levels with lifestyle changes alone, then your doctor should decide whether to add cholesterol-lowering medication based on your risk factors for heart disease. Remember, medications are never a substitute for a healthy lifestyle.

Other Tests You Should Have

Newer, expanded tests can give clues beyond those provided by the basic cholesterol results discussed earlier. You may have to ask your doctor for these tests, but they are well worth it. *Important blood tests for all adults to consider...*

• **LDL-P.** The "P" stands for "particle." It measures the number of LDL particles that carry cholesterol. It's a more effective indicator of cardiovascular risk than LDL cholesterol alone because it shows how likely you are to develop atherosclerosis. Elevated LDL-P means that you are at risk of having a heart attack even if your LDL cholesterol is normal.

My approach: Patients should strive for an optimal LDL-P level of less than 700 nmol/L.

• **Apo-B.** This test measures a protein known as Apolipoprotein-B (Apo-B). It appears on the surface of all cholesterol particles that can enter the artery walls and potentially lead to atherosclerosis.

My approach: Patients should aim for an optimal level of less than 60 mg/dL. Depending upon the profiles offered by the laboratory that is being used, it's appropriate to measure particle number with LDL-P and/or Apo-B to get an accurate assessment of heart attack risk.

•**CRP.** Studies show that elevated C-reactive protein (CRP), which serves as a marker for inflammation, indicates an increased risk for heart disease and stroke. In some cases, a patient can have a normal cholesterol level but an elevated CRP reading.

My approach: Ask for a high-sensitivity CRP (hs-CRP) test (it's more accurate for vascular inflammation than standard CRP tests). Patients should strive for an hs-CRP level of less than 2 mg/L.

•**Vitamin D.** Most people associate vitamin D with bone health—it plays a key role in promoting the absorption of bone-building calcium. But that's not all vitamin D does. Preliminary research shows that correcting a vitamin D deficiency (through foods, such as salmon and vitamin D–fortified cereal, and/or supplements) can significantly lower heart disease risk.

My approach: Ask your doctor to test your vitamin D level. An optimal level is greater than 30 ng/ml.

•**Omega-3 index.** This blood test measures the percentage of healthful omega-3 fat in the membranes of your red blood cells. Low levels of omega-3 are linked to an increased risk for heart attack and sudden cardiac death.

My approach: Patients should aim for an omega-3 level of greater than 8%.

What to Do Next

If one or more results from these tests are not optimal, your doctor may choose from these treatments…*

*Always discuss all heart disease prevention recommendations with your personal treating physician.

•**Go Mediterranean.** Better eating habits (including a Mediterranean diet that consists of plenty of seafood, a minimum of red meat and an abundance of fruits, vegetables, legumes) is the first step.

Although there are various diets that claim to reduce heart attack risk, the preponderance of evidence confirms that the Mediterranean approach does so most effectively. It improves cholesterol levels, reduces inflammation and lowers blood sugar levels.

•**Get off the couch!** There is no way around it. Exercise is essential to becoming heart attack proof. It not only lowers blood pressure, heart rate and body weight, but it also helps control lipid levels, such as total and LDL cholesterol, and reduce inflammation and blood sugar levels.

My approach: Walk 30 to 45 minutes daily. To make sure that you stay on track, buy a pedometer and strive for 10,000 steps each day. Believe it or not, most people walk less than 3,000 steps per day.

•**Consider taking a statin.** These cholesterol-lowering drugs, which include *atorvastatin* (Lipitor), *simvastatin* (Zocor) and *rosuvastatin* (Crestor), can be used if lifestyle measures don't sufficiently improve total and LDL cholesterol. It's not well-known, but statins also can improve LDL-P, Apo-B and CRP levels.

•**Get more omega-3s.** Foods that are rich in omega-3s (such as salmon and sardines) and supplements, including fish oil, boost omega-3 levels, reduce the inflammation marker CRP and lower triglyceride levels.

Skip the Fast Before a Cholesterol Test?

Christopher Naugler, MD, assistant professor of pathology and laboratory medicine at the University of Calgary, Canada, and coauthor of the study, which was published in *Archives of Internal Medicine.*

If you've ever had a cholesterol test scheduled for midday or afternoon, then you know what a pain it can be to have to fast for the usual eight hours beforehand—because in reality, you probably won't have eaten since the previous night's dinner—a lot longer than eight hours.

Fasting doesn't bother some people—lucky them. But lots of us find it very difficult. Many individuals become so hungry and dizzy that the cholesterol test is hard to bear.

So it's good to know that this ironclad fasting rule—which was thought to ensure more reliability in cholesterol test results because eating could make your results spike higher or lower, depending on what you ate—might not be essential. And in fact, as we learned recently from Christopher Naugler, MD, of the University of Calgary in Canada, what you eat before a cholesterol test may not matter much at all. *Here's why…*

Looking for a More Efficient Test

In addition to his work as a professor, Dr. Naugler is zone clinical section chief of general pathology for Calgary Laboratory Services, which processes an average of 36,000 cholesterol tests each month. With such a large volume of work, "we were looking for ways to avoid turning away nonfasting patients," Dr. Naugler explained—nonfasting patients create more work for everyone (including themselves) because their appointments need to be rescheduled.

As there were already several small studies suggesting that fasting had only a modest effect on cholesterol levels, researchers at the lab decided to simply begin processing cholesterol tests for all of its patients, regardless of whether patients had remembered to fast or not. (In case this sounds reckless to you, don't worry. The cholesterol results, as well as the number of hours the patient fasted, were both reported back to the patient's physician, who could then decide whether the result was acceptable or whether the patient needed to return for a repeat test.) "After six months, we had more than 200,000 cholesterol panels, which is a large amount of data," said Dr. Naugler. So Dr. Naugler and

his team decided to analyze those tests to see whether fasting did indeed impact the results of cholesterol tests.

This was what's called an observational study, so the researchers did not directly compare, say, two patients of the same gender and age who had similar risk factors for high cholesterol and then ask one to fast and ask the other not to fast. (Hopefully future studies will.) Instead, these researchers compared groups of thousands of individuals (ones who fasted versus ones who didn't) and then controlled for age and gender. They were curious to see what the broad, overall trends suggested.

Dr. Naugler's analysis found that levels of HDL cholesterol and total cholesterol stayed relatively stable, varying only about 2%, depending on whether patients had or had not fasted. Levels of LDL cholesterol varied by less than 10% and triglycerides (blood fats) by less than 20%. "The levels that varied the least—HDL and total cholesterol—are the ones that matter the most in terms of estimating risk for cardiovascular problems," said Dr. Naugler. "The algorithms commonly used for assessing cardiovascular disease risk (the Framingham Coronary Heart Disease Risk Score and the Reynolds Risk Score) use only HDL and total cholesterol levels (not triglyceride or LDL levels)."

But isn't a variation of 10% and 20% kind of a big difference? Dr. Naugler didn't argue

Lower Bad Cholesterol

Raising HDL ("good") cholesterol levels may not reduce heart disease risk. Studying the genes of about 170,000 people, researchers discovered that the 15 HDL-raising variants did not reduce the risk for heart attack.

Better understood: The link between LDL "bad" cholesterol and heart disease. Decreasing LDL levels through diet, medication and/or other methods clearly lowers risk.

Ronald M. Krauss, MD, senior scientist and director of atherosclerosis research at Children's Hospital Oakland Research Institute, Oakland, California.

that those variations aren't significant—his point is simply that those variations, no matter how big or small, are not as meaningful when it comes to assessing a patient's risk for cardiovascular disease.

"This confirmed similar results that had been reported previously, but ours was the first large-scale North American study to report this finding," Dr. Naugler said. "We suggest that there is now sufficient evidence that most routine cholesterol screening tests can be performed without fasting. This is more convenient for patients and would also benefit labs by transferring some of the morning demand for tests to later in the day."

A Fasting-Free Future?

Ask your doctor whether fasting is necessary before your next cholesterol test. If your doctor allows you to skip the fast, use common sense and avoid eating high-fat foods in the day or two before the screening, advised Dr. Naugler, since those types of foods are likely to cause cholesterol to spike the most.

But don't be surprised if your doctor still asks you to fast before your next cholesterol test (especially if he's ordering other blood work that does require fasting, such as a blood sugar test). "Time will tell," said Dr. Naugler when asked whether his research is likely to shift any of the official recommendations about cholesterol-screening protocols.

What You Need to Know About Cholesterol-Lowering Drugs

Suzanne Steinbaum, DO, director of women and heart disease at the Heart and Vascular Institute, Lenox Hill Hospital, New York City, and a founder of Women's Cardiac Care Network, a citywide public health program. She lectures nationally and on-air. *www.srsheart.com*

Without question, the best way to prevent cardiovascular disease (CVD) is to maintain a diet low in saturated fat (found in red meat and fatty dairy products) and high in fruits, vegetables, legumes and whole grains…and to do aerobic exercise (such as brisk walking) for at least 30 minutes most days of the week.

However: For women at high risk for CVD, even careful adherence to these guidelines is not enough—they need additional protection against heart attack and stroke. So do many women whose CVD risk is borderline (somewhat elevated) and who cannot or do not follow a healthful lifestyle. In such cases, doctors often recommend one of the statin medications, which decrease levels of low-density lipoprotein (LDL) "bad" cholesterol, artery-clogging plaque and inflammation.

Problem: Even though there is now strong evidence that statins protect women against CVD, millions of at-risk women still are not being offered the medication.

Statins can cause side effects, some potentially quite serious—so the advantages must be weighed against the disadvantages. *What you need to know…*

The Big News from a Big Study

A recent study included 17,802 healthy women and men who did not have high LDL. What they did have were high blood levels of the compound C-reactive protein (CRP). This can be a sign of chronic inflammation, which contributes to heart disease. Some study participants took a placebo…others took *rosuvastatin* (Crestor) at 20 milligrams (mg) per day, a typical dose for a person with high cholesterol.

What happened: The study was halted after only 21 of its scheduled 60 months when a mid-study analysis showed that, compared with placebo users, statin users had 54% fewer heart attacks…48% fewer strokes…and 20% fewer deaths. With those results, it became unethical not to offer a statin to the placebo group.

Consequence: In showing that statins prevent heart attack and stroke in women and men at borderline CVD risk, the study altered the balance of pros and cons that doctors use to decide whether to recommend a statin for a specific patient.

Who's at Borderline Risk?

The following are borderline risk factors—not worrisome enough to put you at high risk but still significant for assessing your odds of having a heart attack or stroke…

- **Over age 65**
- **High CRP**
- **Blood pressure of 120/80 mmHg to 130/85 mmHg**
- **High stress levels**
- **Sedentary lifestyle.**

New thinking: If you have two or more of the risk factors above, a statin may be appropriate. In making this determination, your doctor also may check for…

- **High blood levels of apolipoprotein B** (a particle in cholesterol)
- **Coronary artery calcium score (an indicator of plaque) over 400.**

Who's at High Risk?

Having either of the risk factors below puts you at high risk for heart attack and stroke…

- **Confirmed heart disease**—for example, you have angina (chest pain) or have had angioplasty (an artery-opening surgical procedure)
- **Previous heart attack or stroke.**

Also: You are at high risk if you have two or more of the following…

- **Family history of heart attack** (father before age 55, mother before age 65 or sibling at any age)
- **Total cholesterol above 200 mg/dL**
- **LDL above 130 mg/dL**
- **High-density lipoprotein (HDL) "good" cholesterol below 50 mg/dL**
- **Triglycerides (a type of blood fat) above 150 mg/dL**
- **Blood pressure above 130/85 mmHg**
- **Glycated hemoglobin, or HbA1c (a measure of long-term blood sugar levels), above 6%**
- **Type 2 diabetes**
- **Body mass index of 25 or higher**
- **Waist larger than 35 inches**
- **Current or recent smoker.**

If you are at high risk, it is essential to talk to your doctor—a statin is almost certainly best for you.

Concerns About Safety

Statins' side effects may include nausea, headache, muscle aches and memory loss. Rarely, statins cause serious damage to the liver, kidneys and/or muscles. Statins may not be appropriate if you have a problem with your liver, kidneys or thyroid or if you regularly have more than two servings of alcohol daily.

But: Don't let fears of side effects deter you from trying a statin. If you do experience adverse effects, your doctor may suggest taking your statin at a lower daily dose or every other day…or trying a different statin.

Reduce side effects: Many statin side effects are caused by damage to mitochondria, the "engines" of cells. Because statins may deplete coenzyme Q10 (CoQ10)—a vitamin-like substance needed to produce energy in cells—CoQ10 supplements may help by strengthening mitochondria. A typical dose is 50 mg to 100 mg of CoQ10 daily, but some people need more—ask your doctor for guidelines.

Alternatives to Statins

One reason that doctors often recommend statins instead of supplements to reduce cholesterol is that far more research has been done on the drugs. Also, while certain supplements have been shown to lower LDL, no studies have shown that this translates directly to reductions in heart attacks and strokes.

However, some small studies show encouraging results from natural therapies.

Example: In a recent 74-person study, one group took a statin...the other group received diet and exercise counseling, plus daily supplements of fish oil containing almost 3,800 mg combined of the omega-3 fatty acids eicosapentaenoic acid (EPA) and docosahexaenoic acid (DHA), plus red yeast rice at 2,400 mg to 3,600 mg.

After three months: In the statin group, LDL dropped 40% and triglycerides dropped 9%...in the lifestyle/supplements group, LDL dropped 42% and triglycerides dropped 29%. How much of this improvement was due to lifestyle and how much was due to supplements is not known.

More research is needed before recommendations on red yeast rice can be made. However, there is so much evidence for the cardiovascular benefits of fish oil that virtually all women—whether or not they take a statin—should ensure that their intake is adequate. *Best...*

• **If you are at low risk for CVD,** have at least two weekly servings of cold-water fatty fish, such as salmon or mackerel...or take a daily dose of fish oil that provides 500 mg of combined EPA/DHA.

• **If you are at borderline risk,** eat fish four times weekly...or take 1,000 mg of EPA/DHA daily.

• **If you are at high risk,** eat fish four times weekly and take 2,000 mg to 4,000 mg of EPA/DHA daily.

Caution: If you take a blood thinner, such as *warfarin* (Coumadin), ask your doctor before taking fish oil.

Most people who take a statin continue for the rest of their lives. However, it is possible to reduce risk factors and negate the need for a statin through diet, exercise and other lifestyle changes. If there is a significant change in your health status or lifestyle—for instance, you lose a lot of weight or become a vegetarian—ask your doctor to reevaluate your need for the drug.

Statin Dangers Uniqu...
to Women

Beatrice A. Golomb, MD, PhD, professor of medi...cine at the University of California, San Diego School of Medicine and lead author of a research letter published in *Archives of Internal Medicine.* The findings in this study stem from a larger study that focused on statins' effects on thinking, mood and behavior.

Chances are that you or someone you love is taking a cholesterol-lowering statin medication. But these drugs can have numerous side effects, including muscle pain, liver damage, digestive problems, memory loss, even life-threatening muscle damage. Now a recent study adds two more side effects to that list...and, sorry to say, women are particularly likely to be affected.

The study involved 1,016 generally healthy adults who had moderately elevated levels of LDL (bad) cholesterol and no heart disease or diabetes. Participants were randomly assigned to take either a placebo...*simvastatin* (Zocor) at 20 mg...or *pravastatin* (Pravachol) at 40 mg. (These are standard, relatively modest statin dosages.) The capsules, taken daily for six months, looked identical, and neither the participants nor the researchers knew at the time which group was receiving which treatment. At the end of the study, participants reported how much energy they had, comparing how they felt after six months on the pills with how they had felt at the start of the study. They used a five-point scale ranging from "much less" to "much more" to rate their energy level and degree of exertional fatigue (such as fatigue during exercise).

Findings: Statin users were much more likely than placebo users to experience a decrease in energy...worsened exertional fatigue...or both. These side effects were somewhat worse with simvastatin than with pravastatin (though simvastatin was more effective at reducing cholesterol)...and were significantly more pronounced in women than in men. In fact, among female simvastatin users, four out of 10 experienced one *lem for Women*

...hile two out of 10 re-
...ergy loss.

...hers noted that this
...some mechanism by
...ffect cell health.

...ns ages 45 and up
...nong them and you
...g your energy…

**...doctor factor in
...tigue when gauging the drug's
benefits versus its risks.** This is particularly
important for patients for whom statins have
not been shown to prolong life—groups that
include women…people without heart disease…and seniors over age 70, even if they
do have heart disease.

• **Discuss whether you can reduce your
statin dosage or switch to a different medication to see if your side effects lessen.**

• **Ask your doctor about dietary and
lifestyle changes that may help lower your
cholesterol to the point that statins would
no longer be recommended.**

Bonus: Such lifestyle changes should give
you an energy boost, too.

The Vitamin That's Better Than Statins— The Natural Way to Fight Heart Disease

Steven Nissen, MD, chairman of the Robert and
Suzanne Tomsich Department of Cardiovascular Medicine at the Cleveland Clinic main campus. He is editor
of *Current Cardiology Report* and senior consulting
editor to *Journal of the American College of Cardiology*. He is coauthor of *Heart 411* (Three Rivers).

Niacin, a B vitamin, has been known
as the best way to raise HDL "good"
cholesterol, thus helping to reduce
risk for heart attacks. But a recent study has
called this into question—which has made
many patients and doctors wonder just how
effective niacin is. *What you need to know…*

Recent Controversy

A government study, reported in 2011 in *The
New England Journal of Medicine*, involved
3,414 patients who were randomly assigned
to receive either niacin or a placebo. All of
the patients already were taking a cholesterol-lowering statin medication.

The study was stopped early when investigators concluded that patients getting niacin did not have fewer heart attacks or other
cardiovascular events, even though they did
have increases in HDL. The study, taken in
isolation, suggests that increasing HDL with
niacin isn't protective.

However, most authorities believe that
the study, called AIM-HIGH, was seriously
flawed. It involved a relatively small number of patients—the most authoritative cardiovascular studies typically include tens of
thousands of patients. Also, patients in the
control group were given small amounts of
niacin to mimic the side effects of full-dose
therapy. This prevented them from knowing
they were taking a "placebo," but it could
have skewed the results.

This study's findings were sufficiently different from previous research that they have
to be viewed with caution. Additional, larger
studies are needed to determine how much
(if any) benefit patients will get from combining niacin with a statin.

Here's what we do know: Niacin alone
is effective at raising HDL and, based upon
older studies, probably reduces the risk for
heart attack.

A Pharmacological Vitamin

Most people with undesirable cholesterol are
advised to take one of the statin medications,
such as *atorvastatin* (Lipitor) or *simvastatin*
(Zocor). These medications are very effective
at lowering LDL "bad" cholesterol, but they
have only a modest effect on HDL.

Niacin works both ways. It increases HDL
by 15% to 35%. At the same time, it slightly
lowers LDL (by about 10% to 12%) and triglycerides, blood fats that have been loosely
linked to heart disease.

Like other B vitamins, niacin (vitamin B-3) is naturally present in foods, such as meats, leafy vegetables, legumes and whole grains. It also is in multivitamins and B-complex supplements.

When to Use It

Some patients with low HDL who are at moderate risk for heart disease and who don't need statins to lower LDL may be advised to take niacin to reduce their risk. Men with an HDL level substantially below 40 milligrams per deciliter (mg/dL) and women with an HDL below 45 mg/dL might be candidates for treatment. For both men and women, an HDL of 60 mg/dL or higher is ideal.

Important: Niacin is recommended only when these patients have tried, without success, to significantly increase HDL with lifestyle changes.

Examples: Not smoking, regular exercise and eating a healthful diet. When combined, these factors can increase HDL by 10% to 15%. That's enough for some patients—but not for everyone.

Modest amounts of alcohol—no more than two alcoholic beverages a day for men or one alcoholic beverage for women—also have been shown to cause slight increases in HDL.

People who already are taking a statin to reduce LDL may be advised to take niacin to boost HDL. We usually wait for a few months after starting statin therapy before adding niacin because statins slightly increase HDL, which can affect the niacin dose.

Niacin is sometimes used as an alternative treatment for patients who can't tolerate statins (because of muscle pain, for example). Niacin doesn't reduce LDL anywhere near as much as statins, but it can help patients with slightly high LDL who also have low HDL and high triglycerides.

How to Use It

The standard dose of nicotinic acid (the form of niacin used to raise HDL) is one gram to three grams daily. Patients usually are advised to start with the lower dose, increasing it as needed to achieve the recommended HDL level.

In these doses, niacin almost always causes side effects. The main one is flushing, in which the skin (often on the face) reddens and feels hot. Flushing can last anywhere from a few minutes to several hours. It usually becomes less bothersome after patients have taken niacin for several weeks or months.

Other side effects may include an upset stomach, headache or, in rare cases, liver damage. Patients who take niacin or other medications for cholesterol usually are advised to get regular blood tests.

Over-the-counter (OTC) niacin supplements may be just as effective as prescription drugs. However, supplements are more loosely regulated than medications—it's difficult to know if the OTC product that you're taking has the amount of niacin listed on the label. But whether you get it OTC or by prescription, don't take high-dose niacin without a doctor's supervision.

To Reduce Flushing

To alleviate this common side effect, I recommend the following…

•**Use extended-release niacin, such as prescription Niaspan.** This is the only form of niacin I prefer because it causes somewhat less flushing than immediate-release niacin.

Warning: Do not take any product labeled "no flush niacin"—these products do not raise HDL at all.

•**Take it at bedtime.** You still will experience flushing, but you probably will sleep through it.

Also helpful: Don't drink alcohol within an hour of taking niacin. It increases the intensity of flushing.

Take one aspirin, wait an hour and then take niacin. It's an effective way to reduce flushing.

Important: Take 81-mg to 325-mg regular aspirin. Be aware that enteric-coated forms will reduce the antiflushing benefit. Aspirin can cause bleeding and stomach ulcers, so always check with your doctor.

"Grape" Way to Lower Cholesterol

Leo Galland, MD, director of the Foundation for Integrative Medicine in New York City. He is author of *The Fat Resistance Diet* (Broadway). *www.fatresistancediet.com*. Dr. Galland is a recipient of the Linus Pauling award.

Plant foods offer a cornucopia of health benefits, and mounting evidence continues to reveal new plant chemicals that promote health. The latest darling is red grape juice. Recent studies are showing that compounds in the juice actually lower cholesterol and other cardiovascular risk factors.

Grape Juice and Cholesterol

In one recent study in Spain, researchers took a group of 15 healthy subjects and 26 subjects who were receiving dialysis and gave all of them a total of 100 milliliters (ml) of red grape juice concentrate daily (100 ml is a little more than half a six-ounce can of the concentrate). Dialysis patients were chosen for the study because they're at a higher risk for developing cardiovascular disease.

After only two weeks of drinking the juice concentrate, all subjects had reductions in low-density lipoprotein (LDL) cholesterol (the "bad" kind), oxidized LDL cholesterol (the really bad kind) and total cholesterol. As a bonus, their high-density lipoprotein (HDL, or good) cholesterol went up. In addition, an important marker of inflammation, MCP-1, went down by half after three weeks.

What Makes Grape Juice Go?

Red grape juice is a rich source of polyphenols, potent antioxidants that "mop up" harmful free radicals, which are a big part of the aging process and are associated with degenerative diseases. The polyphenols (also known as polyphenolics) include all sorts of plant compounds such as catechins and anthocyanins that have been shown to be protective against various cancers and heart disease. "This is yet another piece of evidence for the importance of consuming fruits and vegetables that are rich in the polyphenolics," says Leo Galland, MD, an expert in nutritional and integrative medicine.

Dr. Galland explains that cholesterol metabolism in the body is influenced by a process known as oxidative stress—the damage that occurs when free radicals attack your cells and DNA, much the way oxygen attacks apple slices left out on your kitchen table and turns them brown. The phenolic compounds in red grape juice—and in other plant foods—work to disarm the free radicals. By preventing the oxidation of LDL cholesterol (which increases the risk for LDL to generate cardiovascular disease), the compounds have strong benefits on heart health.

Good Red Fruit Juices

The good news is that the phenolic compounds that lowered oxidation of LDL cholesterol, prevented oxidation and also lowered inflammation in the study are not specific to red grape juice. "You should be able to achieve similar results with other kinds of red fruit juice, like pomegranate, for example," Dr. Galland said.

Bottom line: Red grape juice contains antioxidant and anti-inflammatory compounds that rank high among the established benefits of other well-known antioxidants such as vitamin E, lycopene and vitamin C. And one of the benefits seems to be a significant improvement in cholesterol. Not only that…it tastes good, too.

Chapter 5

EVERYDAY HEART-HEALTH SECRETS

Five Foods Proven to Prevent Heart Attacks

Cardiovascular disease is still the number-one killer in America. It accounts for about one third of all deaths, according to the American Heart Association.

Most of us know that a diet rich in fruits, vegetables and whole grains and low in saturated animal fats lowers the risk of heart disease. But certain foods have been shown to be particularly beneficial. Of course, no food is a magic bullet—you still need to exercise daily and maintain a healthy weight—but eating the recommended amounts of the following can go a long way toward preventing heart disease…

Spinach

Like most fruits and vegetables, spinach is rich in vitamins and minerals. What makes spinach stand out for keeping the heart healthy is folate, one of the B vitamins. According to several studies, including an extensive report from the Harvard School of Public Health, folate helps prevent the buildup of *homocysteine*, an amino acid in the blood that is a major risk factor for heart disease and stroke.

How much: Two cups of raw spinach (about two ounces) has 30% of the daily value (DV) for folate…one-half cup of cooked spinach provides 25%. Frozen and fresh spinach are both good, but beware of canned spinach—it may have excessive amounts of salt. Too much salt increases blood pressure in certain individuals and high blood pressure is another major risk factor for cardiovascular disease.

Alternatives: Asparagus. Four spears have 20% of the DV of folate. Also, many breakfast cereals are fortified with folate—check the labels.

Salmon

Salmon is rich in omega-3 fatty acids. Omega-3s reduce inflammation and make your blood less "sticky," which prevents plaque—fatty deposits—from clogging your arteries.

Bonnie T. Jortberg, RD, CDE, senior instructor, department of family medicine at University of Colorado at Denver and Health Sciences Center. She was program director of Colorado Weigh, a weight-loss and healthy-living program offered throughout the Denver metropolitan area. She is coauthor of *The Step Diet Book* (Workman).

Having unclogged arteries reduces the risk of heart attack and stroke.

How much: The American Heart Association recommends two to three three-ounce servings of salmon a week. Fresh or frozen, farmed or wild, is fine, but go easy on canned salmon, which may be high in salt.

Alternatives: Other cold-water fish high in omega-3 fatty acids include mackerel, lake trout, sardines, herring and albacore tuna. If you don't like fish, have one teaspoon of ground flaxseeds daily—sprinkle on cereal, yogurt or salads, and drink plenty of water to avoid constipation.

Tomatoes

Tomatoes are loaded with lycopene, a carotenoid that gives them their color. Lycopene reduces cholesterol in the body. Too much cholesterol can lead to atherosclerosis (hardening of the arteries), which decreases blood flow to the heart—and that can lead to heart attack and stroke.

Cooked and processed tomato products, such as spaghetti sauce and tomato juice, provide the greatest benefits. Researchers at Cornell University found that cooking or processing tomatoes boosts lycopene levels and makes lycopene easier for the body to absorb. Look for low-sodium or no-salt-added products.

If you like ketchup, another source of lycopene, buy an organic brand, made with pure cane sugar, not processed high-fructose corn syrup. Organic ketchup can contain up to three times as much lycopene as nonorganic brands, according to a study published by the United States Department of Agriculture. Other organic tomato products weren't studied, so it is not yet known if they're also higher in lycopene.

How much: One cup of tomato juice (about 23 milligrams, or mg, of lycopene) or one-half cup of tomato sauce (20 mg) daily. A medium raw tomato has 4.5 mg.

Alternative: Watermelon (one and a half cups of cut-up watermelon contain 9 mg to 13 mg of lycopene).

Oatmeal

Oatmeal is one of the best and most studied sources of soluble fiber. Soluble fiber absorbs water and turns to gel during digestion. It then acts like a sponge to absorb excess cholesterol from your body. That's good for your heart. Studies show that five grams (g) to 10 g of soluble fiber a day can reduce LDL "bad" cholesterol by about 5%.

Soluble fiber also helps remove saturated fat in your digestive tract before your body can absorb it. That's also good for your heart.

How much: One and a half cups of cooked oatmeal daily. This provides 4.5 g of fiber, enough to lower cholesterol. Rolled oats and steel-cut oatmeal work equally well to help lower cholesterol, but beware of flavored instant oatmeal—it is likely to have sugar added. Too much sugar in your diet increases the chance of inflammation, a risk factor for atherosclerosis. Sugar also can lead to weight gain, which is another risk factor for cardiovascular disease.

Alternatives: Kidney beans and brussels sprouts each have three grams of soluble fiber per one-half cup cooked.

Pomegranates

Pomegranates are loaded with polyphenols, antioxidants that neutralize free radicals, which can damage the body's cells. Polyphenols help maintain cardiovascular health by scooping up free radicals before they damage arteries. They also are believed to reduce LDL "bad" cholesterol. Red wine and purple grape juice are great sources of polyphenols, but pomegranates have the highest amount.

How much: 1.5 ounces of concentrated pomegranate juice daily. This is the amount used in most studies. Look for products that are labeled 100% juice, or concentrated, with no added sugar.

Caution: Pomegranate juice may affect the metabolism of prescription drugs and may cause blood pressure to decrease too much when combined with certain blood pressure medications. Check with your doctor.

Alternatives: Red wine (no more than two five-ounce glasses a day for men and one for women) and purple grape juice (four to six ounces a day).

The Food That Cancels Out Genetic Heart Risk

Sonia Anand, MD, PhD, professor of medicine, Michael G. DeGroote School of Medicine, McMaster University, Hamilton, Ontario, Canada.

If you're one of the millions who have a family history of cardiovascular disease (CVD), then you already know that you're at increased risk for CVD yourself—you might even think that there isn't much that you can do to change your unfortunate genetic fate. But according to a recent study, there is something that you can do—and it won't just reduce your genetic risk, but it can practically cancel it out altogether. Even better, it's something that's so easy to do that it's almost laughable—eat at least five servings of fruits and vegetables a day.

Yep, it's something that you've heard a million times before. But now we have proof that this simple lifestyle change can alter your cardiovascular destiny—and be honest, do you really follow the five servings recommendation? Past research has shown that the vast majority of people don't. For example, in a report on the topic from the CDC in 2010, about two-thirds of people in the US ate fruit less than twice a day and nearly three-quarters of people ate vegetables less than three times a day.

Healthy Foods = A Healthy Heart

Researchers from McMaster and McGill Universities in Canada examined results from two large previous studies. One was the Canadian-led INTERHEART study, which collected information from more than 8,000 men and women around the world—some had had heart attacks and some were controls of similar ages with no history of heart disease. The other was a Finnish study called FINRISK, which followed more than 19,000 Finns (men and women), including more than 1,000 who developed CVD. What the two studies had in common was that they both collected DNA samples from participants as well as self-reported information about their dietary habits.

For the recent analysis, researchers noted whether participants carried a variant in the chromosome 9p21—a known genetic risk factor for CVD—and examined their diets to see if what they ate had any impact on whether or not they developed CVD.

What they discovered: The risk of CVD in people with the gene variant who ate the highest amounts of fruits and raw vegetables was similar to the risk in people without the high-risk gene variant who also ate a diet high in fruits and vegetables. These findings were published in *PLoS Medicine*.

Eat Five to Stay Alive

To find out more about why eating fruits and veggies can make such a powerful difference when it comes to protecting your ticker, we spoke with joint principal investigator of the study Sonia Anand, MD, PhD, professor of medicine and epidemiology at McMaster's Michael G. DeGroote School of Medicine. She said that the plentiful antioxidants in these foods might specifically target the gene variant, turning off its genetic expression and thereby negating the higher risk for CVD.

Berries should be at the top of your shopping list, said Dr. Anand, since they tend to contain the highest amounts of antioxidants—as should raw veggies, since cooking vegetables at high temperatures for long periods of time can destroy important nutrients. "Think of your diet the same way you would think about taking a drug," said Dr. Anand. "You wouldn't skip taking your daily pill, so don't skimp on eating fruits and veggies every day."

Six Ways to Liven Up Your Heart-Healthy Diet

Janet Bond Brill, PhD, RD, an expert in nutrition and cardiovascular disease prevention based in Valley Forge, Pennsylvania. She is director of nutrition for Fitness Together, a franchise company of almost 500 personal fitness-training studios, has served as a nutrition consultant for several corporations and is author of *Prevent a Second Heart Attack* (Three Rivers). *www.DrJanet.com*

Just about everyone knows that a Mediterranean-style diet can help prevent heart disease. Even if you've already had a heart attack, this style of eating—emphasizing such foods as fish and vegetables—can reduce the risk for a second heart attack by up to 70%.

Problem: About 80% of patients with heart disease quit following dietary advice within one year after their initial diagnosis. That's often because they want more choices but aren't sure which foods have been proven to work.

Solution: Whether you already have heart disease or want to prevent it, you can liven up your diet by trying foods that usually don't get much attention for their heart-protective benefits...

SECRET 1: **Popcorn.** It's more than just a snack. It's a whole grain that's high in cholesterol-lowering fiber. Surprisingly, popcorn contains more fiber, per ounce, than whole-wheat bread or brown rice.

Scientific evidence: Data from the 1999–2002 National Health and Nutrition Examination Survey found that people who eat popcorn daily get 22% more fiber than those who don't eat it.

Important: Eat "natural" popcorn, preferably air-popped or microwaved in a brown paper bag, without added oil. The commercially prepared popcorn packets generally contain too much salt, butter and other additives. Three cups of popped popcorn, which contain almost 6 g of fiber and 90 calories, is considered a serving of whole grains. Studies have shown that at least three servings

of whole grains a day (other choices include oatmeal and brown rice) may help reduce the risk for heart disease, high cholesterol and obesity.

SECRET 2: **Chia seeds.** You're probably familiar with Chia pets—those terra-cotta figures that sprout thick layers of grassy "fur." The same seeds, native to Mexico and Guatemala, are increasingly available in health-food stores. I consider them a superfood because they have a nutrient profile that rivals heart-healthy flaxseed.

In fact, chia seeds contain more omega-3 fatty acids than flaxseed. Omega-3s increase the body's production of anti-inflammatory *eicosanoids*, hormonelike substances that help prevent "adhesion molecules" from causing plaque buildup and increasing atherosclerosis.

Scientific evidence: A study published in the *Journal of the American College of Cardiology,* which looked at nearly 40,000 participants, found that an omega-3 rich diet can prevent and even reverse existing cardiovascular disease.

Other benefits: One ounce of chia seeds has 10 g of fiber, 5 g of alpha-linolenic acid and 18% of the Recommended Dietary Allowance for calcium for adults ages 19 to 50.

Chia seeds look and taste something like poppy seeds. You can add them to baked goods, such as muffins, or sprinkle them on salads and oatmeal or other cereals.

SECRET 3: **Figs.** They're extraordinarily rich in antioxidants with an oxygen radical absorbance capacity (ORAC) score of 3,383. Scientists use this ORAC scale to determine the antioxidant capacity of various foods. An orange, by comparison, scores only about 1,819. Fresh figs are among the best sources of beta-carotene and other heart-healthy carotenoids. (For more information about the ORAC scale, see page 311.)

Scientific evidence: In a study published in the *Journal of the American College of Nutrition,* two groups of participants were "challenged" with sugary soft drinks, which are known to increase arterial oxidation. Oxidation in the arteries triggers atherosclerosis, a main risk factor for heart disease. Those who were given only soda had a drop in healthful antioxidant activity in the blood…those who were given figs as well as soda had an increase in blood antioxidant levels.

Bonus: Ten dried figs contain 140 mg of calcium. Other compounds in figs, such as quercetin, reduce inflammation and dilate the arteries. Perhaps for these reasons, people who eat figs regularly have much less heart disease than those who don't eat them, according to studies. Most dried figs contain added sulfites, so it's best to buy organic, sulfite-free dried figs.

SECRET 4: **Soy protein.** Tofu, soy milk and other soy foods are "complete proteins"—that is, they supply all of the essential amino acids that your body needs but without the cholesterol and large amount of saturated fat found in meat.

Scientific evidence: People who replace dairy or meat protein with soy will have an average drop in LDL "bad" cholesterol of 2% to 7%, according to research from the American Heart Association. Every 1% drop in LDL lowers heart disease risk about 2%.

A one-half cup serving of tofu provides 10 g of protein. An eight-ounce glass of soy milk gives about 7 g. Edamame (steamed or boiled green soybeans) has about 9 g per half cup. Avoid processed soy products, such as hydrogenated soybean oil (a trans fat), soy isoflavone powders and soy products with excess added sodium.

SECRET 5: **Lentils.** I call these "longevity legumes" because studies have shown that they can literally extend your life.

Best choices: Brown or black lentils.

Scientific evidence: In one study, published in the *Asia Pacific Journal of Clinical Nutrition*, the eating habits of five groups of older adults were compared. For every 20 g (a little less than three-fourths of an ounce) increase in the daily intake of lentils and/or other legumes, there was an 8% reduction in the risk of dying within seven years.

Lentils contain large amounts of fiber, plant protein and antioxidants along with folate, iron and magnesium—all of which are important for cardiovascular health.

Similarly, a Harvard study found that people who ate one serving of cooked beans (one-third cup) a day were 38% less likely to have a heart attack than those who ate beans less than once a month.

Caution: Beans have been shown to cause gout flare-ups in some people.

Important: Lentils cook much faster than other beans. They don't need presoaking. When simmered in water, they're ready in 20 to 30 minutes. You need about one-half cup of cooked lentils, beans or peas each day for heart health.

SECRET 6: **Pinot Noir and Cabernet Sauvignon.** All types of alcohol seem to have some heart-protective properties, but red wine offers the most.

Scientific evidence: People who drink alcohol regularly in moderation (one five-ounce glass of wine daily for women, and no more than two for men) have a 30% to 50% lower risk of dying from a heart attack than those who don't drink, according to research published in *Archives of Internal Medicine*.

Best choices: Pinot Noir, Cabernet Sauvignon and Tannat wines (made from Tannat red grapes). These wines have the highest concentrations of flavonoids, antioxidants that reduce arterial inflammation and inhibit the oxidation of LDL cholesterol. Oxidation is the process that makes cholesterol more likely to accumulate within artery walls.

Bonus: Red wines also contain resveratrol, a type of polyphenol that is thought to increase the synthesis of proteins that slow aging. Red wine has 10 times more polyphenols than white varieties.

In a four-year study of nearly 7,700 men and women nondrinkers, those who began to drink a moderate amount of red wine cut their risk for heart attack by 38% compared with nondrinkers.

If you are a nondrinker or currently drink less than the amounts described above, talk to your doctor before changing your alcohol intake. If you cannot drink alcohol, pomegranate or purple grape juice is a good alternative.

The Red Wine That Does the Most for Your Health

Ramon Estruch, MD, PhD, senior consultant, associate professor, department of internal medicine, University of Barcelona, Spain, and coauthor of a study published in *Circulation Research*.

Raising a glass of red wine and drinking to your health may give you a sense of satisfaction because you've heard that a bit of wine can be good for your heart.

But: There are downsides, too—alcohol increases the risk for certain cancers, and too much of it can harm the liver and increase blood pressure.

So you'll want to toast a recent Spanish study that reveals how people who enjoy the taste of red wine can indulge in the beverage and get the health benefits—without the health risks.

The secret: Opt for red wine that contains no alcohol.

Raise a Glass!

The study participants included men ages 55 to 75 who were at high risk for heart problems because they had diabetes or various cardiovascular disease risk factors. First, after a two-week period of abstinence from alcohol, each participant's baseline blood pressure was measured and certain blood tests were done.

Then, during one four-week period, each participant drank 9.2 ounces (about two glasses) of regular red wine with dinner each day. During a second four-week period, each man drank 9.2 ounces of nonalcoholic red wine with his evening meal. And during a third four-week period, each drank 3.4 ounces (about two shots) of gin daily with dinner. (The men knew what they were drinking, but this knowledge wouldn't affect results.) Participants all followed a similar diet and drank no other alcohol during the study. At the end of each four-week period, participants' blood pressure readings were compared with their baseline readings.

Results: After drinking regular red wine, the men's blood pressure dropped insignificantly…and after they drank gin, their blood pressure didn't change at all. However, after consuming the alcohol-free red wine, the men's blood pressure dropped, on average, nearly six points for systolic pressure (the top number of a blood pressure reading) and more than two points for diastolic pressure (the bottom number). This represents a significant decrease—perhaps more than enough to reduce heart disease risk by 14% and stroke risk by 20%!

The Real Power in Wine

To discuss how alcohol-free red wine reduces blood pressure, we contacted study coauthor Ramon Estruch, MD, PhD. He said that polyphenols—healthful antioxidants found in fruits, vegetables and wine—in nonalcoholic wine had more potent effects than those in regular wine, probably because alcohol interferes with antioxidant activity. Gin contains no polyphenols and thus does not have antioxidant benefits. While white wine and plain old grape juice do contain polyphenols, red wine contains more, which is why the researchers focused on it.

Dr. Estruch also explained that, when participants were drinking alcohol-free wine, their blood levels of nitric oxide were four times higher than when they were drinking regular red wine. This is an important change—because nitric oxide helps blood vessels relax, thus reducing blood pressure and allowing more blood to reach the heart and other organs. Again, polyphenols get the credit for the improvement in nitric oxide levels.

Would women experience the same effects from drinking nonalcoholic red wine? Researchers are planning to do an all-female study to find out, though they suspect that the benefits will be similar.

Is It Really Wine?

Unlike grape juice, nonalcoholic wine is fermented just like regular wine—in fact, it is regular wine—but then the alcohol is removed. Though the process does not affect polyphenol levels, true wine aficionados may recognize that taking out the alcohol leaves the wine lighter and less robust (and also leaves you without the buzz, of course). Many people find the nuanced taste of alcohol-free wine quite appealing—and perhaps all the more in light of this recent evidence for the beverage's health benefits.

Important: It is impossible to remove all alcohol from wine, though the amount left in is small at less than one-half of 1%. Still, if you are avoiding alcohol completely, nonalcoholic wine may not be appropriate for you. Also, if you have diabetes, keep in mind that alcohol-free wines do contain some sugar, so it is best to check with your doctor to see whether it is OK for you to consume nonalcoholic wine.

There are many types of nonalcoholic wine, including various reds and whites as well. Cabernet sauvignon, petit syrah and pinot noir have the highest levels of polyphenols—and a general guideline is, the drier the wine, the higher the polyphenol content. These days, alcohol-free wines are sold just about anywhere that regular wine is sold— even in many fine wine stores—and you can find them at many supermarkets and health-food stores. They're sold online too (for instance, at *www.ArielVineyards.com*) and typically cost less than $10 per bottle.

Health-Boosting Hot Cocoa Recipes

Janet Bond Brill, PhD, RD, LDN (licensed dietitian/nutritionist), nationally recognized nutrition, health and fitness expert who specializes in cardiovascular disease prevention and weight management. She is author of several books, including *Cholesterol Down: 10 Simple Steps to Lower Your Cholesterol in 4 Weeks—Without Prescription Drugs* and *Blood Pressure Down: The 10-Step Plan to Lower Your Blood Pressure in 4 Weeks—Without Prescription Drugs* (both from Crown/Three Rivers). *www.DrJanet.com*

By the time you're halfway through this article, you should be craving a nice toasty-warm mug of hot cocoa. Not the super-sweet stuff you remember from kidhood—made with sugary fake "chocolate-flavored" syrup or a packet of chemicals —but a palate-pleasing yet calorie-conscious grown-up version.

It's time to head to the stove! Because hot cocoa's key ingredient (the cocoa!) is packed with nutrients that benefit your body and brain.

For instance, recent research suggests that cocoa's antioxidant flavanols and other healthful components may help prevent clogged arteries, improve circulation and reduce blood pressure…combat inflammation…keep your mind and memory sharp…and even make it easier to keep weight under control.

For tips on transforming sticky-sweet kid-style hot cocoa into a super-healthful and tasty beverage with adult appeal, we turned to Janet Bond Brill, PhD, RD, LDN. As a nutrition, health and fitness expert and author of *Cholesterol Down: 10 Simple Steps to Lower Your Cholesterol in 4 Weeks—Without Prescription Drugs*, she had lots of smart suggestions and creative recipes to share.

Choosing the Right Stuff

For the healthiest, yummiest hot cocoa you've ever had, start by selecting the right main ingredients…

• **Cocoa.** Use natural unsweetened cocoa powder. Stay away from "Dutched" cocoa or anything labeled "processed with alkali," Dr. Brill recommended—it undergoes processing, including alkalizing, that depletes disease-fighting antioxidants.

• **Milk.** If you go with cow's milk and want to limit your fat intake, Dr. Brill suggested using 1% or fat-free milk. But cow's milk isn't your only option—there are plenty of unsweetened alternatives to choose from. (If you do choose a presweetened brand of milk for any of the recipes below, eliminate or reduce the amount of sweetener suggested in the recipe.)

Tasty options to try: Almond milk, which has fewer calories than skim cow's milk and is rich in calcium and vitamin E...oat milk, which provides a type of fiber that may help reduce cholesterol...hemp milk (derived from shelled hemp seeds), which contains fatty acids believed to fight heart disease and arthritis...rice milk, which tastes much like cow's milk but can be tolerated by some people who are allergic to cow's milk...or regular or light (reduced-fat) soymilk, which contains heart-healthy soy protein.

• **Sweetener.** Experiment to see how little sugar you can add to your hot cocoa and still satisfy your taste buds. You may be pleasantly surprised at how the other flavors come through when they're not overpowered by sugar. Or swap sugar for a low-calorie sweetener, such as Splenda or stevia.

• **Spices.** Cinnamon, nutmeg and ginger are packed with disease-fighting antioxidants. Experiment with these and other favorite spices and flavorings to put your own personal spin on your cocoa.

Recipes You'll Love

DR. JANET'S QUICK-N-HEALTHY HOT CHOCOLATE

2 Tablespoons natural unsweetened cocoa powder

2 packets (4 teaspoons) Splenda...or other low-calorie sweetener or sugar, to taste

12 ounces soymilk or other type of milk

⅛ teaspoon vanilla extract

Nutmeg, ginger and/or other spices to taste, optional

In a large microwavable mug, mix cocoa powder with sweetener. Stir in milk, vanilla extract and other spices if desired. Microwave on high for 60 seconds. Stir, then microwave for another 60 to 90 seconds or until steaming (do not allow to boil over).

CINNAMON-ALMOND HOT CHOCOLATE

12 ounces almond milk

1 vanilla bean

1 cinnamon stick

2 packets (4 teaspoons) Splenda...or other low-calorie sweetener or sugar, to taste

⅛ teaspoon vanilla extract

2 Tablespoons natural unsweetened cocoa powder

Place almond milk in a small, thick-bottomed saucepan over low heat and bring to a low simmer, whisking as needed so milk doesn't stick to the pan. Add the vanilla bean and cinnamon stick. Remove from heat and steep for 10 minutes. Strain the milk, discarding vanilla bean and cinnamon. Return the milk to the saucepan and place over low heat until simmering. Add sweetener, vanilla extract and cocoa powder. Whisk vigorously until cocoa has blended. Heat over low heat for four minutes or until steaming, constantly stirring.

EUROPEAN-STYLE THICK SOY COCOA

⅓ cup natural unsweetened cocoa powder

2 packets (4 teaspoons) Splenda Brown Sugar Blend...or other low-calorie sweetener or sugar, to taste

2 teaspoons cornstarch

⅛ teaspoon ground cinnamon

12 ounces unflavored or vanilla soymilk or other type of milk

Fat-free whipped topping, optional

In a saucepan, mix cocoa, sweetener, cornstarch and cinnamon. Whisk in six ounces of the milk to dissolve dry ingredients and create a thick paste (like chocolate frosting). Add the remaining six ounces of milk and whisk until smooth. Place over low heat and stir until steaming (do not boil). If desired, top with fat-free whipped topping to complete your guiltless splurge.

Heart-Healthy Ice Pops and Other Treats

Jamison Starbuck, ND, naturopathic physician in family practice and a guest lecturer at the University of Montana, both in Missoula. She is past president of the American Association of Naturopathic Physicians and a contributing editor to *The Alternative Advisor: The Complete Guide to Natural Therapies and Alternative Treatments* (Time Life).

When I see patients during the summer, I love to talk up some of the great fresh foods that they can easily add to their diets. A basic tenet of naturopathy is that nutrient-packed foods can be used as "medicine" to help prevent chronic conditions such as cancer and heart disease. And the summer season—when local fresh fruits and vegetables are readily available in most parts of the country—is perhaps the best time of year to give your diet a "nutrient boost." With a little creativity and a trip to your own garden and/or your local farmer's market or grocery store, you can easily add more foods to your daily diet that not only taste great, but also help protect your health. *My favorite nutrient-packed summer foods…*

•**Fresh flowers.** You may have never thought of this, but fresh blossoms of nasturtium, violet and calendula make a great addition to greens or potato salad. Not only do these flowers make your dish look beautiful, they also contain minerals, such as potassium and magnesium, and beta-carotene—key nutrients that promote heart, bone and muscle health.

My advice: Add six to eight of the fresh flowers mentioned above (look up photos of the flowers online so you don't mistakenly eat a different variety that may not be as safe or tasty). Flowers taste a little bitter but nicely complement certain greens—for example, I like violets on spinach.

•**Heart-healthy ice pops.** You can make your own anthocyanin-rich ice pops by freezing the fresh, unsweetened juice of purple or red fruit. To ensure optimal freshness, make your own juice. *Anthocyanin*, the pigment in grapes, blueberries, raspberries and pomegranates, helps improve blood vessel health, which benefits your entire body. Studies show that anthocyanin can help prevent heart disease and cataracts and reduce inflammation.

My advice: Buy an ice pop tray or use an ice cube tray and add a few frozen cubes to your water or iced tea.

•**Parsley pesto.** Two tablespoons of chopped parsley contain ample vitamin C and all of your daily vitamin K requirement.

Caution: You may need to use less parsley if you take a blood thinner—too much vitamin K may interfere with these drugs. Parsley pesto—a blend of parsley and basil, olive oil, pine nuts or walnuts and Parmesan cheese—is a delicious way to get more of this nutrient-packed food.

My advice: Make a traditional pesto recipe with half parsley and half basil. Serve on pasta or rice or as a dip.

•**Sun tea.** Summer-harvested peppermint, which aids digestion, is delicious prepared as sun tea—a great alternative to sugary beverages.

My advice: In a glass jar filled with three quarts of water, add about 12 well-rinsed six-inch peppermint stalks (leaves and stems)—or eight bags of your favorite herbal tea—and three tablespoons of honey. Seal it and set it out in the sun for six hours.

•**Watermelon.** Watermelon is an absolute nutrient powerhouse. It contains lycopene, vitamin C and beta-carotene—all of which help prevent cancer and promote immune health.

My advice: Choose the dark pink or red-fleshed varieties of watermelon for the greatest nutrient boost.

Amazing Way to Double the Nutrients in Watermelon

Penelope Perkins-Veazie, PhD, plant physiologist, US Department of Agriculture (USDA) Agricultural Research Service in Lane, Oklahoma.

Watermelon, like many fruits today, is in our supermarkets nearly year round, but it's still a hot summer afternoon that makes an ice-cold slice a real taste treat. Beyond being yummy, watermelon is full of healthful benefits—high in the antioxidant lycopene, a carotenoid pigment that produces the deep red color (and recent research has shown may help heart health), and is fairly rich in vitamins C, B-6 and B-1 (thiamine), and beta-carotene. It also has magnesium and potassium—all for just 46 calories a cup. But now researchers at the USDA Agricultural Research Service in Lane, Oklahoma, have discovered a way to improve the melon's health benefits even more.

It's this simple: Just leave the melon out of the fridge for seven to 10 days if fresh-picked and a few days if store-bought before you open it. A watermelon kept at room temperature has double the level of beta-carotene and some 11% to 40% more lypocene.

Maximum Ripeness

Penelope Perkins-Veazie, PhD, was a lead researcher on this study. She says that allowing melons to be at room temperature for several days before eating gives them the chance to reach maximum ripeness. As the melon sits, the color of the red flesh inside becomes more intense and the rind thins, reflecting the fact that the fruit is continuing to ripen. For this study, watermelons were stored at 41° F, 55.4° F and 69.8° F, with 69.8° F repre-

sentative of room temperature. If your room is warmer, keep in mind that increased heat will accelerate the process, she says. When you are preparing to serve the melon it is fine to chill it first, though this will slow any further increase in nutrients. How do you know when a melon is ripe? Completely ripened melon will sound almost hollow when tapped sharply.

Eat When at Peak

Dr. Perkins-Veazie also cautions to refrigerate melon once cut or damaged because yeast organisms, bacteria and mold can easily invade it. But when you do open the fruit, you'll know that you have let the melon ripen too long if the rind is soft, pitted or has dark spots…or if the melon flesh has an orange tint and a pumpkin-type odor (which is not a surprise, since watermelons are in fact related to pumpkins).

While the study was performed on watermelons, tomatoes—another lycopene-rich food—as well as other fruits and vegetables are best eaten at their peak ripeness, and best bought when they have been harvested close to that peak ripeness to maximize their nutritional benefits.

Tasty Way to Lower Heart Attack Risk

In a recent study of 93,600 women, those who ate more than three servings of strawberries or blueberries each week had a 34% lower risk for heart attack compared with those who rarely ate these berries.

Theory: Berries are rich in antioxidant anthocyanins, which have been shown to help regulate blood pressure and improve blood vessel function.

For heart health: Eat a handful of fresh or frozen berries a few times a week.

Eric Rimm, ScD, associate professor of epidemiology and nutrition, Harvard School of Public Health, Boston.

Heart Rx: Hot Peppers

Zhen-Yu Chen, PhD, professor, food and nutritional science, Chinese University of Hong Kong. He is coauthor of a study published in the *European Journal of Nutrition*. Dave DeWitt, coauthor of *The Complete Chile Book: A Gardener's Guide to Choosing, Growing, Preserving, and Cooking* (Timber Press), and publisher of the Fiery Foods & Barbecue Supersite. *www.Fiery-Foods.com*

Some people naturally gravitate toward hot, spicy foods, such as those containing cayennes, jalapeños, habañeros and other chile peppers.

But people who prefer to keep their fare on the mild side may want to rethink their choices, since a recent study shows that these sizzling peppers may provide a key health benefit.

Hot Stuff

Zhen-Yu Chen, PhD, a professor of food and nutritional science at the Chinese University of Hong Kong, wanted to see whether capsaicinoids—pungent compounds found in chile peppers—might boost cardiovascular health, so he tested his theory on hamsters.

Dr. Chen and his team put hamsters (that all had similar cholesterol levels) into five groups. They were all fed a high cholesterol diet, but four of the groups were fed varying amounts of powdered capsaicinoids and the fifth group consumed no capsaicinoids. *After six weeks, researchers discovered…*

Total cholesterol in all of the hamsters went up—but hamsters in the control group that didn't eat capsaicinoids had their total cholesterol rise three times as high (about 28%) as those in each of the other groups (which rose just 10% to 12%).

Hamsters in the control group that didn't eat capsaicinoids also had aortic arteries that were more rigid and less relaxed, compared with the capsaicinoid groups.

In other words, the animals that ate the chile pepper compounds had much healthier cardiovascular systems.

Cranberry Juice for Your Heart

The healthful polyphenols in cranberry juice have been found to improve blood vessel function. When study participants were tested immediately after drinking cranberry juice and then again 12 hours later, they showed a decrease in arterial stiffness, a risk factor for heart disease.

Beware: Some cranberry juice products are blends of multiple fruit juices and may not have enough cranberry content to achieve this benefit.

Best: Because of the natural tartness of 100% cranberry juice, stick with "cranberry juice cocktail." Low-calorie versions contain less sugar and calories than 100% grape juice and 100% pomegranate juice.

Jeffrey B. Blumberg, PhD, director, HNRCA Antioxidants Research Laboratory, Tufts University, Boston, and coauthor of a study published in *The American Journal of Clinical Nutrition*.

Fiery Foods You Can Use

When we spoke with Dr. Chen, he was cautious about how the study's results might apply to humans. It's not yet known whether eating a certain amount of chile peppers would help keep our cholesterol in check or keep our arteries nice and supple. And certainly, eating chile peppers is not a proven substitute—not yet, anyway!—for any medications being taken to maintain heart health.

You say that you dislike spicy food? You don't have to overdo it. In fact, the capsaicinoids in the study made up as little as one tenth of 1% of the weight of the animals' diets—and benefits were still seen.

Here are two easy and delicious ways to use chile peppers in your kitchen from Dave DeWitt, coauthor of *The Complete Chile Pepper Book* and publisher of the Fiery Foods & Barbecue Supersite, *www.Fiery-Foods.com*. (You may want to wear gloves when handling hot peppers, because if there's residue on your hands and then you touch, say, your eye, it might burn!) Add a small amount of the pepper or pepper powder to your meals at first (DeWitt gives you suggested starting points, below) and then take a taste. If you think you'd enjoy a spicier taste, gradually add more. If you overdo it, reduce the spiciness by adding more of the other ingredients.

DeWitt's pepper-picking pointers…

•**If you want just a little spiciness:** Use a jalapeño pepper—and the larger it is, the less hot it will tend to be.

•**If you want medium spiciness:** Use cayenne powder or fresh New Mexican chiles, such as the "Big Jim" variety, but be sure to roast them and peel off the tough skins.

•**If you want a very spicy experience:** Use a habañero pepper—and the smaller it is, the hotter it will tend to be.

SPICED-UP SPAGHETTI SAUCE

This recipe works well with almost any sort of tomato-based spaghetti sauce—and even many creamy or pesto sauces.

28 ounces tomato sauce

1 jalapeño pepper (mildly spicy result)…

or ½ teaspoon cayenne powder (medium-spicy result)…

or ½ habañero pepper (quite spicy result)

If using a fresh pepper, cut it in half vertically, remove the stem and seeds, and then mince. Put the minced pepper or powder and the tomato sauce in a food processor or blender, and then blend them together for 30 seconds, which will chop the pepper into even finer bits.

KICKED-UP VANILLA ICE CREAM

This is a popular dessert in Arizona, said DeWitt. "The butterfat in the ice cream tones down the hotness of the pepper a little, so you're not overwhelmed, but the peppers still add flavor that surprises."

2 scoops vanilla ice cream

½ jalapeño, minced as described above (mildly spicy result)…

or ½ teaspoon cayenne powder (medium-spicy result)…

or ¼ habañero pepper, minced (quite spicy result)

Just mix the minced pepper or powder into the ice cream—that's it! "The cayenne powder works fine," DeWitt said, "but I prefer using peppers to powder because they add a satisfying crunch."

Go Nuts for Almonds!

Andrew L. Rubman, ND, consulting medical editor for Bottom Line's *Daily Health News* and director of the Southbury Clinic for Traditional Medicines in Southbury, Connecticut.

Nuts have gained popularity in recent years as an excellent source of protein and "good fats." One of the best nuts? Almonds. According to our consulting medical editor Andrew L. Rubman, ND, almonds are one of the most nutrient-dense, good-for-you foods there is.

Almonds Benefits

Although Dr. Rubman encourages eating a variety of nuts, just as you do fruits and vegetables, he particularly likes almonds because of their fatty acid content (almonds are high in monounsaturated fats). Furthermore, almonds have many health-promoting minerals, especially magnesium, but also potassium, which means the nuts help other dietary and supplemental sources protect cardiovascular health. Eating almonds with their skins provides significant amounts of vitamin E and flavonoids. Studies have shown that these two work synergistically to help boost low-density lipoprotein (LDL, or bad) cholesterol's resistance to oxidation by more than 50%, important because LDL cholesterol is not dangerous in and of itself. It is oxidation that makes LDL a plaque-building danger.

Protein Provider

Dr. Rubman adds that almonds are also a good source of protein (6 grams per ounce) nearly as much as one egg (6.3 grams of protein/egg)…and they have fiber and assorted vitamins and minerals. Visit *www. almonds.com* for more on their nutritional content.

Don't Add Calories

Still, some are concerned about the high calorie content of almonds and other nuts. Dr. Rubman has counseled many dieters about how to receive the health benefits of almonds without adding extra calories to their diet.

The solution: If you want to lose weight do not eat more than an ounce a day of unsalted almonds. That ounce would come to 23 nuts, he says, and the unsalted type is simpler because it is easier to stop at your limit with unsalted nuts than the salted, tastier form. Another good way to enjoy the health properties of almonds without toting up too many calories is to add them to other foods rather than eating them plain. Nuts toasted in a dry skillet are even more flavorful. Try chopping some into salads, sprinkling them over string beans or white fish. You can also coat fish or chicken with almond flour—make your own by grinding the nuts in a blender, food processor or even coffee grinder.

Pistachios: Good-for-Your-Heart Snack Food

Pistachios are high in mono- and polyunsaturated fats…low in saturated fats…and a good source of phytosterols, which help reduce LDL "bad" cholesterol and prevent plaque buildup in arteries.

Bonus: One ounce of pistachios provides three grams of fiber and about as much protein as an egg. They also are a good source of lutein and zeaxathin, antioxidants that promote good vision.

Jill Nussinow, MS, RD, dietitian, Santa Rosa, California, quoted in Vegetarian Times. *www.Vegetarian Times.com*

The High-Fat Food That's Surprisingly Good for Your Heart

Ivan Petyaev, MD, PhD, CEO and founder of Lycotec Ltd., Cambridge, UK. His study was published in *Medical Hypotheses.*

You dutifully eat your fat-free yogurts, unbuttered veggies and other virtuously low-fat (and low-flavor) fare.

After all, you want to protect your cardiovascular system from harmful saturated fats.

But: What if you were told that a nice chunk of cheese—yes, that deliciously decadent dairy delight that comes in so many mouthwatering varieties—was also good for your heart?

Well, it's true, according to recent research from the UK, which revealed some previously unknown properties of cheese.

And the findings may help explain a mystery that has confounded scientists for decades…the conundrum called the French paradox.

People in France have remarkably low rates of cardiovascular disease despite the fact that their diets typically are quite high in saturated fat. By some estimates, saturated fats contribute up to 40% of their total calories! Based on that, you'd expect Frenchmen to be dropping like flies from heart disease. But they aren't. Instead, they have the third-lowest rate of cardiovascular mortality in the world.

Some people attribute this to French folks' fondness for red wine, which contains the antioxidant resveratrol. But inhabitants of other countries also drink lots of red wine, yet their heart health can't compare to that of the French.

So researchers wondered what other dietary factors might help explain the French paradox. Since cheese consumption in France is among the highest in the world, they took a close look at cheese—not only a laboratory analysis of the biochemical properties of cheese, but also a clinical trial that directly examined how cheese consumption affects people. What they discovered was extremely promising—and startling.

Newly Revealed Health Benefits

We contacted Ivan Petyaev, MD, PhD, founder and CEO of the firm that conducted the research. *He explained that cheese's heart-protective properties may derive from its beneficial effects on…*

- **Inflammation.** A complex enzymatic transformation that occurs as cheese ripens leads to the formation of substances known to reduce inflammatory markers such as C-reactive protein. This is extremely important, Dr. Petyaev said, because high levels of inflammation are closely associated with cardiac and other vascular diseases.

- **Blood pressure.** Cheese contains compounds capable of inhibiting the angiotensin-converting enzyme (ACE) that controls blood pressure. The effects could be similar to ACE inhibitor medications used to control hypertension.

- **Cholesterol and bacteria.** Cheeses with mold (such as Roquefort) may be particularly advantageous to cardiovascular health. When these cheeses are ripened through fermentation with fungi such as *Penicillium roqueforti*, they form substances that combat bacteria. What do these bacteria have to do with heart disease? Dr. Petyaev explained that, in more than half of adults, bacteria acting as "parasites" in the liver and blood vessels are responsible for increases in cholesterol synthesis.

- **Nutrient status.** Cheese also provides numerous nutrients that the body needs for overall good health—including heart health—such as protein, calcium and vitamins A, D, B-6 and B-9.

The Best of the Bunch

The researchers' analysis was quite extensive, encompassing nine blue-veined cheeses from six different countries…eight white fungi-fermented cheeses from three countries…seven bacteria-fermented cheeses from five countries…and two processed "cheeses" from two countries. Most were made from cow's milk, but some were made from ewe's milk or goat's milk. The various cheeses were evaluated for anti-inflammatory activity using a proprietary patented lab test, Dr. Petyaev said.

Based on the researchers' discoveries, some cheeses rate as more heart-healthy than others. Here are the ones that Dr. Petyaev said top the list. All are available at supermarkets, cheese shops and/or online (for instance, *www.MurraysCheese.com*).

- **Blue-veined cheeses**—such as Roquefort…Danish Blue…Gorgonzola…and mature Stilton.

- **White fungi-fermented cheeses**—such as Camembert (from cow's or goat's milk)…and mature Brie.

- **Bacteria-fermented cheeses**—such as mature Cheddar…mature Emmental, which is similar to Swiss and made with two types of bacteria to produce the characteristic holes…and Ossau-Iraty, a ewe's milk cheese with a toasted-wheat aroma and nutty, grassy-sweet flavor. (While all cheeses are bacteria-fermented, Dr. Petyaev's study suggested that these three are among the most beneficial for your heart.)

You'll notice that the processed "cheese" (such as American cheese) so common in the US does not appear on the list above—because it was not found to have heart-healthy properties.

How much cheese should you eat? Dr. Petyaev recommended aiming for a total of 15 to 25 grams (about one-half to one ounce) per day, choosing from the selections above. Don't go overboard—cheese has around 100 calories per ounce.

To keep the calorie count under control, forget about pairing cheese with bread or crackers. Instead, place slivers of cheese on slices of apple or pear…tuck cheese into celery sticks…or sprinkle cheese over a chopped-veggie salad. If you like your cheese melted, go ahead—melting it will not diminish its beneficial properties.

What If Fried Foods Were Healthy?

Pilar Guallar-Castillón, MD, MPH, PhD, associate professor, department of preventive medicine and public health, School of Medicine, Universidad Autónoma of Madrid, Spain.

Let's talk about fried foods—not just fried foods that you buy at fast-food restaurants, but also pan-fried and deep-fried foods that you cook at home using olive oil, vegetable shortening, butter or whatever you choose. There is something surprising to tell about them.

Fried foods have always been considered dietary no-nos because of the concern that they increase your risk for cardiovascular problems. But a recent Spanish study calls that common claim into question.

This research found that frying may not be nearly as bad for you as you might think—as long as only certain foods are fried and the right cooking fats are used.

The Best Foods and Fats

Researchers were curious to see whether eating fried foods would, in fact, raise the risk for cardiovascular problems. So they asked about 40,000 Spanish men and women between the ages of 29 and 69 to fill out detailed questionnaires about their diets, cooking habits, health and lifestyles. Participants reported what foods they had eaten in a typical week during the previous 12 months (either at home or at a restaurant). Subjects weren't able to report on what types of oil were used to cook the fried foods they ate in restaurants, but they did note that they used only two types of oil in cooking—olive and sunflower. Their most frequently consumed fried foods were, from most to least, fish, meat, potatoes and eggs. At the outset, none of the participants had heart disease.

Next investigators divided the participants into four groups, depending upon how much fried food they ate. They followed them for 11 to 12 years and observed whether or not they had events related to coronary heart disease (such as heart attack or chest pain) and/or died. After taking into account variables such as age, exercise habits, blood pressure and smoking, researchers found that there was no association between how much fried food was eaten and having a heart-related event or dying. Those who consumed the most fried food (about nine ounces daily, on average) were no more likely to have a heart-related event or die than those who consumed the least (about two ounces).

Now, this doesn't mean that people who ate the most fried food weren't on their way to a heart-related event…unfortunately, the researchers didn't measure risk factors.

The study authors reported no fiscal support from organizations that had a financial interest in their conclusions. But researchers acknowledge that this study has limitations. People reported their habits in just one initial questionnaire, and self-reporting is not always accurate—not to mention that eating habits can change over time. But the findings, which were published recently in *BMJ,* certainly suggest an interesting concept that needs to be explored further—perhaps not all fried foods are, in fact, bad for us.

Eat Like a Spaniard!

So why no increased risk for heart-related events or death? Study author Pilar Guallar-Castillón, MD, MPH, PhD, an associate professor of preventive medicine and public health at Universidad Autónoma in Spain, told us the following…

• **One potential reason,** she said, is that the oils that these Spanish participants (and most Spanish restaurants, for that matter) use to cook with are olive and sunflower, which are high in heart-healthy mono- and polyunsaturated "good" fats. These fats are quite different from the ones that Americans commonly use to fry, such as butter, margarine, vegetable shortening and lard—all of which contain at least some saturated or trans fats (or both), which are both bad for the heart.

•**Another potential reason,** she said, is that the most common food that these Spanish subjects were frying was fish, and fish are rich in cardioprotective omega-3 fatty acids—even when they're fried.

So if you're going to indulge in a fried food (whether pan-fried or deep-fried), mimic the Spaniards from this study and use olive or sunflower oil—and get your fried-food fix from fish.

Here's a great recipe: Pan-fry fish in olive or sunflower oil and then let it simmer in a "sofrito" sauce made of fresh tomatoes, garlic, onion and olive oil—the more Mediterranean it looks and smells, the better!

Can a Fatty Diet Protect Against Heart Attack?

Lauren Haar, doctoral student, systems biology and physiology graduate program, University of Cincinnati.

Keith Jones, PhD, associate professor, department of pharmacology and cell biophysics, University of Cincinnati.

Jack Rubinstein, MD, health cardiologist, assistant professor of medicine, division of cardiovascular diseases, University of Cincinnati.

How's this for weird? In spite of all the admonitions to eat a low-fat, high-fiber diet, it appears that a quick high-fat splurge actually might protect you from muscle damage caused by heart attack.

Researchers at the University of Cincinnati have discovered that a short-term, high-fat diet helped protect mice against tissue injury from heart attacks. Although the researchers are quick to add that they don't know yet whether the diet will work the same way for human beings, this may someday lead to a change in dietary recommendations.

Unexpected Findings

A large body of research had established that people who have higher cholesterol levels are at increased risk for heart attack—but that's not the whole story. Surprisingly, in people with certain conditions (such as heart failure), having high cholesterol means that they have a better chance of surviving a heart attack.

This seemingly paradoxical bit of information led associate professor Keith Jones, PhD, University of Cincinnati Health cardiologist, assistant professor Jack Rubinstein, MD, and doctoral student Lauren Haar to do their own research on the topic. They designed a study on mice that were fed a menu intended to create cholesterol levels akin to those in humans who eat a high-fat diet. Some were fed the high-fat diet for just one day...others, for one to six weeks. A control group of mice was fed a standard, lower-fat diet. Then the researchers measured the high-fat diet's effect in two ways—over a short period of time and over the long term—as it related to heart attack survival. (Yes, they induced heart attacks in the mice.)

Researchers found that...

•**Heart damage in mice that had been on the high-fat diet** for up to two weeks was, on average, 70% less than in mice on the six-week high-fat diet and the control diet.

•**No cardio protection occurred in mice on the long-term (six-week) high-fat diet.** In a second experiment, the 24-hour high-fat diet was followed by a control diet for 24 hours before heart attacks were induced—and those mice also experienced greater protection from heart attack damage versus mice who were fed regular grain and vegetable-based chow—confirming that it is, in fact, the short-term, high-fat feeding that provided the most protection.

Bring On the Fat? Not So Fast

As intriguing as the study results are, we can't get too carried away by them, caution Dr. Jones and Dr. Rubinstein. For one thing, it's not known how to time a short-term fat splurge for optimal heart attack protection, if indeed that's possible in humans. Also, it's well-known that heavy people with weight-related health issues tend to have more heart attacks, so for this group, any high-fat program must be approached with extreme caution. That said, this research presents an intriguing model for the future, and the researchers intend to continue studying the heart-protective effects of a short-term fat splurge—for now, in animals. In the meantime, don't trade in your poached salmon and spinach for a bacon cheeseburger. Evidence shows that a regular anti-inflammatory diet low in saturated fat and high in healthful monounsaturated fats—from fish, avocados, olive oil, etc.—offers the best long-term protection against heart disease. But we do now know that an occasional indulgence might not harm you at all…in fact, it might help you…but we can't say for sure yet.

The Eskimo Diet for Heart Health

Zeina Makhoul, PhD, a postdoctoral researcher in the Cancer Prevention Program of the Public Health Sciences Division at the Fred Hutchinson Cancer Research Center in Seattle.

N ot surprisingly, the best thing that an overweight or obese person can do to improve his/her health is to lose weight…but it appears that the next best thing might be to take fish oil!

A recent study conducted in the rugged Yukon-Kuskokwim Delta in southwestern Alaska examined the diet of Yup'ik Eskimos, a native American people, many of whom have maintained a traditional lifestyle, including eating a diet that's especially rich in fish. About 70% of the Yup'ik Eskimos in the study were overweight or obese—a percentage that is consistent with the rest of the US. But compared with overweight or obese folks in other parts of our country, these Yup'ik Eskimos have a far lower risk for heart disease and a lower rate for adult-onset diabetes.

Fishing for the Facts

The Yup'ik Eskimos consume about 30 times more omega-3 fats in their diet on average than do other American adults. This led researchers at the Fred Hutchinson Cancer Research Center in Seattle to design a study measuring the association between their fish-rich diet and their good health. Omega-3 fats, found mainly in saltwater fish such as salmon, halibut and herring, include docosahexaenoic acid (DHA) and eicosapentaenoic acid (EPA), which are the components of most fish oil supplements on the market today. If omega-3s help prevent adult-onset diabetes, the researchers figured that they might also reduce the risk for other conditions associated with being overweight, including heart disease, so the study was designed to measure the association between omega-3 fats and blood markers of chronic disease risk, including C-reactive protein (CRP) and triglycerides.

Results of the study were clear: In the 330 Yup'ik Eskimos studied, the more omega-3 fats they ate, the lower the levels of CRP and triglycerides. Importantly, this was so even in participants who were overweight or obese.

Fish Oil for All?

Zeina Makhoul, PhD, lead author of the study that resulted from the Hutchinson Center's research in Alaska explains: "It's very possible that foods rich in omega-3 protect Yup'ik Eskimos from some of the harmful effects of obesity." But, she said, this particular study was designed to measure only the association and it does not establish a cause-and-effect link between omega-3 fats and the levels of CRP and triglycerides. That, she said, would require clinical trials—and, as a result of the study, clinical trials are a likely next step.

If trials confirm what she and other researchers suspect, Dr. Makhoul said, the outlook is good that higher intake of omega-3 fats will be recommended for virtually everyone and most especially for people who are overweight.

A Top Cardiologist Reveals the Best Supplements for Your Heart

Patrick M. Fratellone, MD, integrative cardiologist and executive medical director of Fratellone Medical Associates, and an attending physician at St. Luke's Hospital, Roosevelt Hospital and Beth Israel Hospital, all in New York City. He is coauthor of *You're on the Air with Dr. Fratellone: Answers to Questions Most Frequently Asked About Supplements and Herbs for the Heart* (iUniverse). *www.FratelloneMedical.com*

Put your hand on your heart. How's it doing in there? For too many women, the answer is, "Not so good." Despite the fact that we try to eat right, exercise and watch our weight, heart disease is still the number-one killer of women in America.

What are we doing wrong? For one thing, we're not getting enough of the nutrients that our hearts need to stay healthy. "Much of our food is depleted of life-sustaining vitamins and minerals," explained integrative cardiologist Patrick M. Fratellone, MD. "That's why many people can benefit from specific supplements—whether their goal is to prevent heart disease or to minimize harm from the particular cardiovascular risk factors they already have."

Here's how the various heart-healthy supplements work...and the protocols Dr. Fratellone typically recommends based on patients' particular risk factors.

Important: Check with your doctor before beginning any supplement regimen. Some supplements can interact with other supplements or medications and/or cause side effects for people with certain medical conditions.

How the Heart Helpers Work

• **Coenzyme Q10 (CoQ10),** the energy generator of all cells, enhances the heart's pumping ability.

Caution: CoQ10 may decrease the effectiveness of blood-thinning medication, such as warfarin.

• **Folic acid,** a B vitamin, helps prevent the formation of homocysteine, an amino acid that damages artery linings.

Caution: Avoid folic acid supplementation if you have a history of cancer.

• **Hawthorn,** an herb, may strengthen heart contractions and reduce blood pressure by relaxing blood vessels.

Caution: Don't use hawthorn if you have low blood pressure or take a beta-blocker or calcium channel blocker medication.

• **L-carnitine,** an amino acid, increases the heart's pumping action...and may facilitate weight loss by increasing metabolism.

Caution: Don't use L-carnitine if you have kidney disease.

• **L-taurine,** another amino acid, dilates blood vessels, improves blood flow and helps reduce blood pressure.

Fish Oil Does Help Your Heart

Fish oil can help your heart despite a report to the contrary, says Michael D. Ozner, MD. A recent study found that taking fish oil pills, which are rich in omega-3 fatty acids, didn't appear to prevent heart attacks or stroke. But the study (which was a review of previous studies) actually demonstrated that fish oil was beneficial in preventing death from heart disease.

Bottom line: Fish oil reduces inflammation, a factor in heart disease...is FDA-approved to lower harmful triglycerides...and has a very low risk for side effects.

For more information on how to make sure that you're getting enough omega-3 fatty acids, see page 23.

Michael D. Ozner, MD, is medical director, Wellness & Prevention, Baptist Health South Florida, Miami, and author of *Heart Attack Proof* (BenBella).

Caution: L-taurine may not be appropriate if you take diuretic medication or have stomach ulcers.

• **Magnesium** regulates blood pressure and heart rate.

Caution: Don't take magnesium if your blood pressure is already low.

• **Omega-3 fatty acids,** found in fish oil, increase HDL (good) cholesterol…decrease LDL (bad) cholesterol and triglycerides…slow plaque buildup in arteries…reduce the risk for arrhythmia (abnormal heartbeat)…and reduce blood pressure.

• **Vitamin B-12** inhibits harmful homocysteine formation.

• **Vitamin D-3** helps prevent inflammation…reduces heart attack and stroke risk in people with high blood pressure…and may protect against heart failure.

Next step: To make use of the information above, you need to know which specific nutrients are most beneficial for you—and that depends on your personal health status.

To Prevent Heart Problems…

Below is Dr. Fratellone's heart-protecting supplement protocol (to be taken daily, continuing indefinitely) for the typical perimenopausal or postmenopausal woman who has not been diagnosed with any condition that increases cardiovascular risk. Ask your doctor if you should take any or all of these five supplements. If you take a multivitamin, check which of the nutrients below your multi already provides.

Preventive protocol…

• **CoQ10**—100 mg daily.

• **Magnesium**—350 mg daily.

• **Omega-3s (in the form of fish oil)**—1,000 mg to 2,000 mg daily of combined EPA and DHA, the most beneficial components.

• **Vitamin B-12**—1,000 micrograms (mcg) daily.

• **Vitamin D-3**—1,000 international units (IU) daily.

If You Are Already at Risk…

You may benefit from additional protection if you have a condition that increases cardiovascular risk. Dr. Fratellone said that it is generally advisable to continue taking the five supplements above, though in some cases, a higher dosage is appropriate (as detailed below)…and to consider additional supplements (observing the aforementioned cautions), depending on an individual's particular health problem.

Ask your doctor about modifying your regimen as follows if you have…

ATRIAL FIBRILLATION OR OTHER ARRHYTHMIA

• **Hawthorn (extract ratio 1:2)**—20 drops mixed with water three times daily.

• **Magnesium**—increase to 500 mg daily.

• **Omega-3s**—increase to 1,000 mg three times daily.

CONGESTIVE HEART FAILURE

• **Hawthorn (extract ratio 1:2)**—20 drops mixed with water three times daily.

• **Vitamin D-3**—increase to 2,000 IU daily.

CORONARY ARTERY DISEASE

• **Folic acid**—1,000 mcg daily.

• **L-carnitine**—1,000 mg three times daily.

• **L-taurine**—500 mg three time daily.

• **Omega-3s**—increase to 1,000 mg three times daily.

DIABETES

• **CoQ10**—increase to 100 mg three times daily.

• **L-carnitine**—1,000 mg three times daily.

• **Magnesium**—increase to 500 mg daily.

EXCESS WEIGHT
(Body mass index of 25 or higher)

• **L-carnitine**—1,000 mg three times daily.

HIGH BLOOD PRESSURE

• **L-taurine**—500 mg three times daily.

• **Magnesium**—increase to 500 mg daily.

• **Omega-3s**—increase to 1,000 mg three times daily.

• **Vitamin D-3**—increase to 2,000 IU daily.

HIGH CHOLESTEROL

• **CoQ10**—increase to 100 mg three times daily.

• **L-taurine**—500 mg three times daily.

• **Omega-3s**—increase to 1,000 mg three times daily.

HIGH HOMOCYSTEINE

• **Folic acid**—1,000 mcg daily.

HIGH TRIGLYCERIDES

• **CoQ10**—increase to 100 mg twice daily.

• **Omega-3s**—increase to 1,000 mg three times daily.

The Herb for Clear Arteries

Lewis H. Kuller, MD, DrPH, professor of public health, department of epidemiology, University of Pittsburgh.

When we think about clogged arteries, we generally think about arteries near the heart (coronary arteries).

But leg arteries (peripheral arteries) can also get blocked, triggering peripheral artery disease (PAD). PAD can cause ongoing leg cramps (especially while moving around) and leg numbness. The problem can lead to surgery—to increase blood flow or even to amputate.

Of course, healthy habits such as eating well, exercising and not smoking all can help prevent PAD, but eight to 12 million Americans already struggle with the disease, so clearly many of us could use some extra help preventing it.

So it's encouraging to see that researchers have found that one of the all-time best-selling herbs may be an easy, inexpensive, natural way to prevent this painful problem.

Get a Leg Up

What's the herb in question? It's the well-known ginkgo biloba. Researchers wanted to see whether it would stave off a variety of health problems, including dementia, heart attack, stroke, chest pain and what they classified as a clinical diagnosis of a PAD "event" (any severe problem related to PAD that would bring a patient to the hospital for surgical therapy or angioplasty). Lewis Kuller, MD, DrPH, the study's lead author, explained more about the analysis.

The subjects were split into two groups, with one group receiving a supplement containing 120 milligrams (mg) of ginkgo biloba extract twice a day and the other receiving a placebo. (Those who were taking medications for any cardiovascular health problems continued taking them.) Over the course of the study (a median time frame of six years), the herb showed no tangible benefit in terms of preventing dementia—nor did it significantly prevent heart attack, stroke or chest pain.

But there was one finding that caught the researchers' attention. During the study period, 35 patients had a PAD event. The researchers noticed that among those 35 people, 23 were in the placebo group and only 12 were in the ginkgo biloba group—so those who took the extract turned out to be only about half as likely to have a PAD event. In other words, the ginkgo biloba might have helped prevent PAD.

Granted, this finding is based on a small number of people. And the researchers don't know for sure whether patients had had PAD events that met their criteria before the study began, because they didn't have access to prior medical records. But the result is what scientists call "a statistically significant" difference. In other words, it's a finding that shouldn't be ignored, said Dr. Kuller, and one that should be further studied.

Opening Up Blood Vessels

Dr. Kuller suggested that ginkgo biloba's blood-thinning and vessel-dilating properties—stemming from flavonoid antioxidants—may be what made a critical difference.

But if the supplement is so good at opening up blood vessels and thinning blood, then how come it didn't appear to help prevent other cardiovascular problems—beyond just PAD? Dr. Kuller isn't sure but hopes that new research will answer that question.

Of course, there are foods that are rich in flavonoids, including many fruits and vegetables and even red wine and dark chocolate. But amounts and types of flavonoids in foods vary widely—so, Dr. Kuller said, a ginkgo biloba supplement is the only way, for now, to duplicate what was received by the people in the study.

Prevent PAD

If you are at high risk for PAD (risk factors include a family history of PAD, heart disease or stroke...being sedentary...smoking...diabetes...obesity...high blood pressure...high cholesterol...being over the age of 50 and being African American) talk to your doctor about taking a ginkgo biloba supplement—you might mention Dr. Kuller's study.

While taking ginkgo biloba, any healthy person may experience persistent or temporary side effects, including upset stomach, headaches and dizziness, although these tend to be mild. (The higher the dose, the greater the likelihood of side effects.) However people taking certain drugs—including blood thinners and antidepressants—may suffer serious drug interactions (such as bleeding or serotonin syndrome, which can be fatal) while using ginkgo biloba, and pregnant women should also avoid it. If you're taking an anticonvulsant, ginkgo biloba may make the drug less effective. So, again, talk to your doctor about all of your medications (and other supplements that you take) if you want to try it. Study subjects took 240 mg total per day, split into two doses, but ask your doctor about the best dosage for you.

The Spice That Could Save Your Heart

Wanwarang Wongcharoen, MD, department of internal medicine, faculty of medicine, Chiang Mai University, Chiang Mai, Thailand.

People tend to think that bypass surgery is pretty safe. But the reality is, patients who undergo coronary artery bypass graft surgery—its official name—are vulnerable to an in-hospital heart attack in the first few days after the operation.

Now here's good news: Curcuminoids, chemicals in the spice turmeric (the spice that gives curry its yellow color), may help prevent many of these post-op heart attacks, according to recent research from Thailand.

Heart of the Matter

Here's a natural spice accomplishing something that no drug has yet to do as effectively.

In the study, beginning three days prior to their bypass surgery, participants were given either a placebo or 4,000 milligrams (mg) of a curcuminoid supplement daily. They remained on that dose for five days after surgery, along with any necessary medications that they were given before, during and after surgery. The results were striking—30% of the patients who took the placebo had heart attacks in the 72 hours following the surgery...while only 13% of those who took the supplement had heart attacks.

"We believe that the anti-inflammatory and antioxidative effects of curcuminoids are mainly what helped prevent heart attacks," said the study's lead author, Wanwarang Wongcharoen, MD.

It's possible that curcuminoids might also help patients who aren't undergoing bypass surgery but are at high risk for heart attack, said Dr. Wongcharoen.

Should You Eat More Curry?

Before you head to the nearest Indian or Malaysian restaurant thinking that a great-tasting, curry-flavored meal will help protect your heart, keep in mind that the amount of curcuminoids that you get in such a meal is typically less than 10 mg—which is very, very little compared with the massive amount that patients in the study received (4,000 mg). So it's unlikely that consuming curcuminoids through foods would have anywhere near the dramatic effect seen by the bypass patients in the study. Curcuminoid supplements, however, would be more likely to help because they contain much higher amounts, said Dr. Wongcharoen—usually about 250 mg to 500 mg per capsule.

If you're about to undergo bypass surgery, ask your doctor whether taking 4,000 mg of a curcuminoid supplement daily—for three days before the operation and for five days after it—is a good idea, said Dr. Wongcharoen. Just be sure not to abandon your surgery meds. "I do not recommend replacing any drugs with a curcuminoid supplement," Dr. Wongcharoen said. "But it might be a helpful addition." You can buy a curcuminoid supplement at a health-food store or at many health-food and vitamin Web sites— there are many different types, so just make sure that the word "curcumin" is on the label, said Dr. Wongcharoen.

It's generally considered to be a very safe supplement, said Dr. Wongcharoen. Potential side effects include nausea, dizziness and/or diarrhea, and it can slow blood clotting, so if it's taken with other drugs or supplements that may also slow blood clotting (including *clopidogrel, ibuprofen, naproxen, warfarin,* garlic, ginger, ginkgo and/or ginseng), that could be dangerous. (Dr. Wongcharoen found in his study that the supplement group did not bleed any more than the placebo group, which suggests that the anticlotting effect of these curcuminoids may not be very strong—therefore, in his opinion, the reduction in heart attack risk outweighs an additional risk of bleeding.) Keep in mind that taking any supplement in an extreme amount does raise the risk for side effects and adverse interactions—so definitely check with your doctor first.

And if you had bypass surgery more than 72 hours ago, the danger of having an operation-related heart attack has passed, so Dr. Wongcharoen does not recommend that you take a curcumin supplement to prevent heart attacks until future research shows whether it's helpful.

What Not to Eat Before Surgery

James R. Mitchell, PhD, assistant professor of genetics and complex diseases, department of genetics and complex diseases, Harvard School of Public Health, Boston. His study was published in *Science Translational Medicine*.

If you or a loved one is scheduled for surgery anytime soon, beware. There's a risk for heart attack and stroke during many types of surgery. This risk is generally small during noncardiovascular operations (less than 1%), but during cardiovascular operations, it can be as high as 10%!

What can you do about it? Surprisingly, according to a recent study, the risk may be lowered significantly by simply changing your diet in the week before surgery.

Protein Vs. Carbs

Prior studies on mice and other animals had shown that overall calorie restriction can help the body resist stress, including the stress of surgery, but researchers at the Harvard School of Public Health in Boston wanted to see whether cutting back on certain nutrients—not just overall calories—was the real key. So they gave mice different types of diets to find out. Past research on fruit flies had showed that reducing protein, specifically, from the diet extended their lifespan better than restricting carbohydrates, so researchers made sure that one of the diets eliminated protein.

In the first part of the study, for 14 days, mice ate one of three diets—either an "unlimited" traditional diet (mice could eat as much as they wanted of protein, fat and carbohydrates)…a "limited" traditional diet made of the same nutrients but in a restricted amount…or an unlimited protein-free diet. Then, to mimic the experience of a heart attack or stroke mid-surgery, researchers blocked blood flow to the kidneys of the mice for 35 to 45 minutes and then abruptly restarted the blood flow. Next, they examined the mice to see how each fared after the "surgery."

The protein-free group…

• **Had a strikingly better survival rate.** In the week following surgery, 100% of the protein-free group survived…25% of the unlimited traditional group survived…and none of the limited traditional group survived.

• **Had about 70% less waste in their blood than both traditional groups,** which indicated that their kidneys were functioning better.

• **Had a better appetite and did not lose any weight after surgery,** whereas surviving mice from the unlimited traditional group lost about 6% of their weight.

So eliminating protein before the "surgery" was a big help!

In the second part of the study, the researchers wondered if the mice could get the same protection in less time. The great news is that it came very close—six days of a protein-free diet before surgery was nearly as effective as one that was two weeks long.

Eat the Right Things Before Surgery

So what is it about eliminating protein that helped the mice? Coauthor James Mitchell, PhD, assistant professor of genetics and complex diseases at Harvard School of Public Health, explained that when mice (and humans) don't consume the essential amino acids that protein contains, their bodies go on an alert that prepares them to resist stress—including the stress of surgery. "We can't say for sure whether removing protein from a human's diet before surgery will provide the same results, but we're hopeful."

Heartbreaking News for Folks Who Love Diet Soda

Some diet soda lovers close their eyes to the beverage's known potential dangers, such as an increased risk for kidney disease. But if they care about their health, they'll want to take an honest look at worrisome new research linking diet soda to heart attacks and stroke.

The 10-year study involved more than 2,500 participants.

Recent finding: People who reported drinking diet soda daily were 48% more likely to have a heart attack or stroke than participants who rarely or never drank any soda. The results held even after researchers took into account age, physical activity, smoking, calorie consumption, history of heart disease and other cardiovascular risk factors.

The study does not actually prove that consuming diet soda causes stroke or heart attack. For instance, it could be that people who regularly drink diet soda also tend to have other unhealthy dietary habits that contribute to cardiovascular problems. Researchers noted that more study is needed to determine what it is about diet soda—or about people who consume a lot of diet soda—that is responsible for the increased risk for heart attack and stroke.

In the meantime: Just drink water! It's still calorie-free—and if you like a little flavor, squeeze a lemon or lime into it.

Hannah Gardener, ScD, epidemiologist in the department of neurology at the University of Miami Miller School of Medicine and lead author of a study on diet soda and cardiovascular problems.

There are, of course, some downsides to not eating any protein. For example, protein deficiency can lead to side effects that may include feeling tired and weak, losing muscle, losing hair, recovering more slowly from injury, gaining weight and potentially experiencing a spike in blood sugar (if you replace protein with carbs). But it's unknown yet if those side effects would be evident and/ or severe after just one week of going protein-free. Plus, those problems are reversible once a person starts eating protein again.

Dr. Mitchell isn't ready to recommend any particular presurgery dietary restrictions for humans. But based on these results, if you have to go under the knife, you might want to talk to your doctor about steering clear of protein in the one week before the operation.

Which Carbs Place an Unhealthy Load on Your Heart?

James Shikany, DrPH, associate professor in the division of preventive medicine at the University of Alabama at Birmingham (UAB) School of Medicine and an associate scientist with the Nutrition Obesity Research Center at UAB. His work focuses on the association between diet and chronic diseases, including cardiovascular disease and cancer.

Some research indicates that carbohydrates may be as dangerous to our hearts as the dreaded saturated fat.

However, a recent study in *Archives of Internal Medicine* confirmed that we needn't renounce all carbs, just those with a high glycemic index (GI)—meaning those that cause rapid spikes in blood sugar and insulin levels, which can be hard on the body.

Study finding: Compared with women whose diets included the fewest high-GI carbs, women whose diets included the most carbs with a high GI were about twice as likely to develop coronary heart disease (narrowing of the blood vessels that supply blood and oxygen to the heart).

Surprising: High-GI foods include not only the usual carbo culprits (white bread, sweets) but also some foods that we normally think of as healthful, such as brown rice.

James Shikany, DrPH, of the University of Alabama at Birmingham School of Medicine, has studied the connection between GI and chronic diseases for many years. He explained that, over time, a diet full of high-GI foods can lead to chronic high blood levels of insulin. This can have multiple adverse metabolic effects—for instance, on cholesterol levels, blood clotting factors and body weight—potentially increasing heart disease risk.

Here's what women need to know about GI to keep their hearts healthy or to minimize the danger if they already have heart disease…

Demystifying the Glycemic Index

Scientifically speaking, the glycemic index is a measure of how quickly and dramatically equal amounts (usually 50 grams) of various carbohydrate foods will raise blood sugar levels. Based on that, a food is ranked on a scale ranging from 0 (meaning it causes no alteration in blood sugar) to 100 (reflecting an extreme spike in blood sugar equal to that of pure glucose). A GI of 70 or more is considered high.

Tricky: Some high-GI foods don't really deserve a bad rap. For instance, although watermelon is a healthful fruit, it rates a high GI of 72. Dr. Shikany said that this stems from a glitch in the GI concept that arises with foods that are relatively low in carbohydrates—because you would have to eat almost five cups of watermelon to consume 50 grams of carbs! To get around that problem, you also should consider the newer concept of glycemic load (GL), which takes into account a food's GI and its standard portion size. A report from the Harvard School of Public Health classifies a high GL as 20 and up…a GL of 10 or less is considered low. Watermelon's GL is a very reasonable four.

It would be convenient if we could just check product labels to learn a food's GI or GL, but unfortunately such information is not listed. What's more, food processing and preparation methods can affect those numbers.

For example, cooking carrots increases their glycemic ratings because heat breaks down the cell walls, making the carbohydrate more available, Dr. Shikany said. Thus, we must dig deeper to figure out which foods are best and worst for our hearts.

You might assume that you can just follow the often-heard advice to stick mostly to complex carbohydrates, such as whole grains. Yet when it comes to GL, that doesn't necessarily hold true. For example, the GL of mass-produced whole-wheat bread tends to be only slightly lower than that of white bread.

What matters more, Dr. Shikany said, is to have soluble fiber in your food. Soluble fiber slows digestion and absorption and thus helps keep blood sugar levels more stable. Good sources include barley, oats and wheat bran…beans of many types…certain fruits (apples, citrus fruits, mangoes, pears, strawberries)…some vegetables (asparagus, Brussels sprouts, turnips)…flax and psyllium seeds.

Low-Glycemic Guidelines

A great way to be sure that you're eating a low-glycemic diet is to look up favorite foods at www.glycemicindex.com. This database from the University of Sydney in Australia lists the GL (and GI) of many foods. If a food has a GL of 20 or more, instead eat something similar that has a lower GL.

Example: Rather than white rice (with a GL as high as 43, depending on brand) or even brown rice (with a GL as high as 33), eat pearled barley (with a GL of nine to 12).

Of course, you won't always have time to check the database, so Dr. Shikany offered these simple low-GL strategies…

• **Eat foods that are as close to their natural states as possible.** For instance, the GL of apple juice is about 13, whereas raw apples have a GL of just four to six.

• **Breakfast cereals in particular have a wide GL range.**

Rule of thumb: Anything puffed, ground or flaked tends to have a higher GL than oatmeal or All-Bran.

• **Whenever you eat carbs, have some protein and a bit of fat at the same time.** This slows carbohydrate absorption, keeping blood sugar levels more stable…and keeping your heart healthier.

Sunlight Helps Prevent Heart Attacks

Tobias Eckle, MD, PhD, associate professor of anesthesiology, cardiology, and cell and developmental biology, University of Colorado School of Medicine, Denver. His study was published in *Nature Medicine*.

Ah, sunlight. There's nothing like being outdoors on a summer morning.

What you may not know is that sunshine doesn't just boost your mood and your vitamin D level—it also may help you ward off a heart attack or minimize the damage that one can cause, according to a recent first-of-its-kind study.

We spoke to the researchers to find out more about how we can all harness the power of light to brighten our heart health.

According to the study's lead author, Tobias Eckle, MD, PhD, an associate professor of anesthesiology, cardiology and cell and developmental biology at the University of Colorado School of Medicine in Denver, our circadian rhythm—the physical, mental and behavioral changes prompted by light and darkness that occur over each 24-hour period—helps determine the level of a certain protein that can minimize the cell damage and cell death caused by a heart attack. This protein might even stop a heart attack in its tracks. So Dr. Eckle and his colleagues were eager to see whether exposure to certain kinds of light at a certain time might be effective at boosting levels of this protein.

In the study, researchers divided mice into two groups. One group was exposed to light boxes emitting light that was the same level

Just a Little Bit Will Help Your Heart

A little exercise helps the heart a lot. *Recent finding:* Exercising for just 10 to 15 minutes a day (a total of 75 minutes a week) reduces risk for coronary artery disease—the leading cause of death in the US. But the American College of Sports Medicine still recommends at least 150 minutes of moderate-intensity exercise each week for heart health.

Jacob Sattelmair, DSc, product manager, RunKeeper, a personal fitness application company, Boston, and leader of a study that analyzed the results of 33 studies that assessed the health benefits of exercise, published in *Circulation*.

of brightness as daylight ("bright light"), and others were exposed to regular room lighting ("regular light"). Both groups were exposed to the light first thing in the morning at 6:00 am.

Then the mice were given anesthesia and heart attacks were triggered in them. Researchers found that mice that had been exposed to three hours of "bright light" had three times the amount of the protective protein as the mice that had been exposed to "regular light"—and, incredibly, the "bright light" mice's hearts had experienced only one-fifth as much damage!

How Sunny Are the Findings?

There are, of course, unanswered questions—for example, how the findings might apply to humans and how lasting the benefit of the protein might be.

That said, the results are promising. What's especially interesting is that it's the light exposure on the eyes—not the skin—that affects the protein levels, said Dr. Eckle. So humans wearing sunscreen or long sleeves wouldn't blunt the effect.

Safe Ways to Let In the Light

Several forces have conspired over recent decades to keep people out of the sun during the day, such as indoor work and fear of skin cancer. But many people would be likely to benefit from getting more sunlight exposure as early in the morning as possible.

Here are some safe ways from Dr. Eckle to shed more light on your daily routine…

1. Take a daily walk outdoors, and keep wearing sunscreen. Even 10 to 20 minutes a day is better than nothing. Since, as mentioned earlier, it's the way that light affects your eyes (not your skin) that matters, apply sunscreen—that won't dampen the benefits. The added exercise will boost your heart health, too.

2. Get sunlight while indoors. Sit near large, bright windows.

3. Use a light therapy box. If you can't follow either of the first two tips, or if you're at high risk for skin cancer and want to avoid UV rays at all costs, this may be the best option for you. Available online for about $50 and up, light therapy boxes mimic the brightness of sunlight while filtering out most damaging UV rays.

Exercise Is Not Enough to Keep Your Heart Healthy

No matter how much you exercise, avoid sitting for long periods of time as well.

Recent finding: People who sat at a computer or in front of a TV screen for four or more hours a day were 48% more likely to die during the four-year study regardless of how much they exercised. Also, some type of cardiovascular event, such as a heart attack, was twice as likely in those who spent at least two hours a day sitting in front of a screen—compared with those who had less than two daily hours of screen time.

Self-defense: Take frequent breaks from the computer or TV to get up and walk around.

Study of 4,512 adults by researchers at University College London and University of Queensland, Baker IDI Heart and Diabetes Institute and Edith Cowan University, all in Australia, published in *Journal of the American College of Cardiology.*

The Right Exercise If You Have Heart Disease

John P. Porcari, PhD, program director of the Clinical Exercise Physiology (CEP) program at the University of Wisconsin–La Crosse. A past president of the American Association of Cardiovascular and Pulmonary Rehabilitation, he has authored or coauthored more than 350 abstracts and 150 papers on exercise physiology.

Jennifer Cummings, MD, associate professor of medicine at Northeastern Ohio Universities College of Medicine in Rootstown, Ohio, and a cardiologist with City Cardiology Associates in Akron. She serves on the American College of Cardiology's Committee for Clinical Electrophysiology and is an ad hoc peer reviewer for *Journal of Cardiac Electrophysiology, Annals of Internal Medicine* and *Circulation.*

Everyone agrees that exercise is good for you. The goal for most people should be at least 150 minutes of moderate aerobic activity a week, plus strength training two days a week, according to the Centers for Disease Control and Prevention.

But what if you have heart disease, a condition that can make exercise seem dangerous and difficult?

While exercise is helpful for most chronic health problems, some activities are likely to be easier, more beneficial and less risky than others if you need to watch your heart health.* *Best workout if you have cardiovascular disease…*

A key benefit of exercise is reduced heart attack risk. But if you have already had a heart attack or undergone bypass surgery…or have symptoms, such as chest pain (angina),

---

*Always talk to your doctor before starting a new exercise program. If you have a chronic illness, it may be useful to consult a physical therapist for advice on exercise dos and don'ts for your particular situation.

---

that signal established heart disease, you may worry that physical exertion is too risky.

For the vast majority of people with heart disease, it's not—if it's supervised. This usually involves initial and periodic testing to establish safe levels of exercise and monitoring of heart rate and blood pressure for some sessions. Once you're cleared, you can do most sessions on your own.

When performed at the proper intensity, standard aerobic activities are usually suitable. This means you can most likely walk, jog, use a stationary bike or treadmill (or even participate in aerobic dance) as long as you do it at a moderate level that doesn't raise your heart rate too high. Talk to your doctor about the heart rate you should strive for.

Once you have that number, you may want to wear a heart rate monitor—several models are widely available for under $100.

Another option: Use the "Talk Test." If you can talk while exercising, this will indicate with 95% accuracy that your heart rate is in a safe range.

If you have hypertension: Higher-intensity exercise may trigger potentially dangerous

Transcendental Meditation (TM) Improves Heart Health

A recent study of patients with heart disease, funded by the National Institutes of Health, found that practicing transcendental meditation (TM) regularly reduced risk for heart attack and stroke by 48%. TM produces a state of restful awareness—a settled mind in a settled body. The technique must be taught—there is a standard seven-step course that takes about 10 hours over six days. Once learned, TM should be practiced for 20 minutes twice a day. To find a certified TM instructor, go to *www.TM.org.*

Joan-Ellen Macredis, ND, naturopathic physician and licensed acupuncturist based in Stamford, Connecticut.

spikes in your blood pressure—talk to your doctor about appropriate heart rate goals, and remember to breathe (do not hold your breath) and stay away from heavier weights when doing strength training.

Important: Be sure to ask your doctor to reevaluate your target heart rate if you change blood pressure medication—some drugs, such as beta-blockers, will affect your heart rate.

Heart Rate: Why It Matters More Than You Might Think

Wayne Westcott, PhD, a certified strength and conditioning specialist, is the fitness research director and an instructor of exercise science at Quincy College, in Quincy, Massachusetts. He is author or coauthor of numerous books on fitness.

Most of us grew up in the days before gym teachers talked about resting heart rates and target heart rates. When coaches at school wanted us to work harder, they would just yell, "Hustle!" When we overdid it, we would flop down onto the ground for a few minutes until we felt better.

But now that we're older, the whole heart rate business is not something we can ignore. *Recent research reveals the reasons…*

A study of 50,088 adults found that for women under age 70, every increase of 10 beats per minute (bpm) in resting heart rate (number of heartbeats per minute while at rest) boosted the risk of dying from a heart attack by 18%. (No such association was found among women 70 or older.)

In a study of 129,135 postmenopausal women, those whose resting heart rate was above 76 bpm were 26% more likely to have or to die from a heart attack than those whose resting heart rate was below 63 bpm.

A strong heart pumps blood more efficiently, so it doesn't need to beat as fast. Regular aerobic exercise can lower your resting heart rate—but only if you work out at the right intensity. According to Wayne Westcott, PhD, a Quincy College exercise science instructor, if you go too easy during workouts, you miss out on cardiovascular benefits…but if you push too hard, you might experience light-headedness, nausea and a higher-than-normal rise in blood pressure that could dangerously overwork your heart if you have hypertension. Here's how to gauge the right workout intensity for you…

•**Find out your current resting heart rate.** First thing when you wake up, take your pulse at your wrist or neck for one minute.

What resting heart rate suggests about fitness level for women in midlife and beyond…

Excellent	Below 60 bpm
Very good	60 to 65 bpm
Good	66 to 70 bpm
Average	71 to 75 bpm
Worse than average	Above 75 bpm

•**Plan to do a cardio workout at least three times per week.** Good options include brisk walking, running, dancing, cycling and swimming, Dr. Westcott said. (Get your doctor's OK before beginning or intensifying any exercise regimen.)

•**Determine your target heart rate.** Your ideal heart rate while exercising depends on two factors—your age and current fitness level. Dr. Westcott explained that the problem with the target heart rate charts often seen online or at gyms is that they generally are based only on age, not on fitness level, so you could wind up working out too hard or not hard enough. And though one target heart rate formula (called the Karvonen method) does account for resting heart rate, it requires more complicated calculations and, in Dr. Westcott's opinion, yields guidelines that may be too high.

Better: Follow the guidelines in the charts on page 95. To track heart rate during your workout, use a heart rate monitor (about $100 at sporting-goods stores).

Remember: Your warm-up and cool-down do not count as time in your target range.

If your resting heart rate currently is above 70 bpm…

In your	Your target heart rate is	Your cardio workout should last
40s	120 to 130 bpm	15 to 20 minutes
50s	110 to 120 bpm	15 to 20 minutes
60s	105 to 115 bpm	15 to 20 minutes
70s	95 to 105 bpm	15 to 20 minutes
80s	80 to 90 bpm	15 to 20 minutes

If your resting heart rate is 60 to 70 bpm…

In your	Your target heart rate is	Your cardio workout should last
40s	130 to 140 bpm	20 to 25 minutes
50s	120 to 130 bpm	20 to 25 minutes
60s	115 to 125 bpm	20 to 25 minutes
70s	105 to 115 bpm	20 to 25 minutes
80s	90 to 100 bpm	20 to 25 minutes

If your resting heart rate is below 60 bpm…

In your	Your target heart rate is	Your cardio workout should last
40s	135 to 145 bpm	25 to 30 minutes
50s	125 to 135 bpm	25 to 30 minutes
60s	120 to 130 bpm	25 to 30 minutes
70s	110 to 120 bpm	25 to 30 minutes
80s	95 to 105 bpm	25 to 30 minutes

Adjust your workout intensity as needed. Check your resting heart rate monthly—as it improves, intensify your workouts according to the guidelines above.

For safety: Reduce workout intensity and/or duration if you feel exhausted rather than invigorated after exercising…your muscles feel sore for more than a day after working out…you are recovering from an illness…you feel stressed…or the pollen count or air pollution index is high.

Don't Work So Long

Long work hours may harm your heart. *Recent study:* People who worked more than 11 hours a day had 67% higher risk for heart disease than people who worked seven to eight hours a day.

If you work long hours: Decrease your risk for heart disease in other ways, such as eating a healthy diet, exercising and maintaining healthy blood pressure, blood sugar and cholesterol levels.

Mika Kivimaki, PhD, professor, department of epidemiology and public health, University College London, England, and leader of a study that followed 7,095 workers for 11 years, published in *Annals of Internal Medicine.*

Extreme Exercise Hurts the Heart

Marathon runners who were followed over three decades had a 19% lower rate of death than nonrunners—but those who ran more than 20 to 25 miles each week ended up with the same risk as the couch potatoes in the study.

Self-defense: Exercise vigorously for no more than one hour a day.

James O'Keefe, MD, head of preventive cardiology at Mid America Heart Institute at Saint Luke's Health System, Kansas City, Missouri, quoted at Today.com.

Chapter 6

LIFESAVING TREATMENTS

Did You Have a Heart Attack—And Not Know It?

When you have a heart attack, you know it, because the main symptom—crushing chest pain—is overwhelmingly obvious. That's what most of us believe about heart attacks. But it's not always true.

What few people realize: Studies show that 20% to 60% of all heart attacks in people over age 45 are unrecognized or "silent." And the older you are, the more likely it is that you've already had a silent heart attack. In a study of 110 people with a mean age of 82, an astounding 68% had suffered a silent heart attack.

What happens during a silent heart attack? You may have no symptoms at all. Or you may have symptoms that are so mild—for example, a bout of breathlessness, digestive upset or neurological symptoms such as fainting—that neither you nor your doctor connects them with a heart attack.

Scientists don't know why some people have unrecognized heart attacks. But they do know that a silent heart attack is a real heart attack and can cause as much damage to heart muscle as a nonsilent heart attack. And just like a person with a known heart attack, anyone who has had a silent heart attack is at higher risk for another heart attack, heart failure, stroke…or sudden death from an irregular heartbeat.

Recent scientific evidence: In a six-year study by cardiologists from the University of California in San Diego and San Francisco—published in *Clinical Research in Cardiology*—people who were diagnosed with a silent heart attack at the beginning of the study were 80% more likely to have another "cardiovascular event," such as a heart attack or stroke, by the end of the study period.

In a five-year study by cardiologists at the Mayo Clinic, people with an unrecognized heart attack were seven times more likely to die of heart disease than people who didn't have an unrecognized heart attack.

Wilbert Aronow, MD, professor of medicine in the divisions of cardiology, geriatrics and pulmonary/critical medicine, and chief of the cardiology clinic at Westchester Medical Center/New York Medical College in Valhalla, New York. Dr. Aronow has edited eight books and is author or coauthor of more than 2,250 scientific papers, abstracts and commentaries that have appeared in *The Lancet, The New England Journal of Medicine, Circulation* and other medical journals.

If you have risk factors for heart disease, it is vitally important to your health that you find out if you have had a silent heart attack. *Here's how…*

The Key to Detection

If you're at high risk for heart disease, your primary care physician should perform an electrocardiogram (EKG)—a test that checks for problems with the electrical activity of your heart—every year during your regular checkup. If the EKG reveals significant "Q-waves"—markers of damaged heart tissue—you have had a silent heart attack.

"High risk" means that you have two or more risk factors for heart disease. These risk factors include a family history of heart disease (in a first-degree relative such as a sibling or parent)…high blood pressure…smoking…inactivity…obesity…high LDL "bad" cholesterol…low HDL "good" cholesterol…high triglycerides…and type 2 diabetes.

The groups at highest risk for having an unrecognized heart attack are adults over age 65…women…and people of any age with type 2 diabetes.

The Treatment You Need

If your EKG reveals a previously unrecognized heart attack, it's wise to see a cardiologist and receive the exact same treatment that you would get if you had a recognized heart attack. *Elements of that treatment should include…*

•**Treadmill stress test.** The cardiologist will check for and interpret many variables, such as your symptoms (if any), the electrical patterns of your heart rhythms and your blood pressure while you are on a treadmill.

Important: Be sure to get your cardiologist's advice on special steps to take to ensure accurate results. For example, you should have no caffeine within 24 hours of the test.

If the results of the stress test indicate "severe myocardial ischemia"—poor blood flow to the heart muscle—it may be necessary to have a coronary angiogram (X-rays of the heart's arteries) to accurately diagnose the degree of blockage and decide whether you should pursue such options as angioplasty (in which a balloon is inserted into the coronary artery and inflated to restore normal blood flow) or coronary bypass surgery (in which a blood vessel is grafted from another part of the body to give blood a new pathway to the heart).

However, in most cases, heart disease that is associated with a silent heart attack can be managed with lifestyle changes, such as not smoking…losing weight if you're overweight…and getting regular exercise. *In addition, medications may include…*

•**Aspirin.** A daily dose of 81 mg of aspirin is the best choice for an antiplatelet drug to reduce the risk for blood clots.

Very important: A higher dose does not increase the cardiovascular benefit—but does increase the risk for gastrointestinal bleeding.

•**Beta-blocker.** This class of drugs slows the heart rate, relaxing the heart and helping to manage high blood pressure.

•**Angiotensin-converting enzyme (ACE) inhibitor.** These drugs expand blood vessels, improving blood flow and lowering blood pressure—thus allowing the heart to work less.

•**Statin.** If you have heart disease, this cholesterol-lowering medication reduces your risk for another heart attack or dying from heart disease—regardless of whether your levels of LDL "bad" cholesterol are high or low.

In addition, statin use should be accompanied by a diet that is low in cholesterol (less than 200 mg per day) and low in saturated fat (less than 7% of total calories).

Also important: It's crucial that people with diabetes maintain tight control of their HbA1C levels. This measure of long-term blood sugar control should be less than 7%.

However, HbA1C levels should not be aggressively lowered below 6.5% in diabetes patients with cardiovascular disease, according to the Action to Control Cardiovascular Risk in Diabetes study—that increases the risk for death because it would indicate that blood glucose is at times too low.

In general, the best way for people with diabetes to protect against heart attacks and strokes is to give up cigarettes if they smoke… lose weight if necessary…reduce blood pressure to 130–139/80–89 mmHg…and reduce LDL cholesterol to less than 70 mg/dL.

If these lifestyle measures do not also sufficiently lower the person's HbA1C level, standard antidiabetes medication can be used.

Think Twice About Heart Treatments

Larry Allen, MD, MHS, assistant professor of medicine in the division of cardiology at the University of Colorado. He is also co-chair of the 15-member panel that wrote the American Heart Association's statement titled "Decision Making in Advanced Heart Failure" and appeared in the journal *Circulation*.

Surgical treatments for advanced heart failure have come a long way—scientists have made major improvements that can help patients live longer than ever before.

But many of these therapies come with a risk for serious complications and can negatively impact quality of life—so they may add more years to a patient's life, but will they be pleasant ones?

A panel of doctors supported by the American Heart Association recently published a statement regarding treatment decisions for advanced heart failure, including defibrillators, artificial heart pumps and bypass surgery.

They argue that these decisions are complex and need to be discussed in detail between patients and their health-care providers. So before you say "yes" to a new heart failure surgical treatment, there is important information to factor into your decision…

More Years Don't Always Mean Good Years

After reading the American Heart Association's statement, we spoke with the cochair of the panel, Larry Allen, MD, MHS, a cardiologist at the University of Colorado School of Medicine in Denver. *He briefly described some issues that patients will want to consider before proceeding with the following surgical treatments…*

• **Implantable Cardioverter Defibrillator (ICD).** This device helps prevent sudden death by using an electrical shock to get the heart out of a dangerously fast rhythm. But contrary to what you might think, it won't ease the symptoms of heart failure, such as shortness of breath, excessive tiredness and swelling in the belly, legs, ankles and feet. The device can get confused (such as when a patient is exercising) and shock a patient when he doesn't need to get shocked, which can be painful. It also can get infected and need to be replaced. And even if things go well, you still need to see your doctor at least a few times a year to make sure that the device is working properly.

Anemia and Heart Attack

In a recent study, researchers reviewed the medical records of 17,676 heart attack patients for nine years and found that 20% developed moderate-to-severe anemia while in the hospital. Those who developed anemia had more blood drawn for laboratory testing than those who did not develop the condition—an average of 174 ml versus 83.5 ml over a period of 10 days. For every 50 ml drawn, anemia risk increased by 18%. Blood tests are necessary to diagnose conditions and guide treatment, but daily monitoring is sometimes unnecessary in patients who are stable.

If you are hospitalized: Ask your doctor whether frequent blood tests are necessary. These study findings are likely to apply to all hospitalized patients.

Mikhail Kosiborod, MD, cardiologist, Saint Luke's Mid America Heart Institute, Kansas City, Missouri.

• **Coronary Bypass Surgery.** This open-heart surgery is designed to restore blood flow to the heart muscle, with the goal of reducing chest pain and/or improving heart-pumping function. Possible complications during surgery include bleeding, infection, heart arrhythmias, heart attack, kidney failure, temporary memory loss or trouble thinking, and stroke. Recovery tends to take six to 12 weeks, so you may have to take a few months off from working or doing most activities. And it doesn't necessarily prevent arteries from clogging in the future.

• **Left Ventricular Assist Device (LVAD).** This artificial heart pump, which helps the heart deliver oxygen-rich blood to the body, contains external cords and batteries, which typically need to be charged daily. The cords and the spot on the stomach where the main cord comes out of the body can't be pulled on or gotten wet, so that means no contact sports, limited ways to bathe (only sponge baths or showers with precautions to keep the external cord dry) and no sleeping on your stomach. There can be malfunctions with the device after it's implanted. Plus, it puts you at higher risk for internal bleeding and stroke (from blood thinners or from clots), both of which could cause death.

Making Tough Decisions Easier

The challenge, Dr. Allen said, is weighing the benefits versus the risks and annoyances. *Here's what he recommends to any patient with heart failure…*

• **Ask questions.** If your doctor emphasizes only the potential "pros" of a treatment, ask that he or she detail all the potential "cons," too.

• **Whether you go through with a surgical treatment or not, consider palliative care.** When people hear the term "palliative care," they typically relate it to "at death's door." But that is not always true. What palliative care for heart failure really means is managing (but not necessarily trying to cure) the symptoms of the condition and helping patients and families deal with the disease.

Methods vary, depending on symptoms, but a heart failure patient receiving palliative care might be given a diuretic, antidepressant, pain reliever and/or other medications. Health-care providers might also arrange talk therapy, provide assistance with bathing and dressing, and/or give the patient an oxygen tank and/or a motorized wheelchair.

• **Get a second opinion.** Most decisions about heart failure treatment are not unforeseen emergencies. Patients often have time to consult two doctors…or even three…before making a decision. Different doctors may be more "for" or more "against" certain treatments, and it's helpful to hear their reasons. Hear them all out and decide for yourself.

• **Meet other patients.** Having face-to-face conversations with patients who have undergone the same type of treatment that you're considering is invaluable because you'll get a realistic sense of what life after surgery might be like. Ask your doctor to introduce you to patients who have had the treatment and who are willing to meet with you. If your doctor can't or won't make such referrals, find a doctor who will. Online patient support groups are also available.

How the Right Heart Surgeon Can Save Your Life

Albert J. Miller, MD, recently retired professor of clinical medicine (cardiology) at Feinberg School of Medicine of Northwestern University, and a clinical cardiologist at Northwestern Memorial Hospital, both in Chicago. He is author of *Chest Pain—When & When Not to Worry* (Selfhelp Success).

Sometimes research affirms what makes sense anyway—but still is compelling and important.

Case in point: Recent research published in *Journal of the American Medical Association* concluded that patients who need an implantable cardioverter defibrillator (ICD)—an implanted electronic device to correct heart rhythm problems—do better when a board-certified electrophysiologist performs the procedure.

Wiring Experts

An electrophysiologist is basically a cardiologist who specializes in the electrical behavior of the heart and who has undertaken specialized training (usually two years) in this field. In this study of patients at risk of life-threatening arrhythmias, the overall complication rate (meaning any complication from the surgery) with electrophysiologists was 3.5%, and the major complication rate (meaning serious medical events, ranging from cardiac arrest and cardiac-valve injury to death) was 1.3%. This is notably better than the complication rates when the devices are implanted by other types of doctors, such as non-electrophysiologist cardiologists, thoracic surgeons or other specialists, which average 5.8% (any complication) and 2.5% (major complication).

Another advantage—the electrophysiologists were more likely to also use cardiac resynchronization therapy (CRT-D) in heart failure patients who could benefit from this treatment. CRT-D uses a special pacemaker to synchronize the action of the left and right ventricles of the heart. Though the reasons for the difference in application rates of this therapy weren't explored in the study, it's likely that electrophysiologists are more up-to-date on the latest technology.

So what does this mean for you? If you're a candidate for a cardiac implant of any kind—whether it's a pacemaker, ICD or CRT-D—consider a board-certified electrophysiologist. There are about 1,000 in the US. To find the one nearest you, call the membership services hotline of the Heart Rhythm Society at 202-464-9855. When it's your heart, any edge you can get is worth the trouble.

Blood Type Can Affect Heart Bypass Surgery

Researchers examined data on more than 15,000 patients (ages 60 and older) who had undergone coronary artery bypass graft (CABG) surgery.

Result: Patients with AB blood type were 20% less likely to die in the eight years after surgery than those with type O, A or B.

Theory: People with AB blood have the highest levels of certain blood-clotting proteins and, as a result, receive fewer blood transfusions after surgery. Blood transfusions have been linked to higher risk for death.

Ian Welsby, MD, associate professor of anesthesiology, Duke University Medical Center, Durham, North Carolina.

Considering Heart Surgery? Do This First

Erik Hulzebos, PT, MSc, PhD, clinical exercise physiologist and physical therapist at the University Children's Hospital and Medical Center Utrecht in Utrecht, the Netherlands, and lead author of a review on preoperative respiratory physical therapy published by *The Cochrane Library*.

It's scary to think about having your chest cut open and your heart operated on. But someday you may find yourself in that situation, given that cardiac surgery is among the most common surgical procedures in the world. In the event that your doctor recommends elective heart surgery, of course you'd want to do whatever you could to ensure an easy recovery.

Well, now there is an important step you can take before elective heart surgery to speed your recovery afterward, a recent study reveals. The key is respiratory physical therapy, which helps prepare your lungs to withstand the stress of surgery.

Why worry about your lungs when it's your heart that is going under the knife? Potentially life-threatening pulmonary complications, such as pneumonia and collapsed lungs, are estimated to occur after at least 20% of cardiac surgeries. This may be due to the effects of anesthesia on lung gases, use of cardiopulmonary bypass (heart-lung machine), chest incisions, diaphragm problems, etc.

Respiratory physical therapy is routinely recommended after cardiac surgery—but researchers wanted to know whether it would confer additional benefits if also provided before surgery. So they reviewed data from eight studies involving a total of 856 adults who were awaiting elective cardiac surgery, such as valve replacement or coronary artery surgery.

Each study included a control group that got no preoperative respiratory therapy...plus a treatment group that, prior to surgery, received regular sessions of respiratory therapy of at least one type. Therapy techniques included incentive spirometry (with lips sealed around the mouthpiece of a handheld device, you try to keep a little ball afloat within the contraption by taking long, deep inhalations)...specially designed breathing and coughing exercises...and aerobic exercise training.

Encouraging findings: Compared with patients in the control groups, those in the presurgical respiratory therapy groups were only about half as likely to develop postsurgical pneumonia or to suffer a collapsed lung... and their average hospital stay after surgery was reduced by more than three days.

What explains the results? Researchers suggested that it was the improved strength and endurance of the respiratory muscles due to the breathing exercises. Because this study focused exclusively on cardiac surgery, it's unclear whether patients anticipating other types of chest or upper abdominal surgery also might benefit from preoperative respiratory therapy—but it makes sense that they would. More research is needed to confirm that.

Pre-op pulmonary prep: If you are anticipating heart surgery, talk to your doctor about presurgical respiratory physical therapy. Improving your lung health now could be your key to a faster, easier recovery.

Breakthrough Treatment for Heart Valve Problems

Michael Chu, MD, assistant professor in the division of cardiac surgery at University of Western Ontario and associate researcher at Lawson Health Research Institute, both in London, Ontario. He is the lead author of a recent review on transcatheter heart valve replacement published in *Canadian Medical Association Journal.*

Here is potentially life-saving news for people with severe aortic stenosis, a narrowing or obstruction of the heart's aortic valve (which connects the left ventricle of the heart to the body's main artery). Many patients who have been told that they are too old or too sick to risk traditional valve-replacement surgery—despite having a poor prognosis without it—are able to get that much-needed new valve with a safer, less invasive procedure called *transcatheter heart valve-replacement surgery.*

To learn more about this breakthrough, we called University of Western Ontario cardiac surgeon Michael Chu, MD, one of the pioneers of this technique. But before we convey the details on the procedure—let's cover some basics.

The heart has four valves. Each valve has flaplike doors called leaflets that open and close in a coordinated rhythm with every heartbeat. When the aortic valve develops stenosis—for instance, from a buildup of calcium deposits—it stiffens and narrows and its leaflets do not open far enough. Less blood is pumped through with each heartbeat, so the heart must work harder to pump normal amounts of blood. Over time, the heart muscle compensates by getting thicker—and eventually the heart begins to fail.

Early on, people with aortic stenosis may have no symptoms. But as the disease progresses, they experience shortness of breath, muscle weakness, chest pressure or pain, dizziness and/or loss of consciousness. Aortic stenosis can lead to congestive heart failure and, in some cases, to sudden cardiac death. Dietary and lifestyle changes, such as eating less salt and getting more aerobic exercise, may help manage some symptoms of aortic stenosis—but they cannot cure it. There are no medications to treat severe aortic stenosis.

When symptoms are severe and cardiac function declines, surgery is needed—and therein lies the problem for many patients. Dr. Chu said that conventional aortic valve replacement is routinely performed in younger, low-risk patients with excellent results. However, for patients over age 75 or those with other health problems (such as a history of stroke, lung disease or kidney disease), conventional surgery can be very risky. Yet without a replacement valve, only about half of such patients survive for more than a year. The procedure offers hope for high-risk patients who otherwise would not be candidates for surgery. *By way of comparison…*

•**Conventional valve-replacement surgery is open-heart surgery done under general anesthesia.** The breastbone is cut open—the patient is put on a heart-lung bypass machine—and the heart is stopped while the new valve is put in place. The patient typically spends seven days in the hospital. Recovery takes about three months.

•**Transcatheter heart valve-replacement surgery also is done under general anesthesia or under a lighter form called sedation.** The surgeon makes a small incision in the groin, then threads a catheter through the femoral artery and up to the heart. A balloon is fed through the catheter and then inflated to widen the constricted valve area. The new valve is pushed up the catheter and into the heart, then implanted within the old valve. The breastbone is not cut, and no heart-lung bypass is needed—because all the while, the heart keeps beating and supplying oxygenated blood to the body. The procedure typically requires a three-to-four-day hospital stay and a one-to-two-week recovery period.

With conventional valve surgery in these high-risk patients, stroke rates as high as 20% have been reported—and 10% to 15% of patients die within 30 days of the procedure,

Epilepsy Drug Protects Heart

An enzyme present in blood vessels dissolves blood clots.

Recent finding: Compounds in some epilepsy and cancer medications increase levels of these enzymes and could prevent heart attack–producing clots.

University of Gothenburg.

Dr. Chu said. By comparison, in a study of patients ineligible for the conventional surgery (average age in the early 80s) who instead had transcatheter surgery, only about 4% had a stroke—and 5% to 10% died within 30 days of the procedure. Long-term results for transcatheter surgery are not yet known, but early data is promising, Dr. Chu said.

More than 10,000 transcatheter heart valve replacements have been done worldwide.

Infection Protection for Cardiac Implant Patients

Bruce Wilkoff, MD, director of Cardiac Pacing and Tachyarrhythmia Devices at the Cleveland Clinic and a professor of medicine at Cleveland Clinic Lerner College of Medicine at Case Western Reserve University in Ohio. He is also the president of the Heart Rhythm Society. *www.HRSonline.org*

There's a good chance that you know (and love) someone who has a pacemaker. Or you have one yourself. No doubt, it's a life-saving device, but you'll want to pay attention to recent research on cardiac implantable electronic devices (CIEDs), such as pacemakers and cardioverter defibrillators. What we have learned has alarmed us. You should know about a potentially deadly problem that is becoming increasingly common—CIED-related infection.

Between 1993 and 2008, the number of CIEDs in use doubled while the number of infections associated with the devices more than tripled, reaching 2.41%, according to a recent study in the *Journal of the American College of Cardiology*. Sadly, 18% of patients with CIED infections do not survive for a year. For those who live, treatment can be economically devastating, with an average cost of more than $146,000.

Bruce Wilkoff, MD, director of Cardiac Pacing and Tachyarrhythmia Devices at the Cleveland Clinic, discussed protection strategies.

He explained that most CIED-related infections are caused by staphylococcus aureus or staphylococcus epidermidis bacteria. Infection can get started if, at the time of surgery, bacteria contaminate the surface of the device, the patient's skin or the area in the chest beneath the skin where the surgeon creates a "pocket" to hold the CIED. The surgeon's scrupulous attention to proper sterile techniques can greatly reduce but not completely eliminate this risk. Sometimes an infection develops soon after surgery, but in other cases it becomes apparent only after a year or more has passed.

We asked Dr. Wilkoff whether staph also can get into the pocket long after the surgery—for instance, by migrating from some other infected site in the body. He said, "It is possible but very uncommon, particularly for these staph bacteria. But about 10% of the time, other bacteria are involved…and 1% to 2% of patients could have the infection occur through another mechanism."

Compared with the infection risk after an initial implantation, the risk is four to six times greater when a patient has another surgery to replace a device (for instance, because its battery is depleted, a component has stopped working or the patient requires a device with additional features).

Reason: Reopening the pocket where the device was placed may allow a colony of bacteria that the body had previously "walled off" to overwhelm the immune system's defenses, Dr. Wilkoff explained. Since a CIED typically lasts about four to eight years, a patient is quite likely to need such repeat surgery.

Warning signs: There is no one symptom that appears in all cases of infection, Dr. Wilkoff said. *But see your doctor quickly if any of the following occur…*

- **You run a fever of 101° or higher.**
- **There is swelling, redness or pain** at the site where the device was implanted.
- **The skin covering the device becomes dimpled or oozes.**
- **The device appears to be shifting position.**
- **Be especially vigilant about watching for such signs if you have diabetes or compromised kidney function.** Either of these conditions can increase your susceptibility to CIED-related infection.

If you do get a CIED infection: Both the device and all of its leads (wires that deliver energy from the CIED to the heart muscle) need to be removed and replaced.

Reason: Staph bacteria can bind to a sticky substance called fibronectin that circulates in the blood and clings to the surface of implanted devices. Once this biofilm of persistent bacterial bugs takes hold, it is very antibiotic-resistant and almost impossible to get rid of without removing the device.

Radiation Risk

There is a high radiation risk from post–heart attack cardiac imaging, warns Louise Pilote, MD. Cancer risk rises with cumulative exposure to radiation from catheterization, angioplasty and nuclear scans—and some of these tests may not be necessary.

Self-defense: Ask your doctor which tests you really need.

Louise Pilote, MD, PhD, MPH, professor of medicine—James McGill Chair and director, division of general internal medicine, McGill University, Montreal. She led an analysis of data on 82,861 people, published in *Canadian Medical Association Journal*.

Before and after the surgery, for a period that can range from several days to several weeks, you receive antibiotics through an IV. You may be given a temporary pacemaker or an external defibrillator during this time. When the infection is gone, your doctor will schedule another surgery to implant a new CIED, often before you go home.

To reduce your risk for a subsequent infection: It is best to use an experienced cardiologist who does a high volume of device implantation and device change procedures. Dr. Wilkoff suggested asking the doctor and/or hospital whether they report the number of CIED procedures they do on a Web site or in a booklet—the larger the number, the better the outcomes tend to be. Also, he noted that women sometimes ask to have the CIED implanted underneath a muscle so that it's less visible. But since this makes it more difficult to remove if an infection does develop, it's important to discuss the pros and cons with your doctor before opting for such placement. And, of course, follow your doctor's advice on minimizing CIED infection risk after surgery.

People Who Have Had a Heart Attack Should Avoid Certain Common Painkillers

Nonsteroidal anti-inflammatory drugs (NSAIDs), such as *celocoxib* (Celebrex) and *ibuprofen* (Advil, Motrin), can increase the risk for another heart attack or dying from coronary artery disease. The elevated risk persists for at least five years.

Self-defense: *Naproxen* (Aleve) has the lowest cardiovascular risk of any NSAID. (Aspirin was not studied.) Or talk to your doctor about alternative painkillers.

Anne-Marie Schjerning Olsen, MD, research fellow at Gentofte Hospital, University of Copenhagen, Denmark, and lead author of a study published in *Circulation.*

Anticlotting Drug Extends Lives

Heart attack patients live longer with a new anticlotting drug. Patients hospitalized for heart attack or severe angina who were given the drug *Xarelto* (rivaroxaban) for an average of 13 months, along with standard anticlotting medicines, were 34% less likely to die from a heart-related problem during that time. Xarelto has not yet been approved to prevent recurring heart attacks and strokes—but the FDA currently allows its use to prevent blood clots and strokes in people with abnormal heart rhythms.

C. Michael Gibson, MD, interventional cardiologist and chief of clinical research, division of cardiology, Beth Israel Deaconess Medical Center, Harvard Medical School, Boston. He led a study of 15,526 people, published online in *The New England Journal of Medicine.*

Heart Attack and Insomnia

Roger Godbout, PhD, professor, department of psychiatry, University of Montreal, Montreal, Quebec, Canada.

As though people who have survived a heart attack don't have enough to worry about, they often find themselves experiencing relentless insomnia. Sleep is key to healing, and a lack of it can substantially slow recovery—all the more reason for anxiousness and stress. Until now, there's been no scientific explanation for the onset of insomnia, although mental stress has been under suspicion as the primary cause.

So here's a surprise—it isn't just stress that keeps heart attack survivors awake at night. Canadian scientists believe that they have found a genuine physiological basis for the sleeplessness. As it turns out, they say, the physical damage of a serious heart attack extends beyond the cardiovascular system all the way to the brain stem where important aspects of sleep are controlled.

The Heart-Brain Connection

In earlier research at the University of Montreal, Roger Godbout, PhD, and his colleagues had performed a series of studies with rats, demonstrating that heart attacks affect the limbic system—the part of the brain that controls your mood—which explains why so many people experience depression after acute myocardial infarction. "Since depression is frequently accompanied by insomnia, we wanted to verify whether the neurons in the brain stem were also affected," Dr. Godbout explained.

Dr. Godbout's theory proved to be right. In his latest study (also done with rats and reported in a recent issue of *Sleep*), he demonstrated that within a few hours of a serious heart attack, the study subjects lost neurons in the brain stem, and within two weeks, it was taking them twice as long to get to sleep. The disturbing effect on their sleep didn't end there. When they finally did fall asleep, it took them a shorter time than before to reach the restful state of deep dream sleep—but this stage, which is when memories are believed to be consolidated, was considerably shortened.

"Thanks to this study, we have been able to show that sleep disturbance following an acute heart attack is not a psychological phenomenon. In fact, there is a clear physiological explanation that the death of cells play a key role in difficulty with sleep," says Dr. Godbout.

Poor quality of sleep is a known risk factor for people with cardiovascular disease. Since insomnia can increase the chances of relapse after heart attack, the risk for complications rises—and a vicious cycle can easily be set in motion.

While there is no specific sleep therapy for those who have lost sleep neurons, Dr. Godbout says, this recent study illustrates the importance of "rapid intervention" in the days following a heart attack, before the first signs of insomnia and depression are even apparent...and before recurring patterns have a chance to set in. You can do much of this intervention yourself. For some, it will mean consulting with your doctor about sleeping medication, and for others, it will simply mean what doctors call good "sleep hygiene"...

• **Fix a regular bedtime and wake-up hour.**

• **Avoid alcohol, caffeine and spicy foods** for four to six hours before retiring.

• **Get regular exercise (but no evening workouts).** Be sure to check with your doctor, as you may need to pass stress tests, blood pressure tests, etc., to be sure that your heart is strong enough to start exercising.

• **In your bedroom, block out light and noise**...make sure the temperature is comfortable (it's worth the higher heating/cooling bills!)...and use bed only for sleep and sex—no TV watching or computer use, because these activities tend to be stimulating and because the temptation to check one more channel or click on just one more Web site is too great.

If you feel that you need a buffer in between your waking activities and lights out,

Aspirin and Heart Surgery

Taking aspirin before heart surgery saves lives. Cardiac patients on aspirin therapy who continued taking aspirin—instead of stopping one week before surgery, as many doctors recommend—had a significantly lower risk for death in the month after surgery than patients who stopped taking aspirin. The aspirin users had a lower risk for kidney failure and major postsurgical cardiac problems, and they spent less time in intensive care.

Jian-Zhong Sun, MD, associate professor of anesthesiology at Thomas Jefferson University Hospital, Philadelphia, and leader of a study of cardiac patients published in Annals of Surgery.

establish a calm and relaxing presleep ritual that works for you, such as taking a warm bath, reading a relaxing book, praying or listening to soothing music. You can still have sweet dreams!

Sedative Use After a Heart Attack Suggests Trouble Ahead

People who take antianxiety or sleep medications after a first heart attack are 25% more likely to have another attack over the next year than patients who do not use sedatives.

Possible reason: Anxiety and sleep deprivation are associated with elevated levels of hormones that are linked to increased cardiovascular risk.

To help cut risk: Follow a heart-healthy diet…and exercise regularly.

Gunnar H. Gislason, MD, PhD, senior consultant scientist and senior research scientist at Gentofte University Hospital, Hellerup, Denmark. He is lead author of a study presented at a recent American Heart Association scientific session.

New Tools to Repair Arteries

Ross Milner, MD, associate professor, Stritch School of Medicine, Maywood, Illinois, chief of vascular surgery and endovascular therapy, Loyola University Hospital, Chicago.

There's yet another deadly medical condition that involves your heart—it's called abdominal aortic aneurysm (AAA), which in simple terms is a weak spot in the main blood vessel that carries blood from the heart to the rest of the body. In the last 40 years or so, this kind of problem has become potentially much more controllable, thanks to sophisticated imaging technology. With ultrasound in particular, doctors can now identify and monitor this killer of 15,000 Americans annually—so that when an AAA grows to the point of being dangerous (typically, larger than five centimeters in diameter), it can be repaired. Improved monitoring and developments make treating an AAA much less difficult and risky.

Taking Some of the Pressure Off

A little background: The aorta is the master artery, conducting blood from the heart to vessels leading to the rest of the body. Occasionally an area of the vessel's wall weakens and begins to bulge—and this is what's known as an aneurysm. People most at risk are men older than age 60, anyone who smokes (or used to) and people with a history of atherosclerosis. Age plays a role, with about 8% of people over age 65 being affected by AAAs. Four times as many men as women have AAAs. And when the condition runs in families, especially if there's been a female relative with an AAA, the risk is higher.

For decades, the only solution to the problem had been dramatic and dangerous surgery. The late 1990s brought a new option—a procedure using a catheter to place a stent inside the aorta (similar to a surgeon using an angioplasty stent to unblock an artery). But one significant problem remained—the surgeon had only one chance to position the stent as accurately as possible, something that can be very difficult to achieve when the AAA is in certain locations.

Now we have more recent news—a second generation of aortic stents that allow for easy repositioning once or even several times during the procedure until the doctor finds the absolute sweet spot for aneurysm repair.

Second-Generation Stent Success

We spoke with Ross Milner, MD, chief of vascular surgery and endovascular therapy at Loyola University Hospital in Chicago, who is among the first surgeons to use these second-generation stents. Dr. Milner explained that most AAAs are near the arteries leading to the kidneys from the aorta. Stents are quite large, and if doctors place them too close to the renal arteries, they can do damage by interfering with blood supply to the kidney(s), putting the patient at risk for kidney failure. "The new stent gives us the ability to be particular about how we place it, knowing that if it isn't exactly where we want it we can easily fix it," said Dr. Milner.

Another Breakthrough Coming

On the horizon is yet another positive step in aneurysm control. Today patients must have periodic monitoring postprocedure with CT scans to be sure that the stent is working properly. The problem, of course, is that CT scans involve high doses of radiation and contrast dyes that can hurt the kidneys. A much easier approach is via a tiny sensor placed in the artery but outside the stent. The sensor measures blood pressure within the aneurysm. By putting an antenna over the patient's abdomen, doctors can activate the device for a pressure measurement that then goes to a computer for a readout. If pressure is normal, they know that all is well with the stent. This device enables doctors to ascertain success of stent procedures both during the procedure and for follow-up. The team at Loyola has a clinical trial under way to gain FDA approval for long-term patient monitoring, something, Dr. Milner says will likely take several years.

Abdominal aortic aneurysms have had haunting mortality figures in the past. At least 50% of patients do not survive to make it to the hospital if an AAA ruptures. It used to be that half of the remaining 50% did not make it out of the hospital after surgery—now, about 80% of those who have the surgery survive. Thanks to the techniques available today, the condition is much more treatable, and patients can look forward to long, full lives.

To Heal Your Heart, Work Out Harder

Trine Tegdan Moholdt, PhD, physiotherapist, postdoctoral fellow, K.G. Jebsen Center of Exercise in Medicine, Department of Circulation and Medical Imaging, and Department of Public Health and General Practice, Norwegian University of Science and Technology, Trondheim, Norway.

When it comes to post–heart attack care, extended bed rest is a thing of the past, and today we know it's by far in your best interest to get up and move around again as soon as possible. Yet, it's still quite surprising to see a recent study suggesting that intense exercise may be the best way to recover, as an increasing number of physicians say that a stepped up workout regimen is just what your heart needs.

Latest Research

In a randomized, controlled trial at the Norwegian University of Science and Technology, 107 heart attack patients began to work out just two to 12 weeks after a myocardial infarction. Investigators, including postdoctoral fellow Trine Moholdt, PhD, physiotherapist, randomly assigned the participants to a 12-week program on one of two different exercise regimens—twice weekly conventional cardiac rehabilitation or more intense interval training on the treadmill. *Dr. Moholdt explained the two approaches...*

• **Conventional cardiac rehab.** The conventional rehab group performed aerobic workouts for about 60 minutes per session at moderate intensity under the guidance of a physical therapist. Their heart rates rose to 70% to 80% of the maximum.

• **Aerobic interval training.** A second group started with a 10-minute warm-up followed by 28 minutes on the treadmill jogging or walking uphill. Workouts included four-minute high-intensity intervals at 85% to 95% of maximum heart rate (to the point where participants couldn't say more than a few words while carrying on a conversation, but not to the point where they had chest or leg pain), interspersed with three-minute recoveries and capped off with a final cool down. Both groups were also encouraged to do an additional workout of the same type and intensity at home.

Greater Intensity = Greater Oxygen Uptake

At the end of the 12-week period, Dr. Moholdt and her team found that more intense aerobic interval training was better at raising participants' peak oxygen uptake—the capacity of the body to transport and use oxygen during exercise, which is a key indicator of cardiorespiratory endurance and physical fitness. Specifically, they discovered that…

In people who exercised at moderate intensity, VO2peak (peak oxygen uptake) increased from 32.2 at baseline to 34.7 mL/kg per minute, demonstrating that any exercise is better than none. But in the high-intensity interval group, VO2peak rose more significantly—from 31.6 mL/kg per minute to 36.2.

Over time, once the workout program was completed and the patients were no longer exercising at the same levels, VO2peak declined in both groups—but less so in the high-intensity group, which appeared to retain some health benefits. Thirty months after completing the program, VO2peak dropped to baseline in the aerobic interval trainees, but significantly below baseline in the conventional cardiac rehab group.

At 30 months, only 4% of the high-intensity group reported being physically inactive, in comparison with 20% of the conventional group. Although the reason for this is unclear, it could be that those who had performed at high intensity under medical supervision were more confident about continuing to work out vigorously on their own. (This might also account for their higher VO2peak at 30 months.)

Dr. Moholdt and her colleagues presented these results at an annual congress of the European Society of Cardiology in Stockholm, Sweden.

Safety First

Of course, not all physicians yet agree about the merits of high-intensity exercise post-heart attack, and Dr. Moholdt acknowledges that further research is necessary—noting, however, that in her experience, it is well-tolerated and emphasizing that strict measures need to be put in place to ensure patient safety. In her program, doctors first check all patients' heart function with electrocardiograms during maximum-effort exercise, and patients wear heart rate monitors throughout aerobic sessions. Trained staff members are on hand to operate emergency equipment as needed in exercise labs—which are located within hospitals.

If you have suffered a heart attack, Dr. Moholdt warns that the single most dangerous thing you can do afterward is remain sedentary. Consult your cardiologist, and together you can design the exercise program that is safest and most effective for you.

MRI No Longer Off-Limits to Millions

Saman Nazarian, MD, assistant professor of medicine, and director, ventricular arrhythmia ablation service, The Johns Hopkins Hospital, Baltimore.

Everyone wants a really careful doctor, of course, but now it looks like physicians can afford to relax a bit when it comes to magnetic resonance imaging (MRI) for the approximately two million heart patients in the US with implanted defibrillators (used to prevent sudden cardiac death) and/or pacemakers (used to regulate heart rhythms). Though MRI is often the favored imaging technology for many conditions, from torn ligaments to finding cancer, it has been considered off-limits—at least until now—for patients with these devices because MRI's powerful magnets might cause the devices to malfunction. A recent large study from Johns Hopkins University School of Medicine in Baltimore, published in the *Annals of Internal Medicine*, has demonstrated that there is, in fact, a safe way to use MRI for these patients.

Why Was It So Dangerous?

The fear regarding MRI in people with these medical devices was that the magnetic field might heat up the devices...move them... make them unable to detect the abnormal rhythms that they are supposed to correct... or cause them to mistake MRI activity for heart activity. Heating of the device components may lead to tissue damage in the heart. Additionally, failure to treat an arrhythmia or an inappropriate delivery of therapy (such as if the device were to administer a shock when the patient didn't actually need one) can be uncomfortable and/or life-threatening. As a result, doctors have had to rely on other types of imaging, including CT scans (which use radiation) or ultrasound, even when MRI would have been the optimal imaging choice.

A Safer Option

The study: 555 MRI examinations (scans of the brain, spine, heart, pelvis, abdomen or an extremity) were performed on 438 individuals (men and women, mean age 66) who needed MRI and had either an implanted pacemaker manufactured after 1998 or an implanted defibrillator manufactured after 2000—because those are the years when such devices were changed to have fewer ferromagnetic materials (fewer metal objects that could be affected by the MRI's electromagnetism). Before the MRI exam began, each patient's device was programmed out of "default mode" and into a safer mode, one that either lowered the devices' sensitivity to the magnets or shut them down temporarily during the hour-long exam. To ensure that these patients weren't at risk for a cardiac event during the MRI, a nurse with experience in device programming who was trained in cardiac life support carefully monitored each patient's heart rhythm, blood pressure and oxygen saturation during the exam, and an electrophysiologist (a cardiologist specially trained in the treatment of people with heart rhythm problems) was available in case any patients needed other treatments.

The vast majority of these imaging scans went off without a hitch, with patients experiencing no problems whatsoever. One patient with a defibrillator experienced a temporary "pulling sensation" in the chest, so his MRI was discontinued. And in three patients with pacemakers, the devices' settings reverted to something called "power on reset," which effectively turned off the doctors' programming and put "default mode" back on. Experiencing "power on reset" is serious and warranted close expert monitoring during the exam, but it's not a permanent problem. None of those patients experienced serious problems throughout a long-term follow-up period (a median time of 214 days after the MRI).

What Patients Need to Know

We spoke with Saman Nazarian, MD, an electrophysiologist and assistant professor of medicine at the university, who said that this research demonstrates that it is safe for certain patients with implanted pacemakers and/or defibrillators to have MRI if the safety protocol outlined in this study is followed, meaning a nurse and an electrophysiologist with the appropriate training must be present during the MRI and the device must be programmed appropriately.

Important: Unfortunately, not all imaging centers have the resources or expertise to provide this, so if you have one of these devices and your doctor wants you to have an MRI instead of another type of imaging test, be aware that you may need to travel to a large medical center that can meet the requirements.

Dr. Nazarian said that about 1.8 million of the two million people in the US with cardiac devices have devices similar to those that were studied, so most people could have them reprogrammed using the safety proto-col developed at Johns Hopkins. More than 100 models from the top three manufacturers of pacemakers and defibrillators were tested, but not every single model was tested—so you should still check with your doctor to make sure that you're eligible for MRI. For example, if you have a disconnected lead from a pacemaker that has been removed from your chest, then you should not have an MRI.

What Heart Patients Must Know About PTSD

Donald Edmondson, PhD, MPH, assistant profes-sor of behavioral medicine in the Center for Behav-ioral Cardiovascular Health at Columbia University Medical Center in New York City and lead author of an article on coronary syndromes and PTSD pub-lished in *PLoS ONE*.

There's a recent study linking a histo-ry of heart problems to the develop-ment of the anxiety disorder called post-traumatic stress disorder (PTSD). Al-though people generally think of PTSD as mostly affecting combat veterans, disaster survivors and victims of violence or sexual assault, it turns out to be surprisingly com-mon in people who have had heart attacks. PTSD symptoms include insomnia, night-mares, irritability, anger, tension, emotional numbness, physiological hyperarousal (rac-ing heart, sweating) and/or flashbacks of the traumatic event.

For the new study, researchers combined the results of 24 studies from around the world involving a total of 2,383 patients. Each patient had experienced an acute coro-nary syndrome (ACS) event, such as a heart attack or unstable angina (chest pain due to poor blood flow to the heart muscle, which can lead to a heart attack), at least one month earlier. Researchers limited their analysis to studies that focused solely on PTSD that the patients themselves attributed to ACS, not

to PTSD due to any other type of traumatic event.

Worrisome findings: A startling 12% of ACS survivors developed clinically signifi-cant symptoms of PTSD…younger patients were particularly likely to be affected. What's more, compared with ACS patients who did not develop signs of PTSD, those who did develop the disorder were twice as likely to suffer a repeat coronary event and/or to die within the following one to three years. The possible reason, researchers said, is that PTSD can provoke an inflammatory response that further damages the heart.

Although the medical community has be-come more aware of the common risk for depression among heart patients, awareness of a similar link between heart attacks and PTSD has lagged.

Bottom line: If you or a loved one has had a heart attack or other acute coronary event, be on the lookout for warning signs of PTSD. Psychotherapy, medication and/or other treatments often can provide relief… but first, patients and their doctors must rec-ognize the problem.

For more help: See *http://bit.ly/NGwtoC* for an article on how transcendental medita-tion eases PTSD.

Heart Failure Patients: Pay Attention to Your Bones

Sumit Majumdar, MD, professor, division of gener-al internal medicine, University of Alberta, Canada.

Patients who have heart failure—mean-ing that their blood isn't being efficiently pumped through the body—apparently have something else to worry about in addi-tion to the fatigue, breathlessness and swollen legs and feet that characterize the condition. Canadian researchers recently learned that older adults with heart failure have a higher risk for osteoporotic bone fractures—breaks that may occur even without a major accident or hard fall. That's unnerving, so we spoke with study author Sumit Majumdar, MD, professor of general internal medicine at the University of Alberta, to find out what's going on.

A Bad Break for Heart Patients

This finding came from a preliminary study presented in 2011 at the annual meeting of the American Society for Bone and Mineral Research. Dr. Majumdar and his team examined patient records of more than 45,500 Canadian men and women, all 50 or older. Of this group, 1,841 had been diagnosed with heart failure in the prior two years. When they examined fracture rates after five years, researchers found that those with heart failure were 28% more likely to get fractures in the spine, hip, forearm or upper arm, compared with those who did not have heart failure.

What's the reason? Researchers aren't yet sure why there are so many more broken bones in people with heart failure, but Dr. Majumdar said it is likely a combination of these two factors…

• **To help control the swelling associated with heart failure,** about 4% of people in the US take "loop diuretic" drugs and about 60% of the heart failure patients in the study were taking them. Why the "loopy" name? The drugs work on a particular part of the kidney known as the "loop of Henle"—although they can actually make patients feel less steady on their feet and, well, loopy! They also reduce bone mineral density (BMD), and they've been shown in previous research to be associated with increased fracture risk (probably because they're diuretics, so they make you urinate more, which can cause deficiencies in calcium, potassium and magnesium). So these drugs such as *furosemide* (Lasix), *bumetanide* (Bumex), and *torsemide* (Demadex) and *ethacrynic acid* (Edecrin)—might be a major reason for the fractures.

• **Heart failure itself causes bone to thin, though at present it's not known why.** And that makes bones more likely to break—even without major impact. For example, a spine fracture can occur from simply rolling over in bed, said Dr. Majumdar.

Broken Bones: More Serious Than You Think

Broken bones are problematic at any age, but they're particularly dangerous for older adults. For instance, about 24% of patients age 65 and older die within a year of hip fracture. And Dr. Majumdar said that even a wrist fracture may land a barely coping elderly patient in a nursing home, since that sort of minor break leaves him/her unable to perform basic tasks and may require surgery. "And these problems are magnified in heart failure patients, because they're especially frail—it doesn't take much to launch a downward spiral," he said.

Bone Up on the Basics

One factor we mentioned earlier—bone mineral density (BMD)—is something to keep an eye on. Dr. Majumdar said it's a good idea to take a BMD test because a low BMD measurement is a known risk factor for fracture in patients with or without heart failure. "The BMD test is kind of like a mammogram—it's not a perfect test, but it helps get patients into the doctor's office to figure out whether there might be a problem," he said. Other signs that you might have brittle bones? Dr. Majumdar said that red flags include any fracture after age 40 or a loss in height of two inches or more.

If you're currently taking a loop diuretic to treat your heart failure (especially if you're prone to fractures and/or have a low BMD measurement), you may want to talk to your doctor to see if there are any alternative treatments that you could try instead.

Another tip: Since a patient with heart failure tends to undergo many chest x-rays to keep tabs on his/her condition, a patient can ask his/her doctor to use these x-rays to look for spine fractures, because it's common to have these types of fractures without realizing it, said Dr. Majumdar.

If nothing else, a patient with heart failure should take the same steps that a patient with osteoporosis would take, said Dr. Majumdar. Got milk? Hope so. Through diet, supplements and/or getting a small daily dose of sunlight, make sure that you're getting enough calcium (1,500 mg daily) and vitamin D (800 IU to 1,000 IU daily), and doing regular weight-bearing exercises (like walking, running, dancing or strength training) to build strong bones, said Dr. Majumdar.

CANCER

If you think breast cancer is the most dangerous cancer for women, you're in good company...but you're wrong. Eighty-three percent of women surveyed believe breast cancer has the highest fatality rates. The reality is that even though breast cancer is the most common cancer among women, lung cancer has the highest rate of death.

Lung cancer claims nearly 40% of the women who get it, while breast cancer claims fewer than 25%. From new screening tests for former smokers, to the breakthrough radiation therapy that rivals surgery for treatment, you'll discover the latest research for helping you avoid or survive lung cancer.

If you don pink in October, or have ever walked or donated to breast cancer research, give yourself a pat on the back. Your hard work is paying off, because fatalities from breast cancer have been on the decline for more than two decades.* But our work is not over. Breast cancer is still the most common cancer in women, making screening, detection and treatment as important as ever.

More important than any statistics, is knowing how to win the war against all cancers.

*http://www.cancer.org/cancer/breastcancer/detailedguide/breast-cancer-key-statistics

Chapter 7

WHAT WOMEN NEED TO KNOW ABOUT LUNG CANCER

Lung Cancer Breakthroughs: Prevention and Detection

Men worry about prostate cancer …women worry about breast cancer…everybody worries about colon cancer, skin cancer and brain cancer. But there's another cancer that claims more Americans' lives than those five other types combined. It's lung cancer, the number-one cancer killer in the country, responsible for more than 157,000 deaths each year.

The good news: Recent advances in prevention and detection are helping in the battle against this fearsome disease. For instance, there's a new screening tool that can cut the odds of dying from lung cancer by 20%. Is it right for you or for someone you love? For answers to that question and more, we turned to Peter Bach, MD, an epidemiologist and lung cancer specialist at Memorial Sloan-Kettering Cancer Center in New York City.

Overdue Prevention Tactic

Not all cases of lung cancer are caused by cigarette smoking, but up to 90% are. The percentage of Americans who smoke has declined significantly over the past few decades, from 42% in 1965 to 19% in 2011…but it's still way too high.

Public education campaigns and high cigarette taxes do help reduce smoking, but now the FDA is exploring another tactic—regulating or even banning menthol cigarettes. The reason? Because menthol may make it easier to become addicted to smoking and harder to quit.

Why it has taken the FDA so long to consider regulating menthol is a mystery. Back in 2009, when the FDA banned the candy, clove and fruit flavorings that made cigarettes more palatable to young smokers, it also called for an investigation on the impact of mentholated cigarettes on public health. Two years later, the FDA's advisory committee concluded that it is "biologically plausible" that adding menthol to cigarettes makes them more addictive, and that removing menthol from cigarettes would improve public health.

Menthol's allure: The addition of menthol is a trick used by tobacco companies—in

Peter Bach, MD, epidemiologist and lung cancer specialist, Memorial Sloan-Kettering Cancer Center, New York City. He has done extensive research and development on lung cancer prediction models and has authored numerous articles on lung cancer for medical journals.

fact, the flavoring is added to all cigarettes, not just those marketed as menthol. Menthol-flavored cigarettes have about 10 times more added menthol than regular cigarettes, but even at the lower levels, the menthol helps mask the harshness of tobacco and the irritation associated with nicotine. Without the added menthol, the harshness and irritation could be turnoffs for new smokers—making them less likely to stick with the dangerous habit.

Menthol works by stimulating the cold receptors on nerve endings in the mouth, nose and skin, creating a cooling sensation. When menthol is added at higher levels, the cooling sensation also is felt in the lungs. At the same time, menthol contains substances that enhance nicotine's "bite," a sensation that smokers seem to crave, further reinforcing smoking behavior.

The FDA is considering banning menthol because it lures smokers and keeps them, but other studies suggest that menthol also makes cigarettes more harmful. Smokers of menthol cigarettes have more than twice the risk for stroke as smokers of regular cigarettes. People who smoke menthol cigarettes also show decreased elasticity and increased stiffness of the carotid arteries (the main arteries feeding the brain) compared with smokers of regular cigarettes. In addition, menthol's cooling action slows respiration, increasing breath-holding time and, in turn, leading to greater exposure to the cigarette's toxins. What's more, the cilia (tiny hairlike structures in the airway that move things along) slow down when exposed to menthol, impairing clearance of toxins from the airway.

Our opinion: It's way past time for menthol to be banned from cigarettes.

Lifesaving Screening: For Whom?

Lung cancer has one of the lowest five-year survival rates of all cancers mainly because it usually is diagnosed too late to be cured. About 90% of people who get lung cancer die because of it.

Recently, the US Preventive Services Task Force, an independent panel of experts in prevention and evidence-based medicine, sought to update its previous determination against routine lung cancer screening for smokers. The task force reviewed relevant studies, relying most heavily on the National Lung Screening Trial (NLST).

The NLST included more than 53,000 smokers who were randomly assigned to undergo three annual exams with either chest x-rays or low-dose CT scans.

Findings: In each of the three rounds of screening, CT exams found more cancers than x-rays. In the first round alone, CT scans identified 270 people with lung cancer, compared with 136 in the x-ray group. CT screening reduced lung cancer deaths by 20%.

Based on these findings, a task force recommendation now in draft form advises annual CT screening for people at high risk—those between the ages of 55 and 79 who have a smoking history of at least 30 pack-years. (A pack-year is an average of one pack per day for one year. So, for example, if you smoked two packs each day for 15 years, you have a 30-pack-year history.) The recommendation applies even to ex-smokers who have quit smoking within the past 15 years. (The NLST did not look at ex-smokers who quit more than 15 years ago.)

If you fall in to the high-risk category, should you go get a CT scan? Probably—but there are several factors to consider first, Dr. Bach said, because the benefits to you may not be quite as great as the NLST findings suggest. The NLST was conducted at 33 academic medical centers around the country, all with expertise in diagnosing and managing lung cancer—whereas the same high-quality results may not be found outside of a top-notch academic community. Also, Dr. Bach believes that the task force's estimate of 20,000 lives saved every year from annual CT screening is overly optimistic. He explained that his institution's analysis of the data, using different statistical methods, estimates about 4,000 lives saved each year.

Why does it matter whether the true benefits are somewhat less than the NLST suggests? Because CT scans are not without risk. Although low-dose CT exposes you to much less radiation than a standard chest CT, it's still much higher than the exposure you'd get from a regular chest x-ray. CT scans also may result in false-positive findings or incidental findings (abnormalities that don't cause harm), both of which can lead to unnecessary invasive testing and anxiety.

Bottom line: If you clearly fall into the high-risk category (age 55 to 79 with a smoking history of at least 30 pack-years and less than 15 years since you quit), you should be aware of the screening option and seriously consider the trade-offs of benefits versus risks. "The most aggressive we should be is to suggest that such patients discuss screening with a doctor who is disinterested—meaning someone who is not the owner of a CT scanner or radiology center," Dr. Bach said.

Lower-risk people should not be offered screening, in his opinion. "Outside of the high-risk group, the potential danger of radiation vastly exceeds the possible benefits of screening. That's even more true for women than for men because the radiation also can contribute to breast cancer risk."

Gender Equality?

Speaking of women, let's consider the issue of gender as it relates to lung cancer risk. Lung cancer used to be considered primarily a man's disease. But several years ago, the pendulum swung in the opposite direction when some studies suggested that female smokers were more susceptible to the harms of cigarettes than male smokers…and that women who had never smoked were more likely to get lung cancer than men who had never smoked.

However, those theories did not hold up in more rigorous studies. Most experts agree, Dr. Bach said, that lung cancer is neither predominantly a man's disease nor a woman's disease. Women and men have the same risk of developing lung cancer and dying from

it…and it is the leading cause of cancer death for both men and women in the US.

Help For Smokers and Ex-Smokers

If you smoke or used to smoke, visit these three important Web sites…

• **The CDC's Tips from Former Smokers public service campaign** has been instrumental in convincing more than 100,000 smokers to drop their smoking habit.

• **Calculate your pack-years**—an important number when considering whether CT screening is appropriate for you.

• **Memorial Sloan-Kettering Cancer Center,** one of the nation's top cancer hospitals, has developed its own online tool that can help you decide whether you should be screened. The criteria used are slightly different than those developed by the task force—so it will be helpful to discuss the guidelines with your own doctor.

New Personalized, Precision Approach to Lung Cancer Treatment

Peter Bach, MD, epidemiologist and lung cancer specialist, Memorial Sloan-Kettering Cancer Center, New York City. He has done extensive research and development on lung cancer prediction models and has authored numerous articles on lung cancer for medical journals.

Prasad Adusumilli, MD, thoracic surgeon and researcher, Memorial Sloan-Kettering Cancer Center, New York City. He has researched and published extensively on lung cancer topics, including the personalization of lung cancer surgical resection procedures.

Although the odds of surviving lung cancer admittedly still aren't great, these days a lung cancer diagnosis is not an automatic death sentence—even in the case of late-stage cancer. We have many more options for treating the disease than we did just a decade ago…and treatment today is more personalized and precise than ever.

For instance, doctors now can look at the individual characteristics of a tumor, including particular cell patterns and genetic mutations. This information helps them to set treatment plans that are more likely to work—and to avoid recommending treatments with low chances of success. In fact, Peter Bach, MD, an epidemiologist and pulmonologist at Memorial Sloan-Kettering Cancer Center in New York City, explained that he is "extremely enthusiastic" about the progress that's been made over the past decade.

The problem: Despite the remarkable advances, not all hospitals have the needed tools in their arsenals…and not all doctors understand which patients will benefit from such a personalized approach. That's why it's important to be in-the-know about the newest ways to beat lung cancer—in case you end up battling the country's number-one cancer killer.

Secrets Found in Cell Patterns

The term lung cancer actually is misleading because the disease is not just one entity. Rather, there are two major types of lung cancer, each with different risk factors, probable prognoses and treatments. And then even within one of those types, different tumors can have different characteristics that affect how aggressive the cancer may be and which treatment may work.

The majority of lung cancers fall in to the non–small cell category. Adenocarcinoma is the most common non–small cell cancer, accounting for about half of all lung cancers. It's the type found most often in current and former smokers—and also in people who never smoked.

When adenocarcinoma is detected before it has had a chance to spread, it's treated surgically. Most of the time, the surgeon performs a lobectomy by removing the entire lobe that has the cancer in it (a pair of lungs has five lobes, three on the right side and two on the left). In some cases, the surgeon does a limited resection, removing just part of the affected lobe.

Tricky: The decision about which procedure to do can be a tough one, according to Prasad Adusumilli, MD, a thoracic surgeon and scientist at Memorial Sloan-Kettering Cancer Center. That's because the surgeon wants to remove enough lung tissue to prevent a cancer recurrence, but at the same time leave enough tissue to preserve lung function. Until now, there hasn't been an evidence-based system to guide surgeons, so the size and location of the tumor (for example, how far the tumor is from the edge of the lung) often have been used as criteria in deciding how much to remove.

Breakthrough: Surgeons at Memorial Sloan-Kettering perform about 1,000 of these operations each year. With all the data they have accumulated over the years, Dr. Adusumilli and his research team have developed an algorithm to help surgeons decide which operation is best for patients with adenocarcinoma.

The research that led to the new algorithm was complicated, but basically the researchers performed microscopic examinations of many hundreds of samples of early-stage adenocarcinoma, classifying each according to the proportion of the five major cell patterns (acinar, papillary, lepidic, micropapillary and solid) seen in the tumor. Then they analyzed the follow-up data to determine the chances of cancer recurrence based on the cell pattern and the type of surgery that was done.

Do You Know the Symptoms for Lung Cancer?

Only 13% of people surveyed know that lung cancer symptoms include a cough that won't go away…persistent pain in the back, chest and/or shoulders…shortness of breath…unexplained wheezing…and coughing up blood.

Regina Vidaver, PhD, executive director, National Lung Cancer Partnership, Madison, Wisconsin, which surveyed 1,000 people. *www.NationalLungCancerPartnership.org*

Overall, the five-year incidence of cancer recurrence was 21% for patients who had a limited resection and 15% for patients who had a lobectomy. When the specific cell patterns were analyzed, though, it became clear that tumors with a higher percentage of cells showing a micropapillary pattern had a much higher risk for recurrence within the same lobe if patients underwent limited resection.

Bottom line: Doctors can now use this knowledge about cell patterns to opt for the tissue-sparing limited resection procedure in patients whose tumors do not have the aggressive micropapillary pattern...and save the more extensive lobectomy for patients whose cell pattern indicates a high risk for recurrence.

Only a limited number of hospitals have the expertise needed to determine a lung tumor's cell pattern right on the spot, in the operating room, at the time of the actual surgery. "This requires expert pathological experience and a large volume of tumors for the pathologists to get experienced," Dr. Adusumilli explained. At hospitals that do not currently have this ability, some patients who get a limited resection may end up needing another operation later if their cancer subsequently is found to have the micropapillary pattern...or, worse, they may have a cancer recurrence.

Hopefully, that will change soon. Dr. Adusumilli and his team of researchers are now trying to develop tools that can more easily determine the cell's pattern—preferably before surgery—sparing patients the need to go under the knife a second time.

Secrets Found in Genetic Mutations

When lung cancer is diagnosed after it has spread to the lymph nodes or beyond, as it is most of the time, treatment involves more than just surgery—it also requires medication. Now, in what Dr. Bach refers to as a "very exciting" development, the particular medications that will work best often can be determined based on specific genetic mutations in the tumors.

How it started: About 10 years ago, during clinical trials for two new lung cancer drugs, doctors observed that some people receiving the drugs *gefitinib* (Iressa) and *erlotinib* (Tarceva) had a much better response than others—even though all the patients had advanced adenocarcinoma. This led to the discovery that the patients who responded well had tumors that showed a specific mutation in the epidermal growth factor receptor (EGFR) gene. People with the mutation survived nearly twice as long on the drug regimen as those without it. It turns out that the mutation is present in about 20% of people diagnosed with advanced adenocarcinoma.

A few years later, researchers discovered another mutation on the anaplastic lymphoma kinase (ALK) gene, which is present in 7% of people with adenocarcinoma. A drug that inhibits ALK activity, called *crizotinib* (Xalkori), is very effective in people who have that particular mutation.

All three of these drugs have been approved, and the required genetic testing is available. Many experts now recommend that all patients with advanced adenocarcinoma have their tumors analyzed for mutations of EGFR and ALK—including patients who have mixed cancer types, even with just a small component of adenocarcinoma. Referring to molecular testing in its entirety, not just for EGFR and ALK, Dr. Bach said, "Now, 60% to 70% of adenocarcinomas have important molecular information that affects therapeutic choices. That's huge! Lung cancer might be the poster child for this kind of precision, personalized medicine."

If you are diagnosed with lung cancer: If at all possible, see an oncologist at a hospital associated with a university, Dr. Bach advised. Academic medical centers usually have the technology and expertise to take advantage of these new tests and procedures. If you live too far away to see a doctor there regularly, consider having a consultation with an appropriate expert at such a facility—that person can advise you and your doctor on the best treatment for you.

Nonsmokers' Risk for Lung Cancer

Charles M. Rudin, MD, PhD, associate director for clinical research at the Sydney Kimmel Comprehensive Cancer Center at Johns Hopkins, Baltimore.

It seems somehow unfair when a person who has never smoked gets lung cancer —and unfortunately, it happens more often than you might guess. Here in the US, 10% to 15% of lung cancer cases (translating to about 20,000 cases per year) fall into this category. The notoriety of this disease was raised when the actress Dana Reeve (widow of Christopher Reeve) died from it in 2006. At the time, people were surprised to hear that this could happen.

So where does that put us in terms of risk? And what can be done to avoid this horrible disease? A special report on this cancer in a recent issue of the journal *Clinical Cancer Research*, authored by scientists at Johns Hopkins University, said that the biology, diagnosis and treatment (everything, in other words) of lung cancer can be very different in never-smokers, defined as people who smoked fewer than 100 cigarettes in their lifetimes. When we contacted the study author, Charles M. Rudin, MD, PhD, associate director for clinical research at Johns Hopkins Kimmel Cancer Center, he said that this type of cancer is often completely unrelated to smoking.

Who's In Danger?

The most important avoidable risk factor is exposure to secondhand smoke, but there are several other known causes of "nonsmoker lung cancer" as well. These include radon gas leaking into homes from naturally occurring uranium in soil...exposure to asbestos...emissions from indoor wood-burning stoves...and cooking oil that gets aerosolized and breathed in when we cook. Dr. Rudin said that there is also evidence that genetics makes some people more vulnerable, noting that mutations increasing risk are now being

identified. But he also said that in many cases of nonsmoker lung cancer, it's not really evident precisely what caused the disease.

Never-Smokers Have a Better Prognosis

A problem with lung cancer overall is that there are no early markers, so it's often quite advanced before it is diagnosed. "There's nothing for lung cancer like the PSA for prostate cancer or the Pap smear for cervical cancer," Dr. Rudin explained, "so there is no method of early detection that has an impact on mortality." This is particularly problematic for nonsmokers, he noted—when they seek help for the cough and chest discomfort that are typical symptoms of lung cancer, doctors are more apt to think that there is a benign cause, such as a respiratory infection, than to look for a malignancy. Whereas a heavy smoker might be sent for diagnostic tests immediately, this would rarely be the case with a patient with no smoking history.

Nonetheless, the never-smoker with lung cancer usually has a better prognosis than the smoker. A key reason is that, aside from the lung cancer, these patients are typically healthier than smokers, who often have other issues, such as cardiac problems, that impede treatment.

Some patients who are found to have particular genetic alterations can benefit from targeted drug therapies that offer significantly higher response rates, Dr. Rudin said. "Some of the newer anticancer drugs are designed to specifically inhibit some of the alterations that we think are important in causing lung cancer," he explained. Otherwise, traditional chemotherapy, radiation and/or surgery are the usual treatments for lung cancer in people who never smoked.

If You're Worried...

Everyone should be aware of risk factors for nonsmoking lung cancer, says Dr. Rudin. He suggests avoiding known causes, particularly exposure to cigarette smoke, asbestos (still found in many building products in older homes) and radon (test your home's levels). While some experts think that it would be good to broadly screen people with respiratory problems via CT scan, there are obvious concerns about radiation exposure from such scans themselves.

Meanwhile, if you are a never-smoker with a persistent cough, especially one accompanied by blood, shortness of breath, weight loss or chest pain, be aware that these symptoms might suggest lung cancer—voice your concerns to your doctor and be sure that you get the testing you need to either confirm or rule out such a diagnosis. And, if you have been diagnosed with lung cancer and have never smoked, Dr. Rudin says, it is important to be sure that your oncologist has your tumor examined for genetic alterations. If any are found, you might be a candidate for one of the newer targeted therapies that offer more hope for a good outcome.

Which Non-Smokers Get Lung Cancer?

Michael J. Thun, MD, is vice president of epidemiology and surveillance research at the American Cancer Society.

Lung cancer tops the list both for new cancer diagnoses and cancer deaths here in the US. While smoking is to blame for the overwhelming majority of lung cancers, a significant proportion of lung cancer cases (10% to 15%) are caused by factors other than smoking. The death of lifelong non-smoker Dana Reeve (wife of actor Christopher Reeve) of lung cancer at the age of 44 in 2006 raised public awareness—and worry —that avoiding smoking may not fully protect non-smokers from lung cancer.

Though the media has paid a lot of attention to lung cancer in non-smokers, many questions remain unanswered and misinformation abounds about the disease, according to Michael J. Thun, MD, at the American Cancer Society. He and a team of researchers

set out to learn what they could by combining data on the incidence and mortality rates of almost two million self-reported "never-smokers" with lung cancer, from studies based in North America, Europe and Asia over a 70-year period.

The study measured how frequently lung cancer occurs in or kills lifelong non-smokers —it did not examine why. As such, the analysis did not examine second-hand smoke and other known risk factors of lung cancer, such as radon, asbestos and indoor air pollution. While it is "well established that second-hand smoke increases the risk for lung cancer, we were unable to evaluate it and other risk factors because this data was not available in many of the cohorts (groups) that were studied," explained Dr. Thun.

The Findings

Here's what they learned…

1. Overall incidence of lung cancer among lifelong non-smokers is rare (fewer than 40,000 cases per year), similar to the incidence rate for brain cancer and other nervous system cancers.

2. The risk that a never-smoker will die from lung cancer before age 85 is slightly higher for men (1.1%) than women (0.8%), but quite small for both genders.

3. Overall, incidence and death rates for lung cancer among non-smokers have remained stable over the time period studied.

The findings contradict two long-held assumptions—that non-smoking women have a higher risk of dying from the disease than non-smoking men, and that lung cancer among non-smokers has been increasing over the decades. The study was published in *PLoS Medicine*, a peer-reviewed journal published by the Public Library of Science.

What Else?

Non-smoking Asians living in Asia (not in the United States) and African Americans have higher rates of lung cancer and are more likely to die of the disease compared with non-smokers of European descent. The higher lung cancer risk among Asian women compared with Western women was seen to occur over a wide area that included China, Japan, the Philippines and Singapore. Dr. Thun speculates that one cause may be their tradition of cooking with open woks, which is known to produce carcinogens dispersed through fumes resulting from heating cooking oil at high temperatures.

Clearly there is a need for more information and research about non-smoking-related lung cancer. Dr. Thun acknowledges that this analysis represents an early step.

Cancer from Smoking Once in a While… Yes, it Can Happen!

Stephen S. Hecht, PhD, professor of cancer prevention, Masonic Cancer Center, University of Minnesota, Minneapolis.

Do you know at least a few people who are quite proud of the fact that they smoke only occasionally? A few cigarettes at a party and then no more smoking for weeks—not bad! The idea, of course, is that the occasional cigarette or two will not inflict smoking's terrible toll on a person's health. But, sorry to say, we have bad news for them and, for that matter, anyone who lights up, however often. A study from the Masonic Cancer Center and department of pharmacology at the University of Minnesota discovered that smoking even one cigarette starts to damage the smoker's DNA within minutes…and the news gets worse. The result of this particular damage is a heightened risk for lung cancer.

The Path of Destruction

This study investigated polycyclic aromatic hydrocarbons (PAHs), which are one among the many constituents of cigarette smoke known to cause cancer. (*Note*: We're also exposed to PAHs in our environment from incompletely burned fossil fuels—it's in vehicle exhaust, coal, agricultural burning, grilled meat, etc.)

How the research worked: Using a special device to measure the substance as it passed into circulation, researchers took blood samples to track the PAH in question (called phenanthrene) as it made its way through the bodies of 12 volunteer smokers. They found that within 15 to 30 minutes after the volunteers had smoked a cigarette, the phenanthrene taken into the body had transformed into a form that attacks DNA. That the transformation occurred this quickly surprised even the researchers—in the paper, they noted it was the same rate they would have expected from injecting the PAH directly into a smoker's bloodstream.

"Definitely" Dangerous

We spoke with Stephen S. Hecht, PhD, professor of cancer prevention, the lead author of the study, who said that the damage PAHs cause include cell mutations, loss of tumor-suppressor gene activity and activation of oncogenes (genes that contribute to converting healthy cells into cancer). He also said that other studies have shown that PAHs are one of the most dangerous types of carcinogens—"near the top of the list" he said. When asked whether having a single cigarette, just one a month or so, could possibly be enough to trigger damage that could contribute to lung cancer, he was adamant. "Definitely," he said.

While it's true that occasional smokers do not consume as much poison from smoking as regular smokers do, it is clear that for the sake of their health, giving up whatever pleasure they get from now-and-then smoking is well worth the effort. And, since smoking is so highly addictive, even occasional smoking also increases the chances that what is now an infrequent indulgence will become a steady habit. The message is clear—abstinence is the only way to go.

Study Links Knee Pain to Lung Cancer

Maria Suarez-Almazor, MD, PhD, a rheumatologist at M.D. Anderson Cancer Center in Houston.

It's a common worry—a strange, inexplicable symptom turns out to be the first sign of an undiagnosed cancer. Such tales are understandably frightening—after all, who doesn't suffer arbitrary aches and pains, especially as we age? While these shouldn't be reason to live in fear, a recent Italian study uncovered a connection between certain unusual symptoms and cancer. Fortunately this is a rare occurrence, but nonetheless, important to be aware of.

Lung Cancer and Knee Pain

In the study, rheumatologists reviewed the records of 296 patients who came to a medical center with a painful knee. In five of these patients—all of whom were middle-aged men with a history of heavy smoking—x-rays showed suspicious growths in their lungs. These men had a type of cancer called non-small-cell lung cancer, which surgeons removed…in all five cases, the knee pain went away after their lung cancer was successfully treated. These results led the authors to suggest that after doctors rule out more common causes for arthritis in a painful knee, a chest x-ray is a good idea—especially in people who have smoked heavily.

To learn more, we called Maria Suarez-Almazor, MD, PhD, a rheumatologist at M.D. Anderson Cancer Center in Houston. She has an interest in what's known as "paraneoplastic syndromes" in illness, where seemingly unrelated problems are caused by your body's attempt to heal itself from other diseases. It turns out that sometimes a malignant tumor produces substances that damage tissues in your body, while at other times such symptoms can be the result of your immune system's effort to fight the tumor, which inadvertently harms healthy tissues.

This study is intriguing, she said, while also pointing out that only a tiny percentage of the patients with knee pain actually had cancer. Nonetheless, she agreed that if doctors can't find any reason for pain in one knee, such as an orthopedic cause, it might be reasonable to suspect a paraneoplastic syndrome. More research is necessary, since this is the first study to suggest an association between knee arthritis and lung cancer.

Dr. Suarez-Almazor said that there are other well-known and more common paraneoplastic syndromes that may lead a doctor to test for cancer more quickly. *She listed some examples…*

• **Lung cancer is commonly associated with a problem called hypertrophic osteoarthropathy,** which as cancer progresses can involve pain in many joints and is marked by clubbing of the fingers, with fingertips growing round and bulbous.

• **An early symptom of acute lymphoblastic leukemia in children is joint pain**—particularly in a knee, along with anemia. Arthritis can also be observed in acute myeloid leukemia in adults.

• **Muscle weakness along with a specific type of rash around the eyes is a sign of a condition called dermatomyositis,** which can be associated with a variety of cancers including lung, ovarian, stomach, colorectal and non-Hodgkin's lymphoma.

It's rare that mysterious pain turns out to be caused by cancer—but people who have joint or other pain or rashes of unknown origin should see their doctor. Chances are the problem will be something else entirely or you'll get a clean bill of health and whatever it is will resolve naturally. In any case, you'll likely feel better after ruling out the worst-case scenario.

LAM: The Slowest-Moving Cancer on Earth

Francis X. McCormack, MD, professor and director of the division of pulmonary, critical care and sleep medicine at the University of Cincinnati College of Medicine. A leading LAM researcher, he also is scientific director of The LAM Foundation.

It's as easy as breathing. That expression describes just how much we take our ability to inhale and exhale for granted. Yet breathing is anything but easy for a person who suffers from *lymphangioleiomyomatosis* (LAM). This progressive and potentially fatal lung disease affects women almost exclusively. It typically develops between the ages of 25 and 50 but can appear later. Though long considered very rare, experts now suspect that LAM is more common than generally believed and is often misdiagnosed as asthma, bronchitis or chronic obstructive pulmonary disease.

We spoke with Francis X. McCormack, MD, a pulmonologist at the University of Cincinnati College of Medicine and scientific director of The LAM Foundation.

His good news: The past decade has brought promising advances that offer new hope to patients.

LAM results from an abnormal growth of smooth muscle cells that develop elsewhere in the body and travel to the lungs, destroying normal lung tissue and causing numerous cysts to form. Gradually the lungs become so damaged that oxygen delivery throughout the body is seriously compromised. No one knows what causes LAM, but because it primarily develops in women of childbearing age, estrogen is thought to play a role. Genetics also may influence risk. Though LAM is not traditionally considered a type of cancer, Dr. McCormack said, "Those of us who think about LAM every day have no doubts. It's the slowest-moving cancer on Earth—but it is cancer."

Warning signs: The main symptom is shortness of breath. At first, this occurs mainly upon exertion…but as LAM progresses, even normal daily activities leave patients breathless. Although LAM patients often are misdiagnosed with asthma, the patterns of the diseases are different. "With asthma, you have good days and bad days. But with LAM, there isn't much day-to-day difference—instead, tolerance for physical exertion drops from year to year," Dr. McCormack explained. Other LAM symptoms include chest pain… frequent coughing…wheezing…and fatigue.

Any unexplained, chronic shortness of breath warrants a visit to the doctor and, quite likely, follow-up with a lung specialist. A high-resolution CT scan (unlike a chest x-ray) is sensitive enough to pick up the lung changes and cysts typical of LAM. To help with the diagnosis, a patient also may get a blood test called VEGF-D and/or a lung biopsy. In addition, the patient is checked for common LAM complications, such as accumulation of fluid in the chest…collapsed lung…and/or benign kidney tumors.

Treatment: Though LAM has no known cure, there are ways to improve quality of life. A healthy lifestyle—low-fat diet, tobacco avoidance, exercise appropriate to one's abilities—can help minimize symptoms. Some patients benefit from bronchodilators, medicines that relax muscles around the airways, improving airflow. Given estrogen's possible involvement, LAM patients generally are advised against birth control pills and estrogen therapy. Since pregnancy hormones might worsen LAM, patients who want to get pregnant should discuss the risks with their doctors.

As LAM progresses, patients may need to use an oxygen tank when exercising or full time. Ultimately, a lung transplant often offers the best hope for improved quality of life and longevity. According to The LAM Foundation, there is no evidence that LAM patients benefit from cancer treatments such as radiation or chemotherapy. However, "targeted" cancer drugs—which act specifically on abnormal biochemical pathways in cancer cells—present a promising area of research.

Recent breakthrough: The drug *rapamycin* (Sirolimus), used primarily to prevent rejection after an organ transplant, shows great promise. In a study led by Dr. McCormack, LAM patients who took Sirolimus daily for one year showed significant improvement in lung function, whereas placebo users lost lung function during the study. "The possibility that you could take this drug for life and prevent progression of LAM is intriguing. However, there is concern about cumulative toxicity, so we need more research," said Dr. McCormack. Possible side effects of Sirolimus include mouth ulcers, acne, increased cholesterol, lung injury and susceptibility to infection. Clinical trials are being planned… meanwhile, the drug can be prescribed off-label for LAM patients.

The vast majority of LAM patients live for more than a decade after symptoms first appear and a number live for more than three decades, The LAM Foundation reports. For more information, visit *www.TheLamFound ation.org*…for a list of medical centers that have LAM experts, click on "Patients" and "USLAM Clinics."

Better Lung Cancer Diagnosis

R esearchers studied more than 170 patients who had been told they did not have lung cancer following CT-guided fine-needle aspiration of suspicious nodules in the lungs.

Finding: After an average of 4.5 months following the test, 18 of the patients were diagnosed with cancer—results of the needle biopsy turned out to be false-negative.

Explanation: The patients most likely to have false-negative results had nodules that were large, making malignant cells more difficult to distinguish from inflamed surrounding tissue.

If you've had a benign fine-needle lung biopsy: Continue to have CT scans for at least two years to monitor any further lesion growth.

Brian Gelbman, MD, assistant professor of medicine, Weill Cornell Medical College, New York City.

Lifesaving Screening for Ex-Smokers

Christine D. Berg, MD, chief of the Early Detection Research Group in the Division of Cancer Prevention at the National Cancer Institute in Bethesda, Maryland, and project officer for the National Lung Screening Trial.

M aybe you started as a teen, lighting up to be cool—then got hooked. Hopefully, you put cigarettes aside years ago or are working hard to kick the habit now. But if you have a history of smoking (or if someone you love does), you'll want to know about a painless screening test that significantly reduces the odds of dying from lung cancer. It's a type of computed tomography (CT) scan called a low-dose helical CT (aka spiral CT) of the chest.

Background: The deadliest malignancy, lung cancer claims more lives than breast, ovarian, colon and prostate cancers combined. Lung cancer causes no symptoms in its earliest and most curable stages, and by the time people develop telltale signs (chest pain, wheezing, coughing up blood), it's usually too late. The five-year survival rate for all lung cancer patients is less than 16%…and previous attempts to develop an early-detection test failed to reduce the death rate.

Encouraging: The recent National Lung Screening Trial (NLST) involved 53,454 symptom-free former or current heavy smokers ages 55 to 74. Participants underwent three annual screenings using either standard chest X-ray (which produces a single image in which anatomic structures of the chest overlie each other)…or helical CT (in which a CT scanner rotates around the person for seven to 15 seconds, producing multiple detailed images). Participants were followed for an average of 6.5 years from the first screening, during which time 442 people in the X-ray group and 354 in the CT group died of lung cancer.

Translation: Low-dose helical CT screening reduced lung cancer death risk by 20%.

Explanation: A screening test does not reduce a person's odds of getting lung cancer, of course. What a helical CT can do is find lung abnormalities when they are still so small that they can be completely removed surgically, said Christine D. Berg, MD, chief of the Early Detection Research Group in the Division of Cancer Prevention at the National Cancer Institute and NLST project officer.

Risks: Though the radiation exposure from a low-dose helical CT is significantly less than from a regular diagnostic chest CT, it is about 30 times higher than from a single-view chest x-ray. Another concern is the high rate of false-positive results (37% with helical CT versus 14% with x-ray), which can lead to unnecessary testing and anxiety.

Who should consider testing? Dr. Berg stated that screening with low-dose helical CT is reasonable for anyone between ages 55 and 74 who meets the NLST entry criterion of at least 30 "pack-years." (To calculate your pack-years, multiply the average number of packs smoked per day by the number of years you smoked.) Research is being done to determine whether the test's benefits outweigh its potential harms for younger individuals and/or those with less of a smoking history, such as 20 pack-years. The test is not appropriate for people with a history of light smoking or no smoking, even if they have a family history of lung cancer.

Low-dose helical CT scans of the chest are available at most imaging facilities that provide CTs. Cost ranges from about from $350 to $1,000, depending on location. At present, insurance generally does not cover helical CT lung cancer screening—though Dr. Berg

stated that this may change within the next few years as the US Preventive Services Task Force weighs in based on the recent evidence of the test's benefits. (Editor's note: As of July 2013, the National Lung Cancer Partnership says insurers will be required to cover CT lung scans.)

New Radiation Therapy Rivals Surgery for Lung Cancer

According to a recent study, 875 adults (age 75 and older) with early-stage lung cancer had surgery…a noninvasive therapy known as stereotactic radiation…or no treatment.

Result: While long-term survival rates after surgery mirrored those after radiation, risk for death within 30 days was higher after surgery.

Implication: Surgery may not be optimal for older lung cancer patients, who are at higher risk for complications.

David Palma, MD, radiation oncologist, Ontario Institute for Cancer Research, Canada.

Pistachios vs. Lung Cancer…Ex-Smokers Take Note

Ladia M. Hernandez, PhD, RD, LD, senior research dietitian, department of epidemiology, University of Texas MD Anderson Cancer Center, Houston.

Nuts, nuts, nuts—researchers seem to find more healthful benefits almost every time they study them. Recent nut news involves one of the worst diagnoses anyone can get—lung cancer.

The recent study, from Texas Woman's University-Houston Center, found that eating pistachio nuts daily may help to reduce the

Genetic Trap for Smokers

Smokers who develop lung cancer show activity in a genetic pathway, PI3K, which doesn't occur in cancer-free smokers. In the future, it may be possible to identify at-risk patients and treat them with cancer-preventing drugs.

Boston University School of Medicine.

risk for lung cancer. The heroic nutrient is gamma-tocopherol, a form of vitamin E that has been shown to be protective against lung cancer and that epidemiologists believe may also lower the risk for other types of cancer, including prostate cancer. It is abundant in pistachio nuts.

In this particular study, researchers asked 36 healthy individuals—men and women—to consume their normal diets for two weeks. Then, for four weeks, 18 of the study participants added about 68 grams (about 2.4 ounces) of pistachios to their diets, while the other 18 participants continued eating normally. At the end of the study, individuals on the pistachio diet had indeed accumulated higher levels of gamma-tocopherol in their blood. Since it is an antioxidant that may protect cells from damage caused by free radicals, it's thought this may help prevent lung cancer from developing.

Pistachio Power

Pistachio nuts provide other important nutrients as well, including fiber, vitamin B-6, phosphorus, thiamine (vitamin B-1), iron, magnesium and potassium. And they can also benefit the cardiovascular system by improving lipid profiles, said study author Ladia Hernandez, PhD, RD, LD, a senior research dietician in the department of epidemiology at MD Anderson Cancer Center.

According to Dr. Hernandez, the one downside to eating pistachios (assuming that you aren't allergic to them) is that they have a high calorie content. But she notes that "the results of this study showed that consumption of 68 grams [roughly two small handfuls] per day of pistachios did not lead to significant weight gain." (*Note:* When the nuts were weighed, they were unshelled and roasted, and participants were given the choice of salted or unsalted pistachios.)

Of course, as nuts go, pistachios aren't cheap. But to many people, pistachios are

Herb May Fight Lung Cancer

A substance extracted from the herb milk thistle can help prevent the spread of lung cancer cells in mice. This finding may help scientists develop new treatments for lung cancer.

Molecular Carcinogenesis

very delicious—more so than other nuts—and they can be used in many healthful ways, raw or roasted...in salads, meatloaf and stuffing for chicken and other fowl...ground and used as a crust for fish...combined with fresh fruit in desserts. If you need a healthful snack idea, you might want to add pistachios to your shopping list.

Better Chemo for Lung Cancer Patients

According to a recent study, when 16 newly diagnosed lung cancer patients were given 2.2 g of fish oil a day for 10 weeks, they maintained their weight during chemotherapy, compared with a control group that did not take fish oil and lost an average of five pounds. Cancer patients often lose weight because chemotherapy reduces appetite and tumors lead to muscle wasting.

Theory: Fish oil may reduce the inflammation that causes the muscle degradation associated with weight loss.

Caution: Be sure to speak to your doctor—fish oil may have a significant blood-thinning effect in chemotherapy patients.

Rachel Murphy, PhD, researcher, University of Alberta, Edmonton, Canada.

Chapter 8

BREAST CANCER BREAKTHROUGHS

Get Through the Mammogram Maze

There has been so much controversy about mammography for detecting breast cancer—whether to have a mammogram at all and if so, what type to have and when—that I find a lot of patients are confused about what to do. I understand why they are confused. It is difficult to make sense of these recent studies. Many of you, like many of my patients, see a gynecologist annually for checkups and get advice about breast health from these specialists. But I have been keeping my eye on these studies—and I want to tell you about a more holistic approach.

Risk vs. Benefit

For a long time, the medical establishment believed that regular breast screening with mammography reduced the death rate from breast cancer by almost one-third in women over age 50 and caused them little harm. Then, in 2009, the US government came out with its controversial recommendation that women ages 40 to 49 with no family history of breast cancer and at average risk for the disease should not get routine annual mammogram screenings. Women ages 50 to 74 were advised to get screenings every two to three years...and women over age 74 were told that they do not need routine screening. In late 2011, the Canadian government basically echoed these recommendations.

Reasoning: Research seemed to point to the idea that the risks of testing outweighed the benefits.

One of the risks: Greater lifetime exposure to radiation. Another study, this one from England, published in *British Medical Journal* in 2011, identified a number of other harms associated with mammography, most notably negative effects on quality of life due to false-positive results...overdiagnosis of cancers that would never have caused symptoms and might have gone away on their own...and unnecessary surgeries, such as biopsies. These researchers determined that

Mark A. Stengler, NMD, naturopathic medical doctor and leading authority on the practice of alternative and integrated medicine. Dr. Stengler is author of the *Health Revelations* newsletter, author of *The Natural Physician's Healing Therapies* (Bottom Line Books), founder and medical director of the Stengler Center for Integrative Medicine in Encinitas, California, and adjunct associate clinical professor at the National College of Natural Medicine in Portland, Oregon. *http://markstengler.com/*

having regular mammograms over a 10-year period actually might result in more harm than good. The American Cancer Society (ACS) is one group that does not agree with the government's recommendations. The ACS maintains that all women should have annual mammograms after age 40. In addition, many studies support the idea of more frequent mammograms.

Timing Is Everything

While the benefits and frequency of mammography remain under debate, other researchers are taking a closer look at when mammography is performed during a woman's monthly cycle. A study by researchers at Group Health Research Institute in Seattle, reported in *Radiology*, found that in premenopausal women, mammograms appear to be more sensitive at detecting breast cancer when the screening is performed during the first week of the menstrual cycle (when you have your period). Premenopausal women often have dense breast tissue, which can make detection with mammogram difficult, resulting in a high number of false-positive results. With most women, breast tissue is less dense during the first week of the menstrual cycle. I recommend that premenopausal women who schedule a mammogram do so at that time. Since postmenopausal women don't have many hormonal changes, the timing of their mammograms is not as important.

Which Screening Is Best

Researchers from the University of North Carolina School of Medicine looked at the diagnostic accuracy of film and digital mammography, which are both a form of x-ray. Film mammography has long been the standard, but it is not as good at detecting cancer in women with dense breasts as digital mammography (an electronic image of the breast stored on a computer), which provides doctors with greater detail. Researchers found that digital mammography was more accurate than film in pre- and per-imenopausal women younger than age 50 with dense breasts. There was no difference between the two methods for women ages 50 to 65. For women over age 65 with fatty breasts, film was slightly more accurate because it gave a better view of problem areas.

In a study by Spanish researchers, published in *Radiology*, false-positive results were slightly higher for film mammography (7.6%) compared with digital mammography (5.7%). The researchers found no difference in cancer detection between the two types of mammography. Film mammography exposes women to slightly more radiation than digital mammography.

Other Tests

Other types of tests are sometimes recommended instead of, or to complement, mammography. Not all techniques are covered by insurance. *Basic techniques include…*

• **Digital breast tomosynthesis (DBT).** In 2011, the FDA approved a device that performs DBT, a form of 3-D imaging (mammography is 2-D). Studies show that DBT provides 7% better detection than other methods because it enables radiologists to pinpoint the location, size and shape of tumors more accurately than mammography can. The procedure does use more radiation than mammography—up to twice the amount. Currently available in numerous hospitals around the country, DBT is recommended by some doctors for young women with especially dense breasts.

• **Thermography.** This technique uses infrared technology to assess variations in body heat. Areas of abnormal heat are considered to be areas that may be cancerous. Like many holistic doctors, I recommend that all women use thermography annually to detect any changes in breast tissue. There is no radiation exposure at all.

• **Ultrasound.** This technique, which is commonly used in conjunction with mammography, uses sound waves to make a picture of breast tissue. It emits no radiation.

• **Magnetic resonance imaging (MRI).** This technique provides details of the breast's internal structure. It can help physicians identify abnormalities not picked up by other techniques. There is no radiation exposure at all.

My Advice

In addition to thermography for women with dense breasts, I often recommend ultrasound as a screening test. You can speak to your doctor about the screening test that will provide the clearest view of your breast tissue.

Women of any age who have a family or personal history of breast cancer or other cancer should talk with their doctors about the annual use of thermography, because it can detect early, slight changes in breast tissue. Then, based on your circumstances, you and your doctor can determine if you need a mammogram every one to three years. You and your doctor will also need to discuss the timing and type of mammogram that is best for you.

I offer all other women similar advice. Since there is no one-size-fits-all solution, you have to work with your doctor to make an informed decision about the best breast health care for you.

3D Mammography Finds More Breast Cancers

Diane LoRusso, MD, clinical assistant professor, Weill Cornell Medical College, New York City, and co-founder, Rye Radiology Associates, Rye Brook, New York. *www.RyeRadiology.com*

Breast tomosynthesis, commonly called 3D mammography, is a relatively new imaging technique that catches more breast cancers than regular 2D mammograms—while more accurately identifying harmless spots as benign.

Recent research reveals how well it works…

• **A recent study from Norway included 12,631 women who were screened with both 2D and 3D mammography.** When radiologists had access to both the 2D and 3D exams, they detected 40% more cases of invasive breast cancer (the type that has spread outside the milk duct or lobule and into the breast tissue itself) than when they saw only the 2D exams.

• **In a separate study from Massachusetts General Hospital,** the combination of 2D and 3D mammography reduced false-positive results (when a suspicious-looking abnormality is found but turns out to be benign) by 39%.

Diane LoRusso, MD, a clinical assistant professor at Weill Cornell Medical College who has practiced radiology for nearly four decades, calls 3D mammography a "remarkable breakthrough and a major improvement in our ability to detect breast cancer."

But: There are some downsides to the 3D test. Should you be asking your doctor for a 3D mammogram? *Here's the info you need to decide…*

The Benefits of 3D

A regular mammogram is a two-dimensional picture of a three-dimensional object that's been flattened out by those uncomfortable breast-squishing plates. Because the compressed breast tissue ends up overlapping itself, one feature can hide in the shadow of another, making it difficult to find tiny cancers hidden in the breast. (Imagine a bunch of letters of the alphabet being layered one on top of the other. They'd be hard to read, right? That's similar to what happens with a 2D mammogram image.)

For the 3D mammogram, the breast is still compressed between the plates—but the arm of the x-ray machine rotates in an arc above the breast, taking 15 separate images. Those are then processed on a computer to create a 3D image that the radiologist can manipulate to view 50 to 60 individual millimeter-thin "slices" of breast tissue. By eliminating overlapping structures, abnormalities are more easily seen. (Imagine that pile of alphabet letters being separated layer by layer. You could view each letter individually, so they would be easy to read.)

The 3D images help radiologists pin down the size, shape and precise location of abnormalities—details that tend to be obscured on 2D images. The improved visibility explains why 3D mammograms detect tumors that 2D mammograms miss…and why the new technology is less likely to yield those anxiety-producing false-positive results that lead to unnecessary (and expensive) extra testing.

The Downsides

Currently, 3D mammography is FDA-approved for use only in addition to regular mammography, not instead of it—so even if you opt for the 3D test, you'll still need regular 2D mammograms as well. One reason is that an important aspect of mammogram reading is to compare a patient's new images to her previous images to see whether anything has changed. Since those previous images were all 2D, for comparison's sake, you need a 2D version of your current images, too. Fortunately, both scans can be performed on the same mammography equipment in rapid succession. (In the future, the FDA may approve the use of 3D mammography alone and/or the technology may be available to produce 2D-like images from the 3D scans—but for now, the separate 2D test is required.)

Radiation is another concern. Though the 3D scan uses about the same amount of radiation as the 2D scan, combining the two doubles your radiation exposure. Still, the total radiation dose for the combined test is well below three milligray, which is the FDA limit for a single mammogram—and it's less than the radiation dose from the film (rather than digital) 2D mammograms of the past. As Dr. LoRusso pointed out, because 3D mammograms produce fewer false-positive results, your overall radiation dose may be lower in the long run since you're less likely to be called back for additional mammograms.

The amount of breast compression involved in 3D mammography is no different from that required for a 2D scan. However, to do both the 2D and 3D tests, you have to endure that breast squishing a bit longer—for about six to 12 seconds per breast, compared with the two to four seconds needed for just the 2D test alone. *The good news:* The design of the compression device on the 3D unit is more comfortable for most patients, Dr. LoRusso said.

Another downside is the expense. Insurance companies generally do not cover 3D mammography because they still consider it experimental. Hopefully, this will change in the not-to-distant future (and it certainly couldn't hurt to ask your insurance company to cover your 3D test). For now, though, you'll probably have to pay the extra cost yourself. Typically this ranges from about $50 to $100, depending on your location and your doctor—a small price to pay for improved cancer detection.

Making Your Choice

Dr. LoRusso recommends the 3D test for all her mammography patients because research shows that it benefits women with all breast types. However, it is particularly important for the 30% of women whose breasts are dense (meaning that they contain more glandular or connective tissue than fatty tissue). Mammogram x-rays do not see through dense tissue as easily as they see through fat tissue—cancerous tissue and dense areas both appear white on the mammogram, so identifying cancer is like trying to pick out a particular cloud in a cloud-filled sky.

Ask your local radiology center or hospital whether it provides 3D mammography…or use the manufacturer's locator service. Currently about 300 radiology centers in the US offer this test. To learn more about 3D mammography and see the machine in action, check out a video from Dr. LoRusso's Web site at *www.ryeyradiology.com/3d-digital-mammography/*.

Finally, Dr. LoRusso said, it is very important to realize that 3D mammography should not replace other breast tests that your doctor may recommend. For instance, if you have dense breasts or palpable masses, you also may need breast ultrasound screening…if you are at very high risk for breast cancer due to genetic factors, you also may need a breast MRI. In short, 3D mammography is an important new tool in the fight to detect breast cancer, but it is not the only tool.

The Breast Test Doctors Fight About

Nooshin K. Darvish, ND, is medical director and founder of Holistique Medical Center in Bellevue, Washington. *www.drdarvish.com*

Utter the word thermography in a roomful of breast specialists and you're likely to set sparks flying. Some doctors say that this imaging technique can detect breast cancer sooner and more safely than mammography—but others dismiss the test as unproven and even potentially dangerous because it sometimes is misused.

The FDA, for its part, approved thermography nearly three decades ago as an adjunctive tool to screen for breast cancer. But it recently warned women against using thermography as a substitute for mammography, saying it was "unaware of any valid scientific evidence showing that thermography, when used alone, is effective in screening for breast cancer."

We contacted integrative cancer therapy expert Nooshin K. Darvish, ND, a former Bastyr University faculty member and medical director of Holistique Medical Center in Bellevue, Washington, to discuss this controversial issue. She explained that thermography uses an infrared camera to detect variations in body heat. It is based on the idea that diseased tissues—including infected, inflamed, precancerous and cancerous areas—produce increases in metabolic activity, blood vessel formation and blood flow that, in turn, increase temperature. Thus, these areas appear as "hot spots" on infrared images. *Proponents say that the technique's benefits include…*

• **Early detection.** Thermography can spot areas of abnormal heat before they show up on conventional tests. "Whereas mammography, ultrasound, CT and MRI are used to identify cancer after the tumor has formed, thermography can identify the first thermal and chemical changes that may lead to cancer prior to the existence of a tumor," said Dr. Darvish. This may provide opportunities for early intervention to reverse the abnormality.

• **Effectiveness.** In a small study published in 2008 in *The American Journal of Surgery*, thermography accurately identified 58 out of 60 breast malignancies (as confirmed by biopsy) among 92 patients—an accuracy rate of 97%.

Comparison: According to the National Cancer Institute, screening mammograms miss up to 20% of breast cancers that are present at the time of screening. Inaccurate results occur more often among younger women and those with dense breasts.

• **Safety.** Unlike mammography, which uses X-rays, an infrared thermography camera emits no harmful radiation.

• **Comfort.** Thermography is noninvasive and does not require painful breast compression. However, you do have to spend time in a cold room.

The Controversy

All this sounds encouraging. So why would this test bring doctors nearly to blows? *Several reasons…*

• **Since the technology was first FDA-approved in 1982, there have been advances in infrared camera quality,** computer technology and standards for training thermographers, Dr. Darvish said. However, while some small studies (such as the one cited above) reflect these improvements, there is an admitted shortage of recent large-scale studies on thermography.

• **Many European doctors are clinically trained to use,** and do use, thermography as an adjunct to mammograms, Dr. Darvish said. But, in the US, medical doctors generally are not trained in or experienced with thermography and often dismiss its value.

• **Some conventional doctors complain that thermography has too high a rate of false-positive results.** Thermography proponents argue that many supposed false positives actually indicate precancerous conditions that won't show up on mammograms for years and should be "watched." What's more, mammography also is prone to false positives—a recent study in *Annals of Internal Medicine* concluded that 61% of women who get annual mammograms starting at age 40 are recalled for additional testing due to false-positive results by the time they reach age 50.

• **Some thermography clinics promote the test as a substitute for mammography.** This potentially dangerous misrepresentation leaves some doctors leery of thermography as a whole…and has prompted the FDA to issue warnings to clinics that violate its regulation classifying thermography as an adjunct rather than an alternative to mammography. Most thermographers, however, agree with the FDA that the technique is best used in addition to conventional tests.

Reasons: While thermography can identify general areas of abnormality, it cannot pinpoint an exact area of suspicion the way mammography and ultrasound can…"cold" tumors (ones with low metabolic activity) are difficult to identify on thermal images…and no screening test can actually diagnose breast cancer—for that, a biopsy is needed.

Who Can Benefit

According to Dr. Darvish, all women can benefit from thermography. *The test is thought to be particularly useful for those who…*

• **Are premenopausal.** Younger women generally have denser breasts, so mammograms are less accurate in detecting premenopausal breast cancers—yet these cancers are potentially the deadliest because they tend to grow fastest, Dr. Darvish said. She recommended that women get breast thermograms every two years from age 19 to 30 and yearly thereafter.

• **Have a family history of breast cancer and/or carry the BRCA gene.** Thermography provides an extra layer of precaution for such high-risk women. Dr. Darvish has several patients who've had negative mammograms but whose thermograms found abnormalities that turned out to be cancer.

• **Have breast traits that make mammography less accurate.** Mammograms are likelier to miss masses in breasts that are large, dense, fibrocystic or have implants.

• **Use hormone replacement therapy or birth control pills.** These medications may increase breast cancer risk. Thermography helps monitor the safety of hormone use, Dr. Darvish said.

• **Are undergoing breast cancer treatment.** A patient's response to therapy can be safely assessed with thermography.

A breast thermogram costs about $280, which most insurance policies do not cover.

For the most accurate test results: Use a physician-supervised facility whose images are read by a doctor certified by the International Academy of Clinical Thermology (*www.iact-org.org*) or the American Academy of Thermology(*www.americanacademyoftherm ology.org*).

Testing procedure: You remove your shirt and bra and sit in a cool room for about 15 minutes while your body adjusts to the ambient temperature. Then you hold your arms in varying positions while pictures of your breasts are taken from different angles, which takes five to 10 minutes. Images are sent to the interpreting doctor. If suspicious areas are identified, a follow-up appointment is made to discuss the best course of action.

Bottom line: If you decide in favor of breast thermography, remember that it is best used as a complementary screening tool along with mammography. According to Dr. Darvish, sensitivity for early detection of breast cancer increases to approximately 95% when thermography and mammography are used together.

Do You Need This Breast Test...Or Could It Do More Harm Than Good?

Rachel F. Brem, MD, professor of radiology and director of the Breast Imaging and Intervention Center at The George Washington University Medical Center in Washington, DC. She has published many articles on breast imaging in various journals and has won numerous awards, including the Editor's Recognition Award from *Journal of Women's Imaging.*

A recent study focusing on the breast cancer-screening test called breast-specific gamma imaging (BSGI) has raised some concern. According to a study published in the journal *Radiology,* the lifetime risk of dying from radiation-induced cancer associated with getting BSGI just one time is equal to the risk of getting mammograms every year from age 40 to 80. What's more, while mammography increases a woman's risk only for cancer of the breast, BSGI also increases her risk for cancer of the uterus, ovaries, intestines, colon, kidneys and bladder. With so many risks, why would anyone be getting this test?

We contacted radiologist Rachel F. Brem, MD, director of the Breast Imaging and Intervention Center at The George Washington University Medical Center, to ask if the potential dangers of BSGI overshadowed its benefits. "The answer is no," she said. "While BSGI should not be used for routine screening for everyone, it is a lifesaver for certain women—because it spots cancers that mammograms miss. For high-risk patients, the opportunity to detect early, curable breast cancer is so advantageous that it far outweighs the risks from BSGI."

While the risks certainly should not be ignored, the study statistics ought to be considered in context.

Consider this: Digital mammography carries an average lifetime risk of inducing 1.3 fatal breast cancers per 100,000 women who are age 40 at the time of exposure. The risk from one BSGI exam is about 20 to 30 times greater—about 30 per 100,000, or roughly 0.03%.

How BSGI works: A small amount of a radioactive compound called a radiotracer is injected into your arm and absorbed by your cells, which then give off radiation in the form of gamma rays. Due to their increased rate of metabolic activity, cancerous cells absorb more radiotracer than normal cells do. Breast images are taken with a special camera that detects the gamma rays. (The camera itself does not put out radiation.) When the images are displayed on a computer monitor, cancer cells appear as visible "hot spots." BSGI does not require breast compression. Typically four to eight images are taken during the 30-to-45-minute procedure.

Your doctor may recommend getting BSGI if you have…

• **An "equivocal mammogram"** (in which results are inconclusive and merit clarification). BSGI not only detects cancers that mammograms miss, it also is more accurate than mammography or MRI in ascertaining that a suspicious area is, in fact, free of cancer—and thus it reduces the number of unnecessary breast biopsies. This is significant because currently, in about 80% of breast biopsies, results are negative.

Women who have breasts that are dense (meaning that they contain more glandular or connective tissue than fatty tissue) especially benefit in this regard because they often have equivocal mammograms. Dr. Brem explained, "Cancerous tissue and dense areas both appear white on a mammogram, so identifying cancer is like trying to pick out a particular cloud in a cloud-filled sky. That's why mammography detects only about one-third of cancers in dense breasts. But BSGI accuracy is not affected by breast density—so that is a distinct advantage."

• **A recent breast cancer diagnosis.** In more than 10% of newly diagnosed patients, BSGI detects second, unsuspected areas of cancer—which, of course, impacts the treatment plan. BSGI also helps determine whether tumors are responding to chemotherapy, allowing doctors to customize treatment.

•**A strong family history of breast cancer**—meaning that multiple family members have had breast cancer, particularly if it was premenopausal or in both breasts…or if your father had breast cancer…or if genetic testing has revealed that you carry a breast cancer gene.

•**A history of Hodgkin disease for which you received radiation during adolescence**—because this treatment significantly increases the risk for breast cancer.

Good news: The amount of radiation used for BSGI is continually being reduced in an effort to find the lowest possible effective dose. "The dose we use today is much lower than the dose used just one year ago," Dr. Brem noted. So while the statistics cited in the *Radiology* study mentioned earlier should not be disregarded, the actual risks associated with getting BSGI today are significantly lower than when the study data was collected.

What to Expect with a Breast MRI

Rachel F. Brem, MD, professor of radiology and director of the Breast Imaging and Intervention Center at The George Washington University Medical Center in Washington, DC.

A breast MRI is a noninvasive test that uses a magnetic field, radio waves and a computer to produce detailed images that can reveal lesions not detectable with mammography or ultrasound. For the test, a nonradioactive contrast agent (dye) must be injected into the bloodstream. Since cancerous areas have more blood vessels, more dye goes to those areas, making the resulting MRI images clearer.

A breast MRI may be prescribed if you…

•**Are at high risk because of a family history of breast cancer** or because genetic testing revealed that you carry a breast cancer gene.

•**Have a mammogram with inconclusive results that merit clarification** (as was the case with my coworker).

•**Are undergoing chemotherapy for breast cancer,** since MRI can reveal whether the disease is responding to treatment.

•**Were recently diagnosed with breast cancer**—because MRI may be useful for presurgical planning. In one recent study from the University of Rome involving 164 breast cancer patients, MRI detected 51 additional suspicious lesions not seen on other tests… and changed the proposed treatment for 20% of patients. In a second study from the same researchers, presurgical MRI was associated with a reduced risk for cancer recurrence. According to radiologist Rachel F. Brem, MD, director of the Breast Imaging and Intervention Center at The George Washington University (GWU) Medical Center, all GWU patients with newly diagnosed breast cancer have an MRI or other imaging test, though this is not the standard at all breast centers.

Risks: The MRI scan itself poses no danger. Possible side effects of the contrast agent include headache, nausea, chest pain, skin rash and irregular heartbeat. Your doctor can help you weigh the test's benefits against these risks.

MRI may not be safe or appropriate if you…

•**Have an implanted device** (pacemaker, cerebral aneurysm clip, cochlear implant, plate, screw or rod) made of any metal other than titanium anywhere in your body. Because MRI uses a powerful magnet, a non-titanium metal device could shift position during the test.

•**Are pregnant or breast-feeding** (the contrast agent could be toxic to the baby).

•**Have kidney problems.** Since patients with kidney disease eliminate the contrast agent from their bodies more slowly, they are at increased risk for side effects, including a serious condition that involves thickening of the skin and organ damage.

Note: Before undergoing a breast MRI, women age 50-plus routinely have a blood test to check for kidney problems because decreased kidney function becomes more common with age.

•**Weigh 300 pounds or more**—you might have trouble fitting comfortably inside the MRI apparatus.

Where and When to Schedule Your MRI

Ask your doctor to refer you to an imaging facility that handles a large volume of breast MRIs, so the staff will have extensive experience with the test. GWU, for instance, does four to six breast MRIs daily, Dr. Brem said.

If you are having an MRI for screening purposes only and you are postmenopausal, simply schedule your MRI at your convenience. If you are premenopausal, the ideal time to have your MRI is between day seven and day 14 of your menstrual cycle (with day one being the first day of your period). Because this is when breasts are least affected by your natural hormones, the MRI results will be easiest to interpret. If you have an irregular cycle, just wait until you get your period and then schedule your MRI for day seven to 14.

Exception: If you have breast cancer or an inconclusive mammogram, do not wait for that day-seven-to-14 window—schedule your MRI immediately, Dr. Brem advised.

What Happens On the Day of the Test

You remove any metal you are wearing (jewelry, hairpins, eyeglasses), and an intravenous (IV) line is placed in your arm to deliver the contrast agent. You lie face-down on a padded table, face nestled into a donut-shaped pillow and breasts hanging freely into cushioned openings containing a signal receiver. (It is recommended that you settle yourself into the pads until you're really comfortable because you must remain motionless once the test begins.) Then you are slid into the MRI tube, which encircles your entire body.

Do you get claustrophobic? Tell your physician ahead of time so he or she can prescribe a calming medication if necessary. To relax inside the tube, focus on your breathing (but don't take deep belly breaths, since staying still is paramount) or imagine yourself in a pleasant place (a mountaintop, a beach). Many imaging centers provide headphones so patients can listen to music, which camouflages the MRI machine's knocking and buzzing noises. The technician can see you and speak to you, and if you need to get out, you can signal the technician by squeezing a handheld device. (Be sure to test the device before entering the MRI to make sure it works.)

After some initial images are taken, the dye is injected into your bloodstream via the IV. You may feel a spreading sensation of warmth and/or notice a metallic taste in your mouth. Expect to be in the tube for about 30 minutes as the MRI produces more than 3,000 images, each showing a thin slice of your breasts.

With so many images to interpret, it may take a few days to get your results. At that point, you and your doctor can discuss the appropriate next steps to take to safeguard your health.

Closer to a Breast Cancer Cure

Richard G. Pestell, MD, PhD, director, Kimmel Cancer Center, professor and chairman, department of cancer biology, and associate dean, cancer programs, Jefferson Medical College, Thomas Jefferson University, and vice president, oncology services, Thomas Jefferson University Hospitals, Philadelphia.

You're no doubt familiar with the old saying that if you want to succeed in business, you must "build a better mousetrap." Well, some cancer researchers have taken the concept a step beyond and built what amounts to a better mouse...one that has enabled them to pin down once and for all the connection between inflammation and the growth of cancer cells—in this case, breast cancer, bringing new hope on the road to finding a cure.

That the two are linked has been postulated for years, but proving it has been impossible because researchers were unable to isolate inflammation in the breast tissue of mice (a good starting proxy for human research for this "tissue line"), we learned from Richard G. Pestell, MD, PhD, director of the Kimmel Cancer Center at Thomas Jefferson University in Philadelphia. And, he explained, "If you knock out all of the inflammatory genes in a mouse, the mouse doesn't survive."

So Dr. Pestell and his colleagues approached the problem from a different direction—they created a new breed of mouse in which inflammation could be incited only in the breast tissue. This enabled them to design an experiment in which inflammation in the breast could be blocked in one set of mice but not others. The researchers could then demonstrate that blocking the inflammation in the breasts of these mice reduced the number of breast cancer stem cells…and dramatically reduced the number and rate of onset of breast tumors.

What Happens Next?

Calling this "a very novel finding," Dr. Pestell said that it opens the door to the development of safer therapy that will specifically treat inflammation and can be targeted directly to the breast.

This will be a vast improvement over the current chemotherapy approach for breast cancer, which nonselectively targets all cells that divide rapidly—killing not only cancer cells but also cells in the digestive tract, bone marrow and hair follicles, the reason for the many serious systemic side effects that accompany cancer treatment, including digestive disturbances, immune system suppression and hair loss.

Dr. Pestell notes that these mice also will be helpful in studying the role of inflammation in illnesses such as heart disease and neurodegeneration as well as other cancers.

The study's results appeared in the journal *Cancer Research*.

Do This Now to Fight Breast Cancer

While Dr. Pestell and his researchers continue their lab studies, you can get to work at home to reduce the influence of inflammation on your body. We know what breeds inflammation—poor diet (sugar, highly refined grains, processed foods and inflammatory fats), lack of exercise, stress, chronic infections and exposure to toxins in the environment. *Focus on reducing inflammation by taking the following steps…*

• **Eat more whole foods and fewer processed ones.** Follow a high-fiber, plant-heavy diet based on unrefined foods rich in anti-inflammatory phytonutrients.

• **Embrace healthy fats.** Replace trans fats and saturated fats with olive oil, nuts, avocados and omega-3-packed fish such as wild salmon, sardines and herring.

• **Take a deep breath.** Choose your favorite stress-management strategy—meditation, deep breathing, building model ships, reading (or writing!) poetry—and make room for it in your daily life.

• **Get moving.** Exercise is a cornerstone of a healthy, anti-inflammatory lifestyle.

Advanced Breast Cancer Has Nearly Tripled in Young Women

Over the past 30 years in the US, the rate of metastatic breast cancer in women under age 40 has increased from about 250 cases in 1976 to about 850 cases in 2009. Researchers are now trying to determine why.

Study of 936,497 women who had breast cancer from 1976 to 2009 by researchers at Seattle Children's Hospital, published in *The Journal of the American Medical Association*.

• **Consider supplements.** Take a daily probiotic to improve the balance of bacteria in your gut. Other anti-inflammatory supplements include fish oil, vitamins C and E, selenium, quercetin, flaxseed oil and resveratrol.

A Mind-Set That May Fight Cancer

Kim Allison, MD, director of breast pathology, University of Washington Medical Center, Seattle, and author of *Red Sunshine: A Story of Strength and Inspiration from a Doctor Who Survived Stage 3 Breast Cancer* (Hatherleigh).

Although you are probably inundated with reading material if you've just recently been diagnosed with breast cancer, here's one more book to include—it's quite a story. It's filled with unusual ideas that may help patients with all kinds of cancer—not only breast cancer—beat their disease. What gives the story a unique twist is that the author, Kim Allison, MD, is the director of breast pathology at the University of Washington Medical Center in Seattle... and Dr. Allison had been promoted into this position just a few weeks before learning, at age 33, that she had an aggressive form of breast cancer with an average five-year survival rate of only 40%.

Today, about six years later, she is healthy—and the book, *Red Sunshine: A Story of Strength and Inspiration from a Doctor Who Survived Stage 3 Breast Cancer*, explains how she got that way.

Knowing how serious her cancer was, Dr. Allison says she chose a "take no prisoners" treatment plan that included chemo, radiation and surgery. She decided to have both breasts removed even though she had cancer on only one side. But those aren't the parts of her treatment that make her story so unique and valuable...it's the things that she did in addition to that—which doctors almost never tell their patients to do!

Adding a Second Approach

As a specialist, Dr. Allison knew as much as anyone could about how to treat her disease medically, but she decided to also develop her own "alternative" treatment strategy so she could feel that she was marshaling every possible resource that might improve her odds of survival.

Her approach is inspiring even to individuals without cancer. It's important to note that Dr. Allison isn't sure that any of the following actions helped cure her cancer, but she admits that they made the journey less onerous. "These strategies changed my perspective and helped me get through each day," she said. *Here are some highlights from the book and direct comments from Dr. Allison…*

Three Big Ideas

• **Develop a winning attitude.** Early on, Dr. Allison decided that she wanted to consider her fight an "opportunity to grow and learn about how tough I can be" rather than just questioning why something so bad had happened to her. She decided that the poison being dripped into her veins—a potent drug called *doxorubicin*, nicknamed the "Red Devil" because of its deep, red color and horrible side effects—should be considered her ally, so she renamed it "Red Sunshine." "That was an important mental switch, because it made me want to show up for treatment," she said.

• **Foster several great teams.** As a busy working mother—with a four-year-old daughter, an infant son and a husband who had recently opened a restaurant—Dr. Allison needed all the help that she could get with her disease and her life. She was fortunate to have friends and family members who were available and willing to assist her. This isn't always possible, she said, but it never hurts to ask for help. She appointed these people to be "gurus" of different things. For example, one was in charge of music (downloading tunes onto her iPod for her to listen to during chemo) and another, who still lived near her

Foods That Lower Risk for Breast Cancer

Eating dark green or deep orange vegetables and fruits that are rich in carotenoids reduces the risk for estrogen-receptor-negative cancers by 13%. Eat spinach, broccoli, cantaloupe, carrots, apricots and other dark green or orange fruits and vegetables.

Review of data from 18 studies involving more than one million women by researchers at Harvard School of Public Health, Boston, published in Nutrition Action Healthletter.

parents in California, was assigned the task of helping her parents cope from afar.

Dr. Allison's medical treatment team included a pathologist, an oncologist and two surgeons. But she also worked with a physical therapist, who taught her techniques to avoid complications like lymphedema (swelling in the arms) after surgery…a nutritionist (who helped her eat a well-balanced diet)…a personal trainer (who helped her continue to work out by encouraging her to walk and do strength training and yoga)…a naturopath (who advised her on supplements that might help with treatment side effects)… and an acupuncturist (who helped her keep her stress and pain levels under control). This was an expensive group, no doubt, but Dr. Allison says that many major cancer centers offer some of this support for free—and you often can get insurance to cover at least part of the cost.

• **Believe in "magic."** Though her career is all about science, Dr. Allison said that she was willing to believe in magic, too. She visited a shaman—a spiritual adviser—an experience she found enriching in ways that she never expected. And, with the help of her mother (who visited regularly) and a friend, she created a "healing ritual" in her backyard. "We stated out loud in a united way that I was planning to destroy the cancer that had grown inside of me. Then I burned an image of my cancer in a fire," she said.

Dr. Allison's cancer is now considered "most likely cured," since there was no residual cancer after chemotherapy was completed—and she's feeling great. Only future research can determine whether or not her unusual, two-tiered psychological and medical approach can make a significant difference, in terms of fighting off cancer—but it probably didn't hurt.

Are More Young Women Getting Breast Cancer?

Banu K. Arun, MD, professor of breast medical oncology and clinical cancer prevention and codirector of clinical cancer genetics, The University of Texas MD Anderson Cancer Center, Houston.

If you're a woman and carry a mutation in your BRCA1 or BRCA2 gene, you probably already know that you're more likely to develop breast or ovarian cancer than women who don't carry such a genetic mutation. But what you probably didn't know is that if you have either one of those mutations and your mom or aunt had breast or ovarian cancer, then there's a good chance that you could be diagnosed with cancer nearly eight years earlier than your mom or aunt was, according to a recent study from The University of Texas MD Anderson Cancer Center in Houston. This research adds to the small but growing body of reports about this trend.

We spoke with the lead study author, Banu K. Arun, MD, associate professor of breast medical oncology and clinical cancer prevention and codirector of the Clinical Cancer Genetics program at the university, to talk about the results and what they might mean for my readers.

Dr. Arun and her colleagues analyzed 132 women with breast cancer who tested positive for either a BRCA1 or BRCA2 mutation between 2003 and 2009—these women served as the "younger" generation in the study. (Dr. Arun decided to look at only women in the younger generation who had breast cancer, not ovarian cancer, because she works in the breast department at the university.) Of these women with both breast cancer and a BRCA mutation, 106 had aunts or mothers who had had either breast or ovarian cancer, so their aunts and mothers made up the "older" generation in the study. By analyzing the ages of cancer diagnosis among the families in both generations, Dr. Arun and her team found that the median age of the cancer diagnosis was 7.9 years earlier for women in the younger generation.

Why the Shift?

This type of news is disappointing, especially now, when we think we have made great strides in preventing cancer—or at least in delaying it. We asked Dr. Arun to explain what is going on.

Several relatively recent trends may have helped lead to earlier BRCA-related cancer diagnoses in younger women, said Dr. Arun, including…

•**An increase in BRCA mutation awareness,** plus an increase in the availability of genetic tests (both of which may have led to an increase in genetic testing).

•**Improvements in imaging techniques** (which has likely led to getting more accurate diagnoses).

•**More environmental influences, such as taking estrogen replacement hormone therapy** or exposure to estrogen-like substances in the environment (which some studies have associated with an increased risk for breast cancer).

Another reason that BRCA-related cancer diagnoses are happening earlier in some women's lives, she said, may have something to do with what epidemiologists call anticipation. It's an unfortunate phenomenon in some inherited diseases in which DNA instability causes an illness to strike at a younger age and/or with increased severity in subsequent generations. (This happens with Huntington's disease, for example.)

In other words, these findings are not necessarily dire. They could mean that women are developing the disease at younger ages or that they're simply discovering it sooner—or both. Since all of those reasons listed above probably play a role, said Dr. Arun, the study's findings are likely due to a mixture of factors.

One limitation of the study is that the researchers assumed that the older generation's breast or ovarian cancer was caused by a BRCA1 or BRCA2 mutation—but there was no way to know for sure (because in some cases, the aunts and moms had already passed away and, in other cases, they never took genetic tests). So the younger generation's cancer may have been hereditary or those women may have been the first generation in their families with the mutation.

Know Your Risk

For women who have a BRCA mutation and are therefore at high risk for both breast and ovarian cancer, the question is: How soon and how frequently should you get screened?

•**How soon to start.** The American Cancer Society (ACS) recommends that high-risk women begin getting screened for both types of cancer at age 30, but they caution that it's a good idea to discuss the best age with your doctor—because if your mom or aunt got either disease at a young age, you may want to start getting screened earlier.

•**How often to go.** The ACS recommends that high-risk women get yearly breast screenings that should include a magnetic resonance imaging (MRI) scan, a mammogram and a clinical breast exam (where a doctor examines your breasts). A pelvic exam done by your doctor during your annual gynecological exam is usually the best way to get screened for ovarian cancer—your doctor might also want to give you a CA-125 blood test, which checks for the level of a certain protein found on the surface of ovarian cancer cells.

In spite of the questions this study raises, it is clear on one point—those at high risk for breast cancer must be aggressive in their screening and do all that they can to reduce environmental and lifestyle risk factors for the disease.

Controversy Update: Mammograms Really Do Benefit Women in Their 40s

Hakan Jonsson, PhD, associate professor of cancer epidemiology at Umea University in Umea, Sweden, and leader of a study of more than one million women.

No doubt you recall the recent brouhaha when the US Preventive Services Task Force shocked America by saying that women in their 40s didn't need mammograms to screen for breast cancer. It claimed that the test's downsides—inconvenience, discomfort, risk for false positives—outweighed its benefits because as many as 1,900 women in their 40s would need to be screened to save "just" one life. At the time, many cancer experts denounced the new guidelines, citing research proving that mammograms reduce breast cancer mortality by at least 15%, regardless of age.

Now, a huge Swedish study provides even more evidence that 40-something women should get mammograms. Today, throughout Sweden, mammography screening is standard for women ages 40 to 74—but in the past, individual counties determined whether women ages 40 to 49 should be "invited" to screen for breast cancer. Researchers looked at breast cancer mortality among women in their 40s, comparing death rates in counties that did screening for this group with death rates in counties that did not. Women were followed for 16 years, on average, from the time screening started.

Result: Women who got mammograms in their 40s were 29% less likely to die of breast cancer during the study than women who did not get screened.

Bottom line: This study supports the American Cancer Society and American Congress of Obstetricians and Gynecologists, which recommend annual mammograms starting at age 40.

How Red Wine Affects Breast Cancer Risk

Glenn D. Braunstein, MD, chairman, department of medicine, vice president for clinical innovation, Cedars-Sinai Medical Center, Los Angeles.

If you're a woman, then you already know that one daily drink of alcohol may raise your risk for breast cancer by about 12%, according to some research. But a recent study suggests that not all alcohol is created equal...when it comes to wine, in particular, white wine may be more risky than red.

Now picture a restaurant full of people ordering wine—what are most of the women having? White, of course. What's their risk?

What's In That Glass?

Glenn D. Braunstein, MD, chairman of the department of medicine at Cedars-Sinai Medical Center in Los Angeles, got the idea to study red wine versus white wine because of substances called aromatase-inhibitors (AIs). AIs are naturally present in red grape skins, red grape seeds and red wine—but not in white grapes or white wine—and, in prior studies they have been shown, in drug-form, to decrease the body's production of estrogen (which many breast cancers require to grow). So Dr. Braunstein wanted to see whether the natural AIs found in red wine might help healthy women blunt the added risk of drinking red wine, making it less risky than white wine.

Red Wine Trumps White

In the study, Dr. Braunstein and his team randomly assigned 36 healthy women (average age 36) to drink eight ounces of either red or white wine with food each evening during the first 21 days of their menstrual cycle. They drank either Cabernet Sauvignon or Chardonnay made by the same company in the same year. After the 21st day, they were told to drink no wine (and consume no grape-related products) until their next menstrual cycle began, at which point they were asked to switch to drinking the other color of wine for 21 days. Twice during the same phases of each menstrual cycle, physicians drew blood from the women to measure their levels of estrogen and other hormones.

The results: Researchers found that when the women drank red wine, they had lower levels of estrogen compared with when they drank white wine. When the women drank red wine, they also had higher levels of several other hormones, which are additional indicators that the red wine was acting as an AI. The researchers concluded that given its effect on estrogen and other hormones, drinking red wine may be less risky than drinking white, in terms of breast cancer risk.

In fact, it is possible that a certain amount of red wine reduces breast cancer risk, said Dr. Braunstein, but additional research will be needed to see whether that's true. The the study was published in the *Journal of Women's Health*.

Belly Up

Dr. Braunstein said that although the only red wine tested was Cabernet Sauvignon, it's likely that red wines made from other red grapes would have similar effects. So, he said, if you're a healthy woman with no history of breast cancer and you like to indulge in alcohol on occasion, then you might want to stick with red wine. But he emphasized that if you don't already drink alcohol, this research does not suggest that you pick up the habit, since you can still get the AI benefit from a glass of purple grape juice or a bowl of red grapes. And if you currently have breast cancer or have already had breast cancer, he added, it may also be wise to stay away from alcohol altogether. Talk to your doctor about your particular risk factors.

The Lowdown on Lymphatic Breast Massage

Gwen White, PT, is a physical therapist and lymphedema specialist with Kaiser Permanente in Portland, Oregon, and coauthor of *Lymphedema: A Breast Cancer Patient's Guide to Prevention and Healing* (Hunter House).

Is it true that massaging your breasts helps prevent breast cancer?

There's a technique called lymphatic breast massage, also referred to as manual drainage therapy or manual lymph drainage. Unfortunately, there is no scientific documentation showing that this technique helps prevent breast cancer.

What lymphatic breast massage can do is reduce swelling after breast cancer surgery, a common complication called lymphedema. It works by promoting the proper function of the lymphatic system, which has the job of breaking down cellular waste, removing impurities from tissues and maintaining fluid balance. By encouraging the flow of lymph fluid through the lymph vessels, this special massage technique—which uses a press-and-release pumping action—helps prevent lymph fluid from accumulating in tissues near the surgical site. Lymphatic breast massage also can ease breast swelling and tenderness associated with premenstrual syndrome…and, along with antibiotics, it can help treat mastitis (a painful breast tissue infection).

For lymphatic breast massage treatment and instruction, consult a physical therapist. You can ask your doctor for a referral or find a practitioner through the National Lymphedema Network (*www.LymphNet.org*) or the Lymphology Association of North America (*www.clt-lana.org/therapists/default.asp*).

Carbs Raise Risk for Breast Cancer—But Which Ones?

Jennifer A. Emond, MS, doctoral student, Cancer Prevention Control Program, University of California-San Diego Moores Cancer Center, San Diego, and Graduate School of Public Health, San Diego State University.

A recent study shows that when it comes to preventing breast cancer recurrence, not all carbs are created equal—certain kinds may raise your risk more than others.

To find out more, we spoke with study author Jennifer A. Emond, MS, a public health doctoral student at University of California-San Diego. Emond and her colleagues presented their findings at a symposium in December 2011.

More Starches = More Cancer

Investigators looked at data from 2,651 breast cancer survivors (average age 53). All had been diagnosed with breast cancer within the previous four years. In phone interviews at the beginning of the study and again one year later, the women reported what they had eaten in the past 24 hours. The women were then monitored for about seven years, on average, to see whose breast cancer recurred.

Researchers examined the relationship between breast cancer recurrence and carbohydrate intake—first looking at quantity (did their overall carb intake increase or decrease?) and then at quality (what were the carbs made of?).

Quality is important to analyze, because the fact is, carbs can be made up of varying amounts of many different constituents, including starch, fiber, sucrose and fructose, and each constituent affects metabolism differently. For example, a typical slice of white bread contains 10.4 grams of starch and less than one gram of fiber. In contrast, a cup of raw carrots contains 3.6 grams of fiber and only 1.8 grams of starch.

Emond and her team discovered...

• **Women who experienced a breast cancer recurrence in the seven-year follow-up period** had increased their overall carb intake during that first year by about 2.3 grams a day, on average, while those who did not have a recurrence during that seven-year period decreased their overall carb intake during that first year by approximately 2.7 grams a day, on average.

• **Changes in the amount of starch eaten accounted for the majority of the changes in total carb consumption** (compared with other types of carbs, such as glucose, sucrose, galactose, fructose, lactose and maltose).

"The results show that it's not just overall carbohydrate intake but particularly starch intake that ups the risk for breast cancer," said Emond.

Why Would Starches Be So Dangerous?

Scientists do not understand exactly how starches increase the risk for breast cancer recurrence, but multiple studies indicate that elevated insulin is associated with higher breast cancer risk—and many starches are known to elevate insulin faster and higher than more complex carbs. But Emond cautioned that this is only one study—these findings will need to be replicated by future research.

We'd love to tell you that all you need to do is just avoid starchy carbs, but Emond said it's not that simple. There are different types of starches, and depending on what else you eat with the starch—such as fiber, fat or protein—it can have varying effects on your insulin level. The next step in research, said Emond, is figuring out which types of starches and which food combinations may raise the risk for breast cancer more than others.

Future research will also need to address whether or not cutting back on certain starches might help women who have never had breast cancer reduce their risk for the disease.

In the meantime, Emond recommends that all breast cancer survivors (actually all cancer survivors) follow the dietary guidelines recommended by the American Cancer Society, which include eating mostly plant-based foods and high-fiber foods and avoiding refined grains (such as white bread, white rice, and cereals and crackers that don't say "whole grain" on the package).

Breast Cancer Vaccine on the Horizon

A breast cancer vaccine could be available in the next decade. An experimental vaccine that targets a protein in most breast cancers was found effective in preventing the disease in mice. Researchers need funding and permission from the FDA for clinical trials.

Vincent K. Tuohy, PhD, professor, department of immunology, molecular medicine and pathology, Cleveland Clinic's Lerner Research Institute, and team leader of an animal study, published in *Nature Medicine*.

Shield Your Breasts

Shield your breasts from CT scans to reduce radiation exposure. The shield—a thin piece of heavy metal—can reduce radiation by at least 30%, lowering risk for radiation-caused cancers in breast tissue in men and women. Many doctors, however, don't use them because the shields can cause streaks and lines on the scans.

Reality: These markings do not cause experienced technicians to miss abnormalities—and the markings can be limited by elevating the shield with towels or foam about two centimeters above the chest.

Terrance T. Healey, MD, director of thoracic radiology and clinical assistant professor, Warren Alpert Medical School of Brown University, and a radiologist at Rhode Island Hospital, both in Providence. He led a study presented at a recent meeting of the Radiological Society of North America.

Good News for Women with Breast Cancer— Five Recent Advances Are Dramatically Changing Treatment Approaches...

Jill Dietz, MD, director of the Hillcrest Breast Center, Cleveland Clinic Foundation. She is a fellow of the American College of Surgeons and member of several professional organizations, including the American Society of Breast Surgeons and Society of Surgical Oncology. A researcher and teacher, Dr. Dietz is also program director for the surgical breast fellowship at Cleveland Clinic.

Women who have breast cancer are now living longer than they did only five years ago—and not simply due to improved mammography techniques.

Reason: Scientific evidence is changing the way physicians can treat the disease—making these treatments much more selective and effective. *Key findings breast cancer patients need to know about...*

•**New thinking on double mastectomy.** Many women with breast cancer opt to surgically remove the breast with the malignancy and the healthy breast. Their decision to remove both breasts is driven by the fear that a new breast cancer will develop in the healthy breast. But recent research suggests that double mastectomy for these women may be overused.

Scientific evidence: Researchers who followed up with 1,525 early-stage breast cancer patients four years after they had received mastectomy, double mastectomy or lumpectomy (a breast-conserving procedure that removes only the malignancy and surrounding tissue) found that women who had both breasts removed would have had a very low risk of developing cancer in the healthy breast.

Who should consider having a double mastectomy? According to the Society of Surgical Oncology, it may be warranted for a woman who is at increased risk for breast cancer because she has two or more immediate family members (a mother, sister or daughter) with breast or ovarian cancer…or has tested positive for mutations in the BRCA1 or BRCA2 gene. These criteria apply to women who have early-stage breast cancer as well as those who haven't developed the disease.

Self-defense: If you don't have a family history or genetic predisposition to develop breast cancer, carefully review your reasons for considering a double mastectomy.

•**Better results with *tamoxifen*.** Doctors have long advised certain breast cancer patients to use an estrogen-blocking drug (tamoxifen) for about five years to stave off future breast malignancies.

Scientific evidence: For 15 years, researchers followed 6,846 breast cancer patients who took tamoxifen for an additional five years after five years of initial use while another group stopped the drug at five years.

Result: Those who used the drug for 10 years had a significantly reduced risk for breast cancer recurrence and death.

The benefits of longer-term tamoxifen use apply primarily to premenopausal women. That's because postmenopausal women have the option of taking another class of drugs called aromatase inhibitors, including *letrozole* (Femara), which are slightly more effective than tamoxifen at preventing future breast cancers but do not, for unknown reasons, offer the same benefit to premenopausal women. Research has not yet determined whether postmenopausal women would benefit from taking letrozole for 10 years rather than the standard five-year recommendation.

Self-defense: If you're a premenopausal woman with breast cancer (especially if the tumor was large and/or you had lymph nodes that tested positive for cancer), ask your doctor about the risks and benefits of taking tamoxifen for more than the standard five

years. Using the drug increases risk for endometrial cancer and pulmonary embolism.

•**Less invasive treatment may improve survival for early-stage breast cancer.** Women with early-stage breast cancer perceive mastectomy to be more effective at eliminating their future risk for breast cancer, but research shows that this is probably not true.

Scientific evidence: In an analysis of more than 112,000 women with stage I or stage II breast cancer who were tracked for an average of 9.2 years, those who received lumpectomy plus radiation had odds of survival that were as good as or better than those who underwent mastectomy.

Self-defense: If you are diagnosed with stage I or stage II breast cancer, ask your doctor about lumpectomy plus radiation.

•**More women could benefit from reconstruction.** With breast reconstruction, a woman who has received a mastectomy (or, in some cases, a lumpectomy) can have her breast shape rebuilt with an implant and/or tissue from another part of her body (typically the abdomen, back or buttocks). When a patient opts for reconstruction, it is ideally performed with the initial breast cancer surgery for the best cosmetic result.

Breast reconstruction does not restore the breast's natural sensation or replace the nipple. However, a new "nipple-sparing" mas-

Blood Test for Breast Cancer

Breast cancer may be detected by a blood test that detects prostate cancer in men?

Recent finding: Levels of prostate-specific antigen (PSA) are more than three times higher in women who have breast cancer than in women who do not have the disease.

Chien Chou, PhD, professor, Graduate Institute of Electro-Optical Engineering, Chang Gung University, Taiwan, and leader of a study published in *Analytical Chemistry*.

tectomy, a technically difficult procedure in which the surgeon preserves the nipple and areola (the brownish or pink-colored tissue surrounding the nipple), is gaining popularity with women whose malignancy does not interfere with this type of surgery.

Scientific evidence: Even though breast reconstruction can offer cosmetic and psychological advantages, not very many women choose to have it. In a study of more than 120,000 women who underwent mastectomy, fewer than one in four of the women with invasive breast cancer opted for reconstruction, while only about one in three of those with early-stage disease got it. Almost all women are candidates for reconstruction, which does not impact survival rates. In some cases, women require one or more subsequent surgeries to fine-tune the reconstruction.

Self-defense: Ask about reconstruction before your treatment begins. If you're a candidate, the breast surgeon can coordinate with a plastic surgeon. Breast reconstruction is often covered by insurance, but some insurers may require a co-pay.

•**Targeted therapies save lives.** Until 40 years ago, breast cancer was treated almost uniformly with radical mastectomy, radiation and some form of hormone therapy.

Scientific evidence: Using new genomic DNA–based tests, doctors are now able to customize treatment based on tumor biology, helping them better predict a patient's risk for recurrence and response to particular treatments. This may help thousands of women avoid chemotherapy, including anthracyclines, which are linked to heart damage and leukemia.

Self-defense: Ask your doctor whether you could benefit from genomic testing to help determine which breast cancer therapies would be most effective for you.

Is There Breast Cancer In Your Family? Ask Dad!

J. Leonard Lichtenfeld, MD, deputy chief medical officer of the American Cancer Society in Atlanta. *www.Cancer.org*

When it comes to physical traits, such as eye color or body type, many women are well aware that these can be inherited from either parent—but not so many realize that a genetic risk for breast or ovarian cancer is as likely to be passed down from your dad's side of the family as from your mom's.

Most inherited genetic predispositions to breast and ovarian cancers are caused by mutations in the BRCA1 and BRCA2 genes, and men are just as likely as women to pass on these mutations to their children. Yet, when researchers at Princess Margaret Hospital in Toronto examined records from their cancer clinic, they found that women were five times more likely to be referred for genetic counseling due to having a maternal history of cancer than they were if the disease occurred in their paternal line.

This has important implications—not only for women worried about their own health but also for fathers who want to be sure that their daughters are doing all that they can to protect themselves. J. Leonard Lichtenfeld, MD, deputy chief medical officer at the national office of the American Cancer Society in Atlanta, stressed the importance of learning as much as possible about both parents' family history. "Many fathers don't realize that they can be carrying genes for breast and ovarian cancer," he said, adding the surprising fact that many health-care providers don't know this either!

Of the 700,000 women worldwide diagnosed with breast cancer each year, 5% to 10% have a genetic predisposition, usually a mutation in one of the BRCA genes. Women with these mutations have a 55% to 87% risk for breast cancer and a 20% to 44% risk for ovarian cancer. In a commentary on the study published online in *The Lancet Oncology*, the researchers pointed out that if doctors don't ask about the medical history on the paternal side, women may not realize that they could be at high risk for breast or ovarian cancer—and that could prevent them from seeking genetic testing.

What you can do: Dr. Lichtenfeld urged women to invest some time in learning their family medical history—from both sides of the family tree. Ask questions of your relatives, and follow through to get as much information as you can. Be alert to other cancers connected to breast cancer on your father's side, such as colon and ovarian cancers. "As you get older and relatives pass away, you'll find that the memory of the diseases they had and the causes of death disappear with them," Dr. Lichtenfeld pointed out. "If you discover a history of breast or ovarian cancer, especially premenopausal, on either side of your family, it's very important to get a consultation with an experienced genetic counselor who will discuss whether a test for the BRCA1 or BRCA2 mutation is appropriate and the implications of the results."

To learn more about how to explore your family health history, go to the Web site for the Surgeon General's Family Health History Initiative at *www.hhs.gov/familyhistory*. You will be able to create, store and share an electronic record (and keep it confidential) for free. It may be the best thing you've ever done for yourself—and your family.

Hot Flashes Reduce Breast Cancer Risk

According to a recent study, women who experience intense hot flashes that wake them up at night and other severe symptoms of menopause, such as night sweats, vaginal dryness, bladder problems and depression, have up to 50% lower risk for breast cancer than women who don't have such symptoms. The protective effect increases with the number and severity of menopausal symptoms.

Possible reason: The symptoms occur as hormone levels fluctuate and drop. Women who have the intense symptoms may have lower levels of estrogen. High levels of estrogen are linked to breast cancer.

Christopher I. Li, MD, PhD, breast cancer epidemiologist, Fred Hutchinson Cancer Research Center, Seattle, and leader of a study published in *Cancer Epidemiology, Biomarkers & Prevention.*

Taking Off Just a Few Pounds Protects Your Breasts

Anne McTiernan, MD, PhD, faculty member at the Fred Hutchinson Cancer Research Center and a research professor in the departments of epidemiology and medicine at the University of Washington, both in Seattle. She is the senior author of a study on weight loss and breast cancer risk published in *Journal of Clinical Oncology.*

Have you heard the news about the big payback for shedding just a little extra body baggage?

Here's the scoop: If you're postmenopausal and overweight, dropping just 5% of your body weight—that's a mere nine pounds if you currently weigh 180—can significantly reduce levels of hormones linked to breast cancer, a recent study shows.

Background: Overweight and obese postmenopausal women are considered to be at elevated risk for breast cancer. That's because, after menopause, fat tissue becomes a major source of various estrogens and other sex hormones that are implicated in tumor growth. Overweight women produce more of these sex hormones than thin women because they have more fat tissue.

For the recent study, participants included 439 sedentary, overweight women ages 50 to 75. One group did 45 minutes of aerobic exercise, such as brisk walking, five days a week...a second group was assigned a diet of 1,200 to 2,000 calories a day...a third group followed both the diet and exercise regimens...the control group did not change their usual diet or exercise routines. Blood tests were done at the start and end of the study to measure levels of hormones linked with breast cancer risk.

After one year: In the control group, there was no change in weight, and hormone levels actually worsened…in the exercise-only group, weight loss and hormone reductions were very modest (though of course exercise has other health benefits).

In contrast: Women in the diet-only group lost 11% of their body weight, on average, while those in the diet-plus-exercise group lost 12%. And in both groups, sex hormone blood levels dropped significantly—by 10% to as much as 26%, on average, depending on the hormone. Such changes, according to previous research, suggest about a 50% decrease in breast cancer risk. Generally, the greater the weight loss, the greater the improvement in hormone levels…yet even participants who lost just 5% of their body weight experienced hormone level changes suggestive of a 22% reduction in breast cancer risk, researchers said.

Bottom line: If you are overweight, start today to make the lifestyle changes that will take off some of those pounds. Besides all the other well-known benefits, slimming down a bit may help you avoid breast cancer!

Even One Drink a Day Raises Cancer Risk— Should You Give Up Alcohol?

Samir Zakhari, PhD, director of the division of metabolism and health effects at the National Institute on Alcohol Abuse and Alcoholism in Bethesda, Maryland. He is a leading expert on alcohol metabolism and the effects of alcohol and alcohol by-products on cancer, cirrhosis and other diseases.

Y ou would think from reading the headlines that a glass of red wine is almost as good for your health as a plateful of vegetables. Moderate drinking is good for your heart, but some studies show that it may increase the risk for cancer.

Recent research: The Million Women Study, which followed 1.3 million women for an average of seven years, found that about 13% of cancers—affecting the breast, mouth, throat, rectum, liver and esophagus—could be linked to alcohol. Women who consumed the most alcohol were the ones most likely to get cancer, but even one drink a day increased risk.

The Evidence

Researchers have known for a long time that heavy drinking is linked to cancer.

Examples: At least 70% of patients with mouth cancer are heavy drinkers. People who have five or more drinks a day are more likely to get colorectal cancers and cancers in the upper digestive tract.

Moderation lowers the risks but doesn't eliminate them. Cancers of the mouth and esophagus have been linked to as little as two drinks a day. An analysis in *American Journal of Epidemiology* concluded that men who have three or more drinks daily have a 41% increased risk for cancer-caused mortality. Women who have two or more drinks daily increase their risk by 20%.

How Alcohol Hurts

It's not yet known precisely how alcohol increases cancer risks. A toxic chemical called acetylaldehyde, produced when alcohol is metabolized (broken down) in the body, may damage genetic material and prevent cells from repairing the damage. In addition, alcohol metabolism produces free radicals that cause cell damage and inflammation, which can promote cancer.

There also appears to be a hormonal link. Alcohol may increase levels of estrogen and other hormones. This could be the reason that women who drink have a higher risk for breast cancer than nondrinkers.

Some people may have genetic variations that make them more or less likely to develop alcohol-related cancers. A study of heavy drinkers found that those who did not develop cancer had a genetic variation that enabled them to metabolize alcohol faster than those without the variation.

Is Abstinence Best?

You may ask, "Why drink if it causes cancer?" *To answer that question, it is helpful to understand the following...*

• **The risks overall are small.** Only 3.5% of cancer deaths worldwide (230,000 a year) are attributable to alcohol. But 90% of those deaths in men could be avoided if they drank no more than two alcoholic drinks a day and 50% of the deaths in women could be avoided if they drank no more than one drink a day.

• **Good for the heart.** Alcohol increases levels of HDL "good" cholesterol. It reduces the formation of blood clots and helps dissolve clots that have already formed. Moderate drinking results in a sharp decrease in heart attack risk (40% to 60%).

• **Study limitations.** Most studies that have linked alcohol to cancer are epidemiological studies. Large groups of people fill out questionnaires about their alcohol consumption and other lifestyle factors. Then researchers track their health over time. Answers to this type of questionnaire can be inaccurate. People either don't remember correctly or tell researchers what they think they should say.

Safer Drinking

The type of drink doesn't matter much. Beer, whiskey, vodka and the like have similar effects on cancer risks. However, the resveratrol in red wine, which has been linked to cardiovascular health, also may prevent cancer by repairing cell damage. But you may have to drink more than moderately to get enough resveratrol, and that is not advisable.

All of the benefits of alcohol, including the cardiovascular benefits, evaporate when people drink too much. Even if you drink moderately (no more than two drinks daily for men or one daily drink for women), alcohol might help or hurt, depending on other factors.

Consider...

• **Your personal and family health history.** A vigorous 20-year-old with healthy habits and no family history of heart problems probably won't benefit from drinking. On the other hand, consider a 55-year-old who doesn't exercise or eat a nutritious diet and who also has a family history of heart disease. This person might benefit from a daily glass of wine. The slightly increased risk would be offset by the cardiovascular benefits.

Or a woman with a family history of breast cancer might decide that it's too risky to drink. A woman without this history might feel comfortable having one drink a day.

• **Always talk with your doctor about the potential benefits and risks of alcohol for you.**

• **Drinking patterns.** People who drink a lot at once, and do this consistently over the years, probably have more organ damage and greater cancer risk than those who drink smaller amounts over time. Let's say one woman drinks nothing during the week but has seven drinks on the weekend...and another woman has one drink a day every day. Their weekly average is the same, but the health effects likely will be different.

• **Eat before you drink.** If you have food in your stomach, alcohol is absorbed more slowly and the liver breaks down alcohol at the rate of about one drink per hour. Drinking on an empty stomach causes alcohol to move more quickly into the liver, potentially causing cell damage.

The Breast Cancer Risk That's as Bad as the Gene

Chaya Moskowitz, PhD, associate attending biostatistician at Memorial Sloan Kettering Cancer Center in New York City and lead author of a study on breast cancer risk among childhood cancer survivors presented at a recent meeting of the American Society of Clinical Oncology.

Don't we all want to weep when we think of kids battling cancer…and isn't it great to know that most children now beat the disease? Nevertheless, as they reach adulthood, some childhood cancer survivors need to be extra-wary about yet another cancer threat, a recent study reveals.

Researchers looked at long-term data (the median follow-up period was 26 years) on 1,268 female childhood cancer survivors who had been treated with radiation to the chest. It's not news that radiation raises a person's risk for future cancers—but what was surprising was the degree to which risk increased.

How the numbers stacked up: Among childhood cancer survivors who had received chest radiation, 24% developed breast cancer by age 50…the median age at diagnosis was just 38. Risk was especially elevated among women who as children got high doses of chest radiation to treat Hodgkin lymphoma (cancer of the immune system)—their rate of 30% was comparable to the 31% rate that the researchers estimated for women who carry the BRCA1 gene mutation.

It is worrisome to note that only about half of women treated with chest radiation as youngsters follow the current breast cancer screening guidelines from the Children's Oncology Group, a consortium supported by the National Cancer Institute. Those guidelines recommend that childhood cancer survivors who received 20 Gy (the unit of measure for radiation) or more to the chest area undergo twice-yearly clinical breast exams, annual mammograms and annual breast MRIs starting at age 25 or eight years after radiation,

whichever comes later. And the recent study findings suggest that these same guidelines also may be appropriate for women who were treated with lower chest radiation dosages, researchers said.

Childhood cancer survivors: Talk to your doctor about breast cancer screening—and make sure that he or she is aware of your chest radiation treatment history.

Tender Breasts May Mean Trouble for Women Who Take Hormones

Carolyn Crandall, MD, professor in the department of medicine at the David Geffen School of Medicine, a scientist with the Jonsson Comprehensive Cancer Center and the associate research director of the National Center of Excellence in Women's Health, all at the University of California, Los Angeles, and lead author of a study on hormone therapy published in *Breast Cancer Research and Treatment*.

If you are considering or currently using hormone therapy (HT) to ease menopausal symptoms such as hot flashes and night sweats, you're probably keenly aware of the concerns about a link between HT and breast cancer. So I want to share recent study results that help identify which HT users are and are not at increased risk for this dreaded disease.

The surprising clue: Sore breasts.

Background: There are two basic types of menopausal HT—estrogen alone…and a combination of estrogen plus progestin (a synthetic progesterone-like hormone). A woman who has had a hysterectomy can take estrogen alone. For a woman with an intact uterus, the combination form of HT is given because the progestin protects against uterine cancer. A common side effect of both types of HT is breast tenderness.

Researchers examined the medical records of more than 27,000 postmenopausal participants in a study called the Women's Health Initiative. The women took either estrogen-only HT, combination HT or a placebo for about five to seven years, on average, then were followed up for several more years. They received annual mammograms and breast exams and periodically answered questions about their health and symptoms, including breast tenderness.

Findings: Women whose breasts became tender within a year after starting combination HT were 33% more likely to get invasive breast cancer during the study period than combination HT users who did not develop new breast tenderness. Among women who were already prone to breast tenderness before the start of the study, use of combination HT doubled the risk for breast cancer. However, for women taking estrogen-only HT, no link was found between breast soreness and cancer risk—in fact, women in the estrogen-only group were less likely to develop breast cancer than women in the placebo group.

Explanation: Combination HT use appears to increase breast density (the proportion of glandular or connective tissue to fatty tissue)—and dense breasts are a known risk factor for breast cancer.

Self-defense for women who are using or thinking about starting HT: Alert your doctor to any breast tenderness you may experience and include this factor in your discussion about the risks and benefits of HT...and be extra-sure to get regular mammograms and breast exams.

Surgical Breast Biopsies Overused

Surgical breast biopsies are overutilized, we hear from Stephen Grobmyer, MD. Researchers analyzed data on 172,342 breast biopsies of women with and without breast cancer.

Finding: Thirty percent of the biopsies were surgical as opposed to the less invasive needle biopsy, in which a tissue sample is obtained via a needle and syringe. Current guidelines recommend that only 10% of biopsies should involve surgery.

Theory: Doctors who overrely on surgery, which has a greater risk for infection than needle biopsy, might not have the resources to perform needle biopsies.

If you need a breast biopsy: Seek a doctor who is knowledgeable about surgical and needle biopsy.

Stephen Grobmyer, MD, associate professor of surgical oncology, University of Florida, Gainesville.

Vitamin D Protects Against Breast Cancer

In a recent study, women with the lowest blood levels of vitamin D in the three months before a diagnosis of premenopausal breast cancer had three times as high a risk for the disease as women with the highest vitamin D levels. Women should take at least 1,000 international units (IU) of vitamin D-3 daily.

Cedric F. Garland, DrPH, adjunct professor in the department of family and preventive medicine at University of California, San Diego, and leader of a study of 1,200 women, published online in *Cancer Causes & Control*.

New Key to Surviving Breast Cancer

In a recent study, mid-stage breast cancer patients attended a "psychological intervention program" consisting of 26 counseling sessions in one year. They learned ways to reduce stress, increase social support, improve diet and exercise, and comply with cancer treatment.

Encouraging results: Compared with a control group that did not attend the program, study participants were 45% less likely to have a cancer recurrence and 56% less likely to die from breast cancer during the seven- to 13-year follow-up.

151

If you have cancer: Your doctor or a mental health professional can refer you to a psychological intervention program in your area.

Barbara Andersen, PhD, professor of psychology at the Comprehensive Cancer Center at The Ohio State University in Columbus and leader of a study of 227 patients.

Multivitamins and Breast Cancer Recurrence

Heather Greenlee, ND, PhD, is an assistant professor of epidemiology at the Mailman School of Public Health and an assistant professor of medical oncology at the College of Physicians and Surgeons, both at Columbia University in New York City, and coauthor of a study on multivitamin/mineral use among breast cancer patients.

Any woman who has faced breast cancer wants to do all within her power to prevent a recurrence, of course, and now a recent study suggests a simple step that may be beneficial—taking multivitamin/mineral supplements.

Here's the scoop: 2,239 women who had been diagnosed with early-stage breast cancer between 1997 and 2000 completed questionnaires about their use of multivitamins before and after their diagnoses. By 2010, 363 of the women had had a breast cancer recurrence…202 had died from the disease.

Results: Women who benefited most from taking multivitamin/mineral supplements were those who had radiation to treat their breast cancer. *Details…*

•**Among women who received radiation and chemotherapy,** long-term multivitamin/mineral users (those who took supplements three or more times weekly for at least 12 months in the five years prior to their initial diagnoses and continued after their diagnoses) were about 50% less likely to experience a breast cancer recurrence than women who never took multivitamins.

•**Among women who received radiation treatment only,** long-term users were about 50% less likely to experience a breast cancer recurrence…75% less likely to die from breast cancer…and 46% less likely to die from any cause than women who never took multivitamins.

Using a vitamin product without minerals did not make a difference in cancer recurrence or death rates, though the significance of this result was limited because few participants used that type of multivitamin.

The study does not prove that multivitamins prevent breast cancer recurrence or death—the apparent benefit could be due to the fact that women in the study who took vitamins typically followed a more healthful lifestyle overall. However, researchers noted that, despite the controversial viewpoint that antioxidant supplements may counteract cancer treatment, multivitamin/mineral use did not appear to have any negative effects for these breast cancer patients.

Mighty Mushrooms Combat Breast Cancer

Cynthia Bye, ND, naturopathic physician specializing in complementary cancer care at Journey to Wellness, her private practice in Vancouver, Washington. She is a graduate of the National College of Naturopathic Medicine in Portland, Oregon, a past board member of the American Association of Naturopathic Physicians and a current member of the board of directors of the Ovarian Cancer Alliance of Oregon and Southwest Washington. *www.cynthiabye.com*

Breast cancer. Those two words strike fear into the heart of just about any woman—and with good reason. According to the American Cancer Society, more than 295,000 new cases of breast cancer will be diagnosed in the US in 2014. Such statistics can leave us feeling that it is only a matter of time before breast cancer affects us or someone we love.

Cynthia Bye, ND, a naturopathic doctor based in Vancouver, Washington, often prescribes mushroom extracts for patients who want to be proactive in improving their immune function and reducing their cancer risk. And in fact, a growing body of research suggests that certain mushrooms are powerful weapons in the fight against breast cancer and other cancers. *For instance, various mushrooms...*

• **Contain chemicals (including conjugated linoleic acid) that act as aromatase inhibitors.** Aromatase is an enzyme in fat tissue that converts testosterone to estrogen. Since estrogen fuels many breast tumors, certain mushrooms combat breast cancer by suppressing aromatase activity.

• **Increase apoptosis, the natural programmed death of old, worn-out cells.** This acts as a check against the cells becoming cancerous (since cancer cells proliferate instead of undergoing apoptosis).

• **Stimulate the immune response through the action of beta glucans,** substances that support the production and/or function of various disease-fighting cells, including white blood cells, T-cells and natural killer cells.

• **Simply eating more mushrooms may be good for you**—but for maximum therapeutic effects, consider mushroom extracts.

Reason: The beta glucans are in the mushrooms' cell walls, which you cannot digest. To get the beta glucans, Dr. Bye said, you need mushroom supplements prepared through a process called hot water extraction.

Dr. Bye recommended using mushroom extracts only under the guidance of a naturopathic doctor who is trained in their use, to assure that you receive a formulation specifically tailored to your needs. Mushrooms come in many different varieties—coriolus, crimini, maitake, portobello, reishi, shiitake, white button, etc.—and each has its own distinct health benefits. The extracts best suited to helping a healthy person stay healthy are not the same as those that might be prescribed for a person with compromised immunity...or for a woman at high risk for cancer...or for a woman with a history of breast cancer who wants to reduce the risk for recurrence.

Referrals: American Association of Naturopathic Physicians (866-538-2267, *www.Na turopathic.org*).

Vitamin D Eases Breast Cancer Drug Pain

Antonella Luisa Rastelli, MD, assistant professor of medicine in the section of medical oncology at Washington University School of Medicine in St. Louis, and leader of a study of 60 breast cancer patients.

Drugs called aromatase inhibitors, which are used to treat breast cancer, can make muscles and joints so painful and stiff that some women taking the medications say that they feel like they're 100 years old...many users experience bone loss, too. Yet because the medication is effective at halting breast cancer cell growth, shrinking tumors and reducing recurrence risk when taken for several years or more, discontinuing its use prematurely often is inadvisable.

Recent study: Recognizing that many breast cancer patients have low blood levels of vitamin D, researchers tested a simple potential solution to the problem of drug side effects—vitamin D supplements. For details, we contacted study leader Antonella Luisa Rastelli, MD, an assistant professor of medicine in the section of medical oncology at Washington University School of Medicine in St. Louis.

Participants included 60 early-stage breast cancer patients with low vitamin D levels who had painful side effects from the aromatase inhibitor *anastrozole* (Arimidex). All received a standard daily dose of 400 international units (IU) of vitamin D-3 (the type typically found in supplements) and 1,000 mg of calcium. Half of the participants also received 50,000 IU of vitamin D-2 (a form that leaves the body more quickly than D-3) weekly for eight or 16 weeks, then monthly to the end of the six-month study period. The other half, serving as the control group, got a placebo weekly or monthly.

Results: After two months of weekly supplementation, the high-dose vitamin D groups reported significantly less musculo-skeletal pain than the control group (though pain relief did not continue when partici-pants switched to the monthly regimen).

Also: After six months, the high-dose vi-tamin D users showed no reduction in bone density, whereas the control group did have some bone loss.

Excessive vitamin D can have side effects of its own, including high levels of calcium in the urine that may increase the risk for kidney stones. Risks are thought to be lower with vitamin D-2 than with D-3—but even so, Dr. Rastelli cautioned that all patients tak-ing high-dose vitamin D supplements must be monitored closely, as the study partici-pants were.

What Breast Cancer Patients Need to Know About Alcohol

Marilyn L. Kwan, PhD, research scientist in the di-vision of research at Kaiser Permanente in Oakland, California, and coinvestigator of the Life After Cancer Epidemiology (LACE) Study.

Many experts define moderate drink-ing for women as no more than one serving of alcohol (1.5 ounces of li-quor, four ounces of wine or 12 ounces of beer) per day. However, a recent study pub-lished in the *Journal of Clinical Oncology* suggests that, for breast cancer survivors, even that moderate level of drinking may be too much.

Researchers followed 1,897 early-stage breast cancer patients for an average of 7.4 years, tracking cancer recurrences and deaths.

Findings: Compared with patients who did not drink alcohol, those who consumed at least three to four drinks per week (an average of roughly one-half drink per day or more) were 35% more likely to experience a breast cancer recurrence...and 51% more likely to die of the disease. Recurrence risk was highest among women who were post-menopausal, overweight or obese.

Possible reason: Alcohol increases estro-gen levels, as does obesity, and excess estro-gen is associated with breast cancer.

However: Among study participants, alco-hol was not associated with any increased risk of dying from causes other than breast cancer—in fact, this risk may have been slightly lower among drinkers, possibly due to alcohol's protective effects on cardiovas-cular health.

Bottom line: It is prudent for breast can-cer patients to talk with their doctors about the risks and benefits of consuming alcohol.

The Noncancer Breast Cancer

Irene Wapnir, MD, chief of breast surgery at the Stanford Cancer Institute and an associate professor of surgery at the Stanford University School of Medi-cine, both in California. She also is the co-chair of a multicenter international trial investigating treatment for women who develop a recurrence of breast can-cer after mastectomy or lumpectomy. For information on clinical trials currently recruiting participants, visit *http://med.stanford.edu/profiles/cancer/faculty/ Irene_Wapnir/*.

Patients are confused, and no wonder—because doctors don't even agree on the name, much less on how aggressively to treat the breast condition officially known as ductal carcinoma in situ (DCIS). Some wom-en with DCIS wind up doing nothing, while others opt for extensive surgery and/or years of pharmacological treatment. *Here's why this confounding condition presents such a dilemma...*

DCIS, which develops when genetic mutations occur in the DNA of cells within a milk duct, is generally considered the earliest form of breast cancer. Also called stage 0 breast cancer, it is noninvasive, meaning that the abnormal cells have not spread beyond the milk duct to invade surrounding breast tissue. Because it seldom produces symptoms, it usually is discovered during a routine mammogram. In itself, DCIS is not life-threatening—in fact, some doctors refer to it as precancer rather than cancer.

The concern, of course, is that if these cancer cells do develop the ability to break down the wall of the milk duct and grow, then they will have become invasive cancer—with the potential to spread and be fatal. The local treatments offered to DCIS patients are similar to those for patients with invasive breast cancer. For some women, this may be overtreatment, as their DCIS cells may never develop the capacity to invade or spread. Problem is, as yet there's no way to foretell whose disease will become invasive and whose won't.

We spoke with Irene Wapnir, MD, chief of breast surgery at the Stanford Cancer Institute and a leading breast cancer researcher. Her recent analysis of two long-term studies on the efficacy of various treatments helped bring increased clarity to the question of how to handle DCIS.

An estimated 60,000 US women are diagnosed with DCIS each year. If you are ever among them, remember that DCIS is not an emergency, so you can safely take several weeks or more to investigate your options. *Here are the treatments—from the least to the most aggressive—to discuss with your oncologist…*

•**Lumpectomy** (surgical removal of the abnormal tissue and a surrounding margin of healthy tissue). This preserves the breast, allows a quick recovery and has a minimal effect on appearance. In Dr. Wapnir's study, which followed patients for an average of about 15 years, 19% of DCIS patients who received lumpectomy alone developed subsequent invasive breast cancer. Dr. Wapnir said

that a DCIS patient over age 70 who also has another medical problem that is potentially life-threatening might consider lumpectomy alone rather than lumpectomy plus radiation and *tamoxifen* (described below).

•**Lumpectomy plus radiation.** The goal of radiation is to kill any lingering cancer cells. Compared with lumpectomy alone, the addition of radiation reduced breast cancer recurrence risk by more than half, Dr. Wapnir found. Also, radiation potentially allows for narrower margins—for instance, the surgeon might remove a 1-mm margin of healthy tissue rather than the 2-mm to 5-mm margin recommended with lumpectomy alone—thus allowing superior cosmetic results. *Downside:* Radiation can have long-term side effects at the treatment site, such as skin darkening or thickening and mild shrinkage of breast tissue.

•**Lumpectomy, radiation and tamoxifen.** A "triple therapy" that includes several years of use of the oral drug tamoxifen is appropriate for patients whose DCIS is determined to be hormone receptor positive. The drug blocks the action of estrogen, a hormone that promotes cancer cell growth. Dr. Wapnir found that, compared with lumpectomy plus radiation, triple therapy reduced tumor recurrence by another 32%. *Bonus:* Tamoxifen protects both breasts, not just the DCIS-affected breast…and it reduces the number of new cancers by half, Dr. Wapnir said.

•**Single mastectomy.** Surgically removing the breast with DCIS eliminates nearly all the risk of developing invasive cancer in that breast and also eliminates the need for radiation. However, women may consider mastectomy more disfiguring than lumpectomy…and there is no known survival advantage to mastectomy. Dr. Wapnir said that mastectomy makes most sense for women whose DCIS is large (more than 5 cm) or in multiple sites in the breast. Alternatively, she added, some women may choose mastectomy due to personal preference or because they wish to avoid radiation or tamoxifen therapy.

• **Double mastectomy.** According to a study from the University of Minnesota, the number of patients opting to remove the healthy breast as well as the DCIS-affected breast has soared since 1998. For women at extremely high risk for invasive breast cancer—for instance, because they carry a BRCA breast cancer gene mutation—it may be reasonable to consider this approach to prevention. But otherwise, Dr. Wapnir said, physicians should take care not to foster patients' fears by overemphasizing the dangers of DCIS and thus subjecting women to double mastectomy for a condition that may never become life-threatening.

Bottom line: For most DCIS patients, breast-conserving lumpectomy plus radiation (and tamoxifen, when appropriate) would be Dr. Wapnir's treatment of choice. In her study, fewer than 1% of the 2,612 participants who underwent lumpectomy, with or without radiation and/or tamoxifen, ended up dying as a result of breast cancer recurrence—a very reassuring statistic.

For help making treatment decisions: A second opinion is always a good idea. To find a National Cancer Institute-designated comprehensive cancer center, check *http://CancerCenters.cancer.gov*.

Love Your Post-Cancer Breasts

Frank J. DellaCroce, MD, cofounder of the Center for Restorative Breast Surgery and the St. Charles Surgical Hospital (a hospital dedicated to breast reconstruction), both in New Orleans. A pioneer of the nipple-sparing mastectomy and stacked flap breast reconstruction techniques, Dr. DellaCroce also is an honorary board member of the Susan G. Komen for the Cure foundation and an American Cancer Society Spirit Award Honoree. *www.BreastCenter.com*

Two recent surgical breakthroughs provide good news and new options for breast reconstruction after mastectomy. If a loved one is facing breast cancer surgery, please pass along this information.

Don't assume she already knows—sadly, only 30% of patients are fully informed about their options for reconstruction prior to their breast cancer surgery, according to a study from the University of Michigan.

For details on these surgical advances, we contacted Frank J. DellaCroce, MD, cofounder of the Center for Restorative Breast Surgery in New Orleans, who pioneered the new techniques. *Here's what women should know about...*

• **Nipple-sparing mastectomy.** Traditionally, mastectomy has meant surgical removal of the entire breast...and reconstruction has included the need to rebuild a nipple by grafting skin from elsewhere and tattooing the area to simulate the areola (the colored ring around the nipple). However, with the new nipple-sparing mastectomy (NSM), the surgeon preserves the breast skin and nipple area while removing the underlying breast tissue, including the cancer, through a small incision below the nipple. This is immediately followed with breast reconstruction using either an implant, a "flap" procedure (described below) or another technique to fill the pocket of breast skin—so the woman leaves the operating room with the cancer gone and the reconstructed breast already in place.

While no reconstruction technique can guarantee a breast that looks exactly as it did before surgery, NSM minimizes scarring... provides optimal cosmetic results...and helps women feel more "whole" after surgery, Dr. DellaCroce said. (For before-and-after photos, visit *www.BreastCenter.com/nipple-sparing-mastectomy.php* and click on "Photo Album.") After NSM, sensation in the nipple may be reduced or eliminated, but results vary and many women report a substantial return of touch sensation in the months after surgery. What about the risk for cancer recurrence? "All studies to date, from multiple institutions, have shown equal cure rates with preservation of the nipple as compared with techniques that sacrifice it," said Dr. DellaCroce.

Who can benefit?: While candidates for NSM must be evaluated case by case, the procedure generally is most appropriate for women who have relatively small areas of cancer that are a safe distance away from the nipple, Dr. DellaCroce said. NSM also may be considered when a woman opts to undergo prophylactic mastectomy because she is at very high risk for breast cancer due to a BRCA gene mutation.

●**Stacked flap.** To understand the new "stacked" procedure, you first need to know about the standard deep inferior epigastric perforator flap breast reconstruction technique. With the standard procedure, a flap of complete tissue—blood vessels, skin and fat—is taken from the abdominal area beneath the breast and used as a "donor" to reconstruct a breast of soft, warm, living tissue. But this may not work well for thin women who are full-breasted, as they may not have adequate abdominal tissue to reconstitute their breast volume, Dr. DellaCroce said. In such women, breast implants may be used to supplement the abdominal donor tissue—but implants can lead to complications, such as painful capsular contracture (hardening of tissue), which may require removal of the implant.

This is where the new stacked flap technique comes in—because it enables even thin women to have implant-free reconstruction using only their own natural tissue (without sacrificing abdominal muscle, as some other reconstruction techniques require). The procedure stacks two layers of abdominal fat under the preserved skin envelope by carefully connecting the blood vessels between them using microsurgery, Dr. DellaCroce explained. This allows for full restoration of volume in the new breast.

Who can benefit?: Thin women undergoing mastectomy who prefer not to use implants...and women who have had radiation treatment to the breast, for whom implants generally are not appropriate because of the likelihood of severe capsular contracture. "The stacked flap may be performed at the same time that mastectomy is performed. Or if mastectomy has already been done, the stacked flap can serve as a wonderful way to recreate a breast out of soft, living tissue

Better Breast Cancer Treatment

An analysis of 17 randomized trials involving 10,801 women found that those who had breast-conserving surgery plus radiation had a 10-year recurrence rate of 19.3%, compared with 35% in the group that received surgery but no radiation. Risk for death after 15 years was 21.4% in the radiation group and 25.2% in the nonradiation group. This means that one death is prevented for every four recurrences.

Sarah C. Darby, PhD, professor of medical statistics, University of Oxford, UK.

at any point at which the patient is ready to proceed with restoration," Dr. DellaCroce said.

Finding a surgeon: Because NSM and stacked flap procedures are so new, you will need to hunt to locate a surgeon experienced with the technique you are interested in. To start, get referrals from the American Society of Plastic Surgeons (*www.PlasticSurgery.org*), then interview several candidates. Dr. DellaCroce recommended choosing a surgeon who confirms that he or she has done at least one per week for a full year of the procedure you're considering and whose success rate exceeds 95%. Also, ask to see photos of the surgeon's work...and get contact information for several patients who have undergone the same procedure so you can ask them about their experiences.

Having the option of reconstruction can be an important facet in a patient's full recovery. Dr. DellaCroce said, "When you lose some component of your physical self, you also lose some of your emotional self. To have the breast rebuilt erases some of the injury of a very difficult event." And that makes the victory of surviving breast cancer all the sweeter.

Radiation Has Little Benefit for Some Older Breast Cancer Patients

About 75% of women age 70 and older with early-stage breast cancer receive radiation therapy, even though the National Cancer Institute (NCI) recommends breast-conserving surgery followed by optional radiation. Because many older women have less aggressive tumors, the NCI guidelines were changed after a large clinical trial found that radiation had little benefit for these patients. Radiation also can cause local skin irritation and, in rare cases, pain and fatigue.

Cary P. Gross, MD, associate professor of medicine, Yale University School of Medicine, New Haven, Connecticut.

Chemo Without Hair Loss?

A "cold cap" allowed breast cancer patients to undergo chemo without losing their hair. During chemo sessions, patients wore the silicone cap, which circulates a coolant that brings the scalp's temperature down to 42°F.

Theory: The cap constricts blood flow to hair follicles and reduces exposure to the chemo chemicals. More than 3,000 women in Europe and Asia have used the cap, and about 80% did not suffer significant hair loss. The cap has not yet been approved in the US. However, the Penguin Cold Cap, which uses frozen packs to cool the scalp, can be rented for $580 a month (316-243-4946, *www.MSC-Worldwide.com/indexusa.html*). Insurance does not cover the cost.

Susan Melin, MD, associate professor of hematology and oncology, Wake Forest University School of Medicine, Winston-Salem, North Carolina.

Stress Fuels Cancer Spread

In laboratory studies, stress was shown to increase the spread (metastasis) of breast cancer cells to the bone. Stress-reducing therapies appear to decrease levels of a molecule that promotes cell migration.

PLOS Biology

Denser Breasts May Increase Risk for Aggressive Tumors

Using mammogram data, researchers measured the breast density of 1,042 breast cancer patients (average age 60), comparing them with 1,794 healthy women.

Result: Women whose breast density exceeded 50% had more than three times higher risk for breast cancer than those with less than 10% density.

Also: Greater breast density was associated with more aggressive tumors. The link between breast density and cancer is not yet fully understood.

Rulla May Tamimi, ScD, assistant professor of medicine, Harvard Medical School, Boston.

But...

Women with dense breasts are no more likely to die from breast cancer than women whose breasts are not dense. Recent research shows that dense breasts can make mammograms harder to interpret, but they do not increase risk for premature death.

Gretchen Gierach, PhD, investigator, National Cancer Institute, Bethesda, Maryland, and leader of a study of 9,232 women, published in *Journal of the National Cancer Institute*.

Breast Implants Linked to a Rare Cancer

About 60 women with silicone or saline breast implants have developed anaplastic large cell lymphoma (ALCL). As many as 10 million women have received implants, so any disease risk is very low, but removing the implants will eliminate the risk.

Self-defense: See your doctor if you develop persistent swelling or pain around the implant. Symptoms usually appear many years after implantation—eight years, on average, and as long as 23 years.

William Maisel, MD, MPH, chief scientist, Center for Devices and Radiological Health, Food and Drug Administration, Silver Spring, Maryland.

Aspirin Fights Breast Cancer

After breast cancer patients receive standard treatment, taking aspirin at least two days a week reduces the risk for having the disease spread by as much as 60%...and risk for death from the disease by as much as 71%. Aspirin and other nonsteroidal anti-inflammatory drugs (NSAIDs) block Cox-2, which has been linked to metastasis of the disease. Further clinical trials are needed to confirm the results.

Michelle D. Holmes, MD, DrPH, associate professor of medicine at Harvard Medical School and associate physician at Brigham and Women's Hospital, both in Boston, and leader of a study of 4,164 women, published in *Journal of Clinical Oncology*.

Estrogen Reduces Breast Cancer Risk for Some Menopausal Women

Recent finding: Women who had a hysterectomy and then took estrogen for six years by itself—not in combination with progestin—had a 23% lower risk for breast cancer than women taking placebos. They also were less likely to die from breast cancer. And those in their 50s had fewer deaths and heart attacks.

Study by researchers at University Hospital of South Manchester and Queen Mary University of London, published in *The Lancet Oncology*.

Surgery Reduces Cancer Risk

More evidence that breast and ovary removal reduces cancer risk for women at high risk for breast and ovarian cancer. For women with the BRCA-1 or BRCA-2 mutations, which increase risk for both types of cancer, surgery is more effective than rigorous screening.

Recent study: Four years after preventive double mastectomy, none of the high-risk women developed breast cancer...but 7% who had intensive screening without surgery did. Only 1% of women at high risk for ovarian cancer who had at least one ovary and fallopian tube removed developed the disease, versus 6% of women who did not have the surgery.

Claudine Isaacs, MD, medical director of cancer assessment and risk evaluation program, Georgetown Lombardi Comprehensive Cancer Center, Washington, DC, and coauthor of a study of 2,482 women at 22 cancer centers in the US and Europe, published in *The Journal of the American Medical Association*.

Something That Can Be Skipped

Some breast cancer patients can skip complete lymph-node removal, we hear from Monica Morrow, MD, FACS.

Recent finding: Node removal, which carries a risk of arm swelling and numbness, does not improve survival in many patients with Stage 1 breast cancer and Stage 2 breast cancer with involved nodes. Following a lumpectomy and sentinel node removal, chemotherapy and radiation treatment generally kill any disease in remaining nodes. Talk to your doctor.

Monica Morrow, MD, FACS, is chief of breast service, department of surgery, Memorial Sloan-Kettering Cancer Center, New York City, and author of a study published in *The Journal of the American Medical Association*.

Super Vitamin!

Vitamin D can prevent cancers of the breast and colon, as well as multiple sclerosis and type 1 diabetes, says Cedric F. Garland, DrPH. Ask your doctor to test your level of 25-hydroxy vitamin D to establish your baseline. If it is below 40 nanograms/milliliter, talk to your doctor about vitamin D-3 supplements totaling 4,000 IU/day. After three months, have the test done again. Under a doctor's care, it should be safe to take up to 8,000 IU daily.

Cedric F. Garland, DrPH, professor, division of epidemiology, department of family and preventive medicine at University of California at San Diego, and leader of a study of the effects of vitamin D, published in *Anticancer Research*.

Radiation After Lumpectomy

Radiation after lumpectomy benefits breast cancer patients, reports Sarah Darby, PhD.

Recent finding: Radiotherapy after the removal of a malignant lump reduces the risk for breast cancer recurrence within the next 10 years by 16%.

Sarah Darby, PhD, professor of medical statistics at Nuffield Department of Clinical Medicine, University of Oxford, England, and coauthor of an analysis of 17 studies involving 10,801 women, published in *The Lancet*.

An Antibody That Shrinks Cancer Tumors Has Been Found

It is effective in fighting seven cancers, including cancers of the breast, colon and prostate. The antibody blocks a protein that cancer cells use to signal immune system cells not to kill them. It will be tested on humans within two years.

Study by researchers at Stanford University School of Medicine, published in *Proceedings of the National Academy of Sciences*.

Better Drug for Breast Cancer

Postmenopausal women with breast cancer do better with the drug *letrozole* (Femara) than *tamoxifen*.

Recent study: Women who had early-stage breast cancer who took *letrozole* were 21% less likely to die than women who took *tamoxifen* during the eight-year follow-up period, which included five years of treatment.

Meredith M. Regan, ScD, biostatistician at Dana-Farber Cancer Institute and associate professor of medicine at Harvard Medical School, both in Boston. She is lead author of a study of 8,010 postmenopausal women, published in *The Lancet Oncology*.

Change in Breast Density Can Predict Cancer

Celia Byrne, PhD, assistant professor in department of oncology, associate director of the Clinical and Molecular Epidemiology Shared Resource at the Lombardi Cancer Center, Georgetown University, Washington, DC.

Nowadays women are far less eager to undergo hormone therapy for severe menopause symptoms than they used to be...and with good reason. We now know that it brings a variety of consequences, including an increased risk for breast cancer. New research has pinned down the reason for that increased risk and also provides a way for women to monitor whether they're nearing the danger zone.

It all has to do with breast density. Whereas it's normal for menopause to bring about a decline in breast density, the opposite occurs when a woman is taking synthetic hormones such as Premarin and progestin, which can propel things in the other direction—density increases, which it appears is what raises a woman's risk for breast cancer.

Why Denser Breasts Are Dangerous

The link between breast density and breast cancer has already been documented. But the study's lead author, Celia Byrne, PhD, an assistant professor in the department of oncology at the Lombardi Cancer Center of Georgetown University, said that this study has now found an association between hormone therapy and breast density.

Dr. Byrne and her colleagues compared breast density in postmenopausal women taking estrogen and progestin therapy with those not taking the hormones. The study, which was presented at the April 2010 meeting of the American Association of Cancer Research, evaluated the women's baseline and one-year follow-up mammograms.

Results: Among the women with the greatest increase in breast density in the group taking hormones, breast cancer risk more than tripled...while in women with the smallest increase in breast density, risk rose by 20%.

Density Should Be Monitored

According to Dr. Byrne, the most important point we can use right now is that women taking hormone therapy should be sure that their breast density is closely monitored. While this therapy is most often given to women with severe menopausal symptoms,

Dr. Byrne said in most cases women need it for only a short period of time. Noting that risk increases even in such a short period as two years, Dr. Byrne suggests having a discussion with your doctor as to what might be appropriate for you and your health. Within three to four months after stopping hormone therapy, breast density typically decreases—bringing down the risk for breast cancer as well.

Breast Implants: Still Questions About Safety

William Maisel, MD, deputy director for science and chief scientist, Center for Devices and Radiological Health, US Food and Drug Administration, Silver Spring, Maryland.

The ongoing debate about the long-term safety of silicone breast implants—which were removed from the US market from 1992 to 2006 (except for breast reconstruction or to replace existing ones)—has reared up again. It was revealed this year that two long-term studies currently addressing the issue have, so far, analyzed only a fraction of the women that they were supposed to be following. The FDA, which regulates the silicone breast implants as medical devices, concluded in August 2011 that they are safe when used as intended. But maybe the more accurate characterization would be: safe enough—as far as we know.

Why the Sudden Worry?

There are two brands of silicone gel-filled breast implants on the market in the US—one is made by a company called Allergan and the other is made by Mentor Corporation. Data on how well women with these implants fare over the long term (for 10 years or longer) is scarce. So when the FDA approved the devices for use in 2006, there was a condition: Each company was required to begin a 10-year study of safety data on

40,000 women who got their silicone gel-filled implants between 2006 and 2016. In 2011—when both companies were supposed to be halfway done with their research—the FDA held a two-day meeting in Washington, DC, to get an update on their progress... and it was not so impressive.

Over the five years, Allergan had collected survey data on only 60% of the women that it was supposed to be following, and Mentor Corporation's patient response rate was even worse—a mere 21%. Therefore many fewer women are being studied than expected. One main problem is that women who were interested in participating in these studies were being asked to complete a massive, 27-page questionnaire each year following surgery.

Making Sense of the Data (Or Lack Thereof)

Silicone implants are quite popular. In fact, in 2010, about 150,000 women got them in the US for cosmetic reasons. Many women obviously feel that the benefits outweigh the risks (or lack of scientific data). William Maisel, MD, deputy director for science and chief scientist with the FDA's Center for Devices and Radiological Health in Silver Spring, Maryland, offered his views on the safety of implants.

Risks vs. Benefits

Many medical devices and drugs that are FDA-approved, as we all know, carry serious risks. In the case of breast implants, Dr. Maisel readily acknowledged that they can cause problems that include scarring, pain, infection, a hardening of the tissue around them, and even rupturing—which can cause silicone to leak into a woman's body (that's one of the reasons that they were removed from the market in 1992). Past research shows that the longer a woman has implants, the more likely she is to experience complications. In fact, one in five women who chooses to get implants for cosmetic reasons will likely need to have them removed within 10

years! But all of those risks are old news and not enough to make the FDA keep silicone implants off the market.

"Not every patient is the same, which is why we always encourage patients to talk to their doctors," said Dr. Maisel. After all, there is evidence supporting patient happiness, too. In the FDA's recent review of research, it found studies that showed that more than 90% of women with silicone implants are satisfied. Plus, body image improves in the majority of women who receive silicone implants, and this feeling lasts for at least two years post-implant. "Based on the total scientific data available right now, we believe that implants are safe and effective," said Dr. Maisel.

Although there is a little bit of long-term data, the thorough research that we thought we were going to have in a few years from Allergan and Mentor Corporation doesn't seem likely to provide the big-picture information that doctors were hoping it would. So what's a woman who is considering getting silicone implants supposed to do, since aspects of the implants' long-term safety are still largely unknown (and may be for a while)?

Simply put: It depends on how much of a risk-taker you are. Are there other implant options to consider getting? Besides silicone, the only other type of implant on the market is saline, but "saline implants have a similar risk profile," said Dr. Maisel.

If you already have silicone implants, said Dr. Maisel, keep a close eye on them and schedule follow-up appointments with your doctor. The FDA recommends that you have periodic MRI scans (three years after your surgery and then every two years after that) to help detect "silent ruptures" that you may not be able to feel. So talk to your doctor about scheduling those tests—especially since Dr. Maisel said that many doctors don't tell patients about this MRI recommendation. Maybe it's because MRIs aren't cheap: An MRI could set you back $2,000 or more—and insurance may or may not cover any of the cost.

Also: Notify your doctor if you develop any unusual symptoms, like pain, asymmetry, lumps, hardness or swelling, because it could mean that your implants have become defective—and you may need to have them removed or replaced.

Shorter Course of Radiation for Breast Cancer

Timothy J. Whelan, BM, BCh, professor and head of the radiation therapy program at the Juravinski Cancer Centre at McMaster University in Hamilton, Ontario, and leader of a study of 1,234 breast cancer patients.

Early-stage breast cancer patients often undergo radiation after a lumpectomy to reduce the risk for recurrence.

Recent study: One group of patients received the standard 25 sessions of radiation, at the typical dose, over 35 days…a second group received 16 sessions of higher-dose radiation over 22 days. Both groups received the same total dose overall and experienced similar side effects during treatment.

Results: Both groups had nearly identical five-year survival rates (96.8% in the standard group and 97.2% in the short-course group)…and approximately the same 10-year recurrence rates (6.7% in the standard group and 6.2% in the short-course group). Radiation toxicity and adverse cosmetic effects (skin changes, breast tissue firmness), were uncommon and were similar in both groups.

Summary: A shorter course of radiation can be more convenient and cost less than the standard course—so ask your oncologist about both treatment options. But note that short-course radiation may not be best for all patients…for instance, women with large breasts are more likely to experience adverse cosmetic effects.

Not All Breast Cancer Radiation Is Created Equal

Benjamin Smith, MD, assistant professor of radiation oncology, The University of Texas MD Anderson Cancer Center, Houston.

Women with early-stage breast cancer who need to undergo lumpectomy must choose one of three types of radiation. If you're ever faced with this difficult decision, weigh your options carefully, because a recent study shows that depending on the type of radiation you choose, the odds of the cancer returning and your having to get a mastectomy can be very different.

One kind, called intraoperative radiation therapy, can be performed during the lumpectomy, but it has yet to gain widespread implementation in the US (there is some data supporting its use, but it's considered controversial). A more traditional approach is whole-breast radiation, which radiates the entire breast after the lumpectomy. The third technique is brachytherapy. Also performed after the lumpectomy, this partial breast radiation delivers a targeted dose of radiation only to and around the tumor(s) through an implanted catheter. Brachytherapy is often an option, though not always, because the tumor has to have a certain geometry to allow for safe placement of the catheter.

To discuss the pros and cons of each type of breast cancer radiation, we called the study's lead author, Benjamin Smith, MD, assistant professor of radiation oncology at The University of Texas MD Anderson Cancer Center in Houston—and he said that even he was surprised by what his study discovered.

Two Types of Treatment

Dr. Smith spoke further about the two main kinds of radiation—whole breast and brachytherapy—and why a woman might choose one over the other. Approved by the FDA in 2002, brachytherapy definitely has its advantages.

While whole-breast radiation typically requires daily hospital visits for three to seven weeks, brachytherapy can be done twice a day over about one week—a big benefit for many women, including those with work or child-care schedules that are hard to alter and older women who are perhaps less mobile than their younger counterparts, Dr. Smith said. This added convenience surely factors into the therapy's increasing popularity.

Which Is More Effective?

Dr. Smith said that his research, which he presented in December 2011 at the San Antonio Breast Cancer Symposium, was the first to amass data comparing whole-breast radiation with brachytherapy from across the US and that it included more women who underwent brachytherapy than any prior study. He and his colleagues looked at the Medicare records of 130,535 women who were all over the age of 66, had been diagnosed with early-stage breast cancer, and had undergone a lumpectomy and then either brachytherapy or whole-breast radiation. (Intraoperative radiation therapy was not part of this study.)

The vast majority of women in the study chose to undergo whole-breast radiation—only about 7,300 of them (or about 6% of them) chose brachytherapy. But of those 7,300 women, the researchers found that 4% of them had mastectomies in the following five years…compared with only 2.2% of the women who chose whole-breast radiation. While the mastectomy percentages in both groups were small, the difference does represent nearly double the risk of having to have a mastectomy within five years of having brachytherapy. When Dr. Smith and his team plucked out only the women who had mastectomies because their cancer had returned (not due to side effects like, say, a radiation burn), they still had double the risk.

So why doesn't brachytherapy appear to be as effective? Since it treats only the tumor and about a centimeter around it, rogue cancer cells lurking in another part of the breast—while uncommon—may be missed, Dr. Smith said.

In terms of complication rates, brachytherapy also didn't fare well. Nearly 16% of women treated with brachytherapy experienced a complication after their procedure, compared with 8% in the whole-breast radiation group. And the infection rates were 16%, versus 10%, respectively. But the complication and infection rates didn't surprise Dr. Smith. "When you have a catheter implanted in your breast, there is a real risk that bacteria will enter the body, especially if patients, physicians and the nursing staff do not pay meticulous attention to keeping the catheter clean," said Dr. Smith.

It's Your Decision

This study certainly suggests that whole-breast radiation has several advantages compared with brachytherapy. But, since life is far from simple, other factors may make brachytherapy the best choice for some women—even those who learn about these statistics, said Dr. Smith. "Some patients might feel that a 4% return rate of cancer is still quite low, and they might be delighted to choose brachytherapy and do one week of radiation rather than suffering through three to seven weeks of it," he said. "But other patients may want to do everything in their power to give themselves the highest chance for a cure—or the idea of having a catheter implanted in their chest, which is more invasive, might really concern them, so those women might opt for whole-breast radiation."

Brachytherapy is still somewhat new, said Dr. Smith, so large, long-term studies haven't been performed until now. As more data emerges, doctors will have an even clearer picture of the benefits and risks.

Chapter 9

LOWER YOUR RISK OF COLORECTAL CANCER

Best Ways to Prevent Colon Cancer

As many as seven out of 10 cases of colorectal cancer could be prevented. While a few risk factors can't be helped—risk rises with age, a personal history of inflammatory bowel disease and/or colorectal adenomas (precancerous polyps), or a family history of adenomas or colorectal cancer—simple steps provide significant protection. *What the studies suggest…*

1. Get screened. A doctor inserts a thin flexible tube with a tiny camera into the colon via the rectum to detect and remove adenomas and cancerous growths.

Problem: Only 43% of US women get the recommended screening.

Best: Get screened every five to 10 years starting at age 50. If you're at elevated risk, ask your doctor about starting earlier.

2. Boost vitamin D. This may inhibit the growth of tumors and the blood vessels that feed them. Many doctors recommend taking at least 1,000 international units (IU) daily.

3. Eat folate-rich foods—cruciferous and dark green leafy vegetables, beans, peas and citrus fruits. Folate promotes DNA replication and repair.

4. Cut back on meat. Increasing consumption of red meat (beef, pork) and processed meat (cold cuts, hot dogs) by four ounces per day boosts colorectal cancer risk by about 28% and 36%, respectively.

Possible culprits: Iron, a pro-oxidant that damages DNA…growth-promoting hormones fed to the animals…carcinogenic compounds created during cooking or processing. Limit red and processed meat to two servings weekly.

5. Limit alcohol. Colorectal cancer is 41% more common among women who consume three or more drinks daily than among nondrinkers. Alcohol may reduce the body's stores of folate.

Best: Have no more than one drink per day.

6. Don't smoke. In a study of 469,019 women, colorectal cancer deaths were about

---

JoAnn E. Manson, MD, DrPH, professor of medicine and women's health at Harvard Medical School and chair of the division of preventive medicine at Brigham and Women's Hospital, both in Boston. She is one of the lead investigators for two highly influential studies on women's health—the Harvard Nurses' Health Study and the Women's Health Initiative. Dr. Manson is author, with Shari Bassuk, ScD, of *Hot Flashes, Hormones & Your Health* (McGraw-Hill).

33% to 51% more common among current smokers who had smoked for 20 years or more than among women who never smoked. The sooner you quit, the sooner your risk will fall. For help, visit *www.smokefree.gov.*

7. Watch your weight. More than 20% of colorectal cancers in US women are due to excess pounds, which contribute to insulin resistance (inability of cells to properly use the hormone insulin), inflammation and overgrowth of cells lining the gut.

8. Move your body. Exercise helps balance levels of insulin and other hormones. It also speeds passage of food and bile salts through the gut, possibly shortening the exposure of intestinal walls to potential carcinogens.

Wise: Exercise 30 minutes or more daily.

9. Consider a daily aspirin. This may reduce colorectal cancer risk when taken at 325 mg daily for 10 years or more. However, aspirin also increases risk for gastrointestinal bleeding—so talk to your doctor about the benefits and risks.

Foods That Fight Colon Cancer

Jung Han Yoon Park, PhD, professor in the department of food, science and nutrition at Hallym University in Chuncheon, South Korea.

Have you ever heard of a nutrient called *luteolin*? It's one of the lesser-known flavonoids, chemical compounds that are found in many vegetables and herbs.

Jung Han Yoon Park, PhD, a professor of nutrition in South Korea recently led a study that showed luteolin's ability to stop colon cancer cells in their tracks. This is potentially big news.

Stopping Cancer in Its Tracks

Dr. Park and her colleagues were eager to study luteolin because colon cancer cells—unlike many other cancer cells—are continually exposed to the foods we eat. Previous studies, she said, had showed that luteolin could cause colon cancer cells to die, but no one knew how it did that. She and her colleagues wanted to find out. Additionally, while they wouldn't expect this to happen, they wanted to make sure that luteolin didn't also cause normal, healthy intestinal cells to die in the process.

Researchers conducted a petri dish study and created three groups. One group contained human colon cancer cells and luteolin...the second group contained human colon cancer cells alone...and the third group contained noncancerous intestinal epithelial cells from rats (because it's difficult to culture healthy human intestinal cells) and luteolin.

The researchers were looking to see whether luteolin affected cancerous and noncancerous cells—and more importantly, how. The results were clear after only one day. By counting the number of cells in the dishes, the researchers found that, as expected, human colon cancer cells that were exposed to luteolin stopped multiplying, while human cancer cells that were not exposed to luteolin kept multiplying. And noncancerous intestinal epithelial cells from rats were not adversely affected by luteolin, which was great news.

So how did plain old luteolin—remember, it's just a natural part of vegetables—have such a large impact on the human colon cancer cells? With more analysis, the researchers discovered that luteolin interfered with an insulin-like growth factor (IGF). Dr. Park said that the study was so encouraging that researchers are expected to test the effect of luteolin on live animals with colon cancer, probably mice. If that goes well, human tests will quickly follow.

Eat It Up

But there's no need to wait for further studies to be done to eat foods containing luteolin, said Dr. Park—especially if you have colon cancer or are at high risk for it. You're probably eating at least a little bit of it already, and there's no harm in eating more by increasing your intake of certain foods and herbs. Parsley and thyme are unusually rich in luteolin (containing more than 50 milligrams per 100 grams). Foods that have 10 to 50 milligrams per 100 grams include peppermint leaves and rutabagas. And others that have small amounts of luteolin include chives, artichokes, broccoli, carrots, peppers (both hot and sweet), beets, Brussels sprouts, cabbage, cauliflower, lettuce, apple skins, basil, chamomile tea and spinach.

Dr. Park said that taking a luteolin supplement right now isn't recommended because more studies need to be done to establish a safe dosage.

Researchers don't yet know how much luteolin-rich food one would have to eat for it to be beneficial, but Dr. Park said, don't be shy about it—fill up your plate because you aren't going to get too much luteolin from food. Because luteolin isn't affected by heat, she said, it doesn't matter whether you eat the vegetables raw or cooked. So serve them up any way you like!

Eat This to Reduce Colon Polyps by 33%

Harvey J. Murff, MD, MPH, associate professor of medicine, Vanderbilt University School of Medicine, Nashville, and leader of a study published online in *American Journal of Clinical Nutrition*.

You don't need to be reminded that it's important to get a periodic colonoscopy starting at age 50 (even earlier if you're at high risk for colon cancer). You already know that's an important way to detect the deadly disease early so that you can treat it quickly and prevent it from advancing.

The great news is that there's something else that women can do to lower their odds of dying from colon cancer—and even reduce the chance of developing it in the first place, according to a recent study.

And it's a lot more enjoyable than getting a colonoscopy! It involves eating a delicious food…

Protection from Polyps

Are you ready to find out what this cancer buster is? It's fish! Salmon, sardines and other oily cold water fish rich in omega-3 fatty acids have been shown to promote brain power, heart health, eye health, clearer skin…and now we can add "may prevent colon cancer" to that list. So we called the researchers to find out why fish may help and how much you need to eat to get the extra protection.

To study the effect of fish on colon health, researchers recruited more than 5,300 men and women between 40 and 75 years old who underwent colonoscopies. After the test, participants—some with polyps and others without polyps (the control group)—answered questions about their diets, general health habits and medical history.

After factoring in variables such as age, race, body mass index and smoking, researchers found that women, in particular, who consumed the most fish (at least three servings a week) were 33% less likely to develop potentially cancerous colon polyps called adenomas than women who ate the least fish (one-half serving or less a week). However, among men, the researchers found no association between eating fish and a reduced risk for potentially cancerous polyps.

While these results don't prove that eating fish definitely prevents colon cancer among women, they do show a strong association, and that is a strong indication that eating fish might help.

Why Fish Helps Females

To discuss why fish may have this effect—and why it has this effect only on women—we spoke to lead study author Harvey J. Murff, MD, MPH, an associate professor of medicine at Vanderbilt University School of Medicine in Nashville.

Healthful omega-3 fatty acids in fish may be what reduce polyp risk because they reduce inflammation throughout the body, including in the colon, Dr. Murff said. But he readily concedes that he and his colleagues were puzzled to see this effect only in women.

He speculates that it may be due to men's diets overall. In the dietary surveys, compared to women, men consumed higher levels of omega-6 fatty acids, which are commonly found in foods such as meat, grains and processed foods, and those can offset the positive impact of omega-3s.

Another possible reason for the disparity: Biological differences between men and women. For example, men and women metabolize fatty acids differently due to having different balances of hormones.

We asked Dr. Murff whether the fact that all women studied were over 40 (and therefore likely either perimenopausal or menopausal) potentially had something to do with the findings. "We are analyzing the data to see whether that made a difference, so we're not sure yet," he said.

Go Fish

Whether you're a man or a woman, you can't go wrong by including more omega-3s in your diet, said Dr. Murff. The American Heart Association recommends eating fish rich in omega-3s at least twice a week, and this study suggests that three servings a week may be even better.

So fill your plate with fish such as salmon, mackerel, herring, lake trout, sardines and albacore tuna. While this study did not examine cooking methods, steaming, baking and broiling are healthier ways to prepare your fish than frying or grilling. You can also get omega-3 fatty acids from nonfish foods, such as flaxseed, walnuts, soybeans and canola oil. Dr. Murff said that getting omega-3s through food is ideal, but if you're interested in taking a fish oil or krill oil supplement, talk to your doctor.

Calcium and Colon Cancer...

In a seven-year study of more than 490,000 adults, women who consumed the most calcium (1,881 mg daily, on average) were 23% less likely to develop cancers of the digestive system (such as colorectal or stomach cancer) than those who consumed the least calcium. Men who consumed the most calcium (1,530 mg daily, on average) had a 16% lower risk.

Self-defense: Aim to eat several servings daily of calcium-rich foods (such as low-fat dairy products, leafy green vegetables, navy beans and calcium-fortified orange juice) and/or take a calcium supplement.

Yikyung Park, ScD, staff scientist, National Cancer Institute, Bethesda, Maryland.

More on Calcium

People with variations in one of two genes have a 39% lower risk for precancerous colon and rectal lesions if they consume at least 1,000 milligrams of calcium a day from food and supplements. People with variations in both genes reduced their risk by 69%.

Caution: Some studies have linked high calcium consumption to increased risk for other health problems. Talk to your doctor.

Xiangzhu Zhu, MD, MPH, staff scientist, division of epidemiology, Vanderbilt Epidemiology Center, Nashville, and leader of a study of 5,810 people, presented at a recent meeting of the American Association for Cancer Research.

Magnesium Reduces Risk for Colon Cancer

For every 100-milligram-per-day increase in magnesium from food (the amount in about one cup of beans or two potatoes), the risk for colon polyps dropped by 19%. Foods high in magnesium include wheat bran, nuts, spinach, soybeans, white potatoes, pinto beans, brown rice, lentils and bananas.

Study of 1,477 people by researchers at Imperial College London, published in *Tufts University Health & Nutrition Letter.*

How to Eat Meat Without Risking Your Health

Barry Popkin, PhD, Carla Smith Chamblee Distinguished Professor in the department of nutrition at the University of North Carolina Gillings School of Global Public Health in Chapel Hill. He is author of *The World Is Fat: The Fads, Trends, Policies and Products That Are Fattening the Human Race* (Avery).

For years, a growing body of scientific evidence has linked diets that contain excessive amounts of red and/or processed meats to health problems ranging from heart disease and cancer (especially of the colon) to diabetes.

Landmark findings: A National Institutes of Health (NIH)-AARP study of about 500,000 adults ages 50 to 71 found that those who ate the most red meat (five ounces daily, on average) had a 30% higher risk for death—mostly from heart disease or cancer—than those who ate the least (two-thirds ounce daily, on average). Those who ate the most processed meat (about one-and-one-half ounces daily) had a 20% higher risk for death than those who ate the least.

In addition, researchers who analyzed data from the Women's Health Study (of about 37,000 women) found that those who ate at least five servings of processed meat (mostly bacon and hot dogs) a week for nine years were 38% more likely to develop diabetes than those who had less than one serving weekly.

Yet scientists point out that it is possible that other factors were responsible for the meat eaters' increased health risks. For example, people who eat little meat may eat large amounts of fruits and vegetables, and those nutrients—not the lack of meat—may be what protects them against heart disease.

Ultimately, you don't have to swear off meat entirely to have a healthful diet. *But before you sharpen the steak knives, consider these six secrets to enjoying meat while staying healthy…*

1. Choose wisely. When shopping for red meat, opt for lean cuts. If possible, choose meat from cattle that are "range-fed"—that is, the animals roam the range and are not confined to small spaces, and they eat grass instead of grain meal.

Animal meat takes on characteristics of the foods eaten by the animal. For example, the muscle tissue of grass-fed animals has levels of beneficial omega-3s that are 10 to 15 times greater than the levels found in grain-fed animals. Plus, the physical activity that occurs with range-fed animals changes the composition of the animals' fat.

Important: Labeling guidelines have been hotly debated in recent years. Many food scientists believe that guidelines have been diluted. For instance, a package labeled "grass-fed" may mean the animal ate grass for only part of its life. In terms of best nutritional value, the best meat is lean and, ideally, range-fed.

Also important: If the meat is marbled or has a large rind of fat, keep looking. Best choices include filet mignon and "loins," such as sirloin and tenderloin, instead of rib eyes, which usually are fattier.

2. Buy meat directly from farms if possible. There are farms across the US that sell range-fed meats. To find a supplier of such meat, consult the Web site *www.EatWild.com*, owned and operated by Jo Robinson, a journalist who has investigated the differences between animals raised in feedlots and range-fed farms for nearly a decade.

3. Eat whole instead of processed meats. Avoid bacon, bologna, deli meats, hot dogs, pepperoni, salami, Spam, canned hash, sausages and other processed meats. These products have little nutritional value and are full of additives, fats, preservatives and salt.

4. Prepare meat wisely. When proteins in meat (found not only in red meat but also in fish, pork and poultry) are exposed to high heat, the carcinogen heterocyclic amine (HCA) forms from a chemical reaction among amino acids (protein building blocks), sugars and creatine (found in muscles).

To avoid this risk, reduce gas heat from high to medium and avoid grilling for long periods of time (the browner the meat, the

169

more likely that HCAs are present). Grill meat over embers instead of flames. Check the meat temperature with a thermometer. Remove beef, pork and lamb from the grill at 160° F, and chicken and hot dogs at 165° F.

One study found that marinating meat before grilling for 40 minutes reduced HCA production by 92%.

Key marinade ingredients: Apple cider vinegar, garlic, lemon juice, mustard, olive oil, salt and spices—especially of the anti-oxidant-rich mint family (thyme, basil and oregano). Reduce the amount of time meat is high-temperature grilled by first heating meat in the microwave. Or instead of grilling, try baking, roasting or stir-frying, all of which create fewer HCAs.

5. Reduce saturated fat intake elsewhere in your diet. It is primarily the saturated fat in red meat that increases blood levels of cholesterol and, therefore, risk for heart disease. If you wish to continue eating red and processed meats (even in limited amounts), reduce your intake of other sources of saturated fat in your diet (such as sour cream, butter and whole dairy products). Generally, you want to limit saturated fat in your diet so that it makes up 10% or less of your total daily calories.

6. Limit meat consumption. Aim to eat no more than an average of one ounce of red meat per day and no more than one ounce of processed meat per week. Keep in mind that red meat includes pork as well as beef.

Also helpful: If you crave the texture of meat, consider replacing some or all red and processed meats with white meat (whole lean chicken, turkey and fish). Fish, in particular, has higher levels of heart-healthy omega-3 fatty acids than red and processed meats.

A surprising finding of the NIH-AARP study described earlier is that regular consumption of white meat did not increase risk of dying at all. In fact, those who ate the most white meat actually had a lower risk of dying than those who ate the least.

Supplements That Reduce Colon Polyps

Most colorectal cancers develop from benign polyps—but a recent study may offer hope for prevention.

For five years, patients who had colon polyps removed took a daily antioxidant combination supplement containing 200 micrograms of selenomethionine (a compound containing the mineral selenium plus an amino acid)...30 milligrams (mg) of zinc...6,000 international units of vitamin A...180 mg of vitamin C...and 30 mg of vitamin E.

Results: Supplement users were 40% less likely than placebo users to develop new polyps during the 13-year follow-up.

Best: If you've had polyps, ask your doctor whether supplementing with antioxidants is appropriate for you.

Luigina Bonelli, MD, head of secondary prevention and screening at the National Institute for Cancer Research in Genoa, Italy, and the leader of a study of 411 people.

Can Aspirin Prevent Colon Cancer?

Andrew T. Chan, MD, MPH, assistant professor of medicine at Harvard Medical School, Boston.

A cursory reading of headlines makes it seem that taking aspirin regularly is a great way to stay healthy. It helps prevent heart disease in men, stroke in women and, according to recent studies, colon cancer, too. All that's true—but it is not all that simple.

We're already quite familiar with both the benefits and associated risks of using aspirin to help prevent cardiovascular problems, but its effectiveness for keeping colon cancer away is newsworthy...or is it? We spoke with one of the country's leading investigators on the matter, Andrew T. Chan, MD, MPH, assistant professor of medicine at Harvard Medical School, to get the whole story.

Does Aspirin Prevent Colon Cancer?

Dr. Chan has led extensive research on aspirin and colon cancer, and has found that long-term aspirin use—taking at least 325 mg (the adult dose) daily for six or more years—significantly reduces risk in both men and women.

As we know, aspirin has many different mechanisms. According to Dr. Chan, in the case of cancer its efficacy relates to the drug's ability to block passages of certain enzymes important in the inflammatory process—in particular cyclooxygenase-2 (COX-2). High levels of COX-2 can be found in most colorectal tumors, but not in colon tissue. COX-2 seems to promote cancer by supporting blood vessels in tumors and may also help tumors spread to surrounding tissues. Aspirin blocks growth pathways.

However colon cancer is a slow-growing disease, generally starting five to 10 years before diagnosis. Dr. Chan's study found that when people stop the daily aspirin therapy, within just four years their risk reverts to its original level. Therefore, Dr. Chan says that for most people, taking aspirin to prevent colon cancer is not a recommendation—you'd need to take a lot in order to decrease your cancer risk, and large doses of aspirin carry a risk for internal bleeding. Furthermore, says Dr. Chan, there are plenty of other things you can do to prevent colon cancer, leading him to conclude that "there are few patients for whom it makes sense to take aspirin as the only means of prevention."

Going Natural

Researchers are always on the hunt for natural ways to decrease risk. A group at the Rowett Research Institute of Nutrition and Health in Aberdeen (Scotland) found in 2006 that a particular curry in India is rich in salicylic acid (the chemical from which aspirin, acetylsalicylic acid, is made), a fact that might help explain low rates of colon cancer in that country. Dr. Chan observes that since aspirin is from a natural product (willow bark), it isn't surprising to find similar compounds and properties in foods. But relying on foods as a source of salicylic acid makes it impossible to know if the amount you're ingesting is too little, too much or just right. In the future, though, he says we may find dietary sources that offer "a little bit of a boost without aspirin's troubling side effect."

A good strategy, says *Daily Health News* contributing medical editor Andrew Rubman, ND, is to limit intake of processed and broiled meats and trans fats, all of which have been linked to increased risk for colon cancer. Dr. Rubman also suggests increasing intake of wheat-bran fiber and fruits and vegetables and taking fish oil, which seems to blunt COX-2 activity and the production of cancer-promoting hormones.

In summary, aspirin therapy isn't for everyone. It can cause internal bleeding that may be dangerous, even lethal. Its preventive properties differ depending on your gender and there are important caveats that apply to its value in holding back colon cancer. If you heard about the benefits but didn't pick up on the risks in the media reports, you may have missed the most important parts of the story.

Dietary Flax May Prevent Colon Cancer

Chandradhar Dwivedi, PhD, currently serves as a distinguished professor and head of the department of pharmaceutical sciences in the College of Pharmacy at South Dakota State University in Brookings, South Dakota. He also serves as a project director of Translational Cancer Research Center, a joint project at South Dakota State University and Sanford Research in Sioux Falls, South Dakota.

While colorectal cancer is the second-leading cause of cancer deaths in the US, it's also one of the most preventable cancers with proper diet and screening. Adding more clout to this statement is

"White Food" Warning

A diet high in white bread, white rice, white potatoes, sugar and other low-nutrition carbohydrates can increase colorectal cancer risk by 25% or more, according to a recent meta-analysis in *The American Journal of Clinical Nutrition.*

Theory: Eating refined carbohydrates increases production of insulin—which feeds the growth of cancerous cells.

Joel Fuhrman, MD, a family physician specializing in natural and nutritional medicine, Flemington, New Jersey. He is author of numerous books, including *Super Immunity* (HarperOne). *www.DrFuhrman.com*

recent research demonstrating that including flax in your daily diet can help prevent colorectal tumor formation.

Flax Facts

We spoke with lead researcher Chandradhar Dwivedi, PhD, who serves as a distinguished professor and head of the department of pharmaceutical sciences in the College of Pharmacy at South Dakota State University. He said that the research, including a study published this year in the medical journal *Nutrition and Cancer,* suggests that by increasing the body's levels of lignans (phytoestrogens found in plants) and omega-3 fatty acids, flaxseed may help inhibit intestinal tumor growth.

Adding just one or two tablespoons daily of flaxseed oil or freshly ground seeds to your diet can lower risk.

Seeds: It's important to note that flaxseeds must be ground to be absorbed (whole flax provides no benefit) and also that the resulting powder should be stored in the refrigerator or freezer in an opaque container, because light facilitates spoiling. You can enjoy ground flaxseed sprinkled directly onto all sorts of cereals and salads or cooked in soups and stews.

Oil: Dr. Dwivedi cautioned against using flax oil for frying, noting that this causes oxidation and blocks the health benefits. Instead, you can take flax oil by the spoonful, whipped into a fruit smoothie or drizzled over cereal or salad.

A growing number of flax-fortified foods are available on supermarket shelves, including breakfast muffins made of flaxmeal and "omega eggs" from flax-fed chickens. Dr. Dwivedi said these are healthful options.

Not everyone can safely take flax—those who take blood-thinning agents should check with their doctor, because flax affects blood clotting. Also, because it is a high-fiber food, flaxseed can be somewhat irritating to people with colitis and hemorrhoids, but adding it in slowly increasing increments often is a good solution.

Get the Best Colonoscopy: Insider Secrets

Brennan M.R. Spiegel, MD, MSHS, assistant professor of medicine, division of gastroenterology, West Los Angeles Veterans Affairs Medical Center, David Geffen School of Medicine at UCLA, chief of education and training, UCLA GI Fellowship Training Program, Los Angeles, California.

Here's some consumer advice that's probably new to you—recent research has found that early morning colonoscopies uncover more polyps than those performed later in the day.

To learn why—and to get other expert tips on how to make sure your colonoscopy is of the best quality—we called Brennan M.R. Spiegel, MD, assistant professor of medicine at the West Los Angeles Veterans Affairs Medical Center, which is part of the David Geffen School of Medicine at the University of California-Los Angeles, where he and his colleagues examined the records of 477 individuals who had colonoscopies during a one-year period. They found that early morning procedures—ones that started at

8:30 or earlier—resulted in the detection of 27% more polyps per patient, on average, than screenings done later in the day…and that as the hours wore on, physicians discovered progressively fewer polyps.

One possible explanation is that patients' self-administered bowel preparation worsens as the day goes on, since there is more time and temptation to eat something while waiting for the procedure—but even after accounting for this and other independent factors, such as age, gender and cancer or polyp history, doctors still detected fewer polyps as the day wore on. Dr. Spiegel speculates that like other professionals, physicians may simply become fatigued or distracted over time.

The findings were published in the journal *Clinical Gastroenterology and Hepatology.*

Got Skills? That Counts, Too

According to Dr. Speigel, skill counts even more than time of day, and your primary goal should be to find an appropriately trained and experienced physician. Dr. Speigel suggests that you should expect your doctor to have performed at least 140 colonoscopies, which is what's required to graduate from a gastrointestinal training program—but 1,000 is the level that he considers to be "fully proficient."

He says it is also a good idea to ask a doctor about his/her outcome history, as follows…

•**How often do you reach the cecum (the very end of the colon)?** The ideal is to get there at least 90% of the time. (Obstruction or poor bowel preparation sometimes makes it impossible, which is why 100% isn't a reasonable expectation.)

•**How often do you detect polyps?**

A good answer would be: In at least 15% of women and 25% of men age 50 and older.

•**How long do you spend examining the colon?** Doctors should take at least six minutes to examine the whole colon—longer for obese patients and for those who are heavy smokers. Those patients require more careful examination, as they are at higher risk for colon cancer.

What This Means to You

On the individual level, Dr. Spiegel says the net effect of the time-of-day study is inconsequential—though 27% is enough of a difference to make anyone schedule a colonoscopy first thing in the morning. Regarding the big picture, Dr. Speigel acknowledges that "multiplying this effect by thousands of patients across the US could mean we're missing lots of polyps, some of which might turn into cancer one day." He emphasizes, however, that this data is from one center only and says the main focus should be on the quality of your doctor. That's because regardless of the hour, an accurate assessment by a skilled and experienced practitioner provides the best odds of preventing colorectal cancer.

Natural Colonoscopy Clean-Out

Leo Galland, MD, director of the Foundation for Integrated Medicine, New York City, and founder of *www.PillAdvised.com,* a Web site devoted to integrated medicine and use of nutritional supplements. The research cited was published in *Gastrointestinal Endoscopy.*

Have you ever met anyone who doesn't hate preparing for a colonoscopy?

Typical doctor's orders let us drink only clear liquids for a day beforehand and then have us downing powerful chemical laxatives that often cause cramping and bloating before causing us to spend the night visiting the bathroom again and again.

Is there a better way? The happy answer is yes.

Though it's not something that your regular doctor is likely to tell you about.

It's a much more natural and pleasant alternative!

People Who Half-Prep

Is there a need for an alternative? Yes...because people aren't properly prepping. Prior research has shown that 25% of colonoscopy patients don't adequately prepare for the procedure—they typically follow some of the prep instructions but not all of them.

A recent study from Washington University School of Medicine in St. Louis showed how dangerous that can be. When average-risk patients didn't do the entire prep, some stool remained in their colons, obscuring the doctor's view by more than 10%, on average. As a result, about one-third of those patients were asked to redo or resume the prep and return for a second colonoscopy. So a good number of patients who didn't properly prep had to have the procedure done all over again. On top of that, these patients may have prevented their doctors from detecting any cancerous polyps early—and that's a scary thought.

Everyone should want to do an adequate job prepping—it's just that the stuff that you have to swallow can make you feel bloated and give you cramps, among other uncomfortable side effects! Are there natural ways to prep that make the process less "cringeworthy"? Yes, said Leo Galland, MD, an internationally recognized leader in integrated medicine. He offers here some dos and don'ts for precolonoscopy cleansing. If his advice differs from what your doctor recommends, bring in this article and have a conversation with him or her about what's best for you.

Natural Ways to Prep

• **Consider using magnesium citrate, a natural mineral laxative.** Magnesium citrate (a magnesium salt of citric acid) is a more reliable purgative than the polyethylene glycol that's often prescribed, Dr. Galland said. "My favorite is called Natural Calm, which is pure magnesium citrate powder with no additives," said Dr. Galland. "Magnesium and citrate are normally found in the body and are also derived from food, so the powder is all natural. Plus, it's no more expensive and

not any harder to find than traditionally prescribed laxatives." How come more doctors don't prescribe Natural Calm? "Marketing," said Dr. Galland. Start drinking it about 5 pm on the day before your colonoscopy is scheduled (you mix three tablespoons of the powder into eight ounces of hot water, then let it cool and drink it). "It goes down best if you add ice and sip it through a straw," said Dr. Galland. Repeat the dose around 10 pm, he said.

Warning: If you have kidney disease, Dr. Galland warned, you shouldn't take a magnesium-based laxative, because excess magnesium can accumulate in tissues, so talk to your doctor about alternative ways to prep for a colonoscopy.

• **Another advantage to Natural Calm is that you may find that it's gentler on your body,** said *Daily Health News* contributing editor Andrew Rubman, ND, medical director of the Southbury Clinic for Traditional Medicines in Southbury, Connecticut. "Because an all-natural laxative has fewer additives, which can act as stimulants and irritants and cause inflammation in the bowel lining, you may experience less bloating and incontinence and fewer cramps."

• **Schedule a morning colonoscopy.** If you're the first or second patient of the day, you'll be more comfortable (read: less hungry) than others scheduled for later, and you're less likely to have a long wait due to earlier appointments taking longer than scheduled.

• **Talk to your doctor about possibly taking an herb hiatus.** Dr. Galland said that some herbs and other supplements have laxative effects, but far more—including fish oils and vitamin E—can interfere with proper blood clotting, which is necessary if any colon polyps are detected and removed during the colonoscopy. Ask your ND and/or your MD whether it's a good idea to stop any herbs and/or supplements (or lower your intake) a week before your colonoscopy is scheduled.

Colon Prep: Pills vs. Liquid

Patients usually take four tablets of bisacodyl instead of the liquid prep before virtual colonoscopy. Could you do the same thing for a regular colonoscopy?

No. Although many people prefer to take pills instead of drinking a liquid laxative, research shows that the tablets do not appear to provide the thorough colon cleansing necessary for a traditional colonoscopy.

Both colonoscopy and colonography (virtual colonoscopy) check for polyps and other signs of colon cancer and require colon cleansing beforehand.

But the two tests are done differently: A tiny camera is inserted into the colon in a colonoscopy, while the less invasive colonography uses a CT scan that provides 3-D images of the colon and rectum.

C. Daniel Johnson, MD, chairman of radiology, Mayo Clinic, Phoenix.

Quick Colon Test Could Save Thousands of Lives

A recent study found that a single flexible sigmoidoscopy test around age 60 can cut colon cancer risk by about one-third. It is cheaper than a colonoscopy (important for people without insurance), takes an average of five minutes and involves no anesthesia. A tiny camera is used to detect any abnormal tissue in the lower-left side of the colon—where about two-thirds of all colon cancers occur—and aid in the removal of precancerous polyps. The test does require a night-before bowel preparation.

Wendy Atkin, PhD, MPH, professor of surgery and cancer, Imperial College London, England, and lead author of an 11-year study of 170,038 people ages 55 to 64, published in *The Lancet*.

The Perfect Colonoscopy Prep—The Accuracy of This Test Depends a Lot on You

Douglas K. Rex, MD, professor of medicine at Indiana University School of Medicine in Indianapolis. Dr. Rex has authored hundreds of papers and book chapters on colonoscopy and was a member of the committee that wrote the guidelines, Screening and Surveillance for the Early Detection of Colorectal Cancer and Adenomatous Polyps, 2008.

It's widely known that colonoscopy is the most effective way to help prevent cancer of the colon and rectum.

What you may not know: The results of some colonoscopies are more accurate than others.

Important recent finding: When researchers reviewed the medical records of nearly 5,000 people diagnosed with colorectal cancer, 8% of the cases—or about one in 13—had malignancies that were not detected during colonoscopies performed within the prior three-year period.

Of course, the skill of the doctor you choose to perform your colonoscopy affects whether polyps (growths that are typically benign and can be removed before they turn malignant) and/or cancers are found. But to a surprising extent, the steps you take before your colonoscopy also greatly affect the test's accuracy.

Secrets to a Good Bowel Prep

For most people over age 50, colonoscopy should be performed every three to five years if polyps have been found and up to every 10 years if no polyps have been found.* Perhaps the most dreaded part of the test, however, is the bowel prep.

If the bowel is not cleansed properly, it increases the likelihood that growths will be

*Some people, including those with a family history of colorectal cancer, may be advised to begin regular colonoscopies sooner or get them more often—speak to your doctor.

missed and that the procedure will take longer than it should, thus increasing the possibility of complications, such as perforation of the colon or rectum wall and post-procedure abdominal discomfort. If the test results are questionable, you may also need to repeat the test sooner.

To give yourself the best odds of an accurate colonoscopy…

Secret 1: **Start preparing early.** Review your doctor's instructions on bowel prep one week before the procedure, if possible. You may be told to temporarily avoid certain medications, such as iron-containing drugs or supplements that can color the intestines and make preparation more difficult. If you are taking medications that increase bleeding risk—for example, blood thinners such as *clopidogrel* (Plavix) or *warfarin* (Coumadin)—you should contact your doctor or the colonoscopist for instructions.

If you take medication for a chronic illness such as heart disease, ask your doctor whether you should take it up to and including the day of the procedure. People with diabetes may need to adjust their medication to keep their blood sugar levels normal while they are following dietary restrictions.

Beginning two to three days before the colonoscopy, many doctors advise you to avoid undigestible fiber from foods such as nuts, seeds, corn and bran cereal. Little pockets of residue from such foods may linger in the intestine, obscuring the doctor's view.

Secret 2: **Be clear on what foods you can eat.** For years, the standard instruction was to take nothing but clear liquids by mouth the day before a colonoscopy. But there is increasing evidence that a diet that includes fiber-free solid foods is not only easier to follow, but also may result in better cleansing.

A study in the journal *Endoscopy* found that patients tolerated the laxative better and the bowel was cleaner when they followed a fiber-free diet that included scrambled eggs, cheese and white bread, compared with a clear-liquid diet.

Theory: A liquid diet may decrease intestinal contractions and slow down bowel activity, while a bit of solid food keeps the bowel active so it can empty more completely.

Don't take this step on your own, though—ask your doctor if it's OK to eat light, fiber-free meals the day before your colonoscopy.

Secret 3: **Discuss your options for a laxative.** The most important part of bowel prep is taking a strong laxative, usually starting the afternoon or evening before you're scheduled for the procedure.

This is typically an unpleasant-tasting prescription preparation, such as polyethylene glycol (PEG), dissolved in an electrolyte solution containing sodium, potassium and other minerals. You may also be instructed to take laxative pills, usually *bisacodyl* (Dulcolax), at some time during the prep.

Not long ago, the standard approach called for a "high-volume" solution—four liters (more than a gallon) of liquid consumed over a period of several hours. Now, many doctors prescribe a "low volume" solution—two liters versus four—that most people find easier to consume.

Caution: The low-volume approach usually works well but may fail to cleanse the bowel adequately if you are prone to constipation or take medication that slows down digestion, such as an opioid for pain or a tricyclic antidepressant, such as *amitriptyline* (Elavil).

If you are still passing brown stool when it's time to leave home for your colonoscopy, let the nurse know when you arrive at the colonoscopy center. The doctor may ask you to use an enema for further cleaning before starting the colonoscopy.

Secret 4: **Ask your doctor about splitting the laxative dose.** Whether you go the high-volume or low-volume route, when you take the purgative can make a crucial difference.

Most doctors used to advise drinking all the solution the night before the procedure. But many now counsel dividing the dose—half the night before and half four to five hours prior to the colonoscopy, even if you have to drink it at 3 am. A 2009 study rated the bowel significantly cleaner when less time elapsed between preparation and procedure.

Here's why: The laxative cleans fecal matter out of the colon, but over time, thick digestive mucus will descend from the small intestine, accumulate and obscure the doctor's view of the part of the large intestine where many cancers develop. Studies have shown that seven to eight hours after taking the laxative, the ascending bowel starts to become obscured by mucus. By 15 to 16 hours, it's often covered with mucus.

Secret 5: **Make sure you're not alone during a bowel prep.** It's rare, but some people get shaky or pass out during bowel prep. This may result from the abdominal cramping, vomiting, diarrhea and/or dehydration that can occur in some patients, so have someone with you overnight, particularly if you're an older adult and/or frail. Drink plenty of fluids to help prevent dehydration. Your doctor will tell you when to stop drinking and eating prior to the colonoscopy.

Secret 6: **Schedule early in the day, if possible.** Several studies have shown that some physicians detect fewer polyps as the day wears on, possibly due to fatigue. For this reason, you may want to schedule the procedure for earlier in the day, although time of day makes far less difference than the doctor's skill.

Choose the Right Doctor

Gastroenterologists as well as some family physicians and internists perform colonoscopies, but gastroenterologists typically have more training and experience doing the procedure.**

However, the number of polyps a doctor detects in his patients is a much better measure of competence than his specialty. Look for a doctor who finds growths in 20% or more of patients.

If a doctor does not find precancerous polyps in this percentage of his screening patients, these patients are up to 10 times more likely to develop cancer before their next colonoscopy. If your doctor can't or won't tell

**To find a gastroenterologist near you, consult the American College of Gastroenterology at *www.gi.org* (click on the "Patients" tab).

you the number of growths he finds in his patients, consider looking elsewhere.

Research also shows that doctors who spend more time find more growths. For example, doctors should take at least six minutes to withdraw the scope (that's when the actual inspection takes place). Although taking more time doesn't guarantee a quality examination, it's fair for patients to tell a doctor that they've heard that taking longer increases polyp detection and that they're expecting a slow, careful exam and documentation of how long the procedure took.

Statins May Reduce Colon and Rectal Cancer Risk

The cholesterol-lowering drugs have previously been associated with a decreased risk for breast, prostate, lung, pancreatic and liver cancers. A recent analysis indicates that they also lower colorectal-cancer risk by 12%. The most effective statins for reducing this risk are the lipophilic statins, such as Lipitor *atorvastatin* (Lipitor). Although generally well-tolerated, statins have been associated with muscle pain and liver toxicity.

Niloy Jewel Samadder, MD, MSc, instructor of medicine, Mayo Clinic College of Medicine, Rochester, Minnesota, and leader of an analysis of 22 scientific studies involving more than 2.5 million participants, presented at a meeting of the American College of Gastroenterology.

Colon Cancer in Your Family

Tell your doctor about family cancer diagnoses, we hear from Argyrios Ziogas, PhD. Because having cancer in one's family increases risk for many types of malignancies, researchers analyzed how often this risk factor changes in patients.

Recent finding: Among the types of cancer for which family diagnoses changed in more than 14,000 patients (ages 30 to 50) studied over a 10-year period were colorectal cancer (an increase of 2% to 7%) and breast cancer (7% to 11%).

Self-defense: Be sure to update your doctor about family members, such as parents and siblings, newly diagnosed with cancer.

Argyrios Ziogas, PhD, associate professor of epidemiology, University of California, Irvine.

Many Colonoscopies Are Unnecessary

Kristin Sheffield, PhD, assistant professor, department of surgery, University of Texas, Galveston. Her study was published in *JAMA Internal Medicine*.

Did you have a screening colonoscopy less than 10 years ago, with perfectly normal results? Or are you over the age of 75? If either applies, you should think twice if your doctor recommends repeating the test now.

Reason: A shocking percentage of colonoscopies are done on people who don't need them—and for whom the expense, discomfort and risks are wholly unnecessary—according to a recent study.

To understand the recent research, you first need some facts about colorectal cancer…

The Good, the Bad

Colonoscopies are not inherently bad, of course. To the contrary, they are the undisputed gold standard of colon cancer detection and are proven to reduce the risk for death from colorectal cancer. They also prevent cancers from developing. That's because most colon cancers start out as small polyps (growths) that, over the course of 10 years or so, slowly grow and go through changes that turn them into cancer. Colonoscopy gives doctors a chance to spot and remove potentially dangerous polyps, often before they turn cancerous.

Starting screening at age 50 is important because typically there are no warning signs that can be seen without a colonoscopy. But given how slowly the disease progresses, the current guidelines from the US Preventive Services Task Force recommend that subsequent routine screening colonoscopies be done only once every 10 years for patients who are not at increased risk for colon cancer. For a person who is at increased risk—for instance, due to a family history of the disease or a previous colonoscopy that revealed something worrisome—earlier and more frequent screening is appropriate.

Colon cancer's slow-growing nature is also the reason why the guidelines recommend that doctors stop routine colonoscopy screening once a person reaches age 76 and halt all colonoscopy testing after age 85. By that time, frankly, a person is far more likely to die from something else before colon cancer could turn fatal. This shifts the pendulum, so that the benefits of colonoscopy no longer outweigh its potential harms, such as colon perforation, bleeding and/or temporary fecal incontinence from the procedure…and cardiopulmonary problems from the sedation. Though these complications are not common, they are more likely to occur and harder to treat in older people.

Official guidelines aren't infallible, of course. Recommendations can and do change as new information emerges. For now, though, the guidelines represent the consensus of opinion from top experts in the field—which is why it's worrisome that they are so often being ignored.

Sifting Through the Records

For the recent study, researchers scoured Medicare records for people over age 70 and older from all of Texas and from other areas around the US, trying to determine how many colonoscopies were being done inappropriately. Because they didn't have access to complete medical records, they couldn't say for sure that certain colonoscopies were inappropriate, so they used the term "potentially inappropriate." For instance, colonoscopies deemed potentially inappropriate included screening colonoscopies done less than 10 years after previous colonoscopies that had been completely normal…and screening colonoscopies done on people older than 75.

If the records showed that the patient had had a barium enema or abdominal CT in the preceding three months, the researchers assumed that the patient was having the colonoscopy to diagnose a medical problem rather than to screen for cancer. In a case like that, the colonoscopy was not deemed potentially inappropriate. Similarly, when there was a previous diagnosis of anemia, gastrointestinal bleeding, abdominal pain or some other potentially colon-related problem, the colonoscopy was considered to be diagnostic rather than routine screening and thus was not considered potentially inappropriate.

After reviewing nearly 120,000 records, researchers saw some startling patterns emerge…

• **Roughly 23% of the colonoscopies were potentially inappropriate.**

• **In people between the ages of 76 and 85, a troubling 39% of colonoscopies were potentially inappropriate.**

• **The physicians who were most likely to perform inappropriate colonscopies were gastroenterologists** (as opposed to some other type of specialist)…had graduated from medical school before 1990…and were working in "high-volume" practices (those that performed more than 175 colonoscopies per year).

Just Say No?

The lesson here is that, before you (or a loved one) agree to a screening colonoscopy, ask your physician why it's being recommended. Then visit *www.uspreventiveservicestaskforce. org* (search "screening for colorectal cancer") to see whether the reason given is in compliance with the current guidelines.

If your doctor's recommendation differs from the guidelines, he or she may have a good reason. For instance, if you come a family with great longevity and can fully expect to live into your 90s or even to 100, your doctor may think that it's in your best interest to get a routine colonoscopy in your 80s if you are in good health, particularly if you never had a screening colonoscopy before.

However, if there seems to be no valid reason for another colonoscopy and no reason to classify you as being at increased risk, ask your doctor whether a less invasive screening test, such as a fecal occult blood test, will suffice. If he still insists on the colonoscopy, you may want to seek a second opinion…or simply say no. It's your colon, it's your money, it's your decision.

A New Way of Testing for Colon Cancer

David A. Ahlquist, MD, gastroenterologist and professor of medicine, Mayo Clinic Medical School, Rochester, Minnesota.

Colonoscopy has been the gold standard in colorectal cancer detection and prevention for a very long time—but it's by no means perfect, and some people will do just about anything to avoid keeping that appointment. Now along comes a new, noninvasive way to screen for colon cancer—stool DNA testing—a procedure that remarkably enough promises accurate detection without the discomfort.

More Accurate Detection

We talked with David A. Ahlquist, MD, at the Mayo Clinic to get a better sense of what the new test offers. He first described a little background. Colorectal cancer is the second-leading cause of cancer deaths in the US, and colonoscopy—the examination of your colon through insertion of a long, flexible tube—so far represents our best weapon to catch and treat it early. But, he explained, colonoscopy may miss some cancers and precancerous lesions, particularly those on the right side of the colon, which has more nooks and crannies, making the search for polyps a challenge. The right side also has a greater likelihood of hard-to-detect flat polyps. In addition, colonoscopy is expensive. And, like any invasive procedure, it is associated with a risk for complications—bleeding, perforation or sedation-related heart problems occur in a small percentage of patients.

Dr. Ahlquist and his research team found that this new stool DNA test identifies cells that are continuously shed from the surface of growths. It detects target lesions—precancers and cancers, no matter if they are on the left or right side of the colon and no matter what stage, which has been a problem for colonoscopy. Because stool DNA testing effectively detects precancerous polyps, this test has the potential to prevent cancer, much like Pap smears have done for cervical cancer. Add to that the fact that it can be done at home and mailed in for analysis...and it requires no medication or diet restrictions.

Dr. Ahlquist and his collaborators at Exact Sciences, the company that developed the test, embarked on an FDA validation study across more than 30 medical centers throughout the US.

Is DNA Stool Testing Right for You?

In August 2014, the Food and Drug Administration approved DNA testing for colon cancer under the specific product name Cologuard. Cologuard is available to patients in the US through their healthcare providers. The Mayo Clinic has collaborated with Exact Sciences to develop the test, and that firm is already meeting with Medicare and major third-party payers to pave the way for coverage. Current guidelines call for colorectal cancer screening if you are 50 or older—earlier if you are at high risk. For example, if you have inflammatory bowel disease (IBD), you face a greater risk for colorectal cancer, and Mayo researchers have confirmed that stool DNA testing can detect cancer and precancer in people with IBD.

We asked Dr. Ahlquist if he thought stool DNA testing could ever come to replace rather than complement colonoscopy. He believes the procedure must always be linked to colonoscopy, because those with positive test results will need to undergo colonoscopies both to locate the cancer or polyps that are present, and to remove them as well. But for initial screening, if it works as advertised, the stool test may well become the preferred choice for patients.

Editor's note: Mayo Clinic and Dr. Ahlquist have a financial interest in the technology referenced in this article. In compliance with the Bayh-Dole Act, this technology has been licensed to Exact Sciences, and both Mayo Clinic and Dr. Ahlquist have received royalties. Mayo Clinic holds an equity position in Exact Sciences.

Choose Your Colonoscopy Doc Wisely

Nancy Baxter, MD, PhD, associate professor, division of surgery, St. Michael's Hospital, University of Toronto, Toronto. Her study was published in *Journal of Clinical Oncology*.

Many colonoscopies in the US are not performed by gastroenterologists—physicians who, of course, specialize in the diagnosis and treatment of digestive conditions. Primary-care doctors and general surgeons also are doing these vitally important screenings that can detect and save a patient from cancer.

Do they do as good a job?

A recent study compares how good the colonoscopies are when done by these three types of doctors—and the results may influence the type of doctor you choose to perform your next colonoscopy.

Which Doc Is Best?

In the study, when researchers examined medical data for men and women ages 70 to 89, they found that in comparison to people who did not have colonoscopies...

• **People who had colonoscopies done by gastroenterologists** ended up having a 65% lower risk of dying from colorectal cancer.

• **People who had colonoscopies done by primary-care physicians** had a 57% lower risk of dying from colorectal cancer.

•**People who had colonoscopies done by surgeons** had a 45% lower risk of dying from colorectal cancer.

In other words, a colonoscopy performed by any of these types of doctor reduces the risk for colorectal cancer death—but this study suggests that when it's performed by a gasteroenterologist, specifically, the risk for colorectal cancer death is lowest of all.

Now, is it possible that patients who were at highest risk for cancer, perhaps because of existing illness or family history, tended to choose to go to surgeons for their colonoscopies, and perhaps that's why their survival rates were the lowest? That is a possibility, the researchers noted—although using that logic, you'd think that the healthiest patients would have chosen primary-care doctors for their procedures and that therefore primary-care docs' results would have been the best…but that wasn't true.

The study was a retrospective analysis of medical data, so researchers didn't have any information about the patients' preexisting health. And (unfortunately) they did not analyze how each type of doctor fared in terms of complication rates.

One limitation of the study is that researchers weren't able to assess why the patients were having colonoscopies in the first place. So it's possible that patients who had symptoms that were suggestive of colon cancer were sent to surgeons, and that could have affected the results.

Until more research is done, what we know so far is that gastroenterologists' patients did best in avoiding death from the main disease that colonoscopies are supposed to find.

Training, Experience and Education Count

To learn more about why gastroenterologists may have come out on top, we talked with study coauthor Nancy Baxter, MD, PhD, who cited three potential reasons…

1. More initial training. To become a board-certified gastroenterologist, a doctor must complete a two- to three-year fellowship that includes specific education and training on GI procedures such as colonoscopy.

2. Higher volume. Gastroenterologists tend to perform more colonoscopies than other physicians (one recent study estimates that they perform roughly two-thirds of colonoscopies). The more experience doctors have, the more skilled they tend to become at both performing the procedure and spotting cancerous or precancerous tissues.

3. Continuing medical education. To remain board-certified, gastroenterologists must continue their education and training to remain up-to-date on the latest developments in their field.

Find the Right Doc

This study suggests that, when you are going to have a colonoscopy, your odds of not becoming a victim of colon cancer are highest when choosing a gastroenterologist. So you can start by looking for a board-certified gastroenterologist in your area at the Web site of the American College of Gastroenterology, *http://Patients.GI.org/find-a-gastroenterologist/*.

But is a gastroenterologist always going to be a better choice? Not necessarily, said Dr. Baxter. Remember, this study looks at overall odds in a large group of patients. There are probably many primary-care doctors and surgeons who perform the procedure just as well as gastroenterologists or sometimes better, said Dr. Baxter. It's just that it might take a little work to find them.

The key to a successful colonoscopy is finding a physician with a good track record at detecting adenomas (the most common precancerous polyps). Whichever type of physician you consult, Dr. Baxter suggests asking, "What is your adenoma detection rate?" Current guidelines from the American Gastroenterological Association suggest that for patients older than age 50, doctors should have at least a 15% adenoma-detection rate in females and at least a 25% detection rate in males. Make sure that the physician you choose meets your high standards—because when it comes to your health, you should accept nothing less.

Higher BMI Means Higher Risk of Colon Cancer

Edward L. Giovannucci, MD, ScD, a professor of epidemiology and nutrition at Harvard School of Public Health, and epidemiologist, department of medicine Brigham and Women's Hospital, Boston, Massachusetts.

E vidence continues to accumulate that obesity leads to a higher risk of diabetes, heart disease, stroke and many cancers. Recently, a Swedish study indicated that a high BMI or body mass index is associated with a higher risk of colon cancer. This comes as no surprise to Edward L. Giovannucci, MD, ScD, a professor of epidemiology and nutrition at Harvard School of Public Health and epidemiologist at Brigham and Women's Hospital in Boston, Massachusetts. For more than a decade, he has been looking into the links between physical inactivity, obesity and colon cancer. The good news—losing just 5% to 10% of your body weight can lower your colon cancer risk, says Dr. Giovannucci.

BMI: a Primer

While not a perfect measure, BMI is an easy-to-use tool that quickly screens for excess weight that can correlate with dangerous health conditions. To learn your BMI, simply visit the Web site of the National Heart Lung and Blood Institute at *http://www.nhlbi.nih.gov/* (search "BMI calculator") and plug in your height and weight—your number will appear.

BMI categories are…

- Underweight = lower than 18.5
- Normal weight = 18.5 to 24.9
- Overweight = 25 to 29.9
- Obese = 30 or higher

This latest research demonstrates that people whose BMI puts them in the obese category experience as much as a 20% greater risk of colon cancer—but, of course, it's not about BMI alone. There may well be a connection between the poor digestive and bowel health that results from poor eating habits. Waist circumference is another important risk factor for colon cancer, since abdominal fat or an "apple" shape is associated with obesity-related diseases. It's important to note that while the correlation between BMI and body fat is strong, it is not perfect. Athletes have a high but healthful BMI because of their increased musculature…women tend to have more body fat than men with the same BMI… and older people typically have more body fat than young people with the same BMI.

Lower Your BMI and Maybe Colon Cancer Risk Too

Obviously, for optimal health, your goal should be a BMI in the "normal weight" category. If your BMI is edging up into the overweight or obese categories, make changes in diet and exercise now before it's too late. According to Dr. Giovannucci, it's especially important to prevent or minimize the weight gain that typically creeps up on us in middle age. He notes that even moderate activities such as regular brisk walking can help control weight gain and potentially reduce the risk of colon cancer.

Blood Sugar Danger

T here is a small increased risk for colorectal cancer if you have high blood sugar, according to recent research. If you have high blood sugar, talk to your doctor about ways to maintain a healthy weight by eating a balanced diet, exercising regularly and, if necessary, taking medication.

Elevated blood sugar levels are associated with obesity, which is a known risk factor for colorectal cancer. High blood sugar may also be linked to higher levels of inflammatory factors that spur the growth of polyps that can develop into cancer.

Geoffrey Kabat, PhD, senior epidemiologist, Albert Einstein College of Medicine of Yeshiva University, New York City.

Why Location Matters When It Comes to Colon Cancer

Robert S. Bresalier, MD, professor of gastroenterology, hepatology and nutrition, The University of Texas M. D. Anderson Cancer Center, Houston.

W e've grown accustomed to the idea that there is a difference between the right and left sides of the brain...but the colon? Yes indeed—a bit of a ruckus was raised following publication in late 2008 of a Canadian study on colonoscopies that found that nearly every cancer on the right side of the colon was missed, a big problem since polyps on that side are also more likely to be deadly. This finding got lots of media coverage, but since then questions have been raised about whether this really is happening. If it is, what can we do about it?

Here's What We Know

First, let's understand our terms. If you stand with your hands on your hips, thumbs aimed toward your back, your right index finger will be pointing approximately to the start of your right (also called ascending) colon... your left one will be at the end of the left (descending) colon. And yes, it is quite true that there are both biological and anatomical reasons why doctors have more difficulty finding polyps that are located on the right side of the colon, we learned from Robert S. Bresalier, MD, professor of gastroenterology, hepatology and nutrition at The University of Texas M.D. Anderson Cancer Center. *He explained that specifically...*

New Drug for Colorectal Cancer?

Recent finding: Fingolimod (Gilenya), a drug now used for multiple sclerosis, blocks an enzyme involved in inflammatory bowel disease and colitis-associated cancers. It could someday be used to treat such malignancies.

Cancer Cell

• **The right side of the colon is more likely to have flat polyps.** These types of polyps are harder to see than the others, so they're more likely to be missed and left in place to grow larger. If that happens, they're also more likely to be cancerous by the time they are discovered.

• **The right side of the colon is larger and baggier and has more nooks and crannies than the left.** If the colon hasn't been properly emptied during colonoscopy preparation, remnants of stool may obscure small lesions in the right side of the colon.

The Truth Behind the Research

Dr. Bresalier said that well-trained doctors know to examine the right side of the colon very closely for the above reasons. In his view, the media coverage claiming that doctors were missing many right-sided colon cancers was unnecessarily alarmist, since the research had some important flaws. First, he said, the conclusions were not drawn from a rigorous double-blind, randomized trial, which is the gold standard for such research —and second, the study included colonoscopies that were performed by physicians who are general practitioners not specifically trained in colonoscopy. He believes that these factors may have skewed the results.

So, regarding this particular worry, it appears we can afford to relax a bit. Just be sure that you get your colonoscopy from a physician who has received special training in performing these types of procedures, and follow your prep instructions thoroughly.

In Pursuit of "Perfect" Poo

Alvin Newman, MD, adjunct professor of medicine in the division of gastroenterology at the University of Toronto Department of Medicine and an attending physician at Mount Sinai Hospital in Toronto, Ontario, Canada. He also is the author of *The Essential IBS Book: Understanding and Managing Irritable Bowel Syndrome and Functional Dyspepsia* (Robert Rose).

When you sit on the toilet and do a #2, do you take a quick peek before flushing? Many people do check their poo to make sure everything looks OK—and there's nothing wrong with that.

But some people go overboard, examining each bowel movement as if they were reading tea leaves. They fret, Is it shaped properly? Is the texture all right? What does that color signify? And why does it look so different today compared with yesterday? Some people even take photos of their supposedly substandard stools to show to their doctors!

To allay such concerns, we contacted Alvin Newman, MD, a gastroenterologist at the University of Toronto and author of *The Essential IBS Book*. He said that stool is composed mainly of water, nonabsorbable "food stuffs," bacteria and sloughed-off cells from the intestinal lining. Stool color is derived from bile pigments and food residues, so it can vary significantly—with dark brown, light brown, yellow, greenish and multicolored all qualifying as normal. "Many things can affect stool color. Bismuth (such as in Pepto-Bismol) and iron can turn stools extremely dark. Beets can turn them reddish. Green stool usually means only that intestinal contents have moved through the digestive system quickly," Dr. Newman said.

Solid-waste elimination is a variable process, so there also is a wide range of normal when it comes to stool size, shape and consistency. Even mucousy stools are generally not worrisome, Dr. Newman said. "In the absence of other things like blood or severe pain and a change in bowel habits, mucus in stool is merely the bowel's way of lubricating itself," he said.

Bowel movement frequency can vary greatly, too, from three per day to three per week, yet still be within the normal range—so skipping a day or two does not necessarily signal a problem with constipation. "It is probably fair to say that the fear of constipation is much more intense than the fear of diarrhea, even though very few people have ever died of constipation, whereas diarrhea may be life-threatening," Dr. Newman noted.

Clearly, there is no such thing as "perfect" poo—and no reason to worry over every little change. But that's not to say you should ignore it altogether. *Do see your doctor without delay if…*

• **Your stools are bright red, dark red, burgundy, maroon or black.** Such colors suggest the presence of blood. The source could be something as simple as a small hemorrhoid, but you should be checked for other conditions, such as an anal fissure (a tear in the tissue lining the anus), colon polyp or colorectal cancer.

• **You pass four or more watery or liquid stools per day for several days.** Severe diarrhea can easily lead to dehydration.

• **You have severe constipation**—for instance, only one bowel movement per week plus frequent bloating and abdominal pain. You may need to be screened for slow-transit constipation, a condition in which things move very lethargically through the bowel. One clue to this condition is if adding fiber to your diet, which normally would ease constipation, instead makes your symptoms even worse.

• **Passing stool is consistently painful.** Your doctor will want to investigate possible causes, such as severe hemorrhoids, an anal fissure or anal abscess (a painful boil-like swelling near the anus).

Some years back, the Scandinavian *Journal of Gastroenterology* published the *Bristol Stool Chart*, which showed and described seven different types of stools (you can check it out at *www.IbsGroup.org/bristolstool*). You may find the chart to be a useful communication aid when discussing bowel movement concerns with your doctor. But remember, unless your doctor specifically asks for a photo, there's no need to take your camera into the bathroom.

Procedures Are Not Risk-Free

Colonoscopies and other endoscopic procedures send one in every 100 patients to the emergency room. The most common complaint is abdominal pain, which probably results from air from the procedure working its way out of the intestine.

Daniel Leffler, MD, director of clinical research, division of gastroenterology, Beth Israel Deaconess Medical Center, Boston, and leader of a study of 6,383 endoscopies and 11,632 colonoscopies, published in *Archives of Internal Medicine*.

Colorectal Cancer Deaths on the Downslide

Did you know that colorectal cancer deaths may drop sharply in the next 10 years? Already over the last decade, the death rate from these cancers fell by about 20%, due to changes in health habits, increased screening and better treatment. Further advances could mean that the rate in 2020 will be half what it was in 2000. About 50,000 people will die from colorectal cancers this year.

Elizabeth Ward, PhD, director of epidemiology and surveillance research, American Cancer Society, Atlanta. *www.cancer.org*

Chapter 10

BEYOND THE BIG 3: WINNING THE WAR AGAINST MELANOMA AND MORE

Symptoms That Should Never Be Ignored—Many Seem Harmless, but They Might Mean Cancer

If you are one of the estimated 1.5 million people in the US who will be told "you have cancer" this year, much of your medical fate will depend on how advanced the malignancy is when it is diagnosed.

When cancer is caught early—before the abnormal cells multiply and spread—the odds of defeating the disease improve dramatically.

Problem: Because cancer is tricky—early symptoms most often (but not always) are painless, and they often mimic common noncancerous conditions—many people ignore red flags that could help them get an early diagnosis.

For the best possible chance of beating cancer: Be alert for subtle symptoms of the disease. Here are cancer symptoms that you should never ignore—and how to distinguish them from more benign causes.*

*Important: If you have a troubling symptom that is not listed in this article, see your doctor.

1. Difficulty swallowing. When you swallow, you've probably had the uncomfortable or painful experience of food getting "stuck"—for example, high in the esophagus or in the middle of the upper chest.

It may be cancer if: You have this sensation all or most times that you eat, and it's usually not painful. Difficulty swallowing is common in people with esophageal or stomach cancer and may be a sign that a tumor is obstructing the esophagus or that inflammation and scarring have narrowed the opening. Inflammation can be a precursor to cancer and also can indicate that a malignant tumor has irritated surrounding healthy tissue.

Because problems with swallowing can evolve slowly, many people adjust the way they eat, taking smaller bites, chewing longer and perhaps even switching to a diet that is mostly liquid. If eating becomes difficult—for any reason—see a doctor.

2. Excessive bleeding and/or unexplained bruising. Leukemia causes a shortage of blood platelets (cellular elements

Amy P. Abernethy, MD, program director of the Duke Cancer Care Research Program and associate director of the Cancer Control Program at the Duke Comprehensive Cancer Center, both in Durham, North Carolina. Dr. Abernethy is also an associate professor of medicine in the division of medical oncology at the Duke University Medical Center.

responsible for clotting), which results in easy and excessive bleeding and unexplained bruising. (Normal bleeding, such as that caused by a cut, should stop after application of direct pressure.)

It may be cancer if: You have an unusual number of unexplained nosebleeds (for example, not due to dry air, a common trigger) and/or develop unexplained bruises (a change in frequency or severity from the norm) that tend to be painful when touched, dark purple and large (the size of a fist or bigger).

Important: Bleeding gums may be a sign of poor dental care or a serious medical problem, such as leukemia. If brushing causes bleeding, see your dentist for an evaluation to determine the cause.

3. Exhaustion. Everyone gets tired, but extreme fatigue due to cancer is quite different. Although all cancers can cause fatigue, this symptom is most common with colon cancer, leukemia and other cancers that may cause anemia.

It may be cancer if: For no apparent reason, you experience overwhelming and debilitating fatigue similar to that caused by the flu.

Important: Fatigue due to cancer is sometimes mistaken for depression.

Key difference: A person with depression often lacks the will and desire to perform daily activities, while a person with cancer-related fatigue wants to stay active but lacks the physical ability to do so.

4. Fever and night sweats. The presence of cancer causes a storm of chemical processes as the body ramps up its immune defenses to fight cancer cells. Fever is one indication that your immune system is fending off an illness, such as a cold or the flu, or even cancer.

It may be cancer if: You have fevers (typically 100°F or higher) that come and go over a period of days or weeks. Cancer-related fevers occur most often at night—often along with drenching night sweats.

Important: Menopausal women often have hot flashes that may lead to night sweats—but sweats due to menopause also

occur during the day. Anyone who experiences night sweats—including menopausal women who have night sweats but no daytime hot flashes—should see a doctor.

5. Lumps. Any new, firm, painless lump that is growing in size or that is bigger than a nickel should be immediately examined by a doctor. Worrisome lumps typically feel firmer than the tip of your nose, while spongy or painful lumps are less of a concern. Lumps can be caused by several types of cancer, including breast, testicular and throat malignancies, and melanoma (skin cancer).

The immune response launched by your body when it is fighting a serious disease—including cancer—may lead to enlarged lymph nodes (the small filtering structures that help prevent foreign particles from entering the bloodstream). Painful and/or swollen lymph nodes are common signs of infection and usually return to normal size within a few days of the infection resolving.

It may be cancer if: Enlarged lymph nodes do not return to normal size and/or have the characteristics described above.

Helpful: Lymph nodes can be found throughout the body, but enlarged ones are easiest to feel behind the neck (at the base of the skull or behind the ears)…in the armpit…in the groin (at the junction of the torso and leg)…in the hollowed space above the collarbone (clavicle)…in back of the knee… and at the crook of the elbow.

6. Persistent cough. Longtime smokers get used to coughing, so they tend not to notice this important symptom of lung cancer. Nonsmokers can experience persistent cough as well, which also can be a symptom of other cancers, including malignancies of the throat and esophagus.

It may be cancer if: You have a cough—with or without breathlessness—that persists for longer than one month. Coughing up blood also can be a cancer symptom.

7. Skin changes. Most people know that changes in a mole can be a sign of skin cancer. But the moles that are most prone to cancerous changes are the type that are flat (as opposed to raised or bumpy in shape).

It may be cancer if: You have a mole that becomes darker...changes color...changes shape (especially in an asymmetrical pattern)...or grows larger. Guidelines recommend seeing a doctor if you have a mole that grows larger than a pencil eraser, but don't wait to see your doctor if you have a mole that undergoes any of the changes described above.

Important: A sore that doesn't heal also can be skin cancer. (In healthy people, most superficial wounds heal within days.)

8. Stumbles or falls. If you suddenly become "clumsy," it may signal a neurological problem, such as nerve damage from diabetes or multiple sclerosis, or it could be a sign of a brain tumor.

It may be cancer if: Your clumsiness is accompanied by confusion, difficulty concentrating and an inability to move your arms and/or legs. Although paralysis is an obvious sign that something is wrong, it is rarely the first sign of a brain tumor. Check with your doctor immediately if your body's basic functions change in any way.

9. Unexplained weight loss. If you experience significant weight loss (about 10 pounds or more of your body weight) that is not a result of an intentional weight-loss regimen, it often is a symptom of a potentially serious medical condition, such as cancer or depression.

It may be cancer if: Weight loss is due to a reduced appetite. Always see your doctor promptly if you experience unexplained weight loss.

Melanoma Is On the Rise

Albert Lefkovits, MD, an associate clinical professor of dermatology at Mount Sinai School of Medicine and codirector of the Mount Sinai Dermatological Cosmetic Surgery Program, both in New York City. He is a member of the Medical Advisory Council of The Skin Cancer Foundation and a past-president of the Dermatology Society of Greater New York.

Melanoma is the most dangerous form of skin cancer. It's particularly frightening because it's more likely than other cancers to spread (metastasize) to other parts of the body. More than 76,000 Americans are diagnosed with melanoma each year, and between 8,000 and 9,000 will die from it.

Good news: New technology increases the chances that a melanoma will be detected early—and when it is, you have a 95% to 97% chance of surviving. The prognosis is worse after the disease has spread, but two new drugs can significantly increase survival times—and medications that may be even more effective already are in the pipeline.

Who's at Risk?

A study published in *Journal of Investigative Dermatology* found that melanoma rates increased by 3.1% annually between 1992 and 2004—and the incidence continues to rise.

The increase is due to several reasons. The US population is aging, and older adults are more likely to get melanoma (though it is a leading cause of cancer death in young adults). Public-awareness campaigns have increased the rate of cancer screenings (though officials would like the screening rates to be even higher), and more screenings mean an increase in melanoma diagnoses.

If you are a fair-skinned Caucasian, your lifetime risk of getting melanoma is about one in 50. The risk is lower among African Americans, Hispanics and Asians, but they're more likely to die from it because they often develop cancers on "hidden" areas (such as the soles of the feet), where skin changes aren't readily apparent.

Important: Don't be complacent just because you avoid the sun or use sunscreen. Many cancers appear in areas that aren't exposed to the sun, such as between the toes or around the anus.

State-of-the-Art Screening

Melanomas grow slowly. Patients who get an annual skin checkup are more likely to get an early diagnosis than those who see a doctor only when a mole or skin change is clearly abnormal.

Doctors used to depend on their eyes (and sometimes a magnifying glass) to examine suspicious areas. But eyes-only examinations can identify melanomas only about 60% of the time.

Better: An exam called epiluminescence microscopy. The doctor takes photographs of large areas of skin. Then he/she uses a device that magnifies suspicious areas in the photos. The accuracy of detecting melanomas with this technique is about 90%.

The technology also allows doctors to look for particular changes, such as certain colors or a streaked or globular appearance, that indicate whether a skin change is malignant or benign. This can reduce unnecessary biopsies.

Few private-practice physicians can afford the equipment that's used for these exams. You might want to get your checkups at a medical center or dermatology practice that specializes in early melanoma detection. If this isn't possible, ask your doctor if he/she uses a handheld dermatoscope. It's a less expensive device that's still superior to the unaided eye.

New Treatments

In the last few years, the FDA has approved two medications for patients with late-stage melanoma. These drugs don't cure the disease but can help patients live longer.

•*Ipilimumab* (**Yervoy**) is a biologic medication, a type of synthetic antibody that blocks a cellular "switch" that turns off the body's ability to fight cancer. A study of 676 patients with late-stage melanoma found that those who took the drug survived, on average, for 10 months after starting treatment, compared with 6.4 months for those in a control group.

•*Vemurafenib* (**Zelboraf**) may double the survival time of patients with advanced melanoma. It works by targeting a mutation in the BRAF V600E gene, which is present in about 50% of melanoma patients. Researchers who conducted a study published in *The New England Journal of Medicine* found

that more than half of patients who took the medication had at least a 30% reduction in tumor size. In about one-third of patients, the medication slowed or stopped the progression of the cancer.

•**Combination treatment.** Each of these medications attacks tumors in different ways. They can be used in tandem for better results. For example, a patient might start by taking the first drug, then, when it stops working, he/she can switch to the second drug. This approach can potentially extend survival by up to a year.

Both drugs can have serious side effects. For now, they're recommended only for a select group of patients.

Self-Protection

Take steps to protect yourself…

•**Check your skin monthly.** It's been estimated that deaths from melanoma could be reduced by 60% if everyone would do a monthly skin exam to look for suspicious changes. Look for asymmetric moles in which one part is distinctly different from the other part…moles with an irregular border…color variations…a diameter greater than 6 millimeters (mm), about one-quarter inch…or changes in appearance over time.

•**Get a yearly checkup with a dermatologist.** It's nearly impossible to self-inspect all of the areas on your body where melanoma can appear. I advise patients to see a dermatologist every year for full-body mapping. The doctor will make a note (or photograph) of every suspicious area and track the areas over time.

Important: New moles rarely appear in people over the age of 40. A mole that appears in patients 40 years and older is assumed to be cancer until tests show otherwise.

•**Use a lot of sunscreen.** Even though melanoma isn't caused only by sun exposure, don't get careless. Apply a sunscreen with an SPF of at least 30 whenever you go outdoors. Use a lot of sunscreen—it takes about two ounces of sunscreen (about the amount in a shot glass) to protect against skin cancer.

Reapply it about every two hours or immediately after getting out of the water.

•**Don't use tanning salons.** Researchers who published a study in *Journal of the National Cancer Institute* found that people who got their tans at tanning salons—that use tanning lamps and tanning beds that emit UV radiation—at least once a month were 55% more likely to develop a malignant melanoma than those who didn't artificially tan.

Redheads and Melanoma

Redheads may be at higher risk for melanoma—even if they don't spend much time in the sun.

Recent study: At least 50% of red-furred mice developed melanoma, even though they had not been exposed to ultraviolet radiation...only 10% of similar mice without red fur contracted the cancer. Research has not been conducted on humans, but scientists believe that the body's production of pheomelanin, the pigment in red hair, makes skin cells more vulnerable to DNA damage.

Study by researchers at Massachusetts General Hospital, Boston, published in *BioEssays*.

Face-Saving Skin Cancer Surgery

Margaret W. Mann, MD, assistant professor of dermatology at Case Western Reserve University School of Medicine in Cleveland and director of the Skin Cancer & Mohs Surgery program at University Hospitals/Westlake in Westlake, Ohio.

Basal cell carcinoma (BCC), the most common skin cancer in the US, is rarely fatal but can be disfiguring. Fortunately for BCC patients, there's a treatment called Mohs micrographic surgery, which can literally be a face saver.

BCC develops in the bottom of the epidermis (outermost layer of skin). What is visible on the surface is the "tip of the iceberg," with more tumor cells growing downward and outward into surrounding skin—like the roots of a tree. The cancer most often occurs on the face, scalp or neck but can develop anywhere. Lesions can emerge as red, raised spots that itch, flake, bleed, then heal and return repeatedly. In other cases, BCC appears as a waxy bump...flat, scaly, brown or flesh-colored patch...crusty or oozy lesion... or sore with a sunken center.

If you notice any such spot: See a dermatologist immediately. "The longer you leave it, the larger it grows, so the larger the scar will be when it's removed," cautioned Mohs expert Margaret W. Mann, MD, an assistant professor of dermatology at Case Western Reserve University School of Medicine in Cleveland.

Treatment options for BCC include excision (cutting out the tumor)...curettage and electrodesiccation (scraping off the tumor, then cauterizing the base to destroy any remaining abnormal cells)...cryosurgery (freezing)...radiation...and laser. With these methods, the surgeon must estimate how much tissue to treat, which can lead to unnecessary removal of healthy tissue and/or tumor recurrence if any cancer is inadvertently left behind.

What makes Mohs different is that it allows the surgeon to precisely identify and remove the entire tumor—virtually eliminating the chance that it will grow back and thus providing the highest success rate among treatments—while it leaves surrounding healthy tissue intact to minimize scarring.

How it works: Mohs is usually performed as an outpatient procedure under local anesthesia. The tumor is shaved off in ultra-fine layers, one layer at a time, and each bit of tissue is immediately examined under a microscope. A special dye allows the surgeon to distinguish normal cells from cancer cells. The surgeon can then map the exact location of each projecting "root" of the tumor, so that—layer by layer—every last microscopic portion of cancer can be removed without undue harm to healthy tissue. Although time-intensive, the technique's cure rate is near 99%, Dr. Mann said. For an infographic on the method, visit *http://bit.ly/iKNVMJ* and click on The Mohs Step-by-Step Process.

Another unique aspect of Mohs is that wound reconstruction usually is done immediately because there is no need to wait for a pathologist's report to confirm that the cancer is gone. Depending on the wound's size, it may be stitched…or a graft of skin may be taken from elsewhere…or a flap of living tissue from an adjacent area may be used to fill in the wound. If the treated area is very extensive, plastic surgery may be performed later.

Mohs typically costs more than other types of BCC treatment—and those other methods often work fine, depending on the tumor's extent and location. But Mohs generally is considered the treatment of choice for BCC that is large, deep, fast-growing, irregularly shaped, recurrent, or located near scar tissue or on the face. Discuss your options with your doctor and your insurance company.

Many doctors perform Mohs, but for the best outcome, Dr. Mann recommended using a board-certified dermatologist who is a member of the American College of Mohs Surgery (ACMS). Membership in ACMS requires completion of a one- to two-year fellowship training program and at least 500 supervised Mohs surgery cases—so these physicians are specially trained as cancer surgeons, pathologists and reconstructive surgeons. Visit *www.Mohs College.org* and click on "Find a Surgeon."

Important news: A recent study from Brown University revealed that patients who have had one BCC are likely to have multiple carcinomas over time—suggesting that this type of cancer should be considered a chronic disease. So even after your BCC is successfully treated, it is best to remain on guard for signs of new skin tumors elsewhere on your body.

Calcium + Vitamin D Decreased Melanoma Risk

Jean Y. Tang, MD, PhD, assistant professor of dermatology, Stanford University School of Medicine, Redwood City, California.

If you've had a basal or squamous cell skin cancer removed, as so many people have, you know all about the anxiety that experience leaves you with. Will it come back? Will you get more of them? Or, worst of all, does this mean you are likely to get the far more serious and worrisome melanoma?

Here's the Truth

Sadly, yes, people who have had basal or squamous cell skin cancers are statistically more likely to later develop the deadly skin cancer melanoma than those who haven't had any skin cancers. In fact, a history of any kind of cancer ups your statistical risk for having another—but research suggests that this is especially so with skin cancer.

Now comes the good news. A group of researchers at Stanford University's School of Medicine has found evidence that taking calcium and vitamin D supplements significantly cuts the risk of developing melanoma in a group of women who had previously had nonmelanoma skin cancers.

Research Results

The researchers learned this by analyzing a large pool of data from the 15-year Women's Health Initiative—36,000 women, ages 50 to 79, were followed for an average of seven years. While the study was initiated to investigate the effects of calcium and vitamin D on hip fractures and colorectal cancers, researchers also looked at whether these supplements affect risk for melanoma—and wow, were the researchers surprised by how helpful they are!

Half the women in the study took a daily supplement containing 1,000 mg of calcium and 400 IU of vitamin D, while the other half took a placebo pill.

Findings: Those who took calcium and vitamin D were half as likely to develop melanoma subsequent to their other skin cancers. Surprisingly, the researchers also learned that this protective effect helped only those who had had previous skin cancers. Calcium and vitamin D had no apparent effect on melanoma risk in those who had been skin-cancer free.

On the downside, there was a higher incidence of kidney stones among the calcium/vitamin D takers…and emerging research now suggests that very high levels of supplemental vitamin D may encourage certain skin cancers, so none of us should start gulping vitamin D without speaking to a doctor first. The results were published online in the *Journal of Clinical Oncology.*

What's Up Here?

As noted by lead researcher Jean Y. Tang, MD, PhD, assistant professor of dermatology at the Stanford University School of Medicine, lots of questions remain. For one thing, men weren't included in the Women's Health Initiative, so it's unclear whether they would derive the same benefit from taking the calcium and vitamin D combo. It's also not known whether natural sources of vitamin D (such as sunshine) and calcium (such as from leafy greens and dairy) would have the same effect as the supplements.

Dr. Tang's advice: If you have had basal cell or squamous cell skin cancer…and spend your time indoors for the most part…and/or are a postmenopausal woman (since many are considering calcium supplementation anyway to protect against bone loss), you might discuss a low-dose calcium and vitamin D supplement with your health-care provider. She mentioned also that her team continues to study this issue—focusing particularly on the potential relationship between vitamin D and cancer prevention—with a study that will compare blood levels of vitamin D with the incidence of melanomas. She invited read-ers to participate by contacting her through *http://med.stanford.edu/profiles/Jean_Tang.*

Hidden Melanoma—It Can Strike Where You Least Expect It

Marianne Berwick, PhD, MPH, division chief and head of cancer epidemiology and prevention at the University of New Mexico School of Medicine and associate director of the Cancer Population Sciences Program at the University of New Mexico Cancer Center, both in Albuquerque.

If you spotted a mole on your leg that had changed colors or grown larger or asymmetrical, chances are that you would do the right thing and make an appointment to see your doctor. But melanoma, the deadliest of all skin cancers, often doesn't follow the rules and can develop in an unexpected place, such as the sole of your foot, under a fingernail or even in your eye.

The hidden threat: Even though we don't hear much about it, up to 30% of melanomas have an almost normal appearance or develop in areas where most people—including many doctors—don't think to look.

Good news: The overwhelming majority of patients will survive if the melanoma is detected early. *Where to look—and what to look for…*

A Lump or Unusual Patch

About 15% of all melanomas diagnosed in the US are due to so-called *nodular melanomas.* They can occur anywhere on the body, and they don't necessarily arise from pre-existing moles. These melanomas are particularly dangerous because they grow *into* the skin more rapidly than they expand in width. That's why most people don't notice them until they've already spread.

What to look for: Nodular melanomas can appear as a lump (usually black, red or skin-colored) that may be firm and dome-shaped or as a dark- or light-colored patch of skin that does not quite resemble the surrounding area.

Self-defense: When you examine your skin, make note of any unusual lump...or area that doesn't resemble the surrounding skin, and see a dermatologist promptly.

Under the Nails

About 5% of all melanomas—and the most common form in Asians and people with dark skin—appear under a fingernail or toenail or on the palms of the hands or the soles of the feet. They also can occur in mucous membranes in the nose, mouth or other areas. This cancer, *acral lentiginous melanoma*, is dangerous because most people don't recognize it.

What to look for: A melanoma under a nail often appears as a brown or black streak that grows larger over time. If a melanoma affects the mucous membranes in the nasal passages, it can cause persistent congestion or nosebleeds.

Self-defense: See your dermatologist right away if you notice a nail streak that's getting bigger and is not due to an injury. Go to your doctor if you have nosebleeds for no obvious reason or develop unexplained chronic congestion. Ask your dentist to check your mouth at routine dental exams.

"Age" Spots

These flat areas of sun-damaged skin vary in size, are gray-brown or black and usually appear on the face, arms, shoulders and/or hands. If a spot changes over time, it could be *lentigo maligna melanoma*.

What to look for: A flat "spot" that gradually spreads and develops an irregular shape. It will be a brownish color and usually appears on the face, neck or other sun-exposed areas.

Self-defense: Have a dermatologist check age spots when they first appear. If an area changes quickly (over a period of about two weeks) or has irregular borders, see a dermatologist promptly.

Scalp Changes

Unless you have thinning hair or you are bald, your scalp isn't an area that's easy to see. That's why melanomas on the scalp are so dangerous—most people don't notice them until they're already advanced.

What to look for: Scalp melanomas usually follow the normal rules of ABCDE—Asymmetry...Border irregularities...Color changes...Diameter (larger than about one-quarter inch)...and Evolving (changes in appearance over time). Areas that itch or bleed persistently also should be checked promptly.

Self-defense: Once a month, take a few minutes to examine every part of your scalp. You can use a comb and/or hair dryer to move your hair out of the way. Use a mirror to help you see the top and back of your scalp and/or ask a family member or your hairdresser to check those places for you.

Below and More

Melanomas can occur in areas that have never been exposed to sun.

What to look for: Any sensation (such as itching or bleeding) in the vulvar area or vagina...or anus that doesn't seem normal (or for a man, around the testicles or penis). You might notice a mole or a discolored area that's changing.

Self-defense: See your doctor right away if you experience unexpected vaginal bleeding or discharge or blood in the urine. Blood that appears during bowel movements is sometimes caused by hemorrhoids but may also indicate cancer, so see your doctor promptly.

Vision Changes

You aren't likely to see an *ocular melanoma* (a rare type of eye cancer), because it's usually not apparent when you look in a mirror.

What to look for: See an eye doctor if you notice a scratchy sensation under the eyelid or possibly changes in vision, such as blurring or a loss of peripheral vision.

Self-defense: There is little evidence that wearing sunglasses will prevent eye melanomas. The best way to protect yourself is with an annual eye exam from an ophthalmologist or optometrist.

More from Dr. Berwick...

The Ultimate Skin Exam

All adults should see a dermatologist at least once a year for a skin exam...or promptly if you notice a change in your skin, including any of those described in the main article. A *thorough* skin exam from a dermatologist—of every *inch* of your skin including areas of the body that do not receive sun exposure—is one of the best defenses against melanoma. You might also be checked with a device called MelaFind, which takes digital pictures of abnormal areas and analyzes them for signs of cancer. It can help your doctor decide if a biopsy is needed.

The first step of a skin exam is to take off all your clothes (and jewelry) and slip into a gown that's open at the front. *See graphic for important areas that are sometimes missed...*

To protect yourself further: Examine every inch of your skin once a month. Don't forget to use a hand mirror to check your buttocks, between the buttocks and the backs of both legs. While sitting, use the mirror to also check the area around (and under) the genitals.

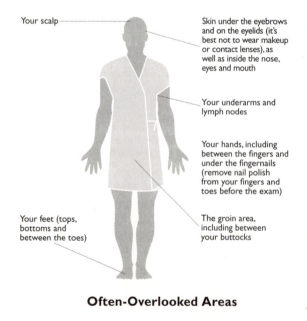

Your scalp

Skin under the eyebrows and on the eyelids (it's best not to wear makeup or contact lenses), as well as inside the nose, eyes and mouth

Your underarms and lymph nodes

Your hands, including between the fingers and under the fingernails (remove nail polish from your fingers and toes before the exam)

Your feet (tops, bottoms and between the toes)

The groin area, including between your buttocks

Often-Overlooked Areas

Women Get Skin Cancer Where?!

Andrew Bronin, MD, associate clinical professor of dermatology at Yale School of Medicine in New Haven, Connecticut. A dermatologist in private practice in Rye Brook, New York, he also is editor in chief of DermClips, an American Academy of Dermatology (AAD) continuing medical education publication.

Remember back in the 1960s, at the height of the feminist movement, when women were encouraged to look at their vulvas (external genitalia) in a hand mirror so that we could learn about our bodies? Turns out there's a medical rationale for this, too—because such self-exams help detect genital skin cancer.

Are you surprised to learn that women can get skin cancer "down there"? Though men also get genital skin cancer, a recent study found that women are almost three times more likely to die of the most common type of this disease. It's not clear why women's mortality rates are higher—it might be that women are more susceptible or that this cancer is more aggressive in women...or just that growths are easier to find on male genitalia, so men get treated earlier in the progression of the disease.

The vulva includes the clitoris, labia (vaginal lips) and opening to the vagina. There are several types of vulvar cancer. To find out how to guard against these potentially deadly cancers, we spoke with Andrew Bronin, MD, associate clinical professor of dermatology at Yale School of Medicine in New Haven, Connecticut, and a dermatologist in private practice in Rye Brook, New York. *Here are the prevention and early detection strategies he recommended to protect yourself from...*

• **Squamous cell vulvar cancer.** This skin cancer arises in the squamous cells (the layer of cells on the surface of the skin) and accounts for nearly 90% of vulvar cancers. Risk factors include age (85% of women who contract the disease are over age 50)…chronic vulvar or vaginal inflammation…infection with HIV (the AIDS virus)…or a history of cervical cancer or lichen sclerosus (a disorder characterized by thin, itchy vulvar tissues).

• **Squamous cell cancer can be linked to certain strains of human papillomavirus (HPV).** The HPVs are a group of more than 100 related viruses, some of which are also associated with genital warts and cervical cancer. The sexually transmitted strains of HPV usually spread during vaginal, anal or oral sex via skin-to-skin contact (rather than via bodily fluids). Though the virus sometimes clears up on its own, there is no sure-fire way to eradicate HPV—so prevention is important. *To reduce your risk…*

• Get tested for HPV. Like a Pap smear, the HPV test analyzes cervical cells. If you are not infected, ask your doctor whether you should get the Gardasil vaccine, which protects against four of the most troublesome strains of HPV. "Although the vaccine is currently FDA-approved for women age 26 and under, it also may benefit older women," Dr. Bronin said. "Even if you are infected with one strain of HPV, consider vaccination—because it may protect you against three other strains."

• Even if a man has no visible genital warts, he could have a "preclinical" HPV infection—meaning that the virus is present and contagious but hasn't yet produced visible symptoms. So if you enter a new relationship, have your partner use condoms. But understand that this is not foolproof since it protects you from infections only in areas covered by the condom.

Also: Be aware that the more sexual partners you've had—and the more partners your partner has had—the higher your likelihood of having been exposed to HPV.

• Don't smoke! Smoking increases vulvar cancer risk, especially if you have HPV.

• **Vulvar malignant melanoma.** This type accounts for only about 4% of vulvar skin cancers, but it is the most deadly because it spreads rapidly. Melanoma develops in the melanocytes, the skin's pigment-producing cells. You probably know that sun exposure increases the risk for malignant melanoma—but sun is not a requirement for the development of this disease. In fact, melanoma has the potential to occur anywhere that you have pigment cells… and that's every square inch of your skin, including your vulva. You can get malignant melanoma even where the sun never shines.

"Having moles that are atypical—in other words, funny-looking to the eye and under the microscope—anywhere on your body increases your risk for vulvar malignant melanoma. So does a personal or family history of any malignant melanoma," Dr. Bronin said. Unfortunately, vulvar melanomas have some of the worst prognoses of all malignant melanomas, with a five-year survival rate of only 50%…precisely because they often are not caught until it is too late.

• **Vulvar adenocarcinoma.** This type begins in the gland cells just inside the vaginal opening or in the top layer of vulvar skin. It accounts for about 8% of vulvar cancers. Though less deadly than melanoma, it has a relatively high recurrence rate.

Concern: Diagnosis often is delayed because a cancerous growth may be easily mistaken for a cyst.

Key: Early Detection

Catching vulvar cancer early offers the best chance for a good outcome. *Potentially life-saving strategies…*

• **Give yourself periodic vulvar self-exams.** The frequency depends on your personal risk factors, so ask your gynecologist to recommend a schedule.

What to do: "Use a mirror to check the inner and outer labia, vaginal opening, clitoris and perineal area between the vagina and anus. Look for abnormal lumps or growths… red, white or grayish lesions…changes in pigmentation… swelling…or sores that don't heal," Dr. Bronin suggested. If you spot any such signs, see your gynecologist or dermatologist as soon as possible.

• **Also be on the lookout for unexplained itching, tenderness, pain or nonmenstrual bleeding**—and again, alert your doctor without delay.

• **Get an annual gynecologic checkup.** Your doctor will be watching for the disease (among other things)—but it doesn't hurt to ask, "Do you see any signs of vulvar cancer?"

Diagnosis and treatment: When suspicious growths are found, the tissue is biopsied. If the precancerous condition *vulvar intraepithelial neoplasia* is diagnosed, laser therapy or surgery can keep it from turning into a squamous cell cancer. If the biopsy does reveal squamous cell cancer, treatment options include laser therapy, surgery, radiation and/or chemotherapy.

If a pigmented skin lesion is suspected of being malignant melanoma, it should be surgically removed by a dermatologist or gynecologist and examined at a pathology lab. Early recognition and removal of a malignant melanoma can be lifesaving.

For vulvar adenocarcinoma, treatment also is surgical, with the extent of the surgery depending on the extent of the disease. Again, Dr. Bronin emphasized, early detection offers the best chance for limiting the necessary surgery and enhancing the prognosis.

Contraceptives Do More Than Just Prevent Pregnancy

Birth control pills reduce by 50% the risk for cancer of the uterine lining (endometrium), and women taking the Pill for at least 10 years have nearly half the risk for ovarian cancer as women who do not take the Pill. Intrauterine devices (IUDs) help protect against cervical cancer by triggering an immune response to HPV, the virus that causes the cancer.

University of California, *Berkeley Wellness Letter.* www.WellnessLetter.com

---

Good Buzz: Coffee Helps Protect Against Endometrial Cancer

Youjin Je, ScD, nutrition researcher in the department of nutrition at Harvard School of Public Health in Boston and leader of a meta-analysis on coffee and endometrial cancer risk published in *International Journal of Cancer.*

J ava lovers, rejoice—recent research reveals yet another potential health perk from drinking coffee. We already have evidence that coffee can reduce the risk for diabetes, stroke and Parkinson's disease, and perhaps for Alzheimer's, depression and basal cell skin cancer, too. And now it appears that coffee also reduces a woman's odds of getting cancer of the endometrium (uterine lining), the most common gynecologic cancer in the US.

What we all want to know: How much joe would we need to drink to help guard against endometrial cancer? To get the answer, Harvard researchers analyzed data from 16 studies involving a total of 369,004 women (including 6,628 endometrial cancer patients) who were followed for up to 26 years.

Findings: Women who drank the most coffee—an average of three to four cups daily—were 29% less likely to get endometrial cancer than women who drank little or no coffee. Overall, each eight-ounce cup of coffee consumed per day reduced a woman's endometrial cancer risk by 8%. (These stats were for women who drank regular coffee or regular as well as decaf…there was not enough data on decaf alone to draw firm conclusions about its effects on endometrial cancer risk.)

Drink think: Coffee is an excellent source of chlorogenic acid, an antioxidant that helps prevent the damage to cells' DNA that triggers the cancer process. Also, caffeine and/or other bioactive compounds in coffee may have favorable effects on hormones, including estrogen and insulin, thus inhibiting cancer cell growth.

Downside: For some people, excess caffeine can cause irritability, anxiety, restlessness, headaches, sleep problems and/or abnormal heart rhythms.

Is black best? This study did not specifically assess the effects of drinking coffee black versus adding cream and/or sugar. But researchers cautioned that consuming lots of cream or sugar could contribute to insulin resistance and excess weight gain—both of which can increase endometrial cancer risk.

Bottom line: Go ahead and enjoy your java (provided the caffeine doesn't bother you), but don't go too light or too sweet.

The Truth About HPV

Sin Hang Lee, MD, pathologist at Milford Hospital and director of Milford Medical Laboratory (a subsidiary of the hospital that provides comprehensive testing), both in Milford, Connecticut. Dr. Lee is an internationally recognized expert in the area of human papillomavirus and has developed a DNA sequencing test to identify specific HPV genotypes.

Each year in the US, 55 million women receive a Pap test to check for abnormal cells that might be an early sign of cervical cancer. Of these, 3.5 million tests show abnormalities that require medical follow-up, and about 12,000 women are diagnosed as having cervical cancer.

Recent development: Since 2006, when the pharmaceutical company Merck began TV and print advertisements for Gardasil, a vaccine against the mainly sexually transmitted human papillomavirus (HPV), which is present in up to 99% of cervical cancer cases, many women have been increasingly confused about their real risks for the disease and what role a vaccine may play in preventing it.

Gardasil is also FDA-approved for preventing certain vulvar and vaginal cancers in females and for preventing genital warts in males and females. It was recently approved to prevent anal cancer in males and

females. Cervarix, another HPV vaccine, was approved by the FDA in 2009.

For the facts that every woman should know about HPV and cervical cancer, we spoke with renowned HPV expert Sin Hang Lee, MD, a pathologist who has studied cervical cancer for more than 50 years and trained in the laboratory of Dr. Georgios Papanicolaou, the scientist who developed the Pap test to detect cervical cancer. *Dr. Lee's most important insights…*

FACT 1: **There is no cervical cancer crisis.** Thanks to regular use of the Pap test, the incidence of cervical cancer has been dramatically reduced. Of the Pap tests performed annually in the US, only about 0.02% result in a diagnosis of cervical cancer when a biopsy is performed.

If all women got annual Pap tests—and the tests were analyzed properly (not all HPV tests distinguish between benign HPV strains, or genotypes, and those that may cause cancer)—death from cervical cancer would be extremely rare. The disease is highly preventable if lesions are detected in a precancerous stage.

Note: The American College of Obstetricians and Gynecologists (ACOG) revised its recommendations for Pap tests in 2009. For women ages 21 to 30 without symptoms or risk factors, the ACOG recommends the test every two years…and every three years for women age 30 and older who have had three consecutive normal tests. Discuss the frequency of your Pap tests with your doctor.

FACT 2: **The concern over HPV infection is overblown.** While HPV can cause cervical cancer, the story is more nuanced than people are led to believe from public service announcements and vaccine ads.

There are about 200 known genotypes of HPV, but only 13 are considered "high risk" for causing cervical cancer—HPV-16, 18, 31, 33, 35, 39, 45, 51, 52, 56, 58, 59 and 68. Of these, HPV-16 and HPV-18 are believed to cause 70% of all cervical cancers. That means that you can have any of the 187 other genotypes without having an increased risk of developing cervical cancer. The prevalence of high-risk genotypes varies worldwide and depends in part on a woman's level of sexual activity.

Important: Nearly all cases of genital warts are caused by two low-risk genotypes, HPV-6 and HPV-11. This means that warts you can see and feel are annoying but usually not dangerous.

Even better news: Even though there is no treatment for HPV infection, women's immune systems are typically effective at fighting HPV. More than 90% of HPV infections disappear on their own and do not progress to precancerous stages or cancer. In fact, the average HPV infection lasts only about six months. This means that a woman who receives testing when the infection is active may be HPV-negative within a matter of months.

The women who should be most concerned about cervical cancer are those infected with a high-risk genotype in which the infection is persistent (lasting more than six months). Women typically undergo repeat testing every six months until the infection clears, and a biopsy may be recommended if an infection of the same genotype persists while the Pap test is still abnormal or questionable.

FACT 3: **HPV vaccines don't guarantee cancer prevention.** Gardasil prevents infection with four genotypes—the high-risk HPV-16 and HPV-18 and the low-risk-for-cancer, genital wart–causing HPV-6 and HPV-11. (Cervarix prevents only HPV-16 and HPV-18.)

Some women consider it useful to be protected against two of the 13 cancer-causing genotypes. However, most women are unaware that there is no evidence showing how long the vaccine will remain effective.

Important: I recommend that women who want to get the HPV vaccine ask their gynecologists to make sure that they are not already infected with HPV-16 or HPV-18. There is some evidence that women who get the vaccine when they are infected with HPV—especially HPV-16 and HPV-18—have an increased risk of developing cervical cancer.

Reported side effects of the Gardasil and Cervarix vaccines include temporary pain and swelling at the injection site and headache.

FACT 4: **Not all HPV testing is adequate.** Historically, HPV tests have not distinguished between benign and specific cancer-causing genotypes. Newer HPV tests, including Cervista HPV HR, are designed to detect when any of the 13 cancer-causing genotypes or the intermediate-risk genotype HPV-66 is present, but they do not identify the specific genotype. To identify the specific HPV genotype—with virtually no risk for false-positive results or misidentification—physicians can request a DNA sequencing test. This test is available from the nonprofit organization SaneVax, Inc., *www.SaneVax.org*, for $50.

New HPV Test for Cervical Cancer Saves Lives

Mark H. Stoler, MD, professor of pathology, cytology and gynecology, associate director, surgical pathology and cytopathology and director, gynecological pathology fellowship program, University of Virginia School of Medicine, Charlottesville, Virginia.

There's good news for more than 12,000 American women who develop cervical cancer each year. On a global scale, the World Health Organization estimates that there are 528,000 new cases of cervical cancer annually—a figure that translates into 266,000 deaths. Now, finally, a significantly more sensitive version of the test—called cobas HPV—has arrived, and it is sure to bring about a major reduction in those frightening numbers.

The cobas HPV test, developed by Roche, identifies 14 strains of the human papillomavirus (HPV), the sexually transmitted virus that causes nearly all cervical cancers. In combination with regular Pap smears, this test can help you get an earlier and more accurate diagnosis.

A More Sensitive HPV Test

A single Pap test can detect a precancerous lesion only 50% to 80% of the time. In contrast, current HPV tests can tell us whether or not a woman has one of a dozen cancer-linked HPV strains (indicating a possible pre-cancer) but is not able to specifically identify the strains. This new level of analysis afforded by the cobas HPV test detects more than 90% of existing precancers, notes Mark H. Stoler, MD, a professor and associate director of surgical pathology and cytopathology at the University of Virginia Health System. He said that the test specifically identifies the HPV-16 and HPV-18 viruses—the two highest-risk varieties of HPV that are responsible for seven out of 10 cervical cancers. The test can also identify 12 other high-risk types as well (31, 33, 35, 39, 45, 51, 52, 56, 58, 59, 66 and 68).

While doctors have successfully used Pap tests to detect the possibility of cervical cancer for more than a half-century, cutting its incidence rate by up to 75% in the past 50 years, the new cobas HPV test provides even greater accuracy in detection (and thus protection) because it analyzes specific HPV genotypes that put women at highest risk. In their analysis of data from the Roche ATHENA trial (Addressing THE Need for Advanced HPV Diagnostics), the largest registration study ever conducted for cervical cancer screening and encompassing more than 47,000 women in the US, Dr. Stoler and his colleagues found that 25% to 30% of women who tested positive for HPV-16 or HPV-18 had a precancerous lesion even though their Pap test results were only minimally abnormal. In other words, these women were at a much more significant risk than was previously appreciated. These results were published online in a recent issue of the *American Journal of Clinical Pathology*. This was just the first in a series of reports to be published from the large-scale ATHENA study.

Get an Early and More Accurate Diagnosis

The cobas HPV test is widely available. Contact your insurer to see if it covers the cost ($50-$100).

At present, the FDA has approved the cobas HPV test for adjunctive use with Pap smears in women 30 and older and to help sort quickly through those Pap tests that appear abnormal. If you test negative on both the Pap and the cobas HPV, Dr. Stoler says you can wait at least three years to be screened again. If you test positive for HPV—especially HPV-16 or HPV-18—your doctor will order further testing, such as a cervical exam (colposcopy) or a cervical biopsy, to confirm or rule out the possibility of cervical cancer.

Many advances in cancer screening have disappointed in recent years. By combining the cobas HPV test with a Pap, we have what seems to be a safe, accurate and reliable tool that represents a real step forward in cervical cancer screening practice.

Cervical Cancer in Your Past? Here's How to Protect Your Future

It's a huge relief for any woman to put cervical cancer behind her and get on with life, of course.

But: Even more than four decades after being successfully treated, women who have undergone radiation therapy for cervical cancer have a 30% increased risk of developing a second cancer. The most vulnerable areas are those near the cervix—including the colon, rectum, anus, bladder, ovaries and genitals.

Cancer defense: Researchers urge cervical cancer survivors to scrupulously adhere to their oncologists' recommendations for getting periodic follow-up cancer screenings of organs near the cervix.

Anil K. Chaturvedi, PhD, MPH, researcher in the infections and immunoepidemiology branch of the National Cancer Institute in Bethesda, Maryland, and lead author of a study of 104,760 cervical cancer survivors.

No More Yearly Gyno Visits?

Diane M. Harper, MD, MPH, vice-chair for research and a professor in the departments of community and family medicine, obstetrics and gynecology, and biomedical and health informatics at the University of Missouri–Kansas City School of Medicine. She is one of the country's leading cervical cancer researchers and experts on HPV.

According to current cervical cancer screening recommendations from the American College of Obstetricians and Gynecologists (ACOG) for women age 30 and older, if a woman's last three consecutive Paps were negative (meaning that her cervix showed no abnormal cells or potentially cancerous changes) or if her HPV tests did not detect any of the human papillomavirus types that can cause cervical cancer, she can wait three years before seeing her gynecologist again for additional cervical cancer screening.

It could be argued that most women age 30 and older do not need to have both an HPV test and a Pap—and in fact, the HPV test may one day replace the Pap as the initial screening for cervical cancer. But for the time being, either the Pap alone or both the HPV test and Pap are recommended by ACOG.

From the patient's point of view, an HPV test is performed just like a Pap and both can easily be done at the same time. A gynecologist sweeps the cervix with a soft brush to collect the cells that are shedding from the cervix, then places the sample in a vial of liquid and sends it to a lab. For the Pap, the cells suspended in the liquid are examined under a microscope to analyze their shape. For the HPV test, DNA from the cells is separated from that same liquid sample and tested for the presence of the 14 high-risk types of HPV associated with cervical cancer. Insurance typically covers the Pap and may cover the HPV test.

Important: If you use your gynecologist as your primary care provider, as some women do, you will still need to see him or her annually or as often as the doctor recommends for your regular checkup, even if you don't get a Pap or HPV test at those visits.

Be On the Alert for Ovarian Cancer

Alexi Wright, MD, medical oncologist, Dana-Farber Cancer Institute, instructor in medicine, Harvard Medical School, both in Boston.

The pink ribbons we see everywhere in October make it seem like breast cancer is a woman's worst nightmare. But, in fact, we know that there is another even more insidious cancer to fear—ovarian cancer. It's true that this type of cancer is rarer, but it can be more lethal and harder to detect, in part because its symptoms are commonplace and dismayingly vague, including abdominal bloating, digestive difficulties and fatigue. While not as public, researchers are working hard on understanding and beating ovarian cancer, and there is news—some good, some bad.

Screening Tests Don't Deliver

The disappointing results are now in from a National Cancer Institute and National Institutes of Health study that began in 1993, evaluating the effectiveness of early screening for ovarian cancer using a combination of ultrasound imaging and a blood test looking for the presence of CA-125 (a protein associated with the cancer). The study split 80,000 women ages 55 to 74 into two groups—one group was screened yearly from 1993 to 2001, and the other group was not. It then followed the women until 2010.

The findings: The number of women in each group who developed ovarian cancer and the deaths from it were nearly identical—in both groups, more than three-quarters of the diagnoses were at stage III or IV. The screenings arguably even made matters worse, since they also yielded 3,000 false-positives, leading 1,000 of those women to have surgery to remove ovaries that were ultimately found to be cancer-free.

Hard to Detect

We spoke with Alexi Wright, MD, medical oncologist at the Dana-Farber Cancer Institute in Boston and an expert on this subject, for help putting this information in perspective. *She explained that there are several reasons why this disease is so hard to detect, including a few that are actually quite basic…*

•**A typical early-stage ovarian cancer tumor is too small to be picked up with screening technology currently available.**

•**The tumor is somewhat diffuse.** Unlike most other cancers that start out contained in an organ such as the uterus, liver or lungs, ovarian cancer spreads over organs like a thin film or may be scattered all over the abdomen like grains of rice.

•**It grows really fast.** Once this cancer develops to an advanced stage, its assault is incredibly rapid. "The size of the cancer doubles roughly every two months," Dr. Wright said.

Then, as far as the blood test goes, researchers initially believed that testing for the presence of higher-than-normal levels of CA-125 would reliably reveal ovarian cancer at an earlier stage but, alas, this didn't prove to be true. It turned out to be a "limited screening test," Dr. Wright said, because researchers have since learned that ovarian cancer isn't the only problem that causes a high level of CA-125—there are lots of other things that raise the level, too, including inflammation in the abdomen, which could also be caused by diverticulitis, pelvic inflammatory disease and even pregnancy and menstruation. This test is now sometimes used to monitor treatment of ovarian cancer but, Dr. Wright explained, its value in that context is being questioned as well.

A Brighter Note

Now for some good news…scientists have recently announced a genetic finding that offers some hope. In addition to the BRCA genes that increase a woman's risk for both breast and ovarian cancer, there is a gene called RAD51D that runs in a small number of families and creates ovarian cancer susceptibility. Knowing this may help doctors create new and better treatment options.

In addition, Dr. Wright said that there has been considerable improvement in the treatments we already have. With more than a dozen different chemotherapy medicines now available, doctors can determine the genetic defect causing the disease in each patient and then use the best available drug to kill cancer cells more precisely without harming as many healthy ones.

Ultimately, though, it remains true that the best advice any woman can be given is to have a high index of suspicion when it comes to symptoms of ovarian cancer, since finding it early can make the difference between life and death. In women whose cancers are diagnosed at the earliest possible stage (1A), the five-year survival rate is 87%, whereas in women whose cancers are advanced (stage IV), that number plummets to just 11%. Relatively early symptoms of ovarian cancer may include bloating, constipation, abdominal pain, gas, getting full easily when eating, abdominal swelling, urinary frequency and unexplained weight gain. If you have any of these symptoms, particularly for more than a few weeks, Dr. Wright urges you to visit your gynecologist for an ultrasound and/or CT scan immediately. If you think that the doctor isn't hearing your concerns, speak up and insist on being paid attention to…or consider getting a second opinion.

Better Ovarian Cancer Detection

According to a recent finding, among 37,000 healthy women (average age 57) who took part in studies to investigate the effectiveness of transvaginal ultrasound screening, 72 ovarian cancers were detected. Of these, 70% were early stage, and 88% of these women had a five-year survival rate, compared with about 50% of unscreened women who were diagnosed with ovarian cancer.

Theory: Ultrasound detects changes in size and structure of the ovary. Women at risk for ovarian cancer (due to family history, for example) should discuss transvaginal screening with their doctors.

Edward J. Pavlik, PhD, director, Ovarian Screening Research Program, University of Kentucky, Lexington.

A Simple Question That Could Save Your Life

M. Robyn Andersen, PhD, MPH, cancer researcher at the Fred Hutchinson Cancer Research Center and an affiliate associate professor of health services and epidemiology at the University of Washington School of Public Health, both in Seattle. She is the lead author of a study on an ovarian cancer screening questionnaire published in *Open Journal of Obstetrics and Gynecology.*

Belly bloat, abdominal discomfort, the feeling of a too-full tummy. It's easy to dismiss such vague complaints as simple digestive upset or some other minor malady. So it's no wonder that many women don't bother to mention such symptoms… and doctors often don't think to inquire about them.

Problem: These subtle symptoms also can be warning signs of ovarian cancer—and ignoring them can be a potentially deadly mistake.

When ovarian cancer is caught and treated early, while still confined to the ovary, the cure rate is about 90%…but when diagnosis is delayed until after the cancer has spread, the five-year survival rate plunges to just 20% to 30%. So even though ovarian cancer is relatively uncommon, affecting fewer than 2% of women, its deadly nature makes it a formidable foe.

Can't screening tests be given to all women to help detect the disease early on? Not a good idea. Currently available tests—the CA-125 blood test (which measures markers

for ovarian cancer) and ultrasound scan of the ovaries—unfortunately have high rates of false-positive results. Since an operation is needed to confirm the diagnosis, these screening tests can lead to unnecessary surgeries in which healthy ovaries are removed and women are placed at risk for surgical complications such as infections and blood clots. That's why the US Preventive Services Task Force recently reaffirmed its recommendation against routine ovarian cancer screening.

Encouraging news: In response, researchers have been working to develop a simpler, safer screening tool that could be used for all women, with the goal of identifying those who truly are most likely to benefit from further testing. And now a recent study, though small, suggests a simple step in the right direction.

The key is a single-question patient questionnaire that typically takes less than two minutes to complete and can be done right in the doctor's office. It gets patients and doctors thinking about the warning signs that merit further investigation.

Study participants included 1,200 women ages 40 to 87 who happened to have appointments at a Seattle clinic (for instance, for routine mammograms or follow-ups to previous appointments). While they were there, the women wrote their answers to the question, "Are you currently experiencing any of the following symptoms frequently?" *The symptoms listed…*

- **Pain.** Abdominal/pelvic pain
- **Eating.** Feeling full quickly or unable to eat normally
- **Abdomen.** Abdominal bloating or increased abdomen size

Women who answered yes to the question further indicated how many days per month they were experiencing the symptom and how long they had had the symptom. Participants were considered to be "positive for symptoms" if any of the above signs were currently occurring more than 12 times per month and were present for less than one

Symptoms of Ovarian Cancer

Know the symptoms of ovarian cancer: Bloating…increased abdominal size…pelvic or abdominal pain…difficulty eating…and/or feeling full quickly. Consult your physician if you begin to experience one or more symptoms every day or two—or more than 12 times in a month. Though most likely the symptoms are caused by a noncancerous condition, they should not be ignored.

M. Robyn Andersen, MPH, PhD, member, public health sciences division, Fred Hutchinson Cancer Research Center, Seattle, and coauthor of a study of an ovarian cancer symptoms index, published in *Open Journal of Obstetrics and Gynecology.*

year. (Past symptoms that disappeared do not suggest ovarian cancer.)

Results: 5.5% of the women were positive for symptoms, and most of these patients chose to go on with further testing. During the one-year follow-up period, one woman was diagnosed with ovarian cancer—and she was among those who had answered yes to the questionnaire. Importantly, among the women who reported no symptoms, none ended up being diagnosed with the disease during the follow-up—a testament to the accuracy of the questionnaire as a screening tool.

Researchers hope that primary-care doctors will soon begin using this simple questionnaire to identify patients who may have ovarian cancer.

In the meantime: If you develop any of the above symptoms and they are new to you and occur frequently, you can help protect yourself by immediately alerting your doctor. In most cases, they will not signal ovarian cancer—but women who do have such symptoms are at higher risk than other women and may benefit from follow-up with the currently available tests.

Should You Be Screened for Uterine Cancer?

Debbie Saslow, PhD, director, Breast and Gynecologic Cancer, American Cancer Society, Atlanta.

A test for an insidious, lethal cancer isn't used very much even though it has been around for years and has a very high success rate of detecting risk. Why is that?

The cancer is uterine cancer, which sometimes can progress quickly and dangerously. So why isn't this test being recommended as a screening for all postmenopausal women, who are the most likely to get uterine cancer?

And who should get the test? For answers to these questions, we turned to Debbie Saslow, PhD, director of breast and gynecologic cancer at the American Cancer Society in Atlanta.

Thick and Thin

Also known as endometrial cancer, since it begins in the endometrium (the lining of the uterus), uterine cancer is the most common gynecological cancer, affecting more than 43,000 women and causing nearly 8,000 deaths in this country each year.

You may not realize that one physiological characteristic that a gynecologist is attuned to is the thickness of your uterine lining. It's normal for the lining of a woman's uterus to atrophy and grow thin with menopause, Dr. Saslow explained. There are several reasons why a woman might have a thickened uterine lining, but cancer is one of them, so the condition should be monitored. A test called transvaginal ultrasound (TVS) is one way this can be done.

How it works: A technician inserts a specially designed ultrasound probe into a woman's vagina and captures an image, which is sent to a display, enabling the technician to measure the thickness of the uterine lining. Though it can be somewhat uncomfortable, this test is not painful.

Researchers in the UK administered TVS to nearly 37,000 postmenopausal women, measuring the thickness of their uterine linings and then following them for a year to see how many developed cancer. The study, which was published in *The Lancet*, found that women with a uterine lining that was 5 mm or thicker were indeed at about 80% higher risk for uterine cancer within a year.

Even so, the study authors oppose using TVS for mass screening and, said Dr. Saslow, so does the American Cancer Society. One reason, she said, is that the risk of a false-positive result is high. Nearly 15% of women who undergo TVS and are found to have abnormally thick uterine linings will then end up having to endure an uncomfortable (and expensive) biopsy, with all the accompanying mental turmoil that brings—but they will not have cancer. Meanwhile, she said, the vast majority (90%) of women who do have endometrial cancer also will have abnormal bleeding as an early warning sign. These factors have led the researchers and other experts to conclude that it is unlikely there will be much benefit to screening asymptomatic women. "We found that there is no proof that detection through screening improves outcome over detection from symptoms (vaginal bleeding)," Dr. Saslow explained.

Are You a Candidate?

While TVS is not a routine test, it is widely available. Risk factors for uterine cancer include obesity…never having been pregnant…and exposure to synthetic estrogens, such as hormone replacement therapy, or *tamoxifen* (for breast cancer). Dr. Saslow said that at present the American Cancer Society is focused on limiting the number of false-positives and therefore recommends screening only for women with a rare hereditary disease called Lynch syndrome that increases the risk for both uterine and colorectal cancers.

Cancer screening tests remain a controversial topic, and this story sheds light on the complexities that make it so difficult—the risk-versus-benefits equation does not

always present a clear case for making a recommendation. The one thing that every woman absolutely should know is that the most important warning sign of uterine cancer is vaginal bleeding after menopause—if you experience this symptom, call your doctor immediately.

Thyroid Cancer: The Fastest-Increasing Cancer in America— Could You Be a Victim?

Michael G. Moore, MD, FACS, assistant professor of otolaryngology, head and neck surgery and director of head and neck surgery at Indiana University School of Medicine, Indianapolis, and a physician and researcher at the University of Indiana Melvin and Bren Simon Cancer Center in Indianapolis.

More and more Americans are getting thyroid cancer. The incidence of new cases has doubled in the last 40 years, making it the fastest-increasing cancer in the US. In the years between 1997 and 2006, the incidence of thyroid cancer increased by 6.5% per year, according to data from the National Cancer Institute.

Here, who gets thyroid cancer and why it's on the rise…

Who's at Risk?

You can feel the outline of the thyroid gland by touching the area on the neck just below the Adam's apple. It's an endocrine (hormone-producing) gland that secretes triiodothyronine (T3) and thyroxine (T4), hormones that regulate metabolism, heart rate and many other functions.

The most common type of thyroid cancer, papillary thyroid cancer, accounts for about 80% of all cases. It usually is diagnosed when patients are in their mid-40s, and women get it about three times more often than men.

In the majority of cases of thyroid cancer, there are no obvious causes. *However, there are some exposures and conditions that have been identified as risk factors…*

• **Radiation exposure.** Exposure to high levels of radiation from fallout from nuclear power plant accidents and weapons testing has been linked to thyroid cancer.

Also at risk are adults who were treated with radiation during childhood for chronic conditions, such as acne and enlarged tonsils and adenoids. Radiation was used excessively from the 1940s through the 1960s for benign conditions of the head and neck before the risks were fully understood.

Important: Routine exposures during regular X-rays and CT scans at the dentist's or doctor's office have not been shown to result in higher rates of thyroid cancer. In addition, higher treatment doses, such as external beam radiation used to treat head and neck cancer, also have not resulted in increased risk.

• **Hashimoto's thyroiditis is an auto-immune disease that affects the thyroid gland.** It greatly increases the risk for thyroid lymphoma, a less common form of thyroid cancer. Patients with Hashimoto's thyroiditis also have a significantly greater risk of getting papillary thyroid cancer. So if you have Hashimoto's thyroiditis, you should see your doctor regularly to be monitored for thyroid deficiency.

• **Goiter.** This is an enlarged thyroid gland, commonly caused by low dietary iodine or other environmental factors.

• **Being overweight increases the risk for thyroid cancer by about 20%.** Patients who are obese are even more likely to get it.

• **Genetics.** While the majority of thyroid cancers do not run in families, there are specific genetic syndromes, including multiple endocrine neoplasia, that increase the risk for thyroid cancer. If you have a strong family history of thyroid cancer, you should ask your doctor if further testing is desirable.

Keep in mind that the total number of thyroid cancer cases is relatively low. It is estimated that there will be about 60,000 new cases in 2014. (For comparison, about 232,000 new cases of breast cancer and 137,000 new cases of colorectal cancer will be diagnosed this year.)

Why the Increase?

Specialists who treat thyroid cancer agree that they're seeing more cases in recent years. But what they don't know is exactly why.

In addition to the risk factors listed above, it's possible that environmental factors, such as exposure to chemical pollutants, are involved. No definitive study, however, has confirmed environmental agents are responsible.

Also, because women and obese individuals have higher levels of estrogen, it has been suggested that estrogen may be an additional risk factor.

Another factor: Improvements in diagnosis. With the development of ultrasound in the 1980s, it's now possible to detect thyroid nodules that are smaller than one centimeter (cm) across.

A study in *The Journal of the American Medical Association* found that much of the increase in reported cases of thyroid cancer was due to small tumors that might never have been discovered in the past. Many of these tumors are unlikely to grow large enough to cause symptoms.

If You Have It

A typical symptom of thyroid cancer is a painless lump in the gland. Advanced cases may result in enlarged lymph nodes, changes in the voice (hoarseness), difficulty swallowing or breathing, or even coughing up blood.

Most thyroid nodules are discovered by palpation—doctors feel them when they check the neck during routine exams. Or an abnormality might be discovered when you have an ultrasound or other imaging test for an unrelated condition, such as neck pain after a car accident.

If a nodule is detected, you will be scheduled for blood tests (to check levels of thyroid hormones) and an ultrasound. Then if the nodule still seems suspicious, your doctor may order a fine-needle biopsy to look for cancer cells.

The odds are in your favor: About 95% of thyroid nodules are not cancer. And if it is cancer, it's likely to be among the most treatable, with a long-term survival rate of about 97%.

If you do have cancer…

•**Surgery is the main treatment.** Most patients will have a total thyroidectomy, the removal of the entire gland. Patients who have this procedure are less likely to have a recurrence of the cancer than those who have just part of the gland removed.

Exception: Some patients with a microcarcinoma—a tumor that is smaller than 1 cm—are good candidates for a lobectomy, the removal of approximately half of the gland.

•**Radioactive iodine often is given to destroy any thyroid tissue that remains after thyroid surgery,** as well as residual microscopic cancer cells. Thyroid tissue is the only tissue in the body that readily absorbs the iodine, which releases radioactivity and kills the cells.

Radioactive iodine has little effect on healthy cells, so patients experience fewer side effects than they might with other forms of radiation treatment. Some patients, however, will experience side effects, such as nausea or dryness of the mouth or eyes. While the side effects will improve over time when the treatments stop—usually after about six weeks—some effects may persist.

•**Other types of radiation therapy,** along with chemotherapy, may be needed for certain types of thyroid cancer or if the cancer has spread.

•**Supplemental thyroid hormone.** Virtually all patients who have had surgery for thyroid cancer will need the medication *levothyroxine* (Synthroid or Levoxyl, among

Oral Cancer Epidemic

In the past 20 years, there has been a dramatic increase in cancer in the tonsil region and back of the tongue. Though this type of cancer typically has been associated with cigarettes and alcohol, many of today's patients never smoked and do not drink to excess—instead, their cancer is caused by human papillomavirus (HPV).

Before you panic, understand that the vast majority of HPV infections go away on their own with no further ramifications. And the number of people who do get oral cancer from HPV is still relatively small. In the US, about 30,000 nonsmokers are diagnosed with oral cancer each year.

The following symptoms should be evaluated by a doctor—an unexplained lump in the neck, discomfort on one side of the throat, subtle changes in voice, unexplained and persistent ear pain, or difficulty or mild pain with swallowing.

Good news: Cure rates for HPV-related oral cancers are much better than for smoking-related oral cancers.

Ted Teknos, MD, director of head and neck surgery at the Arthur G. James Cancer Hospital and Richard J. Solove Research Institute at The Ohio State University Comprehensive Cancer Center and a professor of otolaryngology—head and neck surgery at The Ohio State University Medical Center, all in Columbus.

others) to replace the hormones that were naturally produced by the gland. An additional benefit of levothyroxine is that it suppresses production of thyroid-stimulating hormone (TSH) from the pituitary gland. High TSH levels could stimulate growth of any remaining cancer-producing cells.

Throat Cancer Is On the Rise—Here's What You Can Do to Protect Yourself...

David M. Cognetti, MD, an otolaryngologist–head and neck specialist at Thomas Jefferson University Hospital in Philadelphia. He is an assistant professor of otolaryngology–head and neck surgery at Jefferson Medical College and codirector of the Jefferson Center for Head and Neck Surgery. He has published numerous articles on oropharyngeal and oral cancers in various professional journals.

Until the 1980s, throat cancers were relatively rare. They mainly affected older men who smoked and drank alcohol heavily.

Now: These same cancers are appearing more frequently, often in healthy men and women who have never smoked or abused alcohol.

Surprising statistic: In the US, oropharyngeal (the part of the throat just behind the mouth, including the tonsils) cancers caused by the human papillomavirus (HPV) increased by 225% between 1988 and 2004. These cancers are now seen more frequently in younger people, but the risk increases with age and peaks between ages 60 to 70. Men are at greater risk than women.

What's the explanation for this dramatic increase?

A Sexually Transmitted Cancer

Research shows that about 60% of oropharyngeal cancers are caused by HPV. This sexually transmitted virus has long been known to cause the majority of cervical cancers—and more recently has been linked to the development of throat and oral (on the tongue or inside the mouth) cancers.

Infections from HPV surged in the 1980s and 1990s, in part because more people were having sex with multiple partners. Since it takes years, or even decades, for the virus to damage the DNA in cells, we're only now seeing an increase in HPV-related cancers, including anal and oropharyngeal cancers. Oral sex is the highest risk factor for HPV-related oropharyngeal cancer.

Every year, approximately 34,000 Americans will be diagnosed with an oropharyngeal cancer, and nearly 7,000 will die from the malignancy.

Most people know that HPV causes genital warts. But only two strains of the virus cause these warts—and if you have them, your cancer risk is no higher because these strains don't cause cancer.

But at least 15 of the other strains—there are about 150 varieties—can potentially lead to cancer.

Important: Although more than half of American adults are believed to have been exposed to HPV, the vast majority of people infected with it clear the virus within a few months. Their risk of developing cancer is the same as if they had never been infected. It's only when the infection is chronic that the risk for cancer rises. Chronic infection with HPV increases risk for cancer at the site of infection, when the virus becomes integrated within the DNA of healthy cells.

Warning Signs

Most patients who are diagnosed with a localized, stage I or stage II (no spread to the lymph nodes) oropharyngeal or oral cancer will survive the disease. Unfortunately, most of these cancers are detected only at a more advanced stage, when the prognosis is poorer for non-HPV-related cancers.

That's why early detection is critical. Check the inside of your mouth every month, and see an otolaryngologist if you have any of the following...

•**Unexplained ear pain.** This is among the most common symptoms of oropharyngeal cancer in adults. It's known as referred otalgia (ear pain) because nerves in the throat that are irritated by cancer cause pain inside the ear.

Note: Adults rarely get ear infections. If you have nagging ear pain and your doctor says that the ear canal looks normal, cancer is a possibility.

• **A lump in the neck, particularly below the ear or on the front of the neck below the jawbone.** In adults, a lump in the neck is often assumed to be cancer until proven otherwise through a biopsy.

• **A sore throat, trouble swallowing and/or hoarseness that does not go away.** See a doctor if these symptoms persist after two weeks.

How to Protect Yourself

All adults should see a dentist at least once a year—especially if you drink alcohol or use tobacco or if you know that you've been exposed to HPV. Dentists routinely check the inside of the mouth for cancer or precancerous changes. They also look at the back of the throat—make sure your dentist looks carefully.

Cervical cancers caused by HPV can be detected by taking a swab of tissue in the cervix (Pap smear) and examining cells under a microscope. There isn't an equivalent test for oropharyngeal and oral cancer, so the exam is crucial. *Also…*

• **Don't use tobacco.** Apart from HPV, smoking and chewing tobacco are the main risk factors for oropharyngeal and oral cancers.

• **If you drink, do so in moderation.** The generally accepted upper safe limit for cancer risk is two alcoholic drinks daily for men and one for women. People who drink heavily are far more likely to get oropharyngeal cancer than moderate drinkers.

In addition…

• **Practice "safer sex."** Using a condom can help prevent infection with HPV. However, it's not a perfect solution because the virus can also be transmitted by unprotected oral sex and even by hand contact with the anal/genital areas.

Two vaccines, Gardasil and Cervarix, prevent infection with cancer-causing strains of HPV. Recommended for preteen girls and boys and young adults prior to sexual activity, either vaccine can prevent the majority of oropharyngeal and oral cancers. However, it's not recommended for people older than age 26.

If You Get Cancer

For reasons that aren't clear, oropharyngeal and oral cancers caused by HPV respond more readily to treatments than malignancies caused by smoking and/or drinking.

The five-year survival rate for smoking/drinking-related stage III or stage IV cancers—the stage at which they're usually diagnosed—is only about 45%. For cancers of the same stage that are caused by HPV, the survival rate is 80%.

Treatment options…

• **Surgery for localized cancer.** When cancers are detected at the earliest stage, they can often be removed by a head-and-neck surgeon or treated with radiation.

• **Surgery plus radiation and/or chemotherapy.** Patients with more advanced oropharyngeal or oral cancer require a combination of treatments. Patients will often get radiation and/or chemotherapy first. If the cancer does not respond, surgery is then performed to remove as much of it as possible. Lymph nodes that harbor cancer cells will also be removed.

Chapter 11

HIDDEN CAUSES OF CANCER AND HOW TO DEFEND YOURSELF

Little-Known Risk Factors for Cancer

What if you were told that your bedside alarm clock —or even your morning glass of orange juice— could possibly increase your risk for cancer?

That would sound pretty far-fetched, right? Believe it or not, scientists in many parts of the world are now making intriguing new discoveries about such surprising and little-known factors that may increase your likelihood of developing, or dying from, cancer.

For example...

Fruit Juice

Fruit is loaded with cancer-preventing antioxidants and fiber. But when you remove the fiber and drink the juice, which is high in sugar, you trigger greater spikes in blood sugar (glucose) and the glucose-regulating hormone insulin. High levels of glucose and insulin, acting as a growth stimulant, can promote more rapid cellular growth and division, which may increase one's risk of developing cancer or promote existing disease.

Scientific evidence: In a study of nearly 1,800 people, those who drank the most fruit juice (more than three glasses a day) were 74% more likely to develop colorectal cancer than those who drank the least, reported researchers in the *Journal of the American Dietetic Association.*

Cancer self-defense: This study, which was based on responses to food-frequency questionnaires, is not definitive, but I believe that the evidence is strong enough to advise people to avoid fruit juice and eat the whole fruit instead. If you don't want to give up fruit juice, mix three ounces of pure fruit juice with three ounces of water. Drink no more than two to three servings of the diluted fruit juice mixture a day.

Also avoid other fast-digesting, glucose-spiking carbohydrates (such as sugar and white flour). Emphasize foods that stabilize blood sugar and insulin, such as whole grains, legumes and vegetables. If you regularly eat pasta, cook it al dente (to minimize blood sugar increases). Choose whole-wheat pasta or brown rice pasta.

Light at Night

Fascinating research is being conducted on possible cancer risks associated with

Keith I. Block, MD, medical director of the Block Center for Integrative Cancer Treatment in Skokie, Illinois. He is author of *Life Over Cancer* (Bantam). *www.BlockMD.com*

a phenomenon known as "light at night" (LAN)—that is, any type of light exposure at night…even from a bedside alarm clock.

Research on the health effects of light exposure began more than two decades ago when scientists first identified an increased risk for breast, prostate, colorectal and other cancers in night-shift workers. Researchers theorize that night-shift work disrupts the body's natural circadian rhythm of daytime activity and nighttime rest, leading to imbalances in the hormones melatonin, estrogen and cortisol, which may play a role in triggering cancer. Now the research extends far beyond night-shift work.

Scientific evidence: Researchers at the University of Haifa in Israel measured light levels in the "sleeping habitats" of 1,679 women. They found that those with the highest "bedroom-light intensity" had a 22% higher risk for breast cancer.

To help protect yourself…

•**Use an alarm clock with a red light.** An alarm clock that's too close to your head and illuminated with any color other than red generates light in the blue spectrum, which may be associated with disruption in sleep and cut the production of melatonin, the circadian-regulating hormone.

In addition, if you need a light to help you find your way to the bathroom, use a dim nightlight. Avoid direct exposure to light.

Helpful: Use a sleep "mask" to cover your eyes when you're sleeping.

Heavy Traffic

It's logical that breathing air pollution from traffic might increase the risk for lung cancer.

Recent unexpected finding: Research published in various peer-reviewed journals in the last year links air pollution from traffic to a higher risk for ovarian, cervical, brain and stomach cancers. Researchers are still studying the association, but it may be due to volatile organic compounds (VOCs), polycyclic aromatic hydrocarbons and other toxic substances in car exhaust that cause cellular damage not just in the lungs but throughout the body. *To avoid exposure to pollution from automobiles…*

•**When driving, maintain a reasonable distance from the car in front of you.** Use the rule of thumb from safety experts—at least one car length for every 10 miles per hour (mph) of speed. So if you're driving 60 mph, there should be at least six car lengths between your car and the one in front of you. And in stop-and-go traffic or at a stoplight, leave one car length of space between your car and the one in front of you.

•**Turn on the air-recirculation system in your car**—and leave it on when you are in heavier traffic. This helps ensure that no outdoor air is circulating in your car.

•**If you live near a busy road, close your home's windows during peak traffic hours** and place one or two air filters in appropriate locations in your home.

•**Avoid driving, bicycling or walking in or near rush-hour traffic whenever possible.**

•**Wear a breathing mask, often used by motorists, joggers and cyclists to filter out noxious odors and fumes,** if you can't avoid areas with high levels of pollution from traffic.

Examples: Filt-R Reusable Neoprene Commuter Pollution Mask (about $30) and Respro Techno Face Mask (about $40)—both are available online. Or, if you can't wear a mask, breathe through your nose instead of your mouth. Breathing through the nose helps filter out particles that get trapped in the mucous membranes.

•**Eat an antioxidant-rich diet with leafy greens, melons and dark-colored fruits** such as plums and berries (for example, blueberries and blackberries)—these protect your body's cells from harmful pollutants.

•**Check the Web site *www.AirNow.gov* for air quality in your area,** and avoid going outside when the air-quality index is higher than the "moderate" range.

Dangerous Plastics

Patricia Hunt, PhD, is a leading BPA researcher, reproductive biologist and geneticist and the Edward R. Meyer Distinguished Professor in the School of Molecular Biosciences at Washington State University in Pullman.

A chemical commonly used in plastics, bisphenol-A (BPA), has powerful hormonelike effects. It is an endocrine disruptor that has been linked to increased risk for a variety of cancers, including breast cancer. A government task force issued a report suggesting that BPA might be an obesogen, a chemical that contributes to obesity.

Worrisome: A study of 2,517 Americans ages six and older found that 93% had traces of BPA in their bodies.

While you may not be able to avoid plastics altogether, you can minimize your risk. *Self-defense…*

•**Do not put plastics in the dishwasher or microwave.** High heat accelerates the migration of chemicals out of household plastics, such as food containers and spatulas.

Caution: Do not assume that products labeled "microwave safe" truly are safe—this label means only that the plastic won't melt in the microwave…it does not mean that it is chemical-free.

•**Don't let plastic wrap touch food.** Seek alternatives to clear plastic wraps (such as foil or glass containers)…or using plastic wrap only to cover containers…or wrapping food in a paper towel or waxed paper before putting it into a plastic bag.

Note: A "wet" food is more likely to absorb toxic chemicals than a "dry" one.

•**Freeze safely.** Cold is less likely than heat to accelerate the migration of chemicals from containers into food. However, even very low levels of BPA can produce profound changes in the body. The longer a food is in contact with any BPA-containing plastic, the greater the risk of exposure, even when frozen.

Recommended: Freeze foods in wide-mouth, dual-purpose, glass jars made for freezing and canning.

•**Replace the plastic you use most often.** Once you realize how much plastic you have in the kitchen, it's tempting to give up on getting rid of it all—so a good first step is to find safer alternatives for the plastic things that you use regularly.

Examples: Replace plastic ice cube trays with metal trays. Use wood cutting boards only. Use waxed-paper bags for sandwiches.

•**Discard damaged containers.** We all have our favorite storage containers that we tend to hang on to even when parts are cracked and the sides are warped. But damaged plastic is breaking down…and when this happens, chemicals are released.

•**Be wary of "BPA-free" plastics.** Some companies have developed plastics that don't contain BPA. Unfortunately, other chemicals in plastics may be just as risky.

Example: Some BPA-free containers use plastics made from structurally related compounds, such as bisphenol-AF or bisphenol-S.

Are they safer? We don't know—but recent studies suggest that bisphenol-AF actually may be more dangerous. Until we know more, use food and drink containers made from glass or stainless steel.

•**Buy from the butcher.** Supermarkets usually have the best prices on meats, but most of those meats are bedded on Styrofoam-like trays and then wrapped in plastic—so the meats are exposed to chemicals from above and below.

Better: Get your meats from a traditional butcher shop and ask to have them wrapped in old-fashioned butcher paper, not the new plastic-coated paper.

•**Opt for opaque.** The food industry prefers clear packaging because it looks "cleaner." But in many cases, clear plastics are more likely to contain BPA than opaque plastics.

•**Check recycling codes.** Some plastic containers are stamped with recycling codes that indicate the types of plastic used. Unfortunately, these codes don't tell very much about how safe a particular plastic is.

Helpful: Use the mnemonic, "5, 4, 1, 2—all the rest are bad for you." The "good" recycling codes may or may not contain harmful chemicals, but the "bad" ones almost certainly do.

• **Watch out for cans, too.** The vast majority of canned foods and beverages come in containers lined with a BPA-containing resin. Eden Foods, ConAgra and Hain Celestial have begun using BPA-free linings in some of their cans. (See a manufacturer's Web site for information on its BPA-free canned products, or contact the company directly.)

• **Skip the receipt.** The thermal paper used for many supermarket receipts (and ATM and other receipts, too) often is coated with BPA to keep the ink from running. If you must handle it, wash your hands afterward—and whatever you do, don't hold that receipt in your mouth while looking for your car keys.

The Sugar–Cancer Link

Patrick Quillin, PhD, RD, CNS, a clinical nutritionist who served for 10 years as director of nutrition for Cancer Treatment Centers of America, *www.Cancer Center.com*. He is author of *Beating Cancer with Nutrition* (Nutrition Times).

With all the negative publicity that high-fructose corn syrup (HFCS) has been getting, an increasing number of food and beverage manufacturers are beginning to replace the processed sweetener with old-fashioned white sugar in products ranging from tomato sauce and soft drinks to salad dressing and bread.

But is sugar really more healthful than HFCS? The truth is, it can be harmful as well.

Latest development: There is growing scientific evidence that consistently high levels of blood sugar may be linked to an increased risk for, and faster progression of, some cancers.

What you need to know: Reducing one's intake of any type of processed sugar and refined carbohydrates could reduce cancer risk and enhance cancer treatments in those battling the disease, according to many experts. Interestingly, the nutrients in fresh and frozen fruit, which are high in natural sugar, have been linked to reduced cancer risk.

Key Research Findings

Important studies have linked high blood glucose levels with…

• **Liver, gallbladder and other cancers.** In a study that appeared in the journal *PLoS Medicine*, Swedish investigators tracked blood glucose and rates of cancer and cancer deaths among more than 500,000 men and women for 10 years.

The researchers found that women with the highest glucose levels had an increased risk of developing cancers of the pancreas and bladder and dying of cancers of the pancreas, uterus, cervix and stomach. In general, cancer risk increased right along with blood glucose readings for both men and women.

These risks were independent of body weight—an important point, since doctors have traditionally attributed any potential link between cancer and high intakes of dietary sugar and other refined carbohydrates to obesity, a known risk factor for various cancers.

• **Pancreatic cancer.** In a study published in *Cancer Epidemiology, Biomarkers & Prevention*, researchers followed more than 60,000 men and women in Singapore for 14 years and found that those who consumed two or more sugared sodas per week had almost twice the risk of developing pancreatic cancer as those who didn't.

The mechanisms linking high sugar intake to increased cancer risk are still being studied. But the likeliest reason is that it leads to higher circulating levels of insulin, as well as a related hormone, known as insulin-like growth factor, both of which scientists think may promote the growth of some cancers, including malignancies of the pancreas and colon. Cancer cells are also believed to feed directly on blood glucose, which means that elevated blood glucose ensures a ready supply of "fuel" for cancer growth.

Cancer-Fighting Action Plan

Even though the scientific evidence linking cancer to sugar consumption is not yet definitive, it's prudent for everyone to take steps to regulate blood glucose levels to reduce cancer risk. It's also wise for cancer patients to follow these steps, as an adjunct to their cancer treatment. *My advice…*

• **Adopt a low-glycemic-index diet.** Glycemic index (GI) indicates how quickly your digestive tract converts a given food into blood glucose. High-GI foods cause blood glucose (and the insulin production that results) to spike sharply, while lower-GI foods produce a more gradual rise. What to do…

• **Reduce your intake of refined simple carbohydrates, most of which have a high GI.** Simple carbohydrates include sugared soda, candy and any other foods containing sugars, such as sucrose, fructose, corn syrup, dextrose and maltose…foods containing refined flour, which includes any type of flour not listed as "whole grain," such as white rice and white bread…processed snack foods… and high-GI vegetables, such as white and red potatoes, corn and turnips.

Important: Do not limit the amount of colorful fruits and vegetables you eat—the fiber in these foods will improve the GI, and their phytochemicals help prevent cancer.

• **Eat more low-GI foods,** which are typically high in protein and complex carbohydrates that produce a mild, gradual rise in blood glucose levels.

Good choices include: Legumes…nuts and seeds…low-fat proteins, such as fish, chicken and lean beef (some fatty fish, such as salmon, have fatty acids that may help guard against cancer)…cheese…nonsweetened yogurt…eggs…low-GI vegetables, such as artichokes, asparagus, bell peppers, broccoli, Brussels sprouts, cabbage, cauliflower and onions…and low-GI fruits, such as cherries, grapefruit, plums, apricots and oranges. To check the GI of various foods, consult the Glycemic Index and GI Database Web site at *www.GlycemicIndex.com.*

My advice: If you have cancer and receive intravenous nutrition at any point during your treatment, ask your doctor about receiving a low-glucose solution (40% glucose) to help control your glucose levels and replacing the calories with protein (amino acids) and fats (lipids). The typical IV solution is 75% glucose.

• **Take nutritional supplements.** If you have cancer or are concerned about your cancer risk, ask your doctor about taking magnesium and chromium supplements to help stabilize your blood glucose levels. Also discuss the dosages he considers most beneficial for you.

Important: If you have a chronic medical condition or take any prescription medication, be sure to consult your doctor before taking these or any supplements.

• **Get serious about exercise.** Regular exercise lowers blood glucose. Exercising (ideally, strength training plus a cardio routine, such as brisk walking) for 30 minutes three times a week will have maximum benefit, but any amount of exercise is better than none.

Medical Conditions That Can Cause Cancer…How to Lower Your Risk

Lynne Eldridge, MD, practiced family medicine for 15 years and now devotes herself full time to researching and speaking on cancer prevention. She is author of Avoiding Cancer One Day at a Time *(Beaver's Pond).*

If you don't have any of the well-known risk factors for cancer, including smoking, a family history of cancer or long-term exposure to a carcinogen such as asbestos, you may think that your risk for the disease is average or even less than average.

What you may not realize: Although most of the cancer predispositions (genetic, lifestyle and environmental factors that increase risk for the disease) are commonly known, there are several medical conditions that also can increase your risk.

Unfortunately, many primary-care physicians do not link these conditions to cancer. As a result, they fail to prescribe the tests and treatments that could keep cancer at bay or reduce the condition's cancer-causing potential. *Medical conditions that increase your risk for cancer…*

1. Diabetes. The high blood sugar levels that occur with type 2 diabetes predispose you to heart attack, stroke, nerve pain, blindness, kidney failure, a need for amputation—and cancer.

New research: For every 1% increase in HbA1c—a measurement of blood sugar levels over the previous three months—there is an 18% increase in the risk for cancer, according to a study published this year in *Current Diabetes Reports*.

Other current studies have linked type 2 diabetes to a 94% increased risk for pancreatic cancer…a 38% increased risk for colon cancer…a 15% to 20% higher risk for postmenopausal breast cancer…and a 20% higher risk for blood cancers such as non-Hodgkin's lymphoma and leukemia.

What to do: If you have type 2 diabetes, make sure your primary-care physician orders regular screening tests for cancer, such as colonoscopy and mammogram.

Screening for pancreatic cancer is not widely available, but some of the larger cancer centers (such as the H. Lee Moffitt Cancer Center & Research Institute in Tampa, Florida, and the Mayo Clinic in Rochester, Minnesota) offer it to high-risk individuals. This typically includes people with long-standing diabetes (more than 20 years) and/or a family history of pancreatic cancer. The test involves an ultrasound of both the stomach and small intestine, where telltale signs of pancreatic cancer can be detected.

Also work with your doctor to minimize the cancer-promoting effects of diabetes. For example, control blood sugar levels through a diet that emphasizes slow-digesting foods that don't create spikes in blood sugar levels, such as vegetables and beans…get regular

exercise—for example, 30 minutes of walking five or six days a week…and consider medical interventions, such as use of the diabetes drug metformin (Glucophage).

2. Helicobacter pylori infection. This bacterial infection of the lining of the stomach can cause stomach inflammation (gastritis) and ulcers in the stomach or upper small intestine. It also causes most stomach cancers.

Startling statistic: An infection with H. pylori triggers a 10-fold increase in your predisposition to stomach cancer. Getting treatment for an H. pylori infection lowers your risk for stomach cancer by 35% but does not eliminate the risk—perhaps due to lingering inflammation. What's most important is to avoid other inflammation-causing habits such as smoking.

What to do: If you are diagnosed with gastritis or a stomach or intestinal ulcer, ask your doctor to check for an H. pylori infection—and to treat it with antibiotics if it is detected. Research shows that a fecal analysis is the most accurate way to detect H. pylori.

3. "Iron overload" disease. This hereditary condition (known technically as hemochromatosis) affects one out of every 200 people, causing them to absorb and store too much dietary iron—in the liver, heart, joints and pancreas. Hemochromatosis also increases a person's risk for cancer (particularly liver cancer).

New research: In a study of more than 8,000 people reported in the *Journal of Internal Medicine,* iron overload increased the risk for any cancer nearly fourfold.

Iron overload should be suspected if you have or had a relative (including a second-degree relative such as a grandparent) with the condition…you have a family history of early heart disease (beginning at age 50 or earlier)…you have a family history of cirrhosis without obvious reasons such as alcoholism or hepatitis…or you have the symptoms of hemochromatosis (joint pain, fatigue, abdominal pain and a bronze appearance to the skin).

What to do: Ask your doctor for a serum ferritin test. If the test confirms iron overload, your doctor can simply and quickly correct the problem with regular bloodletting—a pint of blood once or twice per week until iron levels return to normal, and then three to four times per year.

4. Inflammatory bowel disease (IBD). This autoimmune disease attacks the lining of the intestine, causing symptoms such as abdominal cramping and bloating, bloody diarrhea and urgent bowel movements. The disease takes two main forms—ulcerative colitis (affecting the colon) and Crohn's disease (usually affecting the small intestine). Both forms predispose you to colon cancer.

Recent research: People age 67 and older with ulcerative colitis have a 93% higher risk for colorectal cancer...people of the same age group with Crohn's disease have a 45% higher risk, according to a 2011 study reported in *Digestive Diseases and Sciences*.

Problem: IBD can come and go in flare-ups that occur only once every five or 10 years. This can lead your primary-care physician to underestimate the severity of the problem and your risk for colon cancer.

What to do: IBD usually is diagnosed between the ages of 15 and 30. If you have ulcerative colitis that involves the entire colon, you should have your first colonoscopy eight years after diagnosis or at the standard age of 50 (whichever comes first) and then have another every one to two years thereafter.

If you have ulcerative colitis that involves only the left colon (which represents a somewhat smaller cancer risk than when the entire colon is affected) or Crohn's disease, you should receive your first colonoscopy 12 to 15 years after your diagnosis or at age 50 and then another every one to two years thereafter.

5. Polyps detected in a relative. Most people think that a hereditary predisposition to colon cancer means that you have a first-degree relative (parent, sibling or child) who was diagnosed with the disease.

Surprising fact: If you have a first-degree relative who had a colonoscopy that detected an adenomatous polyp (adenoma)—a type of growth that can turn into cancer within two to five years—you also have a predisposition to colon cancer.

Recent research: Having a first-degree relative with an adenoma appears to make you four times more likely to develop colorectal cancer, according to a report in *Annals of Internal Medicine*.

What to do: Have a first colonoscopy 10 years earlier than the age at which your relative's adenoma was detected and repeat it every five to 10 years (depending on results). That should give plenty of time to detect (and remove) an adenoma so it can never turn into cancer.

Interesting: Some cancer centers also advise earlier screening if a second-degree relative, such as a grandparent, had colon cancer.

Sleeping Pills Are Just Plain Dangerous

Robert Langer, MD, MPH, principal scientist and medical director, Jackson Hole Center for Preventive Medicine, Wyoming.

It's bad enough that people are so desperate for sleep that they resort to taking any of a long list of pharmaceuticals in an effort to help them get a good night's rest. Even worse is that these theoretical helpers come with a long list of associated dangers, including addiction.

Well guess what? The list of dangers just got longer.

Research, conducted by physicians at the Scripps Clinic Viterbi Family Sleep Center in San Diego and Jackson Hole Center for Preventive Medicine (JHCPM) in Wyoming, has shown that use of sleeping pills has been associated with an increased risk for cancer and death.

The most troubling part is that this study found that it's not just daily users who are at risk—those who use them less than twice a month may even be at risk.

It Takes a While for Side Effects to Surface

We spoke with Robert Langer, MD, MPH, principal scientist and medical director at JHCPM, to learn more about these frightening findings. He said that most studies on the safety of sleeping pills last only six months or less. "That's not enough time to examine the risk for many serious health consequences, such as cancer or death," said Dr. Langer. "Our research is more long-term, and we didn't just look at whether or not people were taking sleeping pills. We also looked at which type they were using and how often they were taking the pills."

The researchers looked at the electronic medical records of the population served by the Geisinger Health System (GHS) in Pennsylvania, the largest rural integrated health system in the US. Subjects (mean age 54 years) were 10,529 male and female patients who received prescriptions of sleeping pills as sleep aids (on-label), and 23,676 matched controls with no prescriptions of sleeping pills. They were followed for an average of 2.5 years.

The researchers found that the more sleeping pills that subjects took, the greater their risk for death from all causes and, shockingly, even people who were taking them only sporadically were at higher risk for death. *For example, compared with those who did not take sleeping pills, people who took…*

• **One to 18 sleeping pills a year were 3.6 times more likely to die within the 2.5-year follow-up period.**

• **19 to 132 sleeping pills a year were 4.4 times more likely to die.**

• **133 or more pills a year were 5.3 times more likely to die.**

These results did not differ whether the subjects were using older sleeping pills, such as *temazepam* (Restoril), or newer ones, such as *zolpidem* (Ambien), *eszopiclone* (Lunesta) and *zaleplon* (Sonata), which are marketed as being shorter-acting and safer.

Researchers also found an increased risk for all major cancers among moderate and heavy users of any sleeping pill. There was a 20% increased risk among any users who took 19 to 132 pills a year and a 35% increased risk among any users who took more than 132 pills a year.

It's important to note that none of these results prove cause and effect, but they certainly reveal an unsettling association.

Understanding the Connection

We asked Dr. Langer whether the results could simply be due to the fact that patients who take sleeping pills are usually in worse health—for example, perhaps they don't eat well or exercise as much as they should or maybe they're more stressed. His response was no. "We controlled for every possible variation, matching subjects and controls by age, gender and health history, yet the results remained the same," Dr. Langer said.

So why the increased risk for death and cancer? The authors did not have adequate information to assess possible mechanisms. However, based on prior studies, potential mechanisms include increases in sleep apnea, accidents related to sleep walking/driving, aspiration pneumonia and depression of respiratory function.

Now What?

This is a finding of major consequence, because 6% to 10% of American adults took a sleeping pill in 2010, the most recent year for which statistics are available. But the complicating factor is that sleeping pills do provide health benefits. In other words, not taking a sleeping pill and potentially not getting enough sleep comes with its own set of risks—for instance, insomnia can raise the risk for heart disease, stroke, diabetes, obesity, depression and other serious health conditions. So if you're taking sleeping pills, what do you do?

First, consult your prescribing physician, said Dr. Langer. "Don't stop cold turkey, because that can cause withdrawal symptoms and agitation, as well as sleepless nights. Figure out a plan with your doctor about how to taper off," he said. And then ask your doctor about safer alternatives, such as melatonin or manipulating light exposure, he said. You can also try cognitive behavioral therapy from an informed primary care doctor, behavioral therapist or sleep medicine physician, he added.

Cancer in the Family? Too Few Doctors Recommend Genetic Tests

Katrina Trivers, PhD, MSPH, epidemiologist at the Centers for Disease Control and Prevention in Atlanta and lead author of an article reporting on a survey of 1,878 US physicians.

You are probably aware that if two or more of your close family members (or just one family member for those of Ashkenazi Jewish descent) had breast or ovarian cancer, you are at increased risk for such cancers yourself. That is why various health organizations, such as the US Preventive Services Task Force, issue guidelines on who should consider genetic counseling and possibly be tested for the abnormal genes (BRCA1 and BRCA2) associated with most inherited breast and ovarian cancers. Test results can help determine your risk level and identify appropriate self-defense strategies.

Problem: According to a recent article published in *Cancer*, only 34% of family physicians, 41% of general internists and 57% of gynecologists surveyed reported adhering to guidelines in referring high-risk patients for genetic counseling and testing.

Among the reasons for the low adherence rates: The guidelines are complicated… and the various organizations define high risk differently.

Protect yourself: Visit *www.USPreventiveServicesTaskForce.org/uspstf05/brcagen/brcagenrs.htm* or *www.Cancer.gov/cancertopics/factsheet/risk/BRCA* for more information on genetic risk…then talk with your doctor about your family history of breast and ovarian cancer, including who was diagnosed and at what age, if this information is available.

Reassuring: For women whose genetic test results show that they do carry an abnormal BRCA1 or BRCA2 gene, additional screening tests, medication and/or prophylactic surgery can greatly reduce the risk of succumbing to cancer.

Aspirin for Cancer Prevention

Mario Capecchi, PhD, was awarded the 2007 Nobel Prize in Physiology or Medicine for his research on gene modifications using embryonic stem cells. He is distinguished professor of human genetics and biology at the University of Utah School of Medicine, Salt Lake City, and an investigator at the Howard Hughes Medical Institute in Chevy Chase, Maryland.

Millions of Americans take aspirin to relieve pain, treat headaches and lower fever. It's also among the most effective ways to help prevent heart attack and stroke.

What is less well-known about aspirin is its ability to help lower cancer risk. For example, a study that appeared in *The Lancet* found that low-dose aspirin therapy—75 mg daily, the amount considered "low dose" in Great Britain, where the research was conducted—reduced deaths from colorectal cancer by 40%…from lung cancer by 30%…and from esophageal cancer by 58%.

Simple home remedy: If you're at increased risk for cancer (due, for example, to family history), a daily low-dose aspirin (in the US, 81 mg or one "baby" aspirin) may be worth considering. Just be sure to speak to your doctor before you begin taking aspirin daily—even low-dose aspirin slightly increases bleeding risk.

Six Powerful Moves to Defend Yourself Against Cancer

H. Robert Silverstein, MD, medical director of the Preventive Medicine Center in Hartford, *www.ThePMC. org,* and a clinical assistant professor of medicine at the University of Connecticut School of Medicine in Farmington. He has served on the board of directors of the Connecticut Holistic Health Association and is the author of *Maximum Healing* (North Atlantic).

The average adult produces and removes 250,000 to 500,000 cancer cells every day. In most cases, the body routinely wipes out these cells before they have a chance to multiply. So why do some people still get cancer?

Aside from genetics—which is the cause of 10% of all malignancies—cancer and other inflammatory diseases largely depend on a particular "internal environment" to flourish. People who live a healthy lifestyle have an internal environment that helps prevent inflammatory diseases, such as heart disease, diabetes and rheumatoid arthritis, from progressing. Because inflammation is the underlying cause of many serious diseases, people who avoid and remove inflammatory substances are far less likely to get sick in the first place and more likely to recover when they do. *How to clean up your internal environment...*

Disease-Fighting Mushrooms

It's only in the last decade that scientists have begun to understand the health benefits of Japanese mushrooms, particularly shiitake, enoki, maitake and reishi mushrooms. They have antiviral and antibacterial properties... increase immunity...and reduce the risk for heart disease and cancer.

In a Japanese study, women who ate about three and a half ounces of shiitake mush-

rooms daily reduced their cholesterol levels by up to 12%. The same mushrooms contain the anticancer compound lentinan, which is so potent that it's been approved in Japan as a chemotherapeutic agent.

My advice: Eat shiitake mushrooms (and a variety of the other types described earlier) as often as possible.

Antioxidant Power

The average person's DNA experiences 10,000 daily oxidative "hits," which can eventually lead to cancer and other chronic conditions. To reduce this threat, we must increase our levels of antioxidants (vitamins and other nutrients that remove potentially damaging oxidizing agents from our bodies). *Best antioxidants...*

• **Vitamin C.** Vitamin C is a potent dietary antioxidant. For example, a study at the University of California, Berkeley, found that the oxidation of LDL "bad" cholesterol stopped when people had adequate vitamin C in the blood. This is critical because oxidized LDL is far more likely to accumulate on artery walls and lead to heart disease.

Recommended dose: 500 mg, two to three times daily.

• **Beta-carotene and other carotenoids,** such as lycopene and the "superantioxidant" astaxanthin, are on a par with vitamins C and E for reducing oxidation and inflammation.

Bonus: Foods that are high in carotenoids are also high in other antioxidants.

You don't need carotenoid supplements as long as you include grains, vegetables and/or beans in 19 of 21 meals a week.

Good choices: Whole grains, prunes, blueberries, red beans, broccoli and pecans.

Avoid "Normal Weight Obesity"

Even if you're just a few pounds overweight, your risk of getting cancer can be higher than it should be.

Reason: Fat is a metabolically active substance that increases oxidation and inflammation. It also elevates hormones that increase the risk for cancers of the breast and the prostate.

Important: Many people who think they're lean are heavier than they should be—a condition called "normal weight obesity."

My advice: You don't need "six-pack" abs but should be able to see your abdominal muscles.

Exercise to Prevent Cancer

Everyone knows that exercise is good for the heart. What you might not realize is that regular exercise is among the best ways to prevent cancer.

When researchers at the renowned Cooper Clinic compared exercise with cancer rates, they found that men who didn't exercise had four times more cancer than those who were fit. Sedentary women were found to have 16 times the cancer risk of fit women.

Reason: People who exercise have less inflammation throughout the body and a healthier balance of hormones. Their immune systems are more robust and are more likely to destroy cancer cells as well as viruses and bacteria.

Less is more: Interestingly, the Cooper study found that women who merely walked for 30 minutes a day, five days a week, significantly lowered their risk for breast cancer.

Laugh It Up

A Mayo Clinic study found that optimistic people lived almost 20% longer, on average, than pessimists. People who are upbeat and manage stress appropriately have lower blood pressure, are less likely to be overweight and suffer from fewer autoimmune diseases than those who are tense and angry.

Positive emotions are good medicine—they create a healthy, balanced internal environment without excess levels of damaging stress hormones, such as cortisol, which lead to inflammation.

But how do you relax in a stressful world or make yourself happy when you're feeling down?

Try this: Smile even when you don't feel like it. Facial expressions don't only reflect our feelings, they create them. When you smile, the movement of facial muscles causes blood to circumvent the cavernous sinus cavity, the area where blood is warmed before reaching the brain. Cooler blood in the brain triggers chemical changes that create pleasant feelings.

Breathe Clean Air

Polluted air—from industrial toxins, cigarette smoke, etc.—is a significant cause of disease. The oxidants in pollution, also known as free radicals, damage DNA and trigger inflammation throughout the body, including in and around the blood vessels.

Important: Don't smoke, and avoid secondhand smoke, too. Cigarette smoke contains more than one million oxidants in a single puff of smoke.

Helpful: Use an air purifier to clean indoor air, particularly if anyone in your household smokes. I recommend the Sun Pure Air Purifier SP-20 ($549), 800-469-7583, *www.Natural-Living.com*…and Aireox D-Model 45 ($360), 800-670-7480, *www.Alerg.com*.

Seven Foods Proven to Fight Cancer

David Grotto, RD, LDN, a registered dietitian and former spokesperson for the American Dietetic Association. He is founder and president of Nutrition Housecall, LLC, a Chicago-area consulting firm specializing in family nutrition programs. He writes the "Ask the Guy-a-titian" column for *Chicago Wellness Magazine* and is author of *The Best Thing You Can Eat* (Da Capo) and *101 Foods That Could Save Your Life* (Bantam).

Up to one-third of all cancers could be prevented if people adopted healthier lifestyles, including eating healthier foods. *For even better odds, choose these seven specific foods that have been proven to prevent cancer…*

Cabbage

It's high in anticarcinogenic compounds called glucosinolates. Raw cabbage, particularly when it is fermented as sauerkraut, also is a good source of indole-3-carbinol (I3C), a substance that promotes the elimination of carcinogens from the body.

The Polish Women's Health Study, which looked at hundreds of Polish women in the US, found that those who had eaten four or more servings per week of raw, lightly cooked or fermented cabbage during adolescence were 72% less likely to develop breast cancer than women who had eaten only one-and-a-half servings per week. High consumption of cabbage during adulthood also provided significant protection even if little cabbage was eaten at a young age.

Recommended: Three or more one-half-cup servings per week of cabbage, cooked or raw.

Alternatives: Any cruciferous vegetable, including brussels sprouts, cauliflower, kale and broccoli. A recent study found that men who ate at least three servings per week of broccoli or other cruciferous vegetables were 41% less likely to get prostate cancer than men who ate less than one serving per week. Kimchi, a Korean pickled dish that is similar to sauerkraut, also is a good choice.

Flaxseeds

Little seeds with a nutty flavor, flaxseeds contain lignans, compounds that act like a weak form of estrogen. One study found that women with high levels of enterolactone (linked to a high intake of lignans) had a 58% lower risk for breast cancer. Flaxseeds also contain omega-3 fatty acids, which appear to inhibit colon cancer in both men and women.

Recommended: One to two tablespoons of ground flaxseed daily. You can sprinkle it on cereal or yogurt or add it to soups or stews.

Alternatives: Two or more servings per week of cold-water fish, such as mackerel or salmon, provide cancer-fighting amounts of omega-3s.

For more lignans: Eat walnuts, and cook with canola oil.

Mushrooms

The common white button mushroom found in supermarkets contains anticancer compounds. Scientists who compared vegetable extracts in the lab found that an extract made from white button mushrooms was the most effective at blocking aromatase, an enzyme that promotes breast cancer. Button mushrooms also appear to suppress the growth of prostate cancer cells.

Recommended: One-half cup of button mushrooms, three or four times per week.

Alternatives: Porcinis or chanterelles, wild mushrooms with a nuttier taste.

Olives

A Spanish laboratory study found that two compounds in olives—maslinic acid and oleanolic acid—inhibit the proliferation of cancer cells and promote apoptosis, the death of these cells. Other studies suggest that people who eat olives as part of a classic Mediterranean diet have lower rates of a variety of cancers, including colon cancer.

Recommended: Eight olives a day, green or black.

Alternative: One to two tablespoons of extra-virgin olive oil daily. Drizzle it on salad or vegetables to enhance absorption of their healthy nutrients.

Onions

When researchers compared the 10 vegetables most frequently consumed in the US, onions had the third-highest level of phenolic compounds, which are thought to be among the most potent anticancer substances found in foods.

In a Finnish study, men who frequently ate onions, apples and other foods high in quercetin (a phenolic compound) were 60% less likely to develop lung cancer than men who ate smaller amounts. Quercetin also appears to reduce the risk for liver and colon cancers.

Recommended: One-half cup of onions, cooked or raw, three times per week. Yellow and red onions contain the most cancer-preventing substances.

Alternatives: Apples, capers and green and black tea, all of which are high in quercetin. Garlic, a botanical relative of onions, provides many of the same active ingredients.

Pumpkin

Pumpkin, like all winter squash, is extremely high in carotenoids, including beta-carotene. A long-running Japanese study that looked at more than 57,000 participants found that people who ate the most pumpkin had lower rates of gastric, breast, lung and colorectal cancers. There also is some evidence that pumpkin seeds can help reduce the risk for prostate cancer.

Recommended: Three or more one-half-cup servings per week. Pumpkin can be baked like any winter squash.

Alternatives: Carrots, broccoli and all of the winter squashes, including acorn, butternut and spaghetti squash.

Raspberries

All of the foods that end with "erry"—including cherry, blueberry and strawberry—contain anti-inflammatory compounds that reduce cell damage that can lead to cancer. Raspberries are higher in fiber than most berries and are an excellent source of ellagic acid and selenium, both of which protect against a variety of cancers.

Recent studies have shown that raspberries (or raspberry extract) inhibit both oral and liver cancer cells. The responses in these studies were dose-dependent—the more raspberry extract used, the greater the effect.

Recommended: One-and-a-half cups of raspberries, two or three times per week.

Alternative: Cherries (and cherry juice) contain about as much ellagic acid as raspberries. Frozen berries and cherries, which contain less water, provide a higher concentration of protective compounds than fresh ones.

Chapter 12

CANCER CARE AND REHAB

Getting Ready for Your First Cancer Consultation

When you receive a diagnosis of cancer, you may feel as if you're suddenly on an alien planet, with no map or guidebook to help you find your way to safety. By the time of your initial consultation with an oncologist, you're likely to be frightened and confused—and that can interfere with your ability to take in essential information about your condition and make crucial decisions about your care.

What helps: Knowing how to prepare for and what to expect at that important first visit with your cancer doctor.

To help you get the most out of that meeting, we turned to Stewart B. Fleishman, MD, founding director of Cancer Supportive Services at Continuum Cancer Centers of New York and author of *Learn to Live Through Cancer: What You Need to Know and Do.* Here are his suggestions.

Before your consultation…

•**Contact your insurance company to protect yourself financially.** Find out whether you need an authorization to see the oncologist. If so, ask how long that will take—then schedule your consultation accordingly. It's also a good idea to contact the oncologist's office before your visit to make sure the authorization arrived.

What if your insurance company says that the authorization won't come for a long time—even weeks? Ask to speak to a case-management service representative (sometimes called a disease-management or disease-coordination representative) at your insurance company, Dr. Fleishman suggested—often these people can be very helpful in getting you access to the services you need, especially if you stress the urgent nature of your request for authorization. Or you can pay the oncologist's bill up-front, then file an appeal for reimbursement with your insurance company or through your state insurance ombudsman, again citing the urgency of the situation.

•**Arrange for your test results to be sent to the oncologist.** Due to federal privacy laws, your oncologist's office is not permitted to obtain these test results for you, Dr. Fleishman said. However, the staff at the oncology center will be able to tell you exactly which

Stewart B. Fleishman, MD, founding director, Cancer Supportive Services at Continuum Cancer Centers of New York at Beth Israel Medical Center and St. Luke's-Roosevelt Hospitals, New York City. He also is author of *Learn to Live Through Cancer: What You Need to Know and Do* (Demos).

test results you should have sent in advance and what you should bring with you on the day of your consultation. For instance, you may be asked to arrange for or bring such items as the original glass slides from your biopsy…copies of your x-rays, CT or PET/CT scans…and results of any blood and urine testing.

• **Prepare a detailed personal medical history.** Include current and prior illnesses…surgeries…allergies…and side effects from medication. Also list any prescription or nonprescription medications or nutritional supplements you currently take along with dosages. Be open about all conditions (such as a history of depression) and lifestyle factors (such as whether you smoke or have ever had a problem with alcohol or drugs) that may affect your treatment.

• **Gather info on your family medical history.** Prepare a list of all your close relatives—parents, siblings, children, grandparents, cousins, aunts, uncles, nieces and nephews—on both your mother's and father's sides. For each, record their date of birth and current age or age at the time of death…for any relative who had cancer, list the type of cancer, age at diagnosis and outcome. This information can help your oncologist devise the most appropriate treatment plan, given that some cancers have a strong family pattern, Dr. Fleishman said.

• **Write down all your questions.** Between now and the time of your appointment, carry a notepad or use your smartphone to jot down questions and concerns—about your treatment options and their side effects, complementary therapies, prognosis, etc.—as they come to mind. If you wait until the day of your consultation, you're likely to forget some of the questions you wanted to ask.

• **Arrange to bring a trusted friend or relative to your consultation.** "If you were looking at a new car or considering buying a house, you wouldn't hesitate to ask a friend to come along as an extra pair of eyes and ears. Your initial oncology consultation is no less important—so follow the same principle," Dr. Fleishman said. Patients typically re-

tain less than half the information they hear at an initial consult, so ask your companion to serve as a scribe, taking complete notes on the conversation so you can review the details later. Also, urge your companion to think of questions for the oncologist—he/she might come up with issues that you had not considered but that turn out to be quite important to you.

During the consultation…

• **Arrive early**—you'll need to fill out a lot of paperwork unless the oncology office sent this paperwork to you to complete ahead of time or had you submit the forms online in advance. You will then meet with one of the oncologists, review your own and your family's medical history, and get a full physical exam. After that, you can expect to…

• **Discuss additional needed testing.** Although it may seem redundant, your oncologist probably will want to have your scans and slides reviewed by radiologists and pathologists whom he trusts and is accustomed to working with. This is not an attempt to wrest more money from you or your insurance company. Instead, Dr. Fleishman said, it is an important step in preventing errors. Your oncologist also may refer you to other cancer specialists for specialized blood work…additional scans (for instance, even if you have had a CT scan, the doctor may ask for an MRI)…and/or more sophisticated analysis of the biopsy. These tests help determine whether the cancer has spread and to where.

• **Review your doctor's initial treatment plan.** This will vary depending on the type of cancer you have, of course—but be prepared to hear some unexpected options. For instance, many patients are surprised to be told that surgery is not necessarily their first step. "Until recently, surgery almost always came first. But today, sometimes chemotherapy and radiation are advised right away to shrink the tumor and allow for a smaller surgery," Dr. Fleishman said.

• **Discuss whether a clinical trial is an option for you.** Many patients assume that if an oncologist brings up the idea of participating in a clinical trial that is testing a

America's Top Hospitals for Oncology

Dana-Farber/Brigham and Women's Cancer Center, Boston, 877-332-4294, *www.dfbwcc.org*. One of the outstanding teaching institutions of Harvard Medical School, Dana-Farber offers a roster of subspecialists covering common and rare types of cancer ranging from Hodgkin's disease and lung cancer to skull-base tumors.

Johns Hopkins Medicine, The Sidney Kimmel Comprehensive Cancer Center, Baltimore, 410-955-5000, *www.hopkinsmedicine.org/kimmel_cancer_center*. While this is a large medical institution, the doctors work hard—though not always successfully—to humanize the patient experience. The pathology department is among the best in the US—some say the world—often being called on to offer highly valued second opinions on biopsies.

MD Anderson Cancer Center, The University of Texas, Houston, 877-632-6789, *www.mdanderson.org*. As the largest US cancer center (based on number of patient beds), MD Anderson has many of the assets—and a few of the liabilities—that result from sheer size. Subspecialists in virtually all common and rare cancer types practice here.

Memorial Sloan-Kettering Cancer Center, New York City, 212-639-2000, *www.mskcc.org*. Memorial Sloan-Kettering has some of the country's leading physicians in medical and surgical oncology, hematology and research. Most patients speak favorably of inpatient experiences at Memorial Sloan-Kettering, but outpatients may experience delays and long waiting times.

Other excellent options: Mayo Clinic Cancer Center, Rochester, Minnesota… Duke Cancer Institute, Durham, North Carolina…University of California, Los Angeles, Jonsson Comprehensive Cancer Center… University of Pittsburgh Cancer Institute.

new drug or other type of therapy, it must be very bad news. But this is not the case. "Do not assume that if a clinical trial is mentioned right at the initial consultation it means that your oncologist isn't sure what to do or that standard therapies can't help you," Dr. Fleishman said. In fact, a clinical trial may be a way for you to get access to an effective treatment that is close to FDA approval but that would not be reimbursed by your insurance. Participation may require that certain steps (such as extra processing of a biopsy or special timing of tests) be undertaken right from the start.

•**Ask questions.** Most doctors will invite you to ask whatever questions you may have, but even if yours doesn't, don't be shy or allow yourself to be hurried out the door. If the doctor says something that you don't understand, request clarification. If you still don't understand it, say so and request clarification again. Also, confirm that a copy of the consultation note (a written summary of your visit) will be sent to your primary care doctor and/or the doctor who referred you to the oncologist. You want all your health-care providers to be fully informed about your condition and on the same page with regard to the treatment plan.

After your consultation…

•**Try to be patient.** Ordering additional tests, confirming the presence and extent of the cancer and devising a treatment plan generally will take some weeks. Unless time is truly of the essence—for instance, because you have already been admitted to the hospital or are having trouble breathing well or passing urine or stool—this waiting period is typical and will not negatively affect your health.

•**Get a second opinion from another oncologist.** "If possible, the second-opinion consultant should not work in the same cancer center as the original oncologist. People who work together tend to think through problems in the same way after a while," Dr. Fleishman said. Insurance policies vary, but many do cover that second-opinion consultation, particularly when provided by a doctor within a particular network. Your preparations for and expectations of this second consultation are identical to the first. Afterward, you should ask that the second-opinion information be sent to the first-opinion oncologist and your primary-care doctor. And don't worry about offending the first doctor by seeking that second opinion. As Dr. Fleishman said, this practice is not only routine in the world of cancer treatment, it's a vital step in giving you the very best chance of beating the disease.

Cancer Patients: Where to Find Everything You Need to Know

Patricia Goldsmith, executive vice president and chief operating officer of the National Comprehensive Cancer Network. *www.nccn.org*

At a recent conference on cancer, several oncologists spoke with great enthusiasm about what they described as the patients' very best guide to treatment options—the National Comprehensive Cancer Network (NCCN), an online resource. So we checked it out at *www.nccn.com*, and, yes, it is a treasure trove of information!

NCCN's executive vice president and chief operating officer, Patricia Goldsmith, told us, "Many Americans are probably better equipped to buy a refrigerator or an automobile than they are to make health-care decisions. But when they have access to accurate, up-to-date information, they are empowered—and that is so important when they are battling a life-threatening disease."

NCCN's mission is to offer cancer patients the same information that their health-care professionals get, but in language that patients can understand. *Through NCCN, you can find…*

- **Specific treatment guidelines for dozens of different types of cancer.**
- **Downloadable books** (some of 100 pages or more) called Guidelines for Pa-

tients on breast, ovarian, colon and various other cancers.

- **Conventional and integrative approaches** for managing cancer-related pain, fatigue, distress and other challenges.
- **Information on cancer treatment centers**…cancer drugs (including a section called "no longer recommended uses")…and clinical trials that are recruiting participants.
- **Recommendations on prevention, risk reduction, screening and genetic testing.**
- **Help for caregivers.**

Doctor-patient partnership: One benefit of NCCN is that it helps keep doctors and patients on the same page, Goldsmith said. In fact, two out of three cancer clinicians report checking the NCCN guidelines at least once a month (the clinicians' version of the Web site is at *www.nccn.org*).

Best: If you are a cancer patient, ask your doctor whether his or her recommendations for your treatment are in accordance with NCCN guidelines. If the answer is no, discuss the reasons…and find out how your treatment might vary from the guidelines. "We want patients to be able to have an informed dialogue with their clinicians about their short- and long-term care," Goldsmith said.

Bottom line: Check out the Web site at the time of your diagnosis and periodically as your treatment moves along. If you've already begun treatment or even if you've finished, it's not too late to find information relevant to your care and well-being.

The Anticancer Formula

Raymond Chang, MD, a faculty member at Weill Cornell Medical College, New York City, and a pioneer in the use of complementary and alternative treatments in oncology. He is author of *Beyond the Magic Bullet—The Anti-Cancer Cocktail: A New Approach to Beating Cancer* (Square One).

Researchers are discovering that multiple treatments given simultaneously can be far more effective at fighting cancer than any single treatment. That's because a typical cancer involves an average of 63 genetic mutations, each of which works in different ways. A single treatment is unlikely to affect more than a few of these processes.

Better approach: Cancer "cocktails" that simultaneously attack abnormal cells in a multitude of ways.

Examples: A deadly form of blood cancer, multiple myeloma, now is routinely treated with drug combinations that have doubled survival rates. A French study, published in May 2011 in *The New England Journal of Medicine*, found that patients with pancreatic cancer who were given a combination of four drugs lived about 60% longer than those given standard chemotherapy.

For the most part, the conventional treatment strategy for cancer involves using one or two traditional treatments—surgery, radiation, chemotherapy or hormone therapy—one after the other. Only on occasion are different treatments used in combination simultaneously such as when radiation and chemotherapy are administered following a patient's surgery.

Many oncologists now believe that it's better to hit cancers all at once with a barrage of treatments—including, in some cases, unconventional treatments, such as vitamins, herbs, supplements and medications typically prescribed for other health problems.

Example: I might advise a cancer patient getting conventional treatments to include the arthritis drug *celecoxib* (Celebrex), which makes cancer cells more sensitive to radiation...the hormone melatonin (which decreases the growth of some cancers)...and vitamin D-3 (which may reduce cancer recurrence).

Getting Started

Here's how to make this approach work for you...

• **Keep an open mind.** Ask your doctor if there are safe and effective treatments that he/she recommends that may be unconventional, including "off-label" drugs—medications that haven't been approved by the FDA specifically for your type of cancer.

Doctors often know about new treatments that seem to work for a given cancer. They share stories with their colleagues about treatments that appear to be effective but that haven't yet been completely validated. When you have cancer, there's no reason not to try innovative approaches as long as they are safe.

Important: Don't try any treatment without first checking with your doctor to make sure that it is safe for you. If it is, he can recommend the right dose and tell you when you should take it.

• **Start with conventional care.** I never advise patients to forgo appropriate standard cancer treatments such as chemotherapy and/or radiation. These approaches have been proven to improve survival. You can then supplement these approaches with off-label medications, herbs and/or supplements to help increase effectiveness.

• **Define your goals.** A cure isn't the only reason to use a medley of treatments. The right cocktail also can reduce treatment side effects and improve your quality of life.

Example: Patients with breast cancer may be given hormonal treatments that reduce tumor growth, but in premenopausal women, these treatments also induce early menopause—and the accompanying hot flashes, night sweats and "brain fog." To be more comfortable during the posttreatment period, you can take vitamin E to reduce hot flashes...ginkgo to improve memory...and herbs such as black cohosh to reduce vaginal dryness and night sweats.

Ingredients to Consider

Ask your doctor what you can add to your current treatments to increase their effectiveness. Some of the most common medications in the US have been shown to help cancer patients, as have supplements. *Here, some unconventional treatments that can help...*

• **Vitamin D.** Studies have shown that vitamin D induces apoptosis, the death of cancer cells. This is important because one of the characteristics of cancer cells is the ability to avoid cell death. Using vitamin D along with chemotherapy, surgery and/or radiation could improve your outcome.

• **The ulcer medication *cimetidine* (Tagamet)** strengthens the immune system so that it can fight cancer cells. Studies have shown that patients who start taking cimetidine a few days before colon cancer surgery may be less likely to have a recurrence of the cancer.

• **Aspirin.** An analysis of data from the Harvard Nurses' Health Study found that breast cancer patients who took aspirin reduced the risk of the cancer spreading (metastasis) by nearly 50%.

• **Curcumin,** the active compound in the spice turmeric. Like aspirin, it's an anti-inflammatory that can reduce the invasion and spread of cancer cells. It also can inhibit angiogenesis, the development of blood vessels that nourish tumors.

• **Green tea.** This is one cancer-cocktail ingredient that everyone can "take." One cup of green tea has approximately 45 milligrams (mg) of epigallocatechin 3-gallate (EGCG), a compound that appears to reduce the growth of cancer cells. Dozens of studies have shown that green tea may be effective.

Example: A Mayo Clinic study found that the majority of leukemia patients who took EGCG showed clear improvement. Other studies have shown that it can reduce prostate-specific antigen (PSA), a substance that is elevated in patients with prostate cancer.

I recommend eight cups of green tea a day to fight cancer.

• **Red yeast rice.** This type of yeast, taken in supplement form, contains monacolin K, the same active compound that is used in *lovastatin*, one of the cholesterol-lowering statins. Red yeast rice is an anti-inflammatory that also affects immune response and cell signaling—actions that can help prevent and possibly treat some cancers.

Laboratory studies indicate that red yeast rice (as well as statins) might increase the effectiveness of radiation and chemotherapy.

As for statins, in studies involving nearly a half-million patients, the drugs have been shown to significantly reduce the incidence and recurrence of colon, breast, lung and prostate cancers.

Go Slow

Mix the cocktail slowly. It's not good to start many treatments at the same time. You need to know if a particular ingredient is causing side effects.

Example: I might advise a patient to use Chinese herbs for a week. If he/she is doing well, I might add a second ingredient and then a third.

Cancer Prehab: The First Thing You Need After a Diagnosis

Julie Silver, MD, associate professor, department of physical medicine and rehabilitation, Harvard Medical School, Boston. She also is the founder of Oncology Rehab Partners, creator of the STAR Program Certification and author of *After Cancer Treatment: Heal Faster, Better, Stronger* (Johns Hopkins). *www.JulieSilverMD.com*

If you are facing a cancer diagnosis now—or if you ever face one in the future—the new trend called cancer prehab could be your key to an easier, more complete recovery. According to Julie Silver, MD, a Harvard Medical School associate professor, cancer survivor and author of *After Cancer Treatment: Heal Faster, Better, Stronger,* "From the minute you're diagnosed with cancer, you're considered a survivor of the disease. Survivors need to do whatever they can to improve their health from the very start. Prehab helps you use the time between diagnosis and treatment most effectively by preparing you physically and emotionally."

Cancer prehab services are provided by a range of specialists including physicians, psychologists, social workers, physical therapists, occupational therapists, speech therapists, nutritionists, exercise physiologists and others. The particular types of specialists assigned to your case will depend on your individual needs.

There are certain services that just about all patients can benefit from, regardless of the kind of cancer they have. *These include…*

• **Instruction in coping skills.** Taking classes in deep breathing, progressive muscle relaxation and/or meditation can provide skills that will be invaluable for pain management and for coping with the inevitable fear and anxiety that a cancer diagnosis brings, Dr. Silver said.

• **Evaluation of caregiving needs.** Prehab personnel will advise you on the type of assistance you may need during your treatment and recovery and help you coordinate the practical aspects of your care.

You'll resolve questions such as: Will you be going home or to a rehab center after surgery? Should any temporary changes be made in your home (such as setting up a ground-floor bedroom) to make it easier for you to navigate during your recovery? Who can help with meals, driving and other daily tasks during the weeks while you are healing? Addressing these issues now will save you a lot of stress and uncertainty later.

• **Targeted physical exercises.** These can be hugely beneficial not only for overall health and strength but for helping you survive cancer. "Exercise may reduce the risk for recurrence in some types of cancer, so a prehab program that gets a patient to be more active may increase the length of his or her life," Dr. Silver noted. In some cases, improvements in physical well-being can expand patients' treatment options, too. For instance, Dr. Silver said, "One study showed that prehab improved the respiratory status of lung cancer patients, even making some patients strong enough for surgery that had previously been ruled out."

• **Help with smoking cessation, if needed.** Without a doubt, nonsmokers heal better than those who continue to smoke. Quitting even shortly before cancer treatment begins can make a significant difference in your recovery.

• **Your specific diagnosis and state of health determine what additional services you might need.** That makes sense—a colorectal cancer patient has different concerns than, say, a breast cancer patient. *Examples include…*

• Skin-protection counseling for patients whose treatment will include radiation and/or chemotherapy (since both of these treatments can affect the skin).

• Range-of-motion evaluation and exercises. For instance, postsurgical breast cancer patients often have shoulder pain and limited shoulder movement—so in prehab, patients can work on increasing range of motion prior to surgery so that the aftereffects will be less severe.

• Pelvic-floor strengthening. After surgery and/or radiation for prostate cancer or gynecological cancer, many patients have trouble with urinary incontinence. Doing exercises to strengthen the muscles of the pelvic floor prior to treatment helps reduce the likelihood and severity of posttreatment incontinence.

• Balance and gait evaluation and training. Working with a physical therapist to improve strength, balance and gait skills before cancer treatment helps patients recover mobility more quickly afterward, especially for older people who may already have some subtle balance problems. Yet young cancer patients can benefit, too, because chemotherapy may cause nervous system problems that affect balance and walking.

How to Get Prehab

What comes after cancer prehab and treatment? Ideally, patients then attend cancer rehab—specially designed programs that hasten recovery and improve quality of life for cancer survivors. For more information on cancer rehab, see pages 231-233.

After recovering from cancer herself, Dr. Silver developed something called the STAR Program (Survivorship Training and Rehabilitation) certification for hospitals and cancer centers, which involves a protocol for best practices in cancer rehab—and now prehab, too. Nearly 100 hospitals and cancer centers nationwide have signed up for STAR Program certification so far, and all include some form of prehab. For information and/or a referral to a STAR Program in your area, visit the Web site of Oncology Rehab Partners, an organization founded by Dr. Silver and dedicated to advancing survivorship care.

Alternative: Ask your oncologist about prehab and see if he or she has any suggestions. Fortunately, health insurance and Medicare often cover prehab services.

Complementary Therapies That Ease Cancer Treatment Side Effects

Roberta Lee, MD, vice chair of the department of integrative medicine at the Continuum Center for Health and Healing at Beth Israel Medical Center in New York City. She also is author of *The SuperStress Solution* (Random House).

A diagnosis of cancer presents a difficult battle not only with the disease, but also with the side effects of treatment. To destroy cancer, chemotherapy and radiation basically poison the body—which can bring on a host of miseries. Treatment may be essential, of course...but its side effects can be minimized with natural therapies that strengthen and support the body.

A recent study in *Breast Cancer Research and Treatment* found that 86% of newly diagnosed breast cancer patients incorporated complementary and alternative medicine (CAM) into their treatment. To discuss

which CAM therapies are most effective, we contacted Roberta Lee, MD, vice chair of the department of integrative medicine at the Continuum Center for Health and Healing at Beth Israel Medical Center.

Dr. Lee recommended looking at life after cancer diagnosis as three separate phases—pretreatment, active treatment and posttreatment—because different CAM approaches work best during different phases.

Important: Before trying any complementary therapies, ask your oncologist which ones are safe and appropriate for you.

Before Treatment Begins

The focus now is on ensuring that you will be as healthy and strong as possible, physically and emotionally, when treatment begins...

• **Work with a dietitian who specializes in oncology nutrition.** Visit *www.Oncology Nutrition.org* (a practice group of the American Dietetic Association) for a referral. Dr. Lee recommends lots of fruits and vegetables, whole grains and fish...low-fat organic chicken breast if desired...no red meat...and plenty of water.

• **Consider strengthening supplements.** Dr. Lee suggested folic acid and vitamin B-12, which help with proper cellular division and tissue recovery...vitamin D, which is good for immune regulation, bone health and mood... and probiotics, which help optimize immune function and reduce production of cancer-promoting chemicals. Ask your doctor about dosages.

• **Learn relaxation techniques.** An analysis published in *Psycho-Oncology* found that, when learned prior to rather than during cancer treatment, relaxation techniques were significantly more effective at reducing anxiety. Studies show that progressive muscle relaxation and guided imagery can improve cancer treatment–related nausea, pain, depression and anxiety. Practice a relaxation technique for 15 to 20 minutes daily, Dr. Lee suggested.

• **Exercise appropriately.** Gentle movements (simple stretches, leisurely walks) help you stay calm and centered. As for more vigorous workouts, listen to your body—this is not the time to exhaust yourself.

• **If you work outside the home, plan ahead.** Calculating how long a leave you can afford and making arrangements now for your duties to be covered in your absence will give you less to worry about during treatment and ease your transition back to work afterward.

During Treatment

The primary consideration now is to avoid any CAM therapies that might lessen the effectiveness of your cancer treatment, Dr. Lee emphasized, so your doctor may instruct you to discontinue certain herbs and supplements. *However, the following CAM approaches generally are safe during cancer treatment…*

• **Try acupuncture to minimize hair loss.** Chemotherapy drugs attack cells that are in the process of reproducing—but the drugs can't distinguish between rapidly dividing cancer cells and normal cells. In the body, hair follicle cells are among those that multiply fastest, which is why many patients experience hair loss. Acupuncture helps stimulate hair growth at a cellular level and reduces the stress that can exacerbate hair loss, Dr. Lee said. *Bonus:* Acupuncture can ease chemo-related dry mouth.

• **Drink herbal teas for digestive woes.** Because digestive tract cells also multiply rapidly, chemo patients often develop gastrointestinal troubles. Dr. Lee suggested drinking chamomile tea, ginger tea and/or slippery elm tea as needed to reduce nausea and help smooth over any ulcerations in the intestinal tract. To ease cramping, try fennel tea.

• **For nerve damage, consider glutamine.** Ask your doctor about supplementing with this amino acid to relieve tingling, burning or numbness from chemo-induced neuropathy.

• **Soothe skin with massage.** Skin exposed to radiation treatment often becomes sensitive, warm and red, as if sunburned. For relief, Dr. Lee suggested trying gentle massage with oils…acupressure…reiki

(an energy healing technique in which the practitioner's hands are placed on or above certain spots on the patient's body)…or reflexology (massage of pressure points on the feet). To find a practitioner who works with cancer patients, check the Society for Oncology Massage (*www.s4om.org*).

• **Make each bite count.** You probably won't feel like eating much during treatment, so focus on foods that are easy to digest and nutritionally dense, such as protein shakes, soups and whole-grain breads. Avoid high-fat, spicy or acidic foods likely to aggravate nausea.

• **Do gentle yoga.** An analysis published in *Cancer Control* linked yoga to improvements in sleep quality, mood, physical function and overall quality of life.

• **Ease emotional distress.** Teas made with valerian, chamomile or hops flowers are calming, as are meditation and massage. Also consider hypnosis, which can help you process and release fear.

Referrals: American Society of Clinical Hypnosis (630-980-4740…*www.asch.net*, click on "Public" and "Member Referral Service").

After Treatment

Once chemo and radiation are over, attention shifts to restoring your health…

• **Have your doctor assess your nutrient levels.** Chemotherapy can deplete nutrients… blood tests can reveal whether a special diet and/or supplementation is appropriate to support your recovery. Ask your doctor and/or dietitian about magnesium…vitamin D… folic acid…and vitamin B-12, which, in addition to the aforementioned benefits, helps with mood and memory. Also discuss milk thistle, which helps your liver get rid of lingering toxins from chemotherapy.

• **To encourage hair growth, continue with acupuncture.** Folic acid and vitamin B-12 also can help with this, as can zinc and biotin, Dr. Lee said. Ask your physician about dosages.

• **As strength returns, gradually increase physical activity.** Dr. Lee suggested tai chi, Pilates and yoga, which are not too taxing.

Benefits for recovery: Exercise relieves stress, fortifies your body against further illness and improves overall well-being—all of which make it easier to get on with your life.

After Cancer: You Really Can Get Back to Normal

Julie Silver, MD, associate professor, department of physical medicine and rehabilitation, Harvard Medical School, Boston. She also is the founder of Oncology Rehab Partners, creator of the STAR Program Certification and author of *After Cancer Treatment: Heal Faster, Better, Stronger* (Johns Hopkins). *www.JulieSilverMD.com*

Until relatively recently, there was no such thing as "cancer rehab" to help cancer patients cope with the grueling and sometimes lasting physical and psychological effects of chemotherapy, radiation, surgery or other treatment. Patients, many of whom considered themselves lucky just to be alive, dealt with the problems largely on their own.

Now: Just as patients who have suffered a heart attack or stroke are likely to receive guidance on how to cope with the aftereffects of treatment, more and more cancer patients are beginning to get the help they need to regain the quality of life they had before getting sick.

Who can benefit: Of the 12.6 million cancer survivors in the US, an estimated 3.3 million continue to suffer physical consequences of their treatment, such as fatigue and/or chronic pain…and another 1.4 million live with mental health problems, such as depression and/or a form of mild cognitive impairment known as "chemo brain."

Latest development: As cancer rehab becomes more prevalent throughout the US—hundreds of facilities nationwide offer such programs—there is mounting evidence showing how this type of care can help accelerate recovery, improve a patient's quality of life and perhaps even reduce risk for cancer recurrence (see page 232). In fact, the American College of Surgeons' Commission on Cancer now requires cancer centers in the US to offer rehab services in order to receive accreditation.

When Cancer Rehab Helps

Even though it was first conceived as a resource for patients immediately after their acute phase of treatment, cancer rehab can help long after treatment has taken place. For example, people who were treated years ago and are now cancer-free—but not free of side effects from treatment—can benefit from cancer rehab. Just because you went for, say, physical therapy two years ago after you finished cancer treatment, it doesn't mean that you can't get more help now for the same problem or a different one.

Insurance picks up the tab: Because the benefits of cancer rehab are now so widely accepted, insurance generally covers the cost—regardless of when you were treated for cancer—including consultations with physiatrists (medical doctors who specialize in rehabilitation medicine), physical therapists, occupational therapists, speech language pathologists and others.

Even though cancer rehab therapies tend to be short term (typically requiring two to three sessions weekly in the provider's office for a period of a few weeks), insurance plans often limit the number of visits for such therapies. Be sure to check with your insurer for details on your coverage.

Each cancer patient's situation is different, but here are some common problems and how they are treated with cancer rehab…

Mild Cognitive Impairment ("Chemo Brain")

Cancer patients who have received chemotherapy often complain that they don't think as well and that they have less energy and decreased attention spans. If anxiety or hot flashes due to chemo interfere with sleep, that can decrease cognitive functioning, too.

How cancer rehab helps: A physical therapist might work with a cancer patient by using a specific therapeutic exercise plan. Exercise has been shown to improve cognitive functioning—perhaps by improving blood flow to the brain.

An occupational therapist or speech therapist may recommend strategies to help concentration, attention and memory. This may involve computer-based programs that improve short-term memory.

Anemia and Fatigue

Anemia is common with many hematological (blood) cancers, such as leukemia and lymphomas.

How cancer rehab helps: In a young person who has just undergone a bone marrow transplant, for example, if there is a low red blood cell count (an indicator of anemia) or a risk for infection, a tailored exercise program can build strength and endurance to help fight fatigue.

For an older adult, exercise is also a key part of a fatigue-fighting regimen that improves endurance and overall fitness. If fatigue results in problems with balance and gait, an occupational therapist can help the patient remain independent at home by suggesting a smartphone-based monitoring device such as a motion sensor that notifies a family member or friend if the patient falls.

Breathing Problems

Difficulty breathing and feeling short of breath are common problems in lung cancer survivors. These patients also may experience pain after surgery and have trouble exercising and performing their usual daily activities due to shortness of breath.

How cancer rehab helps: In addition to improving strength and physical performance through targeted exercises, a cancer patient who is having breathing problems would need to improve his/her ability to get more air into the lungs. This may involve "belly

breathing" exercises that will allow him to complete his daily activities without getting out of breath so quickly.

More from Dr. Silver...

Cancer "Prehab" Can Help, Too

C ancer "prehab" is useful during the window after a patient is diagnosed with cancer but before treatment begins to help boost his/her physical and emotional readiness for cancer treatment. For example, a specific exercise program, such as interval training, may be advised to increase strength before surgery. A nutrition program may be used to improve a patient's nutritional status before treatments that may sap appetite or lead to nutrition problems such as anemia. Working with a psychologist can help identify and deal with anxiety and stress before treatment starts. Cancer prehab usually is offered at centers that provide cancer rehab services. (See pages 227-229 for more information).

Also from Dr. Silver...

Cancer Rehab: What to Expect

W hether cancer patients are cured or are living with cancer as a chronic disease, rehab can help them function better, with less pain and more energy. Rehab also is a source of information and emotional support, so patients feel less confused and afraid. That's why Dr. Silver developed the STAR Program® (Survivorship Training and Rehabilitation) Certification for hospitals and cancer centers, which involves a protocol for best practices in cancer rehab.

Progress: Rhode Island is the first state to make cancer rehab services available to every cancer survivor in the state through the adoption of the STAR Program...Massachusetts is not far behind. And the American College of Surgeons' Commission on Cancer recently recommended that, by 2015, every patient treated at an accredited cancer center receive a post-treatment "survivorship care plan." For information and/or a referral to a STAR Program in your area, visit the Web

Ginseng Reduces Fatigue in Cancer Patients

In a recent finding, after eight weeks, cancer patients who had been given 2,000 milligrams of pure ground American ginseng root daily reported feeling less tired than those given a placebo. The same pure ground root used in the study is available through the Ginseng Board of Wisconsin (*www.Ginseng Board.com*). Off-the-shelf ginseng may be processed with ethanol—which can give it estrogen-like properties that may be harmful to breast cancer patients and other patients. Talk to your doctor.

Debra L. Barton, RN, PhD, associate professor of oncology and nurse administrator, division of nursing research, Mayo Clinic, Rochester, Minnesota. Her study was presented at an American Society of Clinical Oncology meeting.

a patient to be more active may increase the length of her life," Dr. Silver noted.

•**Occupational therapy to help with tasks of daily living,** such as bathing, dressing or driving...plus cognitive strategies to ease "chemo brain" and improve concentration, memory and/or organizational skills.

•**Psychological counseling to ease fear, anxiety and a sense of isolation or loss.**

Helpful: Set specific rehab goals for yourself—such as being able to sit comfortably long enough to resume your weekly bridge games—and share them with rehab personnel. Dr. Silver said that she wants to help people return to what they value. For example, one patient longed to return to door-to-door proselytizing with other members of her church, which required stamina to walk long distances, climb stairs and be out in all weather. With help from cancer rehab, Dr. Silver's patient achieved her goal...and with the right support, chances are good that you can, too.

site of Oncology Rehab Partners (*www.On cologyRehabPartners.com*), an organization founded by Dr. Silver and dedicated to advancing survivorship care.

What to expect from cancer rehab: The exact treatment depends on a particular patient's needs. *Typically, cancer rehab includes...*

•**Individualized therapies specific to the type of cancer.** For instance, a lung cancer patient can benefit from improving upper-body strength to help with breathing, plus overall conditioning to assist with walking and other activities that require endurance. For a breast cancer survivor, hands-on therapies can ease pain and minimize scarring and fluid buildup that limit arm movement. A person recovering from head or neck cancer may need speech-language pathology services to help with talking or swallowing.

•**Physical therapy that addresses pain, balance, gait, dizziness and/or exhaustion** ...plus a therapeutic exercise plan that accommodates current limitations while encouraging improvement. "Exercise may reduce cancer recurrence risk, so a rehab program that gets

Fish Oil Helps Chemo Patients Stay Strong

Vera Mazurak, PhD, associate professor of nutrition at the Alberta Institute for Human Nutrition at the University of Alberta in Edmonton, Canada, and coauthor of the two studies on fish oil, published in *Cancer*.

Chemotherapy helps save the lives of cancer patients, but it also causes a host of negative side effects—including loss of muscle mass and malnourishment that can contribute to fatigue, involuntary weight loss, decreased quality of life and even poorer prognoses.

Encouraging: A recent study showed that supplementing with fish oil helps prevent such dangerous side effects.

One group of lung cancer patients who were undergoing 10 weeks of chemotherapy took a daily dose of 2,200 mg of a fish oil supplement containing the omega-3 fatty acid eicosapentaenoic acid (EPA)...a control group underwent the same chemotherapy regimen but did not take fish oil (no placebo was given).

Impressive results: 69% of the patients who took fish oil maintained or even gained muscle mass, as shown on CT scans... only 29% of those who did not take fish oil retained their muscle mass after chemotherapy. Patients whose blood tests revealed the largest increases in EPA levels gained the most muscle mass.

Also: Fish oil users maintained their weight, whereas those in the control group lost weight (a sign of malnourishment).

Reassuring: Patients often are cautioned against supplementing during chemotherapy for fear that supplements could interfere with their cancer treatment—but another recent study from the same researchers found that lung cancer patients who took fish oil actually had increased response rates to chemotherapy and better one-year survival rates.

Fish oil's benefits for chemo patients are especially promising given that no effective treatment for cancer-related malnutrition currently exists. Fish oil also may prove helpful to patients who have other types of cancer or other chronic diseases associated with malnutrition, as well as to seniors at risk for muscle loss, researchers said.

Best: Talk to your oncologist about fish oil. If you take daily aspirin or another blood-thinning medication, be sure that your doctor is aware of this—fish oil can have a blood-thinning effect.

Better Late-Stage Cancer Prognosis

Recent study: When 41 men and women with end-stage cancer added nutritional supplements to their treatment, 76% lived an average of five months longer than expected, with some adding years to their life. The daily regimen included vitamin C, fish oil, selenium, coenzyme Q10, folic acid and vitamin A. The study participants who used the regi-

men had advanced malignancies, including those of the breast, pancreas and prostate.

Theory: Some cancer patients may benefit from antioxidant/vitamin combinations similar to those that have been found to reduce tumor development in animal studies.

If you have cancer: Ask your doctor whether supplements are appropriate for you.

Robert Lister, MD, chairman, Institute of Brain Chemistry and Human Nutrition, London Metropolitan University, UK.

Eat to Beat Cancer Fatigue

Catherine Alfano, PhD, deputy director of the office of cancer survivorship, National Cancer Institute, National Institutes of Health, Bethesda, Maryland, and lead author of a study published in *Journal of Clinical Oncology.*

Battling cancer is hard enough, but many cancer survivors also find that fatigue still plagues them...even years after their diagnosis and often after treatment, too.

And this isn't always just the "I'm a little droopy today" kind of fatigue—some cancer survivors have so little energy that they lose their jobs and stop doing the things that they love.

The fatigue could be due to the cancer, the treatment, the stress of dealing with the disease—or some combination of all three.

What a disappointment, after having faced up to cancer and defeated it!

Fortunately, there's some progress on this front.

Nobody knows for sure why fatigue lasts so long after getting diagnosed with cancer, but one theory suggests that all that systemic inflammation in the body causes an imbalance in the nervous system, making the "fight or flight" sympathetic nerves overactive and the "resting" parasympathetic nerves underactive—which may lead to fatigue.

We've known from past studies that eating certain foods and taking certain supplements can reduce inflammation. So a group of researchers recently studied whether particular foods would help cancer survivors experience less fatigue. They looked at women who had had breast cancer—but there's no reason to think that survivors of other types of cancer wouldn't fall into the same boat.

And the results are very promising!

Who Was Most Tired?

All the cancer survivors in the study had been treated surgically, and some had also had chemotherapy and/or radiation.

Researchers found an interesting connection between their levels of fatigue and their consumption of two sorts of fatty acids—omega-3 and omega-6.

• **The women whose diets had the highest ratios of omega-6s to omega-3s** and who did not take fish oil, cod-liver oil or flaxseed oil supplements (which contain omega-3s) had the most inflammation... and almost half of them were experiencing chronic fatigue.

• **The women whose diets had the lowest ratios of omega-6s to omega-3s** and who had been taking at least one of the supplements listed above had the least inflammation...and only about one-quarter of them were experiencing chronic fatigue.

• **In between these two extremes,** the less omega-6s and the more omega-3s a woman consumed either in her food or from supplements, the less likely she was to have high inflammation and suffer from fatigue.

Which Fats Do You Eat?

This result seems unambiguous. For these cancer survivors, consuming a small amount of omega-6s relative to omega-3s helped them avoid fatigue—the exact amounts they ate weren't as important as the ratio. Researchers aren't sure whether getting omega-3 fatty acids from food versus getting them from supplements made any difference, so for now, "I'd advise cancer survivors to concentrate on increasing their omega-3 fatty acids and decreasing their omega-6 fatty

acids through food," said Catherine Alfano, PhD, the study's lead author and deputy director of the office of cancer survivorship at the National Cancer Institute in Bethesda, Maryland. "Future research will have to test whether taking a supplement that contains omega-3s can help."

Dr. Alfano pointed out that in our bodies, omega-3s are partly responsible for reducing inflammation, and that that function can be overwhelmed by an abundance of omega-6s. If you maintain a favorable omega-3-to-omega-6 ratio, the anti-inflammatory properties of omega-3s can prevail.

Omega-6s are found in abundance in margarine and vegetable oils (including corn oil, canola oil, sunflower oil, safflower oil and soybean oil) and are therefore plentiful in processed food and commercially baked products. If you are a cancer survivor, then these oils and foods containing them should become part of your "eat only a little" list.

Meanwhile, omega-3s, with which you should fill your plate, are found mostly in seafood such as salmon, sardines, halibut, scallops, shrimp and tuna, and in other foods such as flaxseed, walnuts, tofu and soybeans. These are all smart dietary choices in general—and if they can also help you break out of post-cancer fatigue, how terrific is that?

What Your Oncologist Isn't Telling You

Andrea L. Cheville, MD, associate professor of physical medicine and rehabilitation, Mayo Clinic, Rochester, Minnesota. The results of her study were published in the *Journal of Pain and Symptom Management*.

If you have cancer or have had it in the past, then you've already discussed treatments with your oncologist.

During these discussions, has your oncologist ever brought up the topic of exercise and been very specific about it—as in, what types of physical activities you should be doing and how often you should be doing them?

Odds are, he or she hasn't, according to a recent study.

This is alarming, since past research has shown that exercise is associated with improvements in a wide range of cancer-related issues, such as reducing fatigue and enhancing physical quality of life, according to a meta-analysis done by researchers at Duke Cancer Institute in Durham, North Carolina. Exercise may also help prevent cancer recurrence and cancer-related death. One study done by researchers at Harvard Medical School, for example, found that the risks of breast cancer recurrence, breast cancer death and death (from any cause) were 26% to 40% lower in women who exercised most, compared with those who exercised least.

Why are oncologists talking more about pills than Pilates?

And what, specifically, about exercise should cancer patients—and cancer survivors—know?

We spoke with an expert to find out…

Cancer Patients Are in the Dark

In the recent study, researchers interviewed 20 lung cancer patients, and not one participant reported receiving specific instructions from his or her oncologist about exercise—other than a vague suggestion to "stay active."

This is not to say that oncologists don't care about your well-being, emphasized lead study author Andrea L. Cheville, MD. They are simply more apt to zero in on their area of expertise—attacking your cancer and killing it with drugs, radiation, surgery, etc.—as opposed to talking about easing symptoms and preventing recurrence, she said.

It Pays to Get Moving

"We still don't know exactly why exercise helps reduce symptoms and cancer recurrence—it may be that it stimulates metabolism, modulates hormones, boosts immunity and/or reduces oxidative damage to cells (or some combination of these factors), but we do know that it helps," Dr. Cheville said.

It's important for all people to exercise, of course, not only cancer patients. But it's particularly important for cancer patients and cancer survivors to be physically active because having cancer challenges a person's fitness in a variety of ways.

Past research has shown that chemotherapy, for example, is associated with a loss of lean muscle, and it can make patients feel more achy and fatigued than usual. These problems tend to make exercise less appealing, though physical activity actually is what helps solve those problems by building muscle and relieving achiness and fatigue. Cancer patients and survivors are already at a physical disadvantage, and if they exercise progressively less, they will lose even more strength and stamina and be less able to fight off recurrence of the disease.

Exercise That Suits Your Needs

If your oncologist isn't bringing up exercise, Dr. Cheville suggests you should broach the topic yourself. Then, if the doctor doesn't have specific advice about it, ask for a referral to a physical therapist or personal trainer who does have specific experience in working with cancer patients and/or survivors.

Come to think of it, it's a good idea to go see such fitness professionals even if your oncologist did know a bit about exercise—they are the real specialists in it.

Anyone with cancer can exercise, Dr. Cheville said, but the trick is making sure that you go about it safely and effectively. There is no one-size-fits-all workout plan to follow. For example, a woman receiving radiation for breast cancer may be extra tired, so aggressive exercise would not make sense in this context. Instead, she would benefit from gentle, progressive stretching. On the other end of the spectrum, a man who has been in remission from prostate cancer for five years is much better able to handle intense endurance and strength-training exercises, such as weight lifting or jogging. Most patients fall somewhere in between those two examples, so it's usually best to start small—often with light stretches or walking—and then progress gradually into more forceful moves, gauging comfort along the way. And the program should be molded around any targeted problems from the cancer or the therapy, such as not using a sore body part that's healing from an incision or avoiding movements that cause dizziness if a patient is easily nauseated. That's why it's important to ask your physical therapist or trainer for a carefully individualized program.

Also contact your local YMCA or visit *www.livestrong.org* (click on LIVESTRONG at the YMCA), since the Livestrong nonprofit has partnered with YMCAs in 25 states across the country to provide specialized exercise programs for cancer survivors.

Hospice: The Vital Topic Doctors and Patients Don't Discuss

John Ayanian, MD, MPP (master of public policy), professor of medicine and health-care policy at Harvard Medical School in Boston and senior author of a study of 1,517 lung cancer patients.

Too few terminally ill patients who could benefit from hospice care are being apprised of this comforting option, recent research shows. That is sad, because hospice can minimize physical and emotional suffering and improve quality of life in the final weeks. According to the Hospice Foundation of America, the focus of hospice is not to prolong life nor hasten death, but rather to provide "comfort and support to patients and their families when a life-limiting illness no longer responds to cure-oriented treatments." Generally, hospice care becomes an option when a doctor certifies that a patient is expected to survive no more than six months.

But: In a recent study, among patients with metastatic lung cancer who had an anticipated four to eight months to live, only half had discussed hospice care with their doctors. Why the lack of communication? Patients may not bring up the subject because they are unaware of hospice or because they overestimate how long they have to live... while doctors may wait for patients to initiate the conversation because they don't want to intrude.

Helpful: If a loved one's condition is terminal, ask his or her doctor about planning ahead for in-home or residential hospice care.

STROKE

Despite the fact that women are more likely than men to have a stroke—only one quarter of women surveyed could name more than two of the most common symptoms. That puts women at a severe disadvantage because recognizing the signs and getting help quickly are key to surviving a stroke. And, just as with heart disease, the symptoms women experience can be different than what men feel. For example, women may have a sudden onset of hiccups, nausea or general weakness. Read on to uncover the best ways to lower your risk of stroke.

http://www.stroke.org/site/PageServer?pagename=WOMSYMP

Chapter 13

STROKE: THE SIGNS, SYMPTOMS AND SECRETS TO RECOVERY

Women's Fatal Mistake in Seeking Help for Stroke

Imagine this scene: Your husband suddenly feels dizzy, goes numb in one arm or starts slurring his words. Odds are that you would urge him to call 911 or you'd do it yourself without delay, right? Of course. Now suppose you were the one with the symptoms. Would you carry on with your tasks, stoically ignoring the problem and hoping it would just go away? Many woman would. In fact, when it comes to seeking help for possible symptoms of stroke, there's an alarming discrepancy between husbands and wives, a recent study reveals.

Researchers analyzed data on 192 patients with acute stroke symptoms who were brought by emergency medical services (EMS) to the Mayo Clinic in Phoenix. Specifically, they looked at the number of minutes that elapsed between the time a patient first became aware of having symptoms and the time at which 911 was called. They found that, on average, married patients summoned EMS 44 minutes after symptoms were noticed, while single patients called 911 after 46 minutes—so there was no real difference there. And while single men summoned help

quicker than single women did, the difference was not statistically significant.

But: Breaking down the data a different way, researchers discovered that when the patient was a married man, EMS was summoned in an average of just 28 minutes. Yet when the patient was a married woman, the delay between symptom awareness and the 911 call averaged 67 minutes!

Researchers speculate that women are so used to being the caregivers in the family that we put others' needs before our own. When symptoms arise, wives urge husbands to seek care immediately—but we don't take as good care of ourselves. (When we asked whether this also could mean that husbands don't take as good care of us wives as we take of them, the researchers declined to comment…though it's worth talking to our men about!)

Why women's delay in summoning help is so worrisome: With stroke, every minute counts—the earlier patients get help, the more treatment options there are and the less devastating the consequences are likely to

Joyce K. Lee-Iannotti, MD, fellow in the department of neurology at the Mayo Clinic in Scottsdale, Arizona, and lead author of a study on acute stroke symptoms and activation of emergency medical services presented at the recent American Stroke Conference.

be. Also, women have a higher lifetime risk for stroke than men do…and more women than men die of stroke each year, according to the American Heart Association.

Self-defense: Memorize the symptoms of stroke and call 911 immediately if you experience any of the following…

• **Numbness or paralysis on one side of your face or body.** Try smiling into a mirror or raising both arms over your head at the same time—a one-sided smile or an arm that won't stay up could indicate a stroke.

• **Speech problems, such as slurring words or being unable to find the right words.** Try repeating a simple sentence—if you can't, that suggests a stroke.

• **Unexplained dizziness,** loss of balance or difficulty walking.

• **Vision problems,** such as blurred, double or blackened vision.

• **A sudden, severe "bolt out of the blue" headache.**

More info: To see a video about the study and stroke symptoms, go to *http://bit.ly/SLT tUU.*

Catching a Stroke Before It Starts

Fiona Webster, PhD, education scientist and assistant professor in the department of family and community medicine at the University of Toronto in Ontario and lead author of a study on stroke prevention clinics published in *Stroke*.

When you think of saving lives that would otherwise be lost to stroke, you probably imagine frightened but clear-thinking family members calling 911 or efficient ER doctors administering crucial medication just in the nick of time. Those things matter, of course—but a lifesaving approach that often is overlooked is the stroke prevention clinic.

Researchers recently compared the medical records of 16,468 patients who had ex-

perienced either an ischemic stroke (caused when a clot blocks blood flow to the brain) or a transient ischemic attack (TIA), often called a "mini-stroke." TIAs produce symptoms that are similar to stroke—sudden weakness or numbness on one side of the body, slurred speech, dizziness, vision problems—but usually last a much shorter time and often cause no permanent damage. However, the risk of having a full-blown and potentially fatal stroke within three months after a TIA is as high as 20%.

Study findings: TIA and ischemic stroke patients who were referred to stroke prevention clinics that aimed to identify and address risk factors were 26% less likely to die of stroke in the following 12 months than patients who did not attend such programs. These findings underscore the importance of secondary prevention for at-risk patients, researchers said.

Why it works: Many factors that place a person at increased risk for stroke are modifiable. When a patient learns which particular risk factors are putting her in danger and takes steps to control those, her risk is significantly reduced. A stroke prevention clinic is an outpatient program staffed by medical professionals trained to assess, diagnose and treat stroke risk factors. *The treatment duration and exact services provided vary, but typically patients…*

• **Have their blood monitored** to measure how well any medications they take are working to control clotting, modulate blood pressure and/or regulate cholesterol.

• **Receive support to exercise more,** lose weight, reduce stress and/or quit smoking, as needed.

• **Are assessed and treated as necessary for heart conditions,** sleep apnea and other chronic conditions that contribute to stroke risk.

Not all hospitals have stroke prevention clinics—and not all doctors refer their TIA or stroke patients to such programs. If you have had a TIA or stroke, talk to your doctor about whether a stroke prevention clinic could benefit you...and ask your insurer whether your policy covers the cost.

What You Must Know If Your Mother Had a Stroke

Amitava Banerjee, MPH, MRCP (Member of the Royal College of Physicians), DPhil, cardiologist, researcher and clinical lecturer of cardiovascular medicine at the University of Birmingham in the UK.

Here's a man, here's a woman. How likely is either to have a heart attack? No one knows for sure...but what we do know is that the current tools for predicting heart attack risk are less accurate for women than for men. Now a recent study reveals a useful piece of information in this prediction puzzle—a particular type of family history, not of heart attack itself, but of stroke.

Researchers from the University of Oxford analyzed data on 2,210 men and women who had suffered a heart attack or other coronary problem caused by reduced blood flow to the heart.

Findings: About 24% of these patients had one or more first-degree relatives (parent, sibling) with a history of stroke. The female heart patients (but not the males) were more than twice as likely to have a mother who'd had a stroke than to have a father who had suffered a stroke.

What this means: Maternal stroke history may provide a valuable clue in gauging a woman's heart attack risk—even though this factor is not currently included in standard heart attack risk assessments.

Best: Women whose mothers suffered a stroke should be especially careful to minimize heart attack risk by getting blood pressure and cholesterol levels checked regularly, exercising, eating healthfully, losing weight if necessary and not smoking.

Think You Know Your True Risk for Heart Attack and Stroke?

James Ehrlich, MD, clinical associate professor of endocrinology at the University of Colorado, Denver. The chief medical officer of United Cardio Systems, based in Castle Rock, Colorado, Dr. Ehrlich advises physicians on best practices involving biomarkers, imaging technologies and radiation protection.

You may think that you are at low risk for a heart attack because the heart tests that your doctor has ordered had "negative" results. The standard blood test that you received may show that your cholesterol and triglyceride levels are fine. And you may have even received a clean bill of health after taking a cardiac stress test (exercising on a treadmill while heart rhythms are electronically monitored).

Surprising fact: Those two standard heart tests miss many high-risk individuals with early heart disease. For example, a study published in the *Journal of the American College of Cardiology* found that 95% of women who had heart attacks at age 65 or younger were considered low risk.

For the greatest protection: In addition to the standard heart tests, all adults should consider receiving the highly accurate heart tests described in this article, which are not regularly ordered by most physicians but serve as stronger predictors of cardiovascular disease.

Why don't more doctors have conversations with their patients about these important tests? Many physicians closely adhere to the guidelines of the government's Preventive Services Task Force, whose evidence-based recommendations tend to include tests that are less sophisticated and less expensive.

But if your primary care physician or cardiologist does not mention these tests, ask him/her which ones might be right for you. The results will provide the best possible information for your doctor to create a customized medical and lifestyle regimen that can help prevent heart attacks and strokes.

Coronary Calcium CT Scan

This radiological imaging test—also called a CT heart scan—detects and quantifies calcified plaque, a marker for atherosclerosis (fatty buildup in the arteries). This test is up to 10 times more predictive of future heart problems than a cholesterol test and can detect early heart disease that often goes undetected by a stress test.

My advice: Men over age 35 and women over age 40 with one to two risk factors for cardiovascular disease are good candidates for screening with a heart scan. Risk factors include being overweight…having hypertension, diabetes (or prediabetes), high LDL "bad" cholesterol, low HDL "good" cholesterol, elevated triglycerides, a family history of heart disease…and/or smoking.

Risks: Cardiac CT tests expose patients to ionizing radiation (the same type used in x-rays), which has been linked to an increased risk for cancer. Heart scans, such as electron-beam CT scans and late-generation spiral CT scans, now are performed at lower radiation doses—the equivalent of 10 to 25 chest x-rays is typical. These CT scans use faster speeds than standard CT scans to produce the image, are accurate and expose you to less radiation.

Cost and coverage: $150 to $500 and may be covered by insurance.

Carotid Test

An ultrasound test of the carotid (neck) arteries leading to the brain does not involve radiation and measures two important conditions that help predict cardiovascular disease—the dangerous presence of plaque and the thickness of the two inner layers of each artery (the intima and media).

The carotid test is a stronger predictor of a future stroke than coronary calcium and a moderate predictor of heart attack risk.

My advice: I recommend this test for men over age 35 and women over age 40 with one to two risk factors such as hypertension and/or a family history of heart disease or stroke. People with such risk factors as high cholesterol and type 2 diabetes also may benefit from the test.

Results: If there is any noticeable plaque or the thickness of the intima/media is in the top 25% for people of your age, sex and ethnicity, you are at a higher than desirable cardiovascular risk and should pay close attention to all risk factors—especially hypertension.

Cost and coverage: $100 to $500 and often is covered by insurance.

Advanced Lipoprotein Analysis

Advanced lipoprotein analysis includes blood tests that measure hidden risk factors such as…

• **Lp(a),** a dangerous particle that often is elevated in families with a history of premature heart attacks.

• **ApoB/ApoAI,** a ratio of dangerous particles to protective particles.

My advice: This analysis is especially useful for people with heart disease that occurs in the absence of risk factors or who have a family history of premature heart disease (heart attack before age 55 in a father or brother and before age 65 in a mother or sister, for example). Those with type 2 diabetes (or prediabetes) or "metabolic syndrome"—often with a bulging waistline, hypertension, low HDL, elevated triglycerides and/or elevated blood sugar—also are good candidates.

Cost and coverage: Varies widely from as little as $40 to as much as $400—often covered by insurance.

However, not all labs perform these tests.

Labs that perform advanced lipoprotein analysis: Atherotech (*www.atherotech.com*)… Berkeley Heart Lab (*www.bhlinc.com*)…Boston Heart Lab (*www.bostonheartlab.com*)… Health Diagnostic Laboratory (*www.hdlab inc. com*)…LipoScience (*www.liposcience.com*) … and SpectraCell (*www.spectracell.com*).

Other Biomarkers

• **Lp-PLA2 (PLAC test).** This blood test, which measures inflammation in blood vessels themselves, is a powerful predictor of the most common type of stroke (ischemic stroke). The test is more specific for vascular disease than the commonly ordered test for C-reactive protein (which is elevated with any type of inflammation in the body).

Cost and coverage: About $50 to $200 and may be covered by insurance.

• **BNP or NT-proBNP (B-type natriuretic peptide).** This is an early indicator of a weakening heart muscle (even before overt heart failure) and an excellent test for managing patients with heart failure. The test can also be used to help predict risk for heart attack.

Cost and coverage: About $50 to $250 and may be covered by insurance.

Aspirin Resistance Testing

Aspirin helps stop blood components called platelets from sticking together, which reduces the risk for an artery-plugging blood clot. A daily "baby" aspirin (81 mg) or higher doses usually are prescribed for anyone who has had a heart attack or stroke…or for someone who is at risk for either condition.

However, 25% of people are aspirin resistant—the drug doesn't effectively prevent platelet "stickiness."

Aspirin resistance testing measures a urinary metabolite (11-dehydrothromboxane B2), which is high if you are aspirin resistant.

Who should be tested: Anyone taking aspirin to treat or prevent cardiovascular disease.

Cost and coverage: $30 to $150 and often covered by insurance.

Good news: Recent research published in the *Journal of the American College of Cardiology* shows that supplementing the diet with omega-3 fatty acids can overcome aspirin resistance.

Sobering Statistics

About 81 million American adults have cardiovascular disease. This may include narrowed, blocked arteries (coronary artery disease)… irregular heartbeats (arrhythmia)…and/or a weakened heart muscle (heart failure).

Every year, 1.5 million of those Americans have heart attacks and 500,000 of them die. Another 800,000 have strokes, 140,000 of whom die.

Diet Soda Danger

People who drink diet soda have a higher risk for stroke and heart attack.

Recent finding: People who drank diet soda every day were nearly 50% more likely to have a vascular event, such as a stroke, even after accounting for such risk factors as age, gender, smoking and alcohol consumption.

Note: People who drink diet soda every day may have different eating habits than those who don't drink diet soda, which may contribute to cardiovascular problems.

Hannah E. Gardener, ScD, an epidemiologist in the Clinical Research Division, Miller School of Medicine, University of Miami, Florida, and leader of a study of the dietary habits of 2,564 people.

Drink Tea to Guard Against Stroke

Do you love a cozy cup of tea? If not, there is a good reason to develop a taste for it.

Researchers from the University of California, Los Angeles, analyzed data from nine studies involving a total of nearly 195,000 people.

Findings: Compared with people who drank less than one cup of tea daily, those who drank at least three cups daily of green or black tea (both of which come from the Camillia sinensis plant) had a 21% lower risk for stroke…risk dropped 42% for those who drank six or more cups of green or black tea daily. It is the flavonoid epigallocatechin

Stroke Linked to Emotional Neglect

People who reported being emotionally neglected as children were found to be at increased risk for stroke in adulthood, according to recent research.

Neurology

gallate and the amino acid theanine, both of which are found in green and black teas, that might reduce stroke risk, researchers say.

Note: Though not included in the study, oolong tea and white tea (but not herbal teas) also come from the Camillia sinensis plant and therefore may have similar stroke-preventing benefits. There was not enough data on decaffeinated tea to include it in the study.

Lenore Arab, PhD, professor of medicine at the David Geffen School of Medicine at the University of California, Los Angeles, and lead author of a review of studies published in *Stroke*.

"Stroke Belt" Folks: Beware of Fried Fish

Fadi Nahab, MD, assistant professor of neurology at Emory University in Atlanta and lead author of a study involving 21,675 people age 45 and up.

You won't find the stroke belt marked on your typical map of the US. But if you or your loved ones live in any of the eight Southern states with a higher-than-average rate of stroke (Alabama, Arkansas, Georgia, Louisiana, Mississippi, North Carolina, South Carolina, Tennessee), you'll want to know about a recent study that sheds light on a likely reason for this increased risk—fried fish.

Background: We all know that omega-3 fatty acids in fish can protect us against cardiovascular problems by reducing blood clotting and improving blood pressure, blood fats and blood vessel function. When fish is fried,

however, healthful omega-3s are destroyed and unhealthful fats and harmful free radicals are created.

Recent study: Researchers tracked the diets of more than 21,000 people across the country. Compared with people living in other states, those in stroke belt states were 11% to 17% less likely, on average, to eat the recommended two weekly servings of non-fried fish...and 30% more likely to eat fried fish two or more times per week.

Fish highest in omega-3s include salmon, mackerel, herring, lake trout, sardines and albacore tuna. The American Heart Association cautions against shark, swordfish, king mackerel and tilefish, which contain high levels of mercury.

Do You Get Enough of the Anti-Stroke Mineral?

Susanna Larsson, PhD, associate professor at the Institute of Environmental Medicine at the Karolinska Institutet in Stockholm, Sweden, and lead author of a study on dietary magnesium and stroke risk published in *The American Journal of Clinical Nutrition*.

Our moms always told us to eat our greens and beans...and now a new study reveals yet another important reason why these wise women were right. People who consume plenty of foods rich in magnesium—such as leafy green veggies and legumes—appear to have fewer strokes.

Researchers analyzed data from seven studies involving a total of 241,378 people from the US, Europe and Asia who were followed for an average of nearly 12 years.

What they found: For every additional 100 mg of magnesium consumed daily, a person's risk for ischemic stroke (the most common type, which is caused by a blood clot) was reduced by 9%.

Concern: Study participants from the US fell far short of the ideal, consuming foods that provided, on average, just 242 mg of magnesium per day—though the RDA is 320 mg for most adult women and 420 for most adult men.

Because this study focused specifically on food, researchers did not make a recommendation regarding the use of magnesium supplementation. However, it is easy to boost your intake of the brain-protecting mineral with food. *For instance, you can get about 100 mg of magnesium each from…*

- **Beans** (black, lima, navy, white), 1 cup.
- **Beet greens,** 1 cup cooked.
- **Bran cereal,** ½ cup.
- **Brazil nuts,** 1 ounce.
- **Cashews,** 1¼ ounce.
- **Halibut,** 3 ounces.
- **Lentils,** 1¼ cup.
- **Okra,** 1 cup cooked.
- **Spinach,** ⅔ cup cooked.

Eating Oranges May Cut Women's Stroke Risk

Researchers studied the health records of 69,622 women, who reported their food intake every four years for 14 years.

Result: Women whose diets contained high levels of flavanones (found in oranges, grapefruit and other citrus fruit) had a 19% lower risk for ischemic stroke (caused by a blood clot) than those who ate the least amount of flavanones.

Theory: Flavanones are thought to improve blood vessel function and have anti-inflammatory qualities.

Caution: Because grapefruit can interact with some medications, speak to your doctor before increasing your intake.

Aedin Cassidy, PhD, professor of diet and health, Norwich Medical School, University of East Anglia, Norwich, United Kingdom.

Surprising Brain Danger from Drinking

Charlotte Cordonnier, MD, PhD, professor of neurology at the University of Lille Nord de France in Lille, France, and director of a study on alcohol and stroke published in *Neurology.*

You're well aware that overindulging in alcohol is unwise, leading to all sorts of behavior that you'll regret. But you may not realize how much a few extra drinks can place your brain at risk.

And we're not talking just to folks who binge on huge quantities of booze. That's because downing just three drinks a day is enough to drastically lower the age at which you may suffer a stroke!

This disturbing news comes from a French study involving 540 women and men who had experienced an intracerebral hemorrhage (ICH), a type of stroke that occurs when a blood vessel inside the brain leaks or ruptures. Researchers asked the patients or their relatives or caregivers about the participants' drinking habits. Among the ICH patients, 25% regularly consumed 300 grams or more of pure alcohol per week (which by US standards equals about three drinks or more per day) and thus met the study criteria for being "heavy drinkers."

Startling finding: Among the heavy drinkers, the average age at which stroke occurred was 60 years old. That's a full 14 years younger than the average age of the stroke patients who consumed fewer than three drinks per day.

Self-defense: If you drink, do so only in moderation—meaning no more than one drink per day for women or two drinks per day for men. And take note—a drink served in a bar or poured too generously at home may be much larger than the US standard serving size of 12 ounces of beer, five ounces of wine or 1.5 ounces of hard liquor. To protect your brain, don't kid yourself about how much you're actually imbibing.

Mentholated Cigarettes May Increase Stroke Risk

Recent finding: All cigarettes increase stroke risk, but people who smoke mentholated cigarettes have more than double the risk for stroke, compared with people who smoke nonmenthol ones.

Study of 5,167 smokers by researchers at St. Michael's Hospital, Toronto, published in *Archives of Internal Medicine*.

Stroke: It's on the Rise Among Younger People

Brett M. Kissela, MD, professor and vice-chair of the department of neurology at the University of Cincinnati College of Medicine. He was the lead researcher of the National Institutes of Health–funded study, published in *Neurology*, that documented increasing strokes in younger adults.

Few people in their 40s or 50s can imagine having a stroke, particularly if they are generally healthy. But the risk is higher than you might think—dispelling the common belief that stroke is a risk for only the elderly.

An unexpected trend: Over the last several years, there has been an increase in strokes among adults in their 40s, 50s and 60s.What's most alarming about this development is that doctors don't expect to see strokes in these relatively young patients, so the diagnosis sometimes gets overlooked.

Important finding: One in seven young stroke patients was initially misdiagnosed as having another problem, such as a seizure or alcohol intoxication, researchers at Wayne State University–Detroit Medical Center found in a recent study.

What to do: First and foremost, be alert. Stroke can occur at any age, so it's important for all adults to pay close attention to symptoms (see page 242). If you are diagnosed and treated within about four hours of having a stroke, you are far more likely to recover than someone whose diagnosis and treatment are delayed. Unfortunately, only about 20% to 30% of young patients with stroke symptoms go to the emergency room, according to research. The others are likely to shrug off the symptoms (especially if they were relatively minor and/or short-lived) and do not learn that they have suffered a stroke until a subsequent problem is detected later on.

What's Causing Earlier Strokes?

Many of the so-called "age-related" diseases that greatly increase stroke risk, such as high blood pressure (hypertension), diabetes and high cholesterol, are now appearing in patients who are middle-aged or younger—primarily because so many Americans are eating more junk food, gaining too much weight and not getting enough exercise. Family history is also a risk factor for stroke.

But even if you don't have any of these conditions (or a family history of stroke), you are in good physical shape and generally eat a well-balanced diet, do not be lulled into a false sense of security. Anyone can suffer a stroke. That's why it's very important for all adults to be on the lookout for red flags that could signal a stroke.

Stroke Stats

22% to 25%...Decreased risk for stroke among women who drank more than one cup of coffee per day, as compared with women who drank less coffee.

Stroke.

3 to 6 hours...Average delay between the onset of stroke symptoms and the time patients arrive at an emergency department—even though prompt treatment can significantly reduce the debilitating effects of stroke.

American Heart Association

Prevention Works

Stroke is the fourth-leading cause of death in the US. Those who survive a stroke often face a lifetime of disability, including paralysis and speech and emotional difficulties.

Fortunately, younger patients, in general, are more likely to recover than older ones because their brains have greater plasticity, the ability to regain functions after stroke-related trauma. Even so, many young stroke patients will have permanent damage.

Important: Regardless of your age, fast treatment is critical if you experience stroke symptoms. The majority of strokes are ischemic, caused by blood clots that impair circulation to the brain. Patients who are given clot-dissolving drugs, such as tissue plasminogen activator (tPA), within the first few hours after a stroke are far more likely to make a full recovery than those who are treated later.

Up to 80% of strokes can be avoided by preventing or treating the main risk factors, according to the National Stroke Association. For example, not smoking is crucial—people who smoke are twice as likely to have an ischemic stroke as nonsmokers.

Also important…

• **Do not ignore hypertension.** Like stroke, hypertension is often viewed as a problem only for the elderly. But there's been an increase in hypertension in younger patients, who often go undiagnosed.

Warning: Uncontrolled high blood pressure damages the brain—even in patients who haven't had a stroke, according to a recent study published in *The Lancet Neurology.*

If your blood pressure is high (normal is below 120/80), you are two to four times more likely to have a stroke than someone with normal blood pressure.

What to do: All adults should always have their blood pressure taken during routine doctor visits (at least once every two years if your blood pressure is normal…and at least annually if you've been diagnosed with hypertension or prehypertension). You can reduce both blood pressure and the risk for stroke by maintaining a healthy body weight…eating a healthful diet…getting regular exercise…and taking medication if your blood pressure remains elevated despite lifestyle changes.

• **Manage diabetes.** It's second only to hypertension as a risk factor for stroke. Diabetes increases the risk for all cardiovascular diseases, including hypertension. People who have diabetes are up to four times more likely to have a stroke than those without the condition.

What to do: Get tested. The American Diabetes Association recommends that all adults age 45 and older get screened for diabetes every three years.

If you already have diabetes, do everything you can to keep your blood sugar stable—for example, eat properly, get exercise and lose weight, if necessary.

• **Keep an eye on your cholesterol.** It's the third most important stroke risk factor because LDL ("bad") cholesterol can accumulate in the arteries, impede circulation to the brain and increase the risk for blood clots.

What to do: Beginning at age 20, get your cholesterol tested at least every five years. If your LDL is high (less than 100 mg/dL is optimal), you'll want to get the number down by eating less saturated fat…getting more vegetables and other high-fiber foods…and possibly taking a statin medication, such as *simvastatin* (Zocor). Depending on the drug and dose, statins typically lower cholesterol by about 25% to 50%.

• **Pay attention to your alcohol consumption.** People who drink heavily (three or more alcoholic beverages daily for men and two or more for women) are more likely to have a stroke earlier in life than moderate drinkers or nondrinkers.

In fact, in a study of 540 stroke patients, French researchers found that heavy drinkers suffered their strokes at age 60, on average—14 years earlier than patients who drank less or not at all.

Warning: Heavy use of alcohol is also associated with increased risk for hemorrhagic stroke, which is caused by bleeding in the brain (rather than a blood clot). This type of stroke can occur even in patients without a history of serious health problems.

What to do: If you drink, be sure to follow the standard advice for alcohol consumption—no more than two drinks daily for men…or one for women.

Look into the Eyes for an Early Warning Sign of Stroke

Emily Y. Chew, MD, medical officer and deputy director in the division of epidemiology and clinical applications at the National Eye Institute, part of the National Institutes of Health, Bethesda, Maryland.

The eyes may be the windows to the soul, but they also are the windows to the body. Via the eyes, doctors can view internal structures, including nerves and blood vessels. What they learn can provide important clues about your whole body—and your current and future health.

Regular eye exams are obviously important for visual health. But they also can detect conditions that you might not know you have—and that your primary care doctor might have missed.

For example, clots in the retinal blood vessels could mean an increased risk of stroke.

Most strokes are ischemic, caused by blood clots that reduce or stop circulation to parts of the brain. As with other cardiovascular diseases, patients may not suspect that anything is wrong until it's too late.

Your doctor might detect tiny blood clots in the arteries in the retina. Clots in these blood vessels could indicate that there is a similar problem elsewhere in the body, including in blood vessels in the head or neck. Your doctor also might see yellow flecks that indicate high cholesterol, an important stroke risk factor.

Important: See your primary care doctor immediately if you notice a sudden change in your visual field—if, for example, the right side of your field of vision is dark or blurry. Changes in the visual field could mean that you've already had a stroke.

Regular eye exams are critical if you have any stroke risk factors, including diabetes, hypertension, smoking or a family history of cardiovascular disease. The same strategies that can protect you from heart disease also will reduce your risk of having a stroke.

Which Artery-Clearing Procedure Is Safest for Women?

Virginia J. Howard, PhD, associate professor of epidemiology at the University of Alabama at Birmingham School of Public Health, and lead author of a study of 2,502 people.

It's scary to be told that your carotid arteries—the big blood vessels in your neck that supply oxygenated blood to the brain—are dangerously clogged with plaque, leaving you at increased risk for stroke. People with this condition, called carotid artery stenosis, often undergo one of two different surgical procedures… and in men, both surgeries appear to have similar benefits and risks.

But: Among women, one of the procedures seems to be significantly riskier than the other, according to a recent study published in *The Lancet Neurology*.

Researchers recruited more than 2,500 patients from 117 centers in the US and Canada. The two procedures being compared were the traditional carotid endarterectomy, in which a surgeon makes an incision to open the carotid artery, removes the plaque and then stitches up the artery…and the newer carotid artery stenting, a less invasive procedure in which a stent (mesh tube) is inserted into the carotid via a catheter and left in place to keep the artery open.

Results: Compared with women who underwent endarterectomy, women who got stents were more than twice as likely to have a stroke within 30 days after their surgery.

Bottom line: If your doctor recommends carotid artery stenting rather than endarterectomy, be sure to discuss the gender-based differences in stroke risk found in this study.

Breakthroughs in Stroke Recovery

Murray Flaster, MD, PhD, an associate professor of neurology and neurological surgery and director of Loyola Outpatient Clinics at Loyola University Chicago Stritch School of Medicine, where he specializes in vascular neurology and neurological intensive care.

Physician scientists have now discovered that a series of surprisingly simple treatments—performed in the first 24 to 48 hours after a stroke—can prevent additional brain damage and help reduce the risk for disability and complications, including cognitive impairments.

Important: The recommendations described in this article apply only to patients who have had an ischemic stroke (caused by a blood clot). Almost 90% of all strokes are ischemic. Unless it's otherwise noted, these recommendations do not apply to patients who have suffered a hemorrhagic (bleeding) stroke.

Most important treatments following stroke…

• **Maintain or raise blood pressure.** It sounds counterintuitive because high blood pressure is one of the main risk factors for stroke—and because most stroke patients have a spike in blood pressure of about 20 points. But studies have shown that higher-than-normal blood pressure can help patients recover faster, with less brain damage.

• **Giving blood pressure–lowering drugs in the hospital** can cause a decrease in cerebral perfusion pressure (a measurement of blood flow to the brain) that can increase damage.

Recommended: As a general rule, your blood pressure should not be lowered immediately after a stroke, even if you have existing hypertension. As long as your blood pressure reading is below 220/120 (normal is about 120/80), it should be left alone.

In some patients, particularly those with a blockage in a major blood vessel, it might be advisable to actively raise blood pressure with a vasopressive medication, such as *phenylephrine* (Neo-Synephrine).

Exceptions: Blood pressure may still need to be lowered in patients who have had a hemorrhagic stroke (caused by bleeding in the brain) or in those who are taking clot-dissolving drugs. Raising blood pressure in patients who are actively bleeding or at risk for bleeding can potentially cause more bleeding.

• **Reduce body temperature.** Fever is common in stroke patients due to infection or the stroke itself, with up to 25% having a temperature of 100.4°F or higher within 48 hours after being admitted to the hospital. A fever is dangerous because it increases the metabolic demands of damaged brain tissue—energy that should go toward healing. It also triggers the release of inflammatory substances that can cause additional damage.

Recommended: *Acetaminophen* (Tylenol) and hydration. Cooling blankets may be used for fever above 101°F. An experimental treatment called therapeutic hypothermia involves rapidly lowering body temperature with a cooled saline solution given intravenously.

• **Rehydrate.** Dehydration is common in stroke patients because fever and other complications can reduce the body's fluids. If you've had a stroke and are dehydrated, your risk of forming additional blood clots is increased by fivefold.

Reason: Dehydration reduces the volume of blood in the body. This, in turn, reduces blood pressure and increases the tendency of blood to clot.

Recommended: Intravenous (IV) saline solution for at least 24 to 48 hours.

• **Lower the bed.** When the head of the bed is raised, the increased elevation can decrease cerebral blood flow, particularly when the stroke affects the middle cerebral artery, which is common in ischemic stroke.

Important finding: Studies suggest that lowering the head of the bed from 30 degrees to 15 degrees increases blood flow through the middle cerebral artery by 12%. There's an additional 8% increase when the bed is flat.

The trade-off: Many patients aren't comfortable when the bed is completely flat. They also have more trouble swallowing, which increases the risk that they'll get pneumonia after inhaling (aspirating) foreign material from the mouth. Therefore, the head of the bed should initially be elevated to about 15 degrees. If the patient doesn't improve, the bed can be lowered.

• **Use an insulin drip.** It's common for stroke patients to have high blood sugar because of preexisting diabetes or prediabetes. In addition, the stroke itself can temporarily raise blood sugar (in fact, any major stressor in the body can raise blood glucose levels). High blood sugar, or hyperglycemia, is associated with a 2.7-fold increase in poor outcomes following stroke. Poor outcomes could include language difficulties, paralysis, cognitive impairments, etc.

Recommended: Stroke patients should be tested for hyperglycemia immediately after arriving in the hospital emergency department and then as frequently as needed. If blood sugar is higher than 155 mg/dL, insulin should be administered intravenously.

Important: To help prevent stroke-related complications that are worsened by elevated blood sugar, these patients should not be given saline that contains glucose—even if they could benefit nutritionally from the additional sugar.

• **Give a statin quickly.** Stroke patients routinely have their cholesterol tested in the hospital.

Recommended: There's no need to wait for the results before giving patients a cho-lesterol-lowering statin drug, such as *atorvastatin* (Lipitor) or *pravastatin* (Pravachol).

Reason: Even if your cholesterol is normal, statins reduce the inflammatory brain damage that's caused by stroke. Giving these medications quickly can help patients recover more promptly. Continuing statin therapy (if you have high cholesterol and are already taking a statin) can help prevent a subsequent stroke.

• **Start activity early.** Hospitalized patients who are physically active to any degree—even if it is just sitting up in bed—improve more quickly and have fewer complications than those who are initially immobile.

Other benefits: Physical activity also reduces the risk for pneumonia, deep-vein thrombosis, pulmonary embolism and bedsores.

Recommended: Some form of activity within hours after having a stroke if the patient is neurologically stable. Patients should spend as little time in bed as possible even if their mobility is impaired and to do as much as they can tolerate.

Important: Activity should always be carefully guided by nurses, therapists or other members of the hospital team to avoid injury.

Don't Underestimate the Dangers of "Little" Strokes

Shelagh B. Coutts, MD, associate professor of neurology, department of clinical neurosciences, University of Calgary, Alberta, Canada, and lead author of a study published in *Stroke.*

Imagine being rushed to the ER and diagnosed with a "ministroke." You might be told that your symptoms are mild and short-lived and that you can probably expect to be just fine.

A happy ending? Not necessarily—because a recent study has called into question the common assumption that "little" strokes generally have few or no lasting consequences.

In fact, the researchers found that there is a substantial risk for disability after such an event even for patients who do not go on to have another stroke...and they suggested that doctors might not be giving enough patients the special medication that can prevent such disability.

The info you need to protect yourself...

Small Stroke, Big Deal

First, a little bit of background. Ischemic stroke, the most common type, occurs when a blood clot blocks blood flow to the brain. Symptoms include sudden weakness or numbness on one side of the body, slurred speech, dizziness and vision problems. With a major stroke, if the patient survives, such symptoms can be severe and long-lasting, resulting in permanent disability.

In contrast, with a ministroke or transient ischemic attack (TIA), symptoms typically last only a few minutes and might leave no obvious permanent neurological damage. With a minor stroke, which is worse than a TIA but not as bad as a major stroke, symptoms are mild but persistent.

When a patient suffers a major stroke, medication called tissue plasminogen activator (tPA)—which must be administered within a few hours of symptom onset—can break up the clot, opening the blocked blood vessel and restoring blood flow to the brain, minimizing disability. However, in the case of a TIA or minor stroke, doctors often assume that patients will not suffer permanent problems and thus consider the condition too mild to warrant treatment with tPA or another anticlotting therapy. This is the assumption challenged by the recent study.

Surprising Study Findings

Canadian researchers investigated 499 ER patients who had had a TIA or minor stroke, following their progress for 90 days.

What they discovered: Within three months, 15% of these patients developed some form of physical and/or cognitive disability.

Those are not very good odds!

We talked to the lead researcher, Shelagh Coutts, MD. She said that, while the study patients' disabilities weren't necessarily profound, they were severe enough in some cases to interfere with the ability to drive, work, socialize and handle finances.

Ministroke Self-Defense

If you develop possible symptoms of stroke, no matter how mild or temporary, do not brush them off, Dr. Coutts cautioned. Instead, get to an ER right away. You need to be tested immediately to determine whether there has been any damage to your brain. Testing should include a CT scan...and possibly a CT angiography (CTA), a test in which a contrast dye is administered to show any blood vessel blockages or narrowing from the top of the heart to the top of the brain.

You might also want to ask your doctor whether tPA or some other clot-busting thrombolytic drug is appropriate for you. Ministroke and minor stroke patients most likely to develop disabilities—and thus most likely to benefit from such treatment—include those who...

•**Have blocked or narrowed blood vessels in the brain,** as shown on the CTA.

•**Have ongoing symptoms** (rather than symptoms that disappear after a few minutes).

•**Have diabetes.**

•**Are women**—because, for unknown reasons, females are more likely than males to develop poststroke disabilities.

Why not just give tPA to all stroke patients, no matter how minor their strokes? Because tPA is a powerful and potentially risky drug. It has a chance of causing bleeding in the brain, resulting in a hemorrhagic stroke. Dr. Coutts said, "Studies are now needed to see if the risk/benefit balance is in favor of treatment in these patients. In Canada, we are doing a study treating minor stroke patients with blockages within the brain to determine the safety of thrombolysis."

It is also important to note that tPA is not safe for certain patients, such as those taking *warfarin* (Coumadin) or another anticoagulant...those who recently had a head injury, heart attack or surgery...pregnant women...patients with very high blood pressure...or those with any type of bleeding problem.

Mini-Stroke Increases Risk for Heart Attack

A mini-stroke, or transient-ischemic attack (TIA), occurs when a blood clot temporarily blocks a blood vessel to the brain. Symptoms include sudden weakness or numbness of the face, arm or leg...sudden confusion...trouble seeing...and sudden dizziness. Symptoms generally disappear in 24 hours.

Recent finding: Patients who have suffered a mini-stroke are twice as likely to suffer a heart attack within the next five years.

If you have had a mini-stroke: Reduce your risk for heart attack by maintaining healthy blood pressure and cholesterol levels.

Robert D. Brown, Jr., MD, MPH, chair of neurology, Mayo Medical School, Mayo Clinic, Rochester, Minnesota, and leader of a study of 456 TIA patients, published in *Stroke.*

Medication Is Better Than Stents

Medication is better than stents for preventing second strokes, we hear from Marc I. Chimowitz, MD.

Recent study: Half of 451 people ages 30 to 80 who had suffered an ischemic stroke or a mild stroke known as a transient ischemic attack (TIA) were given brain stents to widen a significantly blocked major artery to the brain and an intensive regimen of medications to fight blood clots, high blood pressure and elevated LDL "bad" cholesterol.

The other half received only the medication regimen. After a year, 20% of the people with stents had had a second stroke or died, compared with 12% of the people treated with medication.

Possible reason: Stenting could loosen unstable plaque in the arteries, triggering subsequent strokes.

Marc I. Chimowitz, MD, professor of neurology, Medical University of South Carolina, Charleston.

Vision Rehab: New Hope for Stroke Patients

Krystel R. Huxlin, PhD, neuroscientist and an associate professor of ophthalmology at the Flaum Eye Institute at the University of Rochester School of Medicine and Dentistry in New York. Her research on visual retraining for stroke patients has been published in *The Journal of Neuroscience.*

When you think of all the devastating consequences of stroke, visual impairment may not be one of the first to come to mind...yet about 20% to 25% of stroke victims are left with vision problems. These visual deficits were once thought to be permanent—but now a promising new therapy is helping train the brain to see better again. And even though the software used for this therapy is not yet commercially available, interested patients may be able to benefit from it by participating in ongoing research studies.

We spoke with neuroscientist Krystel R. Huxlin, PhD, an associate professor of ophthalmology at the Flaum Eye Institute at the University of Rochester School of Medicine and Dentistry, who is the researcher at the forefront of the development of the technique. She explained that stroke patients who suffer damage to a part of the brain called the primary visual cortex typically are blind in one-quarter to one-half of their normal visual field.

Reason: The primary visual cortex acts as a gateway for the transfer of information between the eyes and the other brain areas that process visual information. If that gateway is damaged by stroke, patients may have problems with most everyday activities, including reading, driving and even walking.

How Vision Retraining Works

To address the problem, Dr. Huxlin explained, her team first runs tests to map a patient's blind field and understand his or her exact visual impairments. Then, the visual retraining software is customized to address that patient's needs.

On a home computer, the patient uses the specialized software to do targeted visual exercises for about an hour at least five days per week. Dr. Huxlin's patients train for a minimum of three months—and most choose to continue much longer because their blind field continues to shrink and results are so rewarding.

During each training session, the patient fixes her gaze on a small black square in the middle of the screen. Every few seconds, a group of about 100 small dots appears within a circle on the screen that is somewhere in her damaged visual field. The dots appear to move as a group to the left or right, then disappear after half a second. The patient decides which way the dots are moving, indicating her choice with the keyboard. A chime signals whether she has chosen correctly, providing feedback that speeds up learning.

At first, most patients cannot actually see the dots, but nonetheless their brains are able to sense that the dots are moving, Dr. Huxlin said. With practice, a patient's brain eventually recovers the ability to consciously perceive the dots and discern the direction of their movement in the retrained blind field location. Then, the researchers move the dots to another spot in her blind field so the brain can start relearning how to see the new area.

Secret to success: The therapy exploits a phenomenon called blindsight, in which a stroke patient's eyes are able to take in visual information but the damaged brain cannot make sense of it to create conscious vision.

"The training drives whatever spared visual circuitry the person still has, making it work harder, so eventually that visual information is brought into consciousness," said Dr. Huxlin. The 17 patients she has studied so far who trained as prescribed all had significantly improved vision. The improvement seems to be permanent—and some patients have even been able to regain a driver's license.

Who Can Benefit

Visual retraining potentially can benefit patients whose strokes were recent and those whose strokes occurred several years ago, Dr. Huxlin said, provided they are not totally blind. Patients also must be able to complete basic tasks, such as using a computer, fixating points on the screen precisely, pressing keys and following instructions.

Dr. Huxlin's visual retraining software has been licensed by the company EnVision LLC and submitted for FDA approval. It is hoped that the product will be commercially available shortly after FDA approval is obtained. In the meantime, stroke survivors interested in participating in Dr. Huxlin's ongoing research can e-mail her at *huxlin@cvs.rochester.edu* to see if they meet the criteria for study enrollment and, if so, they will be put on a waiting list.

Also helpful: Dr. Huxlin said that, in addition to visual retraining, stroke sufferers can help compensate for vision loss by staying as physically active as possible—for instance, by playing sports such as golf or tennis or by regularly taking walks around the neighborhood or a park. "Those kinds of activities force you to make up for visual deficits by moving your head and eyes more. This pushes your visual system to be more actively engaged—to search for and find the information you need to extract from your environment in order to function," she explained. For patients unable to engage in sports or walk outside, playing action video games would be a reasonable alternative, she added.

Bottom line: For stroke survivors, the future has never looked brighter.

Magnets May Help Stroke Patients

In a procedure called repetitive transcranial magnetic stimulation, electromagnets are strategically placed on a stroke patient's head. The magnets deliver tiny electric currents to the area of the brain affected by the stroke, reducing muscle weakness and improving overall motor function.

Recent finding: Patients given this treatment in addition to physical therapy showed significant improvement in motor function, compared with those who did not receive brain stimulation. Study participants had strokes between one and 36 months before starting this treatment.

Anwar Etribi, PhD, emeritus professor of neurology, Ain Shams University, Cairo, Egypt, and leader of a study published in *European Journal of Neurology.*

When Is It Safe to Drive After a Stroke?

Hannes Devos, PhD, PT, department of rehabilitation science, Catholic University of Leuven, Belgium.

How high on the list of difficult conversations is this one: You're an adult having to tell your mother or father that he/she shouldn't drive anymore...or a spouse having to give your wife or hubby the same message. This is often the case after someone has had a stroke...which doesn't make the conversation (or the decision about whether continued driving is safe) any easier. But there's an interesting recent study that may offer some real practical help in easing you through that tough conversation. Belgian researchers have identified a series of three relatively simple tests—soon to be available in the US. Once that happens, taking them should be quite easy. The estimated time needed is only 15 minutes. The tests can identify who would and who wouldn't be likely to pass a typical driving road test—

a good (but not perfect) indication of who would be a safe driver after a stroke.

Besides sparing you from a wrenching argument with a hurt, defensive and very possibly angry parent or spouse, this might also spare the stroke survivor from having to try to prepare for and get through an official road test—as they may be required to do after a stroke—and ultimately fail it.

How Serious Was the Stroke?

Before we get to these simple new tests, the first thing to know is that for many people, driving is still safe after a stroke—depending, of course, on the amount and type of damage done and the success of rehabilitation therapy.

To find out more, we checked with the lead author of the study, Hannes Devos, PhD, PT, in the department of rehabilitation sciences at the Catholic University of Leuven in Belgium. "Much depends on the area of the brain that's affected," he explained. If the stroke took place in the temporal lobes, which are key to the ability to perceive and understand information, a stroke survivor might see a street sign and be able to read the words...yet not know what they mean. If it's the occipital lobes, which receive and organize input from the eyes, that are affected, then vision might be impaired. And if the stroke occurred in the frontal lobes, where higher organizational function is maintained, then judgment, problem solving ability and motor skills—all obviously vital to safe driving—might be lacking.

Making things even more difficult is the fact that some stroke patients are not aware, or not fully aware, of their deficits, Dr. Devos added. "For example, they may think that nothing serious is wrong with the way their body works even when muscles on one side of the body are barely working at all, so they don't comprehend what's dangerous or what must be avoided," he said. Unfortunately, strokes can be cruel that way...how could all of this—the physical and the psychological—be sorted out in just 15 minutes and tell us who should and who shouldn't be driving?

How the Tests Work

Out of the 1,728 people studied, 54% passed their road tests, the best determinants of success being the following three tests…

• **The road sign recognition test.** In this segment, the person being tested is asked to match 12 road signs, where their meaning must be recognized and matched to cards showing particular driving situations—for example, they might have to match a road sign indicating construction ahead with a card "depicting" men repairing a road.

• **The compass test.** This is a test of perception, attention and mental speed that involves placing cards with "vehicles" on them so that the vehicles are lined up properly according to the directions indicated on a second card—a compass with an arrow showing various directions. This tests the ability to understand directions consistently and under pressure.

• **The trail making test part B (TMT B).** In this segment, participants are asked to quickly connect circles containing numbers or combinations of the numbers one to 12 and the letters A to L, as in 1-A, 2-B, 3-C. What's measured here are visual motor abilities and the ability to shift one's attention.

The tests aren't perfect, but the authors of the study say that they can correctly identify 80% to 85% of those tested who would make unsafe drivers. Importantly, the tests failed to identify 15% to 20% of unsafe drivers—and researchers point out that they may also fail to identify some safe drivers, as well. But post-stroke road tests could make up these gaps.

For families who are sure or fairly sure that driving should no longer be an activity for a loved one, these tests can be a big help in terms of satisfying everyone involved that getting behind the wheel is just no longer a good idea. Dr. Devos says the tests will be available in the US in the very near future and that physicians, neuropsychologists and occupational therapists will be able to help obtain and administer them. Ask your doctor.

The Missing Piece to Stroke Recovery

Michael C. Munin, MD, an associate professor at the University of Pittsburgh School of Medicine and vice-chair for Clinical Program Development in the department of physical medicine and rehabilitation, also at the medical school.

Imagine yourself attempting to open a jar if your hand were bunched in a fist or trying to walk if one of your arms were clenched across your chest.

This type of uncontrollable muscle tightness is a constant challenge for an estimated one million Americans affected by upper limb spasticity. Typically resulting from a stroke, multiple sclerosis, cerebral palsy or an accident that affects the brain or spinal cord, upper limb spasticity most often affects the elbows, wrists and fingers.

Unlike paralysis, which causes loss of muscle function, upper limb spasticity is marked by uncontrollable muscle tightness and/or a lack of muscle inhibition. With upper limb spasticity, a person's elbow might not bend without forcing it down with the other hand, or spasms might cause the arm to recoil as though a spring had been released.

Problem: About 58% of stroke survivors experience upper limb spasticity. Of those, only about half get appropriate treatment—often because the condition develops slowly, and patients assume that it's a complication they have to live with.

Good news: Most people with upper limb spasticity can achieve better muscle control, and even increase their muscle strength, with a combination of medical treatments and specialized physical and/or occupational therapy.

An Undertreated Problem

Upper limb spasticity often goes undiagnosed because it may not develop until weeks, months or even years after a person has a stroke or is diagnosed with a condition that leads to the spasticity.

Best treatment: People with upper limb spasticity have the best chance of regaining mobility and functional ability when therapy combines repetitive task training exercises with injections of botulinum toxin type A (Botox), which was recently approved by the FDA to treat upper limb spasticity. (Botox was approved earlier by the FDA to help remove wrinkles and ease migraine pain.)

Research shows that when used for upper limb spasticity, Botox injections combined with repetitive task training can bring about a 30% improvement, on average, within 12 weeks and, in some cases, an improvement of up to 54%. Benefits typically last about three months. However, patients must have some arm function remaining after a stroke to benefit from the training.

The repetition involved in repetitive task training strengthens the brain's ability to communicate with different muscles. And even though the exercises won't eliminate spasticity, they can make it easier for patients to perform daily tasks, such as cooking meals, buttoning a jacket, even hugging loved ones.

Important: The sooner a person with upper limb spasticity starts the repetitive training, the better—if too much time passes, the muscles atrophy to such an extent that recovery becomes more difficult. Still, it's never too late. What's imperative is to use the affected limb and not ignore it due to disability.

Ideally, patients meet with a physical or occupational therapist at least once a week for about 30 to 60 minutes, often for several months.* Then they practice at home what they've learned.

Important: The goal of therapy is to enable people with upper limb spasticity to do the types of activities that they need to do—for example, watering plants, buttoning clothes, etc.

When starting treatment, it's important to tell the therapist what activities you enjoy most or find most important. You're more

---

*To find an occupational therapist near you, contact the American Occupational Therapy Association, Inc., 301-652-6611, *www.aota.org*. To find a physical therapist, consult the American Physical Therapy Association, 800-999-2782, *www.apta.org*.

Gas May Protect the Brain

Animals that inhaled nitric oxide (NO) after a stroke had better brain function than those in a control group. NO improves brain circulation—important because there still isn't an effective single treatment for the majority of stroke patients.

Circulation Research

---

likely to stay motivated and keep practicing when you see a clear benefit. *Repetitive task training may include…*

• **Stretching exercises.** Spasticity often leads to a shortening of tendons and/or ligaments, which interferes with normal motions. Stretching can lengthen these tissues. Someone with hand spasticity might be advised to open the hand and extend the fingers…hold the stretch for several seconds…and then repeat.

• **Putting lids on jars.** There are more steps to this than you might think. The patient has to expand the fingers to grip the lid…grip the jar with the other hand…then contract the fingers to grip the lid and screw it on.

• **Folding laundry.** This uses muscles in the fingers, wrists, elbows, etc. Studies have shown that many patients who couldn't fold laundry are able to do it on their own, comfortably, after a few months of repetitive task training.

Best Medical Treatments

Recent advances are now making upper limb spasticity more treatable than ever before.

Even though oral medications can be given to treat "global" spasticity that affects multiple regions, such as the arm, head and neck, these drugs often cause unwanted sedation even at low doses. Some of these drugs, such as *tizanidine* (Zanaflex), block nerve impulses. Others, such as *baclofen* (Kemstro, Lioresal) and *diazepam* (Valium), act on the central nervous system to relax muscles.

Newest development: The FDA's March 2010 approval of Botox to treat upper limb spasticity is an important development because Botox reduces muscle tension without the systemic side effects of oral drugs. Botox allows doctors to treat smaller muscle groups in specific areas, such as in the fingers or elbows.

How it works: Botox selectively weakens (it doesn't paralyze) affected muscles. An injection of Botox into a hand, for example, can loosen a clenched fist and allow more normal motions. Someone whose left arm is clenched across his/her body can get an injection of Botox to relax the limb and, say, get his arm into a coat sleeve.

An injection usually starts working within three days but could take up to two weeks. It keeps working for three to four months. The main risk—unintended temporary muscle weakening—is rare and can be corrected with future dose adjustments. *Other approaches…*

•**Phenol injections.** For years, doctors have used a type of alcohol known as phenol to reduce muscle contractions and spasms, but phenol is mainly used to block specific nerves that operate large muscle groups. Because it is a nerve block (injected just above the nerve) rather than a muscle weakener (such as Botox), nerves have to be easily accessible, and these typically are the ones that supply the large muscle groups. Unlike Botox, a phenol injection starts working immediately.

The effects of each phenol injection last four to six months. Patients who get a phenol injection may also be treated with a low dose of Botox. The main side effect of phenol is a burning/tingling sensation at the injection site.

•**Orthotic devices are sometimes used to hold limbs in a desired position.** For example, a patient with hand tightness might wear a "resting splint" at night to keep the fingers open and straight. This may also improve the patient's muscle function during the day. Or a splint might be used to keep the ankle from twisting.

Better Stroke Recovery

Forty-eight stroke survivors underwent conventional gait rehabilitation. Half of them also had 20 sessions of electromechanical robotic gait training. With this therapy, an electromechanical device moves a patient's feet and is controlled by a physical therapist who progressively increases the patient's weight load and walking pace. Among the most severely impaired, five times more patients who received robotic therapy were able to walk unassisted after two years. Robotic therapy made little difference among the less severely impaired.

Giovanni Morone, MD, physiatry specialist, Santa Lucia Foundation, Institute for Research Hospitalization and Health Care, Rome, Italy.

New Types of Surgery

In the past, patients with spasticity often underwent surgery to cut the spinal nerves that caused muscle tightness. This is rarely done anymore.

Now: Surgery is mainly used to lengthen the tendons/ligaments attached to a spastic area. This procedure increases the patient's range of motion.

Surgery also is used to implant a computerized pump that delivers a steady dose of the muscle-relaxing drug baclofen. The pump, which is implanted in the abdomen, can give patients with severe spasticity long-lasting relief. Pump implants are best suited for people who have global spasticity, which covers too many areas to inject. Infection risk is roughly 1%.

Benefit: Because the drug is delivered directly to the spinal area, the required dose can be up to 1,000 times lower than oral medications. This minimizes grogginess and other side effects.

CHRONIC LOWER RESPIRATORY DISEASES

You'd think we could reach gender equality when it comes to breathing, but statistics tell a different story. Women are more likely to be diagnosed with chronic bronchitis than men, and more likely to die from COPD (chronic obstructive pulmonary disorder). For the best ways to keep your lungs healthy, take a deep breath and read on.

According to a study published in *Respirology,* as the rate of tobacco use among men is predicted to decrease, the rate among women is estimated to rise to 20% of the woman population by 2025.

http://www.lung.org/lung-disease/copd/resources/facts-figures/COPD-Fact-Sheet.html

Chapter 14

KEEP YOUR LUNGS
HEALTHY FOR LIFE

How Not to Let Chronic Lung Disease Sneak Up on You

Most people are only vaguely aware of chronic obstructive pulmonary disease (COPD)—even though the Centers for Disease Control and Prevention reports it's now the third-leading cause of death in American adults, after heart disease and cancer. Deaths due to heart disease and cancer have decreased, but that has not occurred with COPD.

An unexpected threat: Even though current or former smokers are at greatest risk for COPD, as many as one out of six people with the condition never smoked.

Good news: COPD can be managed with early diagnosis and treatment. Even those who have had the condition for years can minimize periodic flare-ups by taking the right medications. *What you need to know about COPD...*

Are You at Risk?

Approximately 80% to 90% of all cases of COPD in the US are caused by smoking—primarily cigarette smoking, but long-term cigar or pipe smoking also increases risk.

Secondhand smoke (known as passive smoking) increases the risk for COPD by 10% to 45%, depending on the level of exposure, according to estimates from The World Health Organization. Increased risk can occur with daily exposure to secondhand smoke when living with a smoker.

People with long-term exposure to severe air pollution (as occurs in some big cities) and those who work or worked in the presence of dust, chemical fumes and/or vapors also are at increased risk for COPD.

In addition, some research shows a link between gastro-esophageal reflux disease (GERD) and COPD. The reflux-causing disorder can worsen COPD or, in rare cases, cause it, though researchers are unsure why.

Diagnosis Can Be Difficult

Shortness of breath, a chronic cough, wheezing and excess sputum production (with or without cough) are the main symptoms of COPD.

Roger S. Goldstein, MD, a professor of medicine and physical therapy at the University of Toronto, Ontario, Canada. A respirologist (specialist in lung function) at West Park Healthcare Centre in Toronto, he is also chair of respiratory rehabilitation research at the National Sanitarium Association and past chair of the Canadian Thoracic Society section on COPD rehabilitation.

However, most people with early-stage COPD don't even know that they have it. The symptoms come on so slowly—usually over decades—that people get used to them. They think that it's normal to get short of breath when climbing stairs or to wake up with a mucus-filled cough. Or they attribute the coughing and/or shortness of breath to smoking itself and not to an underlying disease, such as COPD.

Important: The key symptom to watch for is shortness of breath, particularly during exercise or any type of exertion. This often is the first sign of COPD. Other symptoms, such as a chronic cough, usually occur later in the course of the disease.

By the time most people with undiagnosed COPD realize that something's wrong, a significant amount of lung tissue has already been irreversibly damaged.

In the advanced stages of COPD, patients may find that even simple tasks, such as walking to the mailbox or rising from a chair, will leave them short of breath.

Ask for This Test

I suggest that everyone age 45 or older get tested at least once for COPD. Those with COPD risk factors—current or former smokers, for example, or those who are (or have been) exposed to dust/chemicals in the workplace—should be tested annually.

Spirometry is the main test for COPD. It's inexpensive and painless and can be done in the doctor's office in a few minutes. Few doctors routinely test patients with spirometry, but you should insist on it.

What the test involves: You blow into a spirometer, which measures your forced vital capacity (the total amount exhaled) and forced expiratory volume (the amount exhaled in the first second).

A "normal" reading will vary, depending on your age, sex and height. For example, an average, healthy 50-year-old man should be able to exhale about four liters of air in one second. A person with COPD might exhale only about 2.5 liters per second, or less.

Asthma can cause symptoms similar to those caused by COPD. Therefore, if you have asthma, your doctor may have you use an inhaled bronchodilator, then repeat the spirometry test. The spirometry readings will improve immediately in people who have asthma. With COPD, the readings remain the same or improve only slightly.

Insurance typically covers the cost of spirometry.

Best Prevention Strategies

Not smoking is the most important step you can take to protect your lungs. Those at highest risk for COPD have accumulated 20 "pack years"—a measurement calculated by multiplying the number of packs of cigarettes smoked per day by the number of years that you've smoked.

People who quit smoking may regain close to normal lung function if they have very early-stage COPD. Those who quit later can preserve more of their normal lung function and slow the rate at which the disease progresses. Even if you quit smoking years ago, it's possible to have undetected COPD without symptoms.

Since occupational pollutants are the second-leading cause of COPD, people who work in industrial jobs, such as mining or welding, or livestock farming, should always wear the appropriate protective equipment, such as particulate (air-purifying) respirator face masks.

Even in nonwork settings, you should wear a mask if painting, spreading fertilizer or doing any task that may involve dust or fumes.

Caution: Do not wear a mask if you have shortness of breath.

The Right Treatment

If you've already been diagnosed with COPD, your doctor will probably prescribe medications to reduce symptoms—coughing, difficulty breathing, wheezing and/or mucus production—during flare-ups.

Important: Such drugs should be taken at the first signs of a flare-up to minimize lung inflammation and help reduce long-term damage.

An alternative to medication may involve simple breathing exercises and supervised rehabilitation. As the condition progresses, it is customary to use medication and breathing exercises together.

Best COPD medications…

• **Bronchodilators that contain a short-acting beta-agonist,** such as *albuterol* (Proventil) or *tiotropium* (Spiriva), expand and relax muscles around the airways and make it easier to inhale and exhale. Side effects may include vomiting and muscle pain.

• **Inhaled steroids,** such as *fluticasone* (Flovent), reduce inflammation and may improve airflow when used in combination with other medications. Side effects of inhaled steroids may include headache, sore throat and, according to recent research, increased diabetes risk.

During flare-ups, oral steroids may be used for a short course (about 10 days), especially if a bronchodilator alone is not sufficient.

Other treatments…

• **Supplemental oxygen** is sometimes needed to improve breathing and exercise tolerance in those with advanced COPD.

• **Lung volume reduction surgery** may be recommended in rare cases of severe emphysema. It involves removal of the damaged sections of the lungs to allow the remaining lung tissue to work more efficiently. This treatment is effective only when patients have sufficient amounts of healthy lung tissue left after surgery.

Important: If you have COPD, any respiratory illness increases the risk for lung damage and may cause a more rapid decline in lung function. That's why every person with COPD should get an influenza vaccination annually. Your doctor might also recommend a pneumococcal pneumonia vaccination every five years or so.

What Is COPD?

Chronic obstructive pulmonary disease (COPD) is a progressive lung disease that blocks airflow and interferes with a person's ability to breathe. The declining lung function that characterizes COPD is most often caused by emphysema and/or chronic bronchitis.

More than 15 million Americans have been diagnosed with COPD. An additional 12 million may have the disease but not know it.

Vitamin E Prevents COPD (Chronic Obstructive Pulmonary Disease)

Anne Hermetet Agler, Division of Nutritional Sciences, Cornell University, Ithaca, New York.

Chris Burtin, PT, (MSc,), a hospital-based physical therapist in Katholieke Universiteit Leuven, Belgium.

Robert J. Green, ND, naturopathic physician and author of *Natural Therapies for Emphysema and COPD* (Healing Arts Press).

We hear a lot about preventing heart disease, the number-one cause of death in America. And cancer, the number-two cause. And stroke, at number three.

But we rarely hear about preventing the seldom-discussed number-four cause of death in the US—chronic obstructive pulmonary disease (COPD), also known as emphysema and chronic bronchitis, which affects more than 16 million Americans and kills 122,000 yearly.

Now: Results from a recent study provide a nutritional strategy that may help ward off COPD—take vitamin E.

E Is for Easier Breathing

Researchers from Cornell University and Harvard Medical School analyzed data from a seven-year study on nearly 40,000 women aged 45 and older who took either 600 international units (IU) of vitamin E or a placebo every other day.

Results: Those who took the nutrient had a 10% lower risk of developing COPD—even if they smoked, the main risk factor for the disease.

"As lung disease develops, damage occurs to sensitive tissues through several processes, including inflammation and damage from free radicals," says Anne Hermetet Agler, study researcher in the Division of Nutritional Sciences at Cornell University. "Vitamin E may protect the lung against such damage."

"Vitamin E is a powerful antioxidant, which makes it quite useful in counteracting oxidative damage in the lungs," agrees Robert J. Green, ND, a naturopathic physician and author of *Natural Therapies for Emphysema and COPD* (Healing Arts Press).

And Dr. Green says you may want to take vitamin E if you already have COPD.

"Take 400 IU three or four times daily," he advises. "Take it with 50 to 100 milligrams (mg) of vitamin C to enhance absorption. You may need higher doses for therapeutic benefit, but don't exceed 1,600 IU daily without your physician's recommendation and supervision."

Recent Findings

The earliest symptoms of COPD might be a chronic cough and airway-clogging mucus (sputum). Later, you may find yourself unexpectedly short of breath while carrying groceries, climbing stairs or going for a brisk walk. As the disease advances, respiratory difficulties can turn into disasters. Eventually, your best friend could be an oxygen tank.

Good news: Recent research shows there are natural ways to control these and other symptoms of COPD.

•**A more active lifestyle.** In a study reported at an international conference of the American Thoracic Society, researchers found that people with COPD who had a more active lifestyle—more moving around during the day—performed better on a six-minute walk test (the distance they were able to walk in six minutes).

Recommendation: "COPD patients who wish to improve their ability to perform daily tasks may be better served by increasing their normal daily activities, such as walking to the post office, working in the garden, or doing housekeeping, rather than performing intense exercise once in a while," says Chris Burtin, PT, a hospital-based physical therapist in Belgium and the study leader.

"Daily walking is one of the best exercise activities for a person with COPD," adds Dr. Green. "Walking will help build your circulation and increase your stamina, and it will help build activity tolerance. Start out by walking half a block or less. Every other day, you should increase your walking distance a little bit. After a few months, you could be walking up to a mile without gasping."

•**Tai chi.** Researchers at Harvard Medical School studied 10 people with COPD, dividing them into two groups.

Five people took a twice-weekly, one-hour class in tai chi (gentle, meditative exercises that use flowing, circular movements, and balance and breathing techniques). Five didn't.

After 12 weeks, those taking tai chi had improvements in breathing capacity, walking distance and depression compared with those who didn't take the classes.

Recommendation: "Tai chi may be a suitable exercise option for patients with COPD," wrote the Harvard researchers in the journal *Respiratory Care*.

Resource: To find an accredited tai chi teacher near you, visit the Web site www.taichichih.org, and click on "find a teacher."

•**Singing.** "Despite optimal pharmacological therapy and pulmonary rehabilitation, patients with COPD continue to be breathless," noted a team of UK researchers in the journal *BMC Pulmonary Medicine*. "There is a need to develop additional strategies to alleviate symptoms. Learning to sing requires control of breathing and posture, and might have benefits that translate into daily life."

To test their theory, the researchers studied 28 people with COPD—half took twice-weekly singing classes and half didn't.

Results: After six weeks, those taking the classes had better physical functioning and less anxiety about breathlessness, compared with the non-singers.

"Singing classes can improve quality-of-life measures and anxiety, and are viewed as a very positive experience by patients with respiratory disease," concluded the researchers.

Resources: *Ways to learn to sing include…*

•***www.takelessons.com,*** a Web site that connects you to singing teachers in any one of 2,800 cites across the US. 800-252-1508.

•***www.singingvoicelessons.com,*** a Web site that offers the Singing Voice Lessons Series on CD, from voice coach Shelley Kristen.

•***www.easysinginglessons.com,*** a Web site providing downloadable "Singing Is Easy" lessons.

•***Singing for the Stars: A Complete Program for Training Your Voice*** (Alfred Publishing) by Seth Riggs, a book and 2-CD set.

•***Singing for Dummies*** (for Dummies), a book by Pamela S. Phillips.

Herbal Paste Applied in Summer Eases Breathing in Winter

Yongjun Bian, MD, clinical researcher in the respiratory department of Guang'anmen Hospital in Beijing, China, and a research fellow for a study of 125 COPD patients.

For people with chronic obstructive pulmonary disease (COPD), an incurable condition characterized by chronic bronchitis and/or emphysema, winter often brings a worsening of symptoms such as coughing, wheezing, shortness of breath, fatigue and recurrent respiratory infections. Steroids help control symptoms but can have side effects… antibiotics fight infection but increase the risk for antibiotic resistance. So it was welcome news when a recent study provided scientific evidence of the effectiveness of a

Better Lungs Means Better Brain Health

When researchers tracked health data of 832 adults (ages 50 to 85) for nearly two decades, they found that reduced lung (pulmonary) function led to cognitive decline not only in people with chronic obstructive pulmonary disease (COPD) but also in healthy adults.

Theory: Poor lung function reduces oxygen in the blood, which could slow signals between brain cells.

Self-defense: Keep lungs healthy by not smoking, getting regular exercise, eating a healthful diet and avoiding environmental pollutants, including secondhand smoke.

Charles Emery, PhD, professor of psychology, The Ohio State University, Columbus.

topical herbal remedy called Xiao Chuan paste (XCP), which has been used in China for more than 1,000 years to treat COPD and other breathing problems.

Researchers randomly assigned COPD patients to receive either XCP or a placebo paste. As is traditional, the paste was applied to three specific pairs of acupuncture points on the back…the treatment was given four times during an eight-week period in July and August. Then participants were monitored from November through February.

Results: Compared with patients who received the placebo, those who received XCP were significantly less likely to experience an exacerbation of symptoms requiring steroids, antibiotics and/or hospitalization…and they reported a significantly higher quality of life. The only side effect—a mild skin reaction that cleared up without treatment once XCP was discontinued—occurred in just 2% of users.

XCP is made from herbs native to China, including Asarum heterotropoides, Ephedra vulgaris and Acorus gramineus Soland. Researchers theorize that the herbs have properties that affect immune regulation.

You can learn more about XCP by consulting a practitioner of traditional Chinese medicine who is knowledgeable about herbal therapies.

Referrals: National Certification Commission for Acupuncture and Oriental Medicine (*www.nccaom.org*) or American Association of Acupuncture and Oriental Medicine (*www.aaaomonline.org*).

The Supplement for Healthy Lungs—NAC

Richard Firshein, DO, founder and director of The Firshein Center for Comprehensive Medicine in New York City. *www.FirsheinCenter.com*

You know all about the benefits of fish oil...and magnesium...and vitamin D. But here's a supplement that far fewer people are taking—but many could benefit from. It's called n-acetylcysteine (NAC)—and it's especially helpful during cold and flu season since it can combat respiratory ailments. But wait, there's more. NAC also can ease lung and liver problems. To get this amazing remedy on your radar, we turned to Richard Firshein, DO, director of The Firshein Center for Comprehensive Medicine in New York City, and asked him why he recommends NAC to so many of his patients. *Here's what he told us...*

Why It's So Powerful

NAC is an amino acid—and a building block of glutathione, one of the most powerful antioxidants in the body. It helps the body combat damaging free radicals and stimulates other antioxidants in the body to do their beneficial work. In addition, NAC has many uses in the body. *Specifically, it can help you...*

•**Fight colds and flu.** NAC is a remedy often recommended by holistic doctors to prevent—and reduce symptoms of—the flu. A well-known Italian study published in *European Respiratory Journal* found that only 25% of people who took NAC and were injected with a flu virus developed flu symptoms compared with 79% who received a placebo. You also can consider taking NAC when you notice the first signs of a cold.

•**Protect your lungs.** NAC protects the lungs by helping to make glutathione in the lining of the lungs. NAC also can act as a buffer against pollution. When you have a cold, taking NAC can protect your lungs from complications such as bronchitis. In people who have chronic obstructive pulmonary diseases such as emphysema, NAC can help reduce the buildup of mucus and congestion which, in turn, can help relieve the chronic cough that often accompanies emphysema. NAC also is recommended for people with pulmonary fibrosis, since it may slow the disease.

•**Detox the liver.** NAC is known to help cleanse the liver—it helps people whose livers are damaged either because of alcoholism or elevated liver enzymes. Elevated liver enzymes can occur in people who have hepatitis or heart failure or who are obese.

Using NAC

NAC is found in small amounts in some protein-rich foods such as pork, poultry and yogurt. But to really get its health benefits, you have to take it as a supplement. NAC is available at most health-food stores and drugstores.

Dr. Firshein usually recommends that his patients take between 500 mg and 1,000 mg daily of NAC to fight the common cold or flu...protect lungs...and detox the liver. Since every patient is different, it's important to check with your own holistic doctor about the amount of NAC that's right for you. This is especially important for patients with liver or lung diseases.

There are no side effects associated with NAC, although higher doses can cause digestive upset. People with heart or kidney disease should speak to their doctors first before taking NAC.

NAC can be taken on its own, but it's best to take it with other antioxidants, such as vitamin C, since NAC works better in conjunction with other antioxidants. The detoxification process may create toxic by-products that linger in the body. If there's a lot of toxicity, the other antioxidant can lend a hand clearing out the excess toxins.

Better Emphysema Screening

Computed tomography (CT) scans are used to screen for emphysema, a progressive lung disease that enlarges the lung's air sacs, impairing oxygen delivery. In a study of eight nonsmokers and 11 smokers who did not have emphysema symptoms, such as shortness of breath and chronic cough, the patients inhaled "hyperpolarized" helium, a gas used with a new MRI technique that makes the lung sacs easier to view.

Result: The new technique detected signs of emphysema in smokers who were otherwise healthy, while the CT scans did not. To find a medical center that performs this test, contact the International Society for Magnetic Resonance in Medicine, *www.ismrm.org.*

Sean B. Fain, PhD, assistant professor of medical physics and radiology, University of Wisconsin, Madison.

Breakthrough Treatment for Sinus and Lung Problems

Mark A. Stengler, ND, naturopathic physician in private practice Encinitas, California…adjunct associate clinical professor at the National College of Natural Medicine, Portland, Oregon…author of many books, including *The Natural Physician's Healing Therapies* and coauthor of *Prescription for Natural Cures* (both from Bottom Line Books).

I have developed a special treatment for patients with sinus and/or lung problems, including acute sinusitis…asthma flare-ups…and chronic obstructive pulmonary disease (COPD), a condition in which patients have trouble breathing. This incredibly effective treatment involves three natural substances in liquid form administered through a nebulizer, a small machine that transforms liquid medications into mists that can be inhaled through a mouthpiece or mask. *The treatment includes the following…*

•**Glutathione.** This potent antioxidant appears to reduce inflammation of the lungs.

•**N-acetylcysteine (NAC).** This antioxidant thins mucus and stimulates the immune system. It has long been used to treat chronic bronchitis and emphysema. Many doctors know it best as *acetylcysteine* (Mucomyst).

•**Glycyrrhizin.** This is the sweet-tasting compound extract from licorice root. It has anti-inflammatory effects on the respiratory tract.

I first provide patients with this 15-minute treatment in the office to make sure that they can tolerate it, although I've never known anyone to have an allergic or negative reaction to it. If a patient requires further treatments, we send him/her home with vials of the solution and a nebulizer. With reduced dosage, this nebulization therapy also is gentle enough to use with children.

If you are interested in this treatment, your doctor can order these nutrients from a compounding pharmacy. (Because it's prepared in a sterile liquefied solution and tested for microbes, you cannot assemble this treatment on your own.) The solution consists of glutathione (100 mg), N-acetylcysteine (100 mg) and glycyrrhizin (4 mg). One nebulized treatment consists of 2 milliliters (ml) of the nutrient solution combined with 2 ml of distilled water. This nutrient solution can be ordered by your doctor from Downing Labs, LLC. (800-914-7435, *www.downinglabs.com*). Nebulizers can be purchased online or at drugstores for about $40 to $60.

America's Top Lung Centers

John Connolly, EdD, president and CEO of Castle Connolly Medical Ltd., a consumer health research and information company in New York City, and editor and publisher of *America's Top Doctors* (Castle Connolly, *www.castleconnolly.com*). Castle Connolly's physician-led research team has extensive knowledge of the nation's leading medical centers and specialty hospitals.

More than 35 million Americans live with some form of chronic lung disease—asthma, bronchitis or emphysema. Each year, nearly 342,000 Americans die of lung disease, making it the third leading cause of death (following heart disease and cancer).

In the US, there are dozens of specialized lung centers. People who are treated at one of these facilities have the best possible odds of recovering from a serious lung or breathing disorder.

The following lung centers are among the finest in the US. These centers have the greatest number of pulmonary specialists listed in America's Top Doctors (a compilation of the top 1% of US physicians, as rated by their peers) and score high in other well-regarded, independent rankings by related professional organizations and publications. All of the following lung centers also have outstanding lung transplant facilities.

Northeast

•**Brigham and Women's Hospital (Boston).** Surgeons here performed the nation's first triple-organ (two lungs and a heart) transplant in 1995. Cutting-edge care for asthma, lung cancer and chronic obstructive pulmonary disease (COPD), a group of disorders including chronic bronchitis and emphysema. 617-732-5500, *www.brighamand womens.org*

•**Hospital of the University of Pennsylvania (Philadelphia).** Offers an internationally recognized center for the diagnosis and treatment of rare lung diseases. 800-789-7366, *www.pennmedicine.org*

•**Johns Hopkins Hospital (Baltimore).** World-renowned sleep disorders center offers comprehensive testing services for sleep-related respiratory conditions, such as narcolepsy. Also known for its aggressive approach to treating lung cancer. 410-955-5000, *www.hopkinsmedicine.org*

•**Massachusetts General Hospital (Boston).** Noted for asthma diagnosis and treatment. Patients throughout the region are referred to its Pulmonary Vascular Disease Program for pulmonary hypertension (a rare blood vessel disorder of the lungs in which the pressure in the pulmonary artery rises above normal levels). 617-726-2000, *www. massgeneral.org*

•**New York Presbyterian Hospital-Cornell/Columbia (New York City).** Leader in diagnosing and treating asthma. Its Cardiopulmonary Sleep and Ventilatory Disorders Lab provides care for a wide range of sleep disorders related to respiratory conditions. 212-305-2500, *www.nyp.org*

•**University of Pittsburgh Medical Center (Pittsburgh).** Noted for its state-of-the-art Center for Interstitial Lung Diseases (lung disorders caused by inflammation and scarring of the air sacs and their supporting structures). 412-802-3275, *www.upmc.com*

Southeast

•**Duke University Medical Center (Durham, North Carolina).** Known for its interventional pulmonology program, which treats lung cancer and benign airway disorders, such as asthma. 919-416-3853, *http:// pulmonary.duke.edu*

•**Medical University of South Carolina Hospitals (Charleston, South Carolina).** Leader in diagnosing and managing acute and chronic diseases of the chest and allergic diseases. 843-792-3161, *www.musc.edu/pul monary*

•**Shands Healthcare at University of Florida (Gainesville).** Pulmonary specialists offer a wide range of outpatient and inpatient services, including cutting-edge cancer treatments. 855-483-4325, *www.ufhealth.org*

•**University of Alabama Hospital at Birmingham (Birmingham, Alabama).** Highly regarded Pediatric Pulmonary Center offers comprehensive care for children and adolescents with chronic lung disease. 205-939-9583, *http://www.uab.edu/medicine/peds/ppc*

•**University of North Carolina Hospitals (Chapel Hill, North Carolina).** One of the largest clinical cystic fibrosis programs in the country, with more than 500 patients in its pediatric and adult programs. 919-966-6838, *www.med.unc.edu/pulmonary*

•**Vanderbilt University Medical Center (Nashville).** Known for its specialized clinics for lung cancer, adult cystic fibrosis, allergic disorders and pulmonary hypertension. 615-322-2386, *http://medicine.mc.vanderbilt.edu*

Midwest

•**Barnes-Jewish Hospital (St. Louis).** Pioneered lung volume reduction surgery, which removes lung tissue damaged by emphysema. 314-867-3627, *www.barnesjewish.org*

•**Cleveland Clinic Foundation (Cleveland).** Noted for its Sarcoidosis Center of Excellence, and cutting-edge asthma care and research. 866-320-4573, *http://my.clevelandclinic.org/lungs-breathing-allergy*

•**Mayo Clinic (Rochester, Minnesota).** A world leader in lung transplants, and COPD and lung cancer treatment. Surgeons perform more than 1,000 lung cancer surgeries annually. Access to clinical trials of experimental therapies offered for lung cancer. 507-538-3270, *www.mayoclinic.org*

•**University of Chicago Hospitals (Chicago).** One of a handful of US centers with a dedicated interstitial lung disease program. Leader in diagnosing and treating asthma and pediatric lung disease. 888-824-0200, *www.uchospitals.edu/specialties/pulmonary*

•**University of Michigan Health System (Ann Arbor, Michigan).** Leader in diagnosing and managing chronic lung disease, including COPD and asthma. 888-287-1084, *www.med.umich.edu*

•**University of Minnesota Medical Center (Minneapolis).** Its Center for Lung Science and Health specializes in COPD, pulmonary fibrosis, pulmonary hypertension and cystic fibrosis. 612-624-0999, *www.med.umn.edu/pacc*

Southwest/Rocky Mountain

•**National Jewish Health (Denver).** The world's only facility dedicated exclusively to respiratory, immune and allergic disorders. 800-222-5864, *www.nationaljewish.org*

•**University Health System–San Antonio (San Antonio, Texas).** Known for excellence in caring for patients with end-stage lung disease, such as emphysema and pulmonary fibrosis. 210-358-2798, *www.universityhealthsystem.com*

•**University of Colorado Hospital (Denver).** Specializes in cancer prevention and early detection, smoking cessation programs, pulmonary rehabilitation and oxygen therapy. 720-848-0000 *www.uch.edu*

West

•**San Francisco General Hospital (San Francisco).** Recognized for clinical care and research of infectious diseases (such as tuberculosis) and asthma. 415-353-2961, *http://sfgh.medicine.ucsf.edu/divisions/pulmonary*

•**Stanford Hospital & Clinics (Stanford, California).** International leader in cardiopulmonary disease, where the world's first heart-lung transplant was performed. Also has new chest clinic for treatment of adults with lung diseases. 650-725-7066, *www.stanfordhospital.com*

•**UCLA Medical Center (Los Angeles).** State-of-the-art center for asthma, chronic and acute bronchitis, interstitial lung disease, pneumonia, pulmonary vascular disease and sleep-disordered breathing. 310-825-8061, *www.lung.med.ucla.edu*

•**UCSD Medical Center (San Diego).** Recognized worldwide as a pioneer in performing pulmonary thromboendarterectomy (PTE), a type of surgery to open an obstructed artery. Leader in treating chronic thromboembolic pulmonary hypertension (a rare outcome from blood clots in the lungs). 855-355-5864 (LUNG), *http://pulmonary.ucsd.edu*

•**UCSF Medical Center (San Francisco).** Noted center of excellence for adult cystic fibrosis and pulmonary hypertension. Also a leader in treating chest-related cancer, including lung cancer and esophageal cancer. 415-353-2961, *http://pulmonary.ucsf.edu/*

•**University of Washington Medical Center (Seattle).** Known for diagnosing and treating rare lung diseases and genetic lung diseases, including inherited interstitial lung disease. 206-598-4615, *www.depts.washington.edu/pulmcc*

Breathe Easier with Acupuncture

Masao Suzuki, LAc, PhD, associate professor in the department of clinical acupuncture and moxibustion at Meiji University of Integrative Medicine and the department of respiratory medicine at the Graduate School of Medicine at Kyoto University, both in Kyoto, Japan, as well as lead author of a study on acupuncture and COPD published in *Archives of Internal Medicine*.

Imagine being so short of breath that you can barely walk half a block without coughing, wheezing, getting tight in the chest or feeling too fatigued to go on. For people with chronic obstructive pulmonary disease (COPD)—a progressive and incurable lung condition characterized by chronic bronchitis and/or emphysema—such symptoms are a sad fact of life, as are recurrent respiratory infections. Steroids help control symptoms but can have side effects…antibiotics fight infection but increase the risk for antibiotic resistance.

So it was welcome news when a recent study from Japan showed that acupuncture helps relieve symptoms and improve quality of life for COPD patients. Women especially should take note because, despite COPD's reputation as a "man's disease," women account for the majority of US cases.

About the study: COPD patients were randomly assigned to one of two groups. Once a week for 12 weeks, one group received acupuncture at the standard "acupoints" traditionally used for lung problems. The other group got sham acupuncture at the same acupoints, performed with blunt needles that appeared to but did not actually enter the skin. All patients continued with their usual medication throughout the study.

Before treatment began, participants rated their degree of breathlessness after a six-minute walk test, using a scale of zero (breathing very well) to 10 (severely breathless). They also rated their typical level of breathlessness during daily activities…and underwent tests to measure blood oxygenation and other indicators of lung function. Tests were repeated at the end of the 12 weeks.

Results: Breathing scores and test results remained essentially the same for COPD patients who got sham acupuncture. But in the real acupuncture group, the average breathlessness score after the six-minute walk improved from 5.5 to 1.9…tests showed significant improvement in lung function…and patients reported markedly better quality of life. There were no significant adverse side effects. Researchers speculated that acupuncture helps relax the muscles involved in breathing.

Interested patients: It is important to note that the study participants received acupuncture as a complement to, not a replacement for, their usual COPD medication. To find a licensed acupuncturist (LAc) in your area, visit the Web site of the National Certification Commission for Acupuncture and Oriental Medicine (*www.nccaom.org*) or the American Association of Acupuncture and Oriental Medicine (*www.aaaomonline.org*).

Lungs Are More Efficient With Rolfing

Rolfing structural integration, a type of hands-on bodywork, is designed to improve posture, alignment, flexibility and movement as well as to ease tension and pain. A side benefit of the therapy is that it becomes easier to breathe—and typically that occurs after the first session.

Rolfing releases areas of restriction in the myofascial tissue, the weblike connective tissue that wraps around muscles, organs and bones. (Think of the thin white film you see just beneath the skin of a chicken breast as you prepare it for cooking.) Using fingers, hands and elbows, a certified Rolfing practitioner applies firm, steady pressure—slower, deeper and sometimes more uncomfortable than, say, a Swedish massage—to this tissue to stretch and loosen it.

Typically there are 10 hour-long sessions in a Rolfing series. Ida Rolf, PhD, who developed the Rolfing technique more than five decades ago, believed that, to prepare the body for this type of intense therapy, it is important to open up the ribcage. So at the initial appointment, the practitioner applies pressure to the front of the chest and the spaces between the ribs. When that first session is over, clients often find that they can take fuller, deeper breaths because their lungs literally have more room to expand.

To find a certified Rolfing practitioner in your area, contact the Rolf Institute of Structural Integration (800-530-8875, *www. Rolf.org*).

Greg Brynelson, RN, registered nurse and certified Rolfing practitioner based in San Francisco. *www. cityrolfer.com*

How to Travel Comfortably With a Chronic Lung Disorder

Marvin C. Cooper, MD, a New York City–based internist and hematologist who specializes in medical issues related to travel. He is an assistant clinical professor of medicine at the New York University School of Medicine, also in New York City. Dr. Cooper has lectured and published extensively on the topic of travel medicine.

The thought of taking a trip may be daunting if you have lung problems. Will I be uncomfortable or get sick during my trip? These common concerns can be easily managed—if you plan properly.*

Helpful: If you have a chronic lung disease or other condition such as diabetes or heart disease, it's useful to wear a medical identification bracelet or necklace when you travel.**

If you have asthma or severe chronic obstructive pulmonary disease (COPD)—obstruction of the airways due to emphysema and/or chronic bronchitis…

• **Be aware of air quality.** Areas that have high levels of air pollution can create breathing difficulties for people with asthma. Anyone with severe COPD should avoid visiting any destination with an altitude that exceeds 7,500 feet to help prevent shortness of breath.

• **Ask your doctor about oxygen.** If you have COPD and are unable to climb one flight of stairs without suffering shortness of breath, you may need oxygen during a flight. When making your reservation, ask the airline to provide in-flight oxygen (you may need a note from your doctor). Call about 48 hours before your flight to confirm that oxygen will be provided. (Airline customers are prohibited from bringing their own on

*To find a doctor near you who specializes in travel medicine, consult the International Society of Travel Medicine (ISTM). Go to the ISTM Web site at *www.istm.org*.

**These products are available at American Medical ID (800-363-5985, *www.americanmedical-id.com*), starting at about $20.

airplanes.) As soon as you are seated, ask for your oxygen—a small tank with a face mask attached—and use it throughout the flight. Don't wait to experience shortness of breath.

Bring inhalers on the plane. If you have asthma, be sure to bring your inhalers and any other asthma medication with you on the airplane or any other form of transportation you may take.

More from Dr. Cooper...

Travel Savvy for Everyone

Some simple strategies can help keep you well (especially if you plan to fly). These steps are useful even if you don't have a chronic medical condition. *For example...*

• **Observe your seatmates.** High efficiency particulate air (HEPA) filters on airplanes are costly to run, so they typically are not turned on until an airplane has reached a cruising altitude. Even with air filtration, if your airplane seatmate is coughing, sneezing or showing other signs of illness and the flight isn't full, ask the flight attendant to give you a new seat.

• **Drink water and try nasal gel.** The dry air on airplanes often makes people feel dehydrated because the mucous membranes become dry, scratchy and irritated.

Helpful: Drink a glass of water every hour, and consider putting a dab of Ayr Saline Nasal Gel or Rhinaris Saline Nasal Gel (found at drugstores) just inside your nostrils every few hours to help reduce discomfort.

• **Always carry hand cleaners.** Use an alcohol-based hand sanitizer when you're away from a sink.

• **Get up-to-date information on vaccines.** Don't rely on travel agents. Their information is frequently inaccurate or out of date. Instead, ask your doctor and/or check the recommendations at the Web site of the Centers for Disease Control and Prevention, *wwwn.cdc.gov/travel.*

• **Don't count on traveler's insurance.** These policies often have loopholes that exclude the very medical emergencies most likely to arise if you have a preexisting condition. Before buying such a policy, read every clause carefully.

Which Exercises Are Best if You Have Lung Problems?

John P. Porcari, PhD, program director of the Clinical Exercise Physiology (CEP) program at the University of Wisconsin–La Crosse. A past president of the American Association of Cardiovascular and Pulmonary Rehabilitation, he has authored or coauthored more than 350 abstracts and 150 papers on exercise physiology.

Everyone agrees that exercise is good for you. The goal for most people should be at least 150 minutes of moderate aerobic activity a week, plus strength training two days a week, according to the Centers for Disease Control and Prevention.

But what if you have a chronic condition, such as lung disease, that makes exercise difficult—or raises your concern about injury?

While exercise is helpful for most chronic health problems, some activities are likely to be easier, more beneficial and less risky than others.* *Best workouts if you have lung disease...*

• **If you have chronic obstructive pulmonary disease (COPD),** exercise doesn't improve lung function, but it does build muscle endurance and improve one's tolerance for the shortness of breath that often accompanies COPD (a condition that typically includes chronic bronchitis and/or emphysema).

• **Aerobic exercises that work the lower body (like walking or stationary cycling) are good,** but the Schwinn Airdyne or NuStep provides a lower- and upper-body workout with the option of stopping the

---

*Always talk to your doctor before starting a new exercise program. If you have a chronic illness, it may be useful to consult a physical therapist for advice on exercise dos and don'ts for your particular situation.

upper-body workout if breathing becomes more difficult.

•**Asthma,** one of the most common lung diseases in the US, generally does not interfere with exercise unless you are performing an activity that's especially strenuous such as running, which can trigger an attack ("exercise-induced asthma").

With exercise-induced asthma, the triggers vary from person to person. For example, working out in the cold is generally to be avoided (but a face mask or scarf may warm air sufficiently). Very vigorous exercise, such as squash or mountain biking, can cause difficulties for some people with asthma, who may do better alternating brief periods of intense and slower-paced activity (as used in interval training). Know your own triggers.

•**Swimming is also a good choice**—the high humidity helps prevent drying of the airways, which can trigger an asthma attack.

If you use an inhaler such as albuterol to treat an asthma attack: Ask your doctor about taking a dose immediately before you exercise to help prevent an attack, and always carry your inhaler with you throughout the activity.

Natural Help for Asthma

Mark A. Stengler, ND, naturopathic physician in private practice, Encinitas, California...adjunct associate clinical professor at the National College of Natural Medicine, Portland, Oregon...author of many books, including *The Natural Physician's Healing Therapies* and coauthor of *Prescription for Natural Cures* (both from Bottom Line Books).

When she spoke, 53-year-old Shelly made a wheezing sound. She'd had chronic asthma since childhood, and several times yearly suffered acute attacks so severe that she could hardly breathe. Her medical doctor prescribed oral steroids to reduce lung inflammation, but since these can have serious side effects—including immune system suppression, weight gain and hair loss—Shelly asked me for a safer alternative.

For some people, asthma attacks are triggered by sensitivities to dairy products, sugar, gluten (in grains) or other foods. However, Shelly had no major food sensitivities. Certain supplements can ease lung inflammation or reduce the airways' reaction to environmental factors, such as pollen and cold air. Shelly was already taking the supplements that I typically recommend for breathing problems—fish oil, magnesium, lycopene (a plant pigment) and quercetin (a plant compound).

Many asthma patients use a nebulizer, a mechanical device that uses pressurized air to turn liquid medication into a fine mist for inhalation, allowing for a more direct healing effect on the lungs. While nebulized steroids are less toxic than oral steroids, they can cause a sore throat and oral yeast infection.

Natural alternative: Nebulized glutathione (an amino acid) eases congestion by thinning mucous secretions so that they drain more easily. Glutathione is an antioxidant (nutrient that neutralizes harmful molecules called free radicals), so it also may reduce lung inflammation.

Taking this therapy a step further, I combine glutathione with N-acetylcysteine (NAC) and licorice root extract. NAC, an antioxidant amino acid-like substance that thins mucus, often is used in nebulized form (prescription drug name Mucomyst) to treat respiratory conditions. Licorice root, an anti-inflammatory, has been used by herbalists for centuries to ease breathing problems. I believe that these three components, used together, produce a synergistic healing effect.

Over the past two years, I have prescribed this nebulized formula for about 30 patients suffering from bronchitis, sinusitis, emphysema (damaged air sacs in the lungs) and/or asthma. None had an adverse or allergic reaction. Most reported significantly easier breathing—and not one developed pneumonia, a common problem among patients with respiratory ailments.

When Shelly first tried this therapy in my clinic, her wheezing lessened after just five minutes. Thereafter, she used this treatment at home once daily—and within four weeks, her chronic asthma symptoms had improved by 90%. Shelly now uses the nebulizer as needed at the first signs of an acute asthma flare-up, and her asthma attacks are milder and far less frequent.

Important: This prescription formula must be prepared at a compounding pharmacy and used under a doctor's care. To order, your doctor can contact Downing Labs LLC (800-914-7435, *www.downinglabs.com*). When properly prepared, this treatment is quite safe—I even administered it to my four-year-old son for sinusitis with excellent results.

How to Survive an Asthma Attack Without an Inhaler

Richard Firshein, DO, board-certified in family medicine and certified medical acupuncturist and founder and director of The Firshein Center for Comprehensive Medicine, New York City. He is author of *Reversing Asthma: Breathe Easier with This Revolutionary New Program* (Warner).

If you have asthma, then you know how scary it can be when you have an attack and have trouble breathing for anywhere from a few minutes to a few days, depending on its severity.

So you're probably careful to keep your rescue inhaler with you at all times—in case of an emergency.

But what happens if an attack starts and you discover that your inhaler is empty or you don't actually have it?

How can you lessen the severity of an asthma attack and/or stop it altogether without your trusty inhaler?

To find out, we spoke with Richard Firshein, DO, director and founder of The Firshein Center for Comprehensive Medicine in New York City and author of *Reversing*

Asthma: Breathe Easier with This Revolutionary New Program. And he had some very interesting advice…

Do You Need to Go to the ER?

First off, quickly determine whether you're in immediate danger, said Dr. Firshein. If you have a peak-flow meter—a device that measures how much air you can expel from your lungs and that many asthmatics keep around the house—use it. If you're less than 25% off your normal mark, go on to the following steps, but if your number is off by more, get to an emergency room, he said, because this indicates that there is a serious problem—one that could be life-threatening, he said. If you don't have a peak-flow meter, then think about your symptoms. For example, if your lips or fingernails turn blue…if you can't stop coughing…if you feel soreness or tightness around the ribs…if you feel like you're having a panic attack…or if you're so exhausted from the effort of breathing that you can't finish a short sentence or stand up, then you need help fast—get to an ER.

How to Breathe Easier

If you're not in immediate danger, try these tricks, below, from Dr. Firshein. Some of these techniques may help within minutes, while others may take a few hours to kick in, but since it's possible for an attack to last for days, try all of them to play it safe. During a typical asthma attack, the airways are constricted, muscles all over your body become tense and your body produces extra mucus—all of those things make it harder to breathe. So Dr. Firshein's advice addresses all of those problems. You know your body best, so if you try all of these tips but your attack still gets worse, go to a hospital.

•**Change your location.** Asthma is typically triggered by an irritant—either an allergen or toxin—that inflames the airways. So remove yourself from the environment that contains the trigger (if you know what it is) as fast as you can. If you're reacting to dust, pets, mold or smoke, for example, get away from it…or at the very least, breathe through a sleeve, a scarf or your jacket collar to reduce your exposure.

• **Tell someone.** Talking to someone may reduce your anxiety, and that's especially helpful, because anxiety can make your asthma attack worse. Also, if your asthma attack becomes more severe later on, you may need a ride to the hospital, so it's always good to keep someone else in the loop.

Also consider taking an over-the-counter decongestant (such as *pseudoephedrine/* Sudafed) and/or an expectorant (such as *guaifenesin/*Mucinex) or a drug that's a combination of the two (*ephedrine/guaifenesin/* Primatene Asthma), because these loosen mucus and make coughs more productive so you can rid your body of more phlegm.

• **Sip hot coffee or nonherbal tea.** Have one or two cups right away (but no more than that in one sitting, or your heart rate might spike too high—this is true among all people, not just asthmatics). Caffeine is metabolized into theophylline, which is also a drug that's used to prevent and treat asthma by relaxing the airways and decreasing the lungs' response to irritants. Getting caffeine from any source (a soda, an energy drink, a supplement, etc.) will likely help, but tea and coffee have other compounds that act similarly to caffeine (plus, liquids—especially hot liquids—help loosen mucus), so getting your caffeine in this form is best.

• **Practice breathing exercises.** Many people panic when they have an asthma attack and start breathing quickly, but that only restricts the amount of oxygen that the lungs get—in other words, it makes the attack worse. So breathe in through your nose to the count of four and then out to the count of six. Pursing your lips as you exhale will help slow the exhalation and keep the airways open longer. Continue breathing this way for as long as you need.

• **Press on some acupressure points.** The front parts of your inner shoulders (just above the armpits) and the outer edges of the creases of your elbows (when your elbows

are bent) are "lung points." Pressing on one area at a time for a few consecutive minutes may relax muscles that have tightened up.

• **Steam things up.** Take a hot shower or stay in the bathroom with the hot water running from the showerhead or tub or sink faucet. Steam or warm moisture is better than cold moisture because it loosens mucus, so using a cool-air humidifier, although helpful, is not ideal.

• **Ask your doctor about taking magnesium and vitamin C.** Taking 500 milligrams (mg) of magnesium and 1,000 mg of vitamin C during an asthma attack may help if you're an adult. (Children ages 10 to 17 should take half the doses and children between the ages of five and nine should take one-third of the doses.) Magnesium is a bronchodilator that relaxes the breathing tubes, and vitamin C has a slight antihistamine effect.

• **Take medications.** The prescription corticosteroid *prednisone*, available in pill form, is used only for acute problems, such as during an attack, because it helps reduce inflammation—so if your doctor has already prescribed it to you and you have it on hand, use it. "This medication will not work as quickly as an inhaler, but it may prevent the problem from getting out of hand if you're having a lengthy attack," said Dr. Firshein. Just call your doctor and let him or her know that you're taking it, so your doctor can supervise your dosing.

Surgical Cure for Asthma

Sumita B. Khatri, MD, MS, codirector, Asthma Center, The Respiratory Institute, Cleveland Clinic Foundation, Cleveland, Ohio.

A recently developed surgical procedure may be life-changing—even potentially life-saving—for people with chronic asthma who haven't been able to get relief from the standard treatments.

Called bronchial thermoplasty, the procedure was approved by the FDA in 2010. It is worth exploring as a treatment if you or someone you are close to is suffering recurrent asthma attacks that have not been helped by traditional treatments. Thus far, the evidence suggests that this procedure, the first nondrug treatment for asthma, dramatically reduces the occurrence of asthma attacks and improves asthma-related quality of life.

It's estimated that more than 25 million Americans (including seven million children) suffer from asthma, a chronic disease that inflames and narrows airways. Some individuals are born with a predisposition to asthma due to allergies or develop it from exposure to secondhand smoke, while in others the causes may be more unpredictable, such as viral illnesses.

In people with asthma, the layer of smooth muscle that surrounds the airways becomes thicker and more reactive to certain triggers, explained Sumita B. Khatri, MD, codirector of the Asthma Center at the Cleveland Clinic's Respiratory Institute. When a person with asthma has an attack, the muscles around the airways constrict and go into spasms, narrowing the airways and leading to shortness of breath, tightness in the chest and other distressing symptoms.

Reduces Swelling in Airways

In contrast to asthma medications that target inflammation and may secondarily reduce some of the muscle thickening, bronchial thermoplasty treats the airways directly with heat created by radio-frequency waves.

The treatment is apparently quite effective. A randomized, double-blind controlled study of about 300 patients found that those who underwent bronchial thermoplasty experienced vastly improved asthma-related quality of life in the 12 months afterward, including…

•**32% reduction in asthma attacks, on average.**

•**84% drop in visits to hospital emergency rooms.**

•**66% reduction in lost work or school days.**

•**73% decline in hospitalizations for respiratory problems.**

Dr. Khatri said that two years after the first clinical trials, the improvements are still in place—including not only a reduction in symptoms overall but also in the frequency of severe asthma flare-ups and hospitalizations. Many patients also have reduced their need for rescue/emergency medications as well, she said.

Treatments Aren't Painful

Bronchial thermoplasty takes place over three one-hour sessions scheduled three weeks apart. In each procedure, the patient receives light sedation—many actually fall asleep. Each of the three treatments targets a different area of the lungs—in the first session, the airways of the right lower lobe…in the second, the left lower lobe…and in the third, the airways in both upper lobes.

What's involved: The pulmonologist threads a long, flexible tube called a bronchoscope down the mouth or through the nose and into an airway in the lung. Inside the bronchoscope, a special thermoplasty catheter contains electrodes that are heated with radio-frequency energy. This shrinks the muscle, which is believed to prevent the extreme airway muscle contractions during asthma attacks. "This result is expected to be permanent, but there is still not enough data yet to know for sure," Dr. Khatri said.

There are no pain-sensing nerves in the airways, so the application of thermal energy does not hurt, notes Dr. Khatri. Patients are monitored for several hours afterward because symptoms sometimes worsen in the short term. To reduce the likelihood that this will happen, patients take a five-day course of steroids before and after surgery. Though bronchial thermoplasty often is done as an outpatient procedure, Dr. Khatri said that the Cleveland Clinic keeps patients overnight as an added safety precaution. She added that in the immediate post-procedure period,

Asthma and Apnea Danger

Did you know that thunderstorms worsen asthma and sleep apnea? The storms' winds cause pollen to rupture into fragments that can get into the lungs easily, worsening asthma. Falling atmospheric pressure can cause soft tissue in the back of the throat to relax and block the flow of air, increasing the number of apnea events.

Harvard Health Letter, 10 Shattuck St., Boston 02115. www.health.harvard.edu/health

some patients experience discomfort similar to an asthma flare-up, requiring use of rescue/symptom relieving medications. Also, many patients have a sore throat from the bronchoscope, while other possible transitory side effects are chest discomfort or pain, partial lung collapse (serious but treatable), headaches, anxiety and nausea.

Are You a Candidate?

Bronchial thermoplasty is FDA-approved only for people age 18 and older with severe ongoing symptoms from asthma that are not well-controlled with regular asthma medications. It can't be performed on smokers, people with active respiratory infections or people who have heart arrhythmias or have implanted pacemakers, defibrillators or other electronic devices.

Bronchial thermoplasty is expensive—as much as $15,000 or more—but Medicare and some private insurers may cover it.

Asthma Can Come Late in Life

Shortness of breath is not a symptom of aging. Asthma in older patients often is assumed to be bronchitis or emphysema, but at least 40% of patients have their first asthma attack at age 40 or older. Older adults are the only age group in which asthma is getting worse—60% of asthma deaths occur in people age 65 or older.

Self-defense: If you have shortness of breath, get tested for asthma.

Raymond Slavin, MD, allergist and professor of internal medicine, Saint Louis University School of Medicine, and author of a summary of allergic rhinitis, published in *Allergy and Asthma Proceedings*.

Sleep Apnea Solutions— No More Snoring and Snorting

Mark Stengler, NMD, licensed naturopathic medical doctor, founder and medical director of the Stengler Center for Integrative Medicine, Encinitas, California, and associate clinical professor at the National College of Naturopathic Medicine, Portland, Oregon.

Chris Meletis, ND, former chief medical officer for the National College of Naturopathic Medicine and currently the executive director of the Institute for Healthy Aging and a physician on the staff of Beaverton Naturopathic Medicine in Oregon. He is author of 18 books on health and healing, including *The Hyaluronic Acid Miracle* (Freedom Press). *www.DrMeletis.com*

Does your family say you snore so loudly that no one else can sleep? Are you tired despite spending eight hours in bed each night? These complaints come from exhausted patients (or their exasperated spouses). Many of these patients have high blood pressure and/or are overweight, but some are slim and otherwise in good health. Usually they have no idea what is wrong.

In such cases, sleep apnea is usually the cause, a sleep disorder in which a slumbering person's breathing repeatedly stops. It affects up to 24% of adults and 5% of children. Women have apnea half as often as men—until menopause, when women's risk rises (perhaps due to hormonal changes and/or midlife weight gain) to equal men's. Risk rises with age. Untreated, sleep apnea can lead to cardiovascular disease and other serious health problems.

Causes and Concerns

Sleep apnea develops when muscles in the back of the throat, which normally support the soft palate and uvula (a triangular piece of tissue hanging from the soft palate), become flaccid, blocking airflow into the throat. Snoring is produced as the soft palate vibrates. The tongue may slip back, compounding the problem. Throat muscles also may relax, narrowing the breathing passage.

Result: Breathing stops for about 30 to 90 seconds.

Each time this happens, the brain sends out an urgent signal—"Wake up and breathe!" The person does not actually wake up but experiences a partial arousal that prevents deep, restorative sleep. With each arousal, the person gasps and snores as breathing resumes. This happens hundreds of times per night, leading to chronic exhaustion.

Sleep apnea is more than an annoyance—it is dangerous. My colleague Bradley Schnierow, MD, director of the Sleep Disorders Program at the University of California, San Diego, explains that when the body is deprived of oxygen, it triggers a surge in adrenaline. With apnea, this happens many times a night, night after night, sometimes for decades. Repeated adrenaline surges raise blood pressure and limit the oxygen going to the heart—which can eventually trigger a heart attack or stroke. Dr. Schnierow estimates that for about 30% of people with unexplained hypertension, adrenaline surges due to apnea are the cause.

In people with apnea and type 2 diabetes, adrenaline surges make it harder to control blood glucose levels, blood pressure and weight. This increases risk for diabetic coma, kidney disease, atherosclerosis, heart disease and blindness. By raising pressure in the eyes, adrenaline surges can lead to a type of glaucoma (open angle).

People with apnea are chronically sleep deprived, so they are prone to accidents, memory problems and mood swings. In children, apnea can interfere with growth, development and learning, and contribute to behavior problems.

Diagnosis and Treatment

If you suspect sleep apnea, see your doctor. He/she will take a detailed medical history, do a full physical exam and perhaps order an x-ray or magnetic resonance imaging (MRI) scan. If results suggest apnea, you may be referred to a sleep disorder center, where you will spend a night being videotaped... observed by technicians...and monitored by machines that track respiration, blood oxygen, brain waves, eye movements and muscle tone. Although painless, this testing involves having numerous electrodes attached to your body. It usually is covered by health insurance.

There are several downsides to a study in a sleep center...

• **It's expensive,** costing $1,500 to $2,500—which could be out-of-pocket if your insurance has a high deductible.

• **It's inconvenient.** You're spending the night in a strange place with a video camera focused on you and personnel walking in and out.

Instead, you can try a sleep study at home. Using a portable device, it provides the same information as a study at a center—for a fraction of the cost ($450 to $650—check if your insurance covers it). It is becoming the preferred method of testing for many doctors. One brand is the home test by SleepQuest.

For more information: 800-813-8358, *www.SleepQuest.com.*

My advice when the diagnosis is mild apnea...

• **Get blood tests for food allergies.** Food sensitivities may increase production of airway-clogging mucus and trigger respiratory tract inflammation.

Self-care strategies...

• **Sleep on your side.** This helps keep airways open.

• **Lose weight, because extra pounds mean extra tissue in the throat.** Just a 10% weight loss can decrease apnea events by 26%. However, thin people and children can have apnea, too.

• **Don't drink alcohol within three hours of going to bed.** It relaxes the airway.

• **Sing some vowels.** In a study by UK researchers, three months of singing lessons helped decrease snoring, which could in turn decrease apnea.

What to do: Sing the long vowel sounds a-a-a-e-e-e, taking two or three seconds to sing each vowel. Do this once or twice every day for five minutes a session.

• **See a chiropractor.** Neck and spine manipulations improve circulation, reducing airway inflammation and promoting proper nerve impulse flow.

• **Have craniosacral therapy.** Gentle manipulation of the skull and facial bones normalizes the flow of fluids that lubricate the brain and spinal cord, easing sinus and airway inflammation. To find a practitioner, contact the Cranial Academy (317-581-0411, *www.cranialacademy.org*).

• **Get a mandibular advancement device (MAD).** This oral appliance, which resembles a sports mouth guard, brings the jaw forward to open up the back of the throat. About 70% of people who try a MAD like it. A dentist can provide a MAD for about $1,000 (usually not covered by insurance).

For severe apnea, treatment usually involves nightly use of a continuous positive airway pressure (CPAP) machine. This device—a face mask and flexible tube attached to an air pump—provides constant air pressure to keep the airway open. If you have been reluctant to try CPAP or used it years ago and found it uncomfortable, try it now. Today's equipment has a narrower tube and smaller, more comfortable mask (see *www.cpap.com*). Insurance generally covers it.

Occasionally surgery may be warranted. Apnea is now the most common reason for removing tonsils and adenoids. Dr. Mark Stengler (NMD) is reluctant to recommend this, because he feels it reduces immunity to sore throats, but in some apnea cases it may be helpful.

A "last resort" surgical procedure is uvu-lopalato-pharyngoplasty (UPPP), in which a surgeon pares down tissue from the rear of the mouth and top of the throat. This requires general anesthesia and several weeks of recovery. While UPPP helps patients initially, after a few years the buildup of scar tissue may become a significant apnea trigger in itself.

The exciting news is that there's a convenient treatment for sleep apnea called Provent. A small, disposable patch fits over each nostril. The treatment uses your own breathing to create expiratory positive airway pressure (EPAP)—just enough to keep the throat open.

Recent scientific evidence: In a three-month study involving 250 people with sleep apnea, 127 used Provent and 123 used a fake, look-alike device. The people using Provent had a 43% decrease in nighttime apnea events, compared with a 10% decrease for those in the fake group. Over three months, there was also a significant decrease in daytime sleepiness among Provent users.

A 30-day supply of the patches costs about $70. They are prescription-only and currently are not covered by insurance or Medicare.

Expert perspective: Provent is an excellent new option for many people with obstructive sleep apnea, but it is not for mouth breathers, people with nasal allergies or those with severe apnea.

Information: 919-870-8600 ext. 500, *http://Provent.ActiveHealthCare.com*.

Customized Mouth Guard

If the nasal patch is not an option for you, a customized oral appliance may be best. It moves the lower jaw forward, opening the throat. It usually is covered by insurance, either partially or totally.

Dr. Meletis was diagnosed with severe obstructive sleep apnea six years ago—and had very good results with a customized oral appliance. In a recent sleep test, he used CPAP half the night and his oral appliance the other half—his blood oxygen levels were higher while using the appliance.

Do You Have Sleep Apnea?

Suspect sleep apnea—and seek medical evaluation—if you often feel fatigued and have been told that you snore loudly (to check yourself, put a voice-activated tape recorder at your bedside). *Other factors that suggest apnea include...*

● **Excess pounds.** About 80% of people with apnea are overweight.

● **Neck circumference greater than 17 inches** (for a man) or 16 inches (for a woman)—the extra tissue can compress the airway.

● **Enlarged tonsils and/or adenoids** (shown on diagnostic imaging tests).

● **A large tongue, small jaw or pronounced overbite,** which can put pressure on the back of the throat.

● **High blood pressure,** especially when it is unexplained or hard to control even with medication.

● **Being over age 65 and menopausal.** Sleep apnea is two to three times more common among seniors.

● **Having a parent, sibling or child with sleep apnea,** which suggests a genetic propensity toward a narrow airway and/or weak throat muscles.

● **Use of opioid pain medication,** such as *methadone* (Dolophine) or a benzodiazepine tranquilizer, such as *diazepam* (Valium). A study from *Pain Medicine* (published online) found that 75% of patients had sleep apnea while taking these medications.

Mark Stengler, NMD

Red flag: Over-the-counter oral appliances for snoring are available, but for optimal results, you need an oral appliance created for your mouth and jaw by a dentist trained to make such a device.

Important: No matter which device you use, you need to get tested first and then retested after you start using the device to make sure that you are getting the oxygen you need.

Patients with sleep apnea generally report that treatment gives very satisfying results. They feel much better during the day because they sleep more soundly at night—and their spouses do, too.

$50 Fix Reduces Sleep Apnea by 36%

Stefania Redolfi, MD, university researcher, Respiratory Medicine Department, University of Brescia, Italy.

Would you rather wear a strange-looking and uncomfortable mask while you sleep...or tight stockings during the day?

The obvious answer is "um, neither"...but it is entirely possible that people who have a certain type of chronic obstructive sleep apnea may be presented with exactly this choice, based on new European research. A study recently published in the *American Thoracic Society's American Journal of Respiratory and Critical Care Medicine* reports that wearing compression stockings can reduce sleep apnea episodes significantly for one-third of the people whose apnea is caused by chronic venous insufficiency—a pretty dramatic difference for such an easy treatment. Since it was a small, brief and preliminary study focused on just this one cause of obstructive sleep apnea, it's entirely possible that longer treatment may yield even more impressive results that are helpful to even more patients.

Out from Behind the Mask

Even though designers have done their best with continuous positive airway pressure (CPAP) masks and there now are quite a few different models to choose from—there's not a single one that is truly comfortable. They are bulky and uncomfortable on the face and force many wearers to sleep in positions they'd rather not sleep in. Many people who need them refuse to wear them. That's why the news that there is a safe, easy-to-use and inexpensive treatment option for a good portion of people with sleep apnea is quite welcome!

We contacted Stefania Redolfi, MD, of the University of Brescia in Italy, lead researcher of this practical and surprisingly promising study. She explained that chronic venous insufficiency is a vascular problem in which veins (primarily in the legs) can't efficiently pump blood back to the heart. Fluid builds up in the legs during the day and then shifts at night to the neck, bloating tissue there. This causes the person to experience the partial collapse of the pharynx in between breaths during sleep—and so begins the loud, unpleasant "gasp and snore" pattern that characterizes obstructive sleep apnea in these patients.

What does wearing tight stockings during the day have to do with insufficient oxygen at night? It is actually quite ingenious. "Wearing compression stockings during the day helps to reduce the daytime fluid accumulation in the legs," Dr. Redolfi explained, "which in turn reduces the amount of fluid flowing into the neck at night." Absent the pressure created by that fluid, the respiratory system does not narrow as much and, for many people, this intervention is enough to allow them to get adequate oxygen into their lungs by breathing—and sleeping—normally. This is a wonderful thing, because sleep apnea and the constantly interrupted sleep that goes with it can severely undermine a person's health.

What the Right Socks Can Do

The study was small, involving 12 patients—half randomly assigned to wear compression stockings during the day (putting them on as soon as they awakened and taking them off only after getting into bed for the night) for a week, while the other half served as the control, with the two groups switching places after the first week. Subjects spent their nights at a sleep center, where their physiological signs (including brain waves, respiration and eye movements) were measured continuously. Researchers also measured each person's overnight changes in leg fluid volume and neck circumference at the start of the study

Killing You While You Sleep

Close to 30 million Americans have sleep apnea, a sleep disorder in which breathing repeatedly stops and starts. More than 80% of these people don't know they have it. And every year, an estimated 38,000 Americans die in their sleep because sleep apnea has exacerbated a circulatory problem, causing a fatal heart attack or stroke.

For people with sleep apnea, nighttime levels of blood oxygen can plummet from an optimal saturation of 100% to below 65%. This oxygen-robbing disorder can contribute to extreme daytime sleepiness, as well as high blood pressure, heart attack, stroke, congestive heart failure, type 2 diabetes, Alzheimer's disease, erectile dysfunction, depression, anxiety and gastroesophageal reflux disease (GERD). In fact, if you have sleep apnea, you have a nearly five times higher risk of dying overall.

Bottom line: Diagnosing and treating sleep apnea can save your life.

Chris Meletis, ND, former chief medical officer for the National College of Naturopathic Medicine and currently the executive director of the Institute for Healthy Aging and a physician on the staff of Beaverton Naturopathic Medicine in Oregon. He is author of numerous books on health and healing, including *The Hyaluronic Acid Miracle* (Freedom Press). *www.Dr Meletis.com*

and at the end of both the compression-stocking and control periods.

Dr. Redolfi said that the researchers expected the compression stockings would help—but they were somewhat surprised by the degree to which they helped! *Wearing the stockings resulted in…*

•**An average of a 62% reduction in overnight leg fluid volume change,** as compared with when subjects did not wear the stockings.

•**A 60% reduction in neck circumference increase** (used as a proxy measurement to estimate fluid shift into the neck).

•**A 36% reduction in the number of apnea episodes.**

Effective and Inexpensive

This is a very basic intervention that has the potential to make a big difference for patients who are struggling with obstructive sleep apnea. The stockings cost less than $50 and, though they aren't exactly cute or comfortable, Dr. Redolfi said that all the study participants preferred them to the CPAP mask. As simple as it sounds, though, she said that

people with sleep apnea shouldn't try this on their own—it is important to have a sleep study done to measure whether the stockings are making a difference and if so, how much. Talk to your doctor about this. Dr. Redolfi plans further research to ascertain whether wearing the stockings for longer than a week shows more significant results...to learn whether other measures, such as using diuretics or exercises to reduce fluid volume, are useful...and also to examine whether wearing compression stockings can help people with sleep apnea due to other causes, such as obesity.

Chapter 15

STOP SMOKING NOW

Stop Smoking Naturally

Quitting smoking isn't easy. Fortunately, several safe, natural substances can help reduce your cravings. Use these remedies on their own or in conjunction with a smoking-cessation program. I recommend quitting cold turkey—with help from the first two remedies on this list.

• **St. John's wort.** Researchers at Roswell Park Cancer Institute Prevention Center in Buffalo found that 37.5% of participants in a cessation counseling program were smoke-free after taking this herb for 12 weeks, compared with 30.5% who were smoke-free after using prescription drugs. Look for a product standardized to 0.3% hypericin. Take 300 mg three times daily with food.

Best: Take it for four weeks before you stop smoking and then for another two months. Don't use St. John's wort if you are also taking an antidepressant or an oral contraceptive.

• **Caladium seguinum.** This homeopathic remedy can reduce cigarette cravings. Take two pellets, 30C potency, daily for 10 days, beginning the day you quit.

If you still can't quit, add the two remedies below to your regimen—and take all four at once—until your cravings subside.

• **Herbal oat straw (Avena sativa).** This herb can calm the nervous system. Take 20 drops of a tincture in water or juice three times daily at any time of day.

• **5-hydroxytryptophan (5-HTP).** This mood-enhancing amino acid is converted in the body to the neurotransmitter serotonin. It can help reduce the anxiety and irritability associated with nicotine withdrawal. Take 100 mg three times daily on an empty stomach. It is safe when used with St. John's wort, but do not use 5-HTP if you also are taking an antidepressant or medication for Parkinson's disease.

Helpful: Acupuncture can help to reduce cravings. Most qualified acupuncturists will know how to treat smokers who want to quit.

Mark A. Stengler, NMD, licensed naturopathic medical doctor in private practice, Stengler Center for Integrative Medicine, Encinitas, California...adjunct associate clinical professor at the National College of Natural Medicine, Portland, Oregon...author of many books, including *The Natural Physician's Healing Therapies* and coauthor of *Prescription for Natural Cures* (both from Bottom Line Books).

Try hard, and don't stop trying. It takes most smokers about three attempts at quitting before they succeed.

Smart Strategies That Replace Cigarette Cravings With Healthier Habits

Deborah M. Hudson, BS, RRT, program manager, Clarian Tobacco Control Center, Indianapolis, Indiana.

According to some experts, nicotine dependency is one of the most difficult addictions to overcome, even with such aids as nicotine patches, gums and other products. The problem is that those products just replace a drug with a drug. But there is some good news from the natural front—a study from the University of Exeter (United Kingdom) found that just five minutes of isometric exercise (exercises involving pushing against an object that doesn't move, such as doing pushups) was often enough to reduce the need for a cigarette. They also found a 15-minute walk was effective as well. Another study, from Duke University, showed that certain foods—fruits, vegetables, dairy products and non-caffeinated drinks (water and juice)—diminish the palatability of cigarettes.

We spoke with cessation expert Deborah M. Hudson, program manager at the Clarian Tobacco Control Center in Indianapolis to see what other healthful suggestions she might have to help people overcome the urge to smoke. She says anything that is immediately relaxing or distracting will help—deep breathing is first on her list. It offers instant relaxation, while also replacing the deep inhalation smokers perform routinely when lighting up. Best ways to deep breathe—inhale deeply through your nose, to a slow count of three...hold for three... and exhale through your mouth to a count of five. Other effective relaxation techniques include progressive muscle relaxation—tensing and releasing one set of muscles at a time (best done lying down)—and meditation and visualization, which are basic techniques of yoga. Picture yourself strong and healthy, free of "cancer sticks" or "coffin nails." Reinforcing how much easier you will breathe, how free you will feel, how easily you will climb stairs, etc., will help motivate you past the desire for cigarettes, says Hudson.

Eating lots of fruits and vegetables and drinking six to eight glasses of water each day may curb cravings and increase satiety, helping you possibly avoid the six to eight pounds many people gain post-smoking. This partially works by distracting you but also because the healthful carbohydrates supplied by fruits and vegetables are a better alternative to carbs than high-fat and sugary snacks. (However, Hudson says that some people lose weight at this time because they adopt a healthier lifestyle that combines healthful eating as well as exercise.) Chewing on cinnamon sticks may also help put people off smoking. As an alternative, submerge toothpicks in cinnamon oil (available at health stores) and suck on one when a cigarette calls. Wintergreen Lifesavers can be helpful too, says Hudson, especially for former menthol smokers.

Change Up the Routine

For the first few months after quitting, it is absolutely critical to change behaviors and daily routines, avoiding those you associate with cigarettes, says Hudson. Her suggestions include finding new routes to drive to familiar destinations in order to force you to concentrate on driving rather than smoking...fueling up at a different gas station from where you once bought cigarettes...and playing music or books on tape to further occupy your thoughts. At home, Hudson suggests creating an oasis of calm by indulging yourself with whatever soothing, comforting, healthful routines you can, including candles, peaceful music and books (so long as reading isn't associated with your habit). Go out for a brisk walk when the urge strikes, and you will come back with an endorphin high that is far more salubrious than the smoke you thought you needed.

The Truth About e-Cigarettes

Constantine Vardavas, MD, RN, MPH, PhD, visiting scientist at Center for Global Tobacco Control, Harvard School of Public Health, Boston.

I f you've been to a mall lately, chances are you've seen e-cigarettes being sold at a kiosk. Instead of producing smoke, battery-operated e-cigarettes (which have been growing in popularity since they were introduced in 2005) turn a nicotine-filled liquid into a vapor that's inhaled or "vaped."

So using e-cigarettes is often marketed as the "safe" way to smoke and as a healthy way to wean yourself off actual cigarettes— but is it?

A recent study is the first to call that common claim into question.

What "Vaping" Does to You

There has been very little research to date on the safety of e-cigarettes, yet they're still allowed to be sold because they're categorized as "tobacco products," as opposed to "drug delivery" devices. So researchers at the Center for Global Tobacco Control at the Harvard School of Public Health in Boston were eager to get some answers. The study goal was to see whether using an e-cigarette for just five minutes, the average amount of time it takes a person to smoke one regular cigarette, would impact lung health. Results were published online in the medical journal *Chest*. To learn more, we spoke with Constantine Vardavas, MD, RN, MPH, PhD, a scientist at the Center and the study's lead author.

How the study worked: Participants included 30 male and female smokers, ages 19 to 56. Researchers tested participants' lung function and then asked them to "vape" from

an e-cigarette for five minutes, and during that five-minute period the researchers re-tested each subject's lung function.

The results: Researchers discovered that five minutes of vaping increased airway constriction in the lungs by 18%, on average. This result was too small to lead to shortness of breath or breathing difficulties, but the concern is that more frequent or prolonged vaping could potentially lead to those health problems. Even more worrisome, said Dr. Vardavas, was the second finding—use of the e-cigarettes reduced the amount of nitric oxide that was exhaled (by 16%), and that is an indication of inflammation in the lungs.

All after just five minutes!

The study did not examine how long the participants' lungs suffered these effects, Dr. Varadavas said. He suspects that airway constriction likely improved and that inflammation likely subsided relatively quickly. But, he wondered, what if someone "smokes" an e-cigarette multiple times a day, day after day? Would the lungs be able to bounce back as quickly...or at all? The truth is, no one knows, but we do now know that e-cigarettes are not entirely harmless.

The Debate Continues

The FDA is not ignoring the e-cigarette health question. Back in 2010, the FDA tried to categorize them as drug-delivery devices. This would have compelled manufacturers to prove that the devices are safe and effective at helping people quit smoking. But a US Court of Appeals blocked the FDA's attempt because the court didn't agree with the categorization, so manufacturers never had to do any of that.

Supporters of e-cigarettes argue that any toxins in e-cigarettes are present in very small amounts and are found in other FDA-approved products, such as nicotine patches and nicotine gum. They add that the FDA has yet to provide any proof that these contents cause harm. And there is at least one small study that has shown that e-cigarettes may help people quit smoking. The gist of the argument for e-cigarettes is that e-cigarettes might harm you a little bit, but real cigarettes are much, much more harmful.

That may be. But "vape" with caution—they aren't completely benign.

Smoking Promotes Personal Summers

Smoking worsens menopause symptoms. *Recent finding*: Caucasian women who smoke are 56% more likely to have hot flashes than women who don't smoke…and African-American women who smoke are 84% more likely to have hot flashes.

Study of 296 women by researchers at University of Pennsylvania Perelman School of Medicine, Philadelphia, published in *Journal of Clinical Endocrinology and Metabolism*.

Why Some Can't Kick the Habit

Why is it so hard for some people to quit smoking? *There are several reasons…*

• **Dependence.** How long you have smoked matters less than how much you smoke. Typically, people who have more than about 15 or 20 cigarettes daily experience worse withdrawal symptoms than people who smoke fewer cigarettes. Even so, two people who have smoked the same number of cigarettes for the same length of time still can have different degrees of dependence. Heredity may affect dependence and severity of withdrawal.

• **Motivation.** People who have had a heart attack—or other health scare related to smoking—often find it easier to quit.

• **Preparation/practice.** To improve their chances of success, smokers should set a quit date. Before that date, they should start going without cigarettes for part of the day—for example, while driving or watching TV.

Helpful: Most people make five to seven serious attempts before they can remain cigarette-free. With each attempt, they learn which situations make them reach for a cigarette—and what they can do to fight the urge.

Douglas Jorenby, PhD, director, clinical services, Center for Tobacco Research and Intervention, University of Wisconsin, Madison. www.ctri.wisc.edu

What Smoking Does to Your Skin

Dana E. Rollison, PhD, associate faculty member in the department of cancer epidemiology and vice president/chief health information officer at the Moffitt Cancer Center in Tampa, and lead author of a study on smoking and skin cancer published in Cancer Causes & Control.

If you're a smoker, you know the dangers of what you do—lung cancer, throat cancer, heart disease, emphysema and so much more—but because you look healthy (enough) on the outside, it's hard to acknowledge the reality of these potential "inside

Aids Can Be Used Longer

Quit-smoking aids can be used for longer than 12 weeks. The Food and Drug Administration is considering eliminating the current warning on most nicotine-replacement gum, lozenges and patches recommending that people stop using them after 12 weeks. Use of these medications beyond 12 weeks may help some people abstain from smoking. And nicotine itself is not believed to raise the risk for cancer, though it can elevate heart rate, raise blood pressure and may cause adverse skin reactions.

K. Michael Cummings, PhD, chair, department of health behavior, division of cancer prevention and population sciences, Roswell Park Cancer Institute, Buffalo.

problems." Well, a recent study reveals an "outside problem" for smokers—an increased risk for potentially disfiguring skin cancer.

The study focused on two types of non-melamona skin cancer—basal cell carcinoma (BCC), which is rarely fatal but can be disfiguring...and squamous cell carcinoma (SCC), which can cause significant disfigurement and can be deadly. Researchers compared health information on 315 adults who had no history of skin cancer with data on 380 people who had been diagnosed with either BCC or SCC. All study subjects were Caucasian (the group most susceptible to skin cancer) and were asked whether they had ever smoked, for how long and how many cigarettes per day they averaged. In analyzing the data, researchers adjusted for other skin cancer risk factors, such as sun exposure, sunburn history, age, skin tone, and eye and hair color.

Results: Smoking significantly increased women's odds of developing squamous cell cancer—and the more they smoked, the higher their risk. For instance, women who smoked the equivalent of one pack a day for 20 years had three times the risk for SCC as women with no history of smoking. No connection was found between smoking and BCC in women. Male smokers had a modestly increased risk for both types of skin cancer, but the link wasn't strong enough for researchers to definitively declare a connection.

Why female smokers would be at significantly greater risk for skin cancer than male smokers isn't clear, though some studies show that women smokers also are more likely to get lung cancer.

Theory: Estrogen may play a role in the way nicotine is metabolized and in how effectively the body repairs DNA damage caused by smoking, thus influencing a female smoker's cancer risk.

Takeaway message: Everyone should speak to a dermatologist about the warning signs of skin cancer and appropriate screening schedules—but this is especially important if you have a history of smoking. For help in kicking the cigarette habit, contact a free counseling support system that offers information, coaching and/or opportunities to connect with other smokers who want to quit—according to the US Public Health Service, this more than doubles the chances of success. Options include the toll-free quit line 800-QUIT-NOW (800-784-8669), a federal/state partnership...and the interactive Web sites *www.SmokeFree.gov* and *www. Women.SmokeFree.gov* from the National Cancer Institute. Your skin will be the better for it—and so will the rest of your body.

The Most Dangerous Kind of Cigarette

Nicholas T. Vozoris, MD, clinical associate and staff respirologist in division of respirology, St. Michael's Hospital, Toronto, Canada.

Smokers sometimes complain of sore throats from regular cigarettes.

Mentholated cigarettes, on the other hand, seem gentler on the throat because of the cool and soothing sensation of the menthol. And menthol, we all know, is also soothing in cough drops...in chest rubs...and in lots of other drugstore remedies.

So if you're going to smoke, going with menthol makes sense, right?

Sorry, smokers—but if you think that menthol cigarettes are less harmful than regular cigarettes, you're quite wrong.

In fact, recent research shows that people who smoke menthol cigarettes have an even higher risk than other smokers for one particularly dangerous type of cardiovascular event.

Don't Let the Cool Fool You

When the researchers compared the health of smokers of mentholated cigarettes with the health of smokers of regular cigarettes, they found that menthol smokers were more than twice as likely to have had strokes.

When we spoke with the study's author, Nicholas T. Vozoris, MD, a clinical associate

Eating Veggies May Help You Quit Smoking

People who ate the most fruits and vegetables were three times more likely to succeed at stop-smoking programs. *Possible reason:* The high fiber and water content of produce fills the stomach—and because hunger is triggered by hormones such as the ones that cause nicotine cravings, it can be mistaken for the urge to smoke.

Study of 1,000 smokers by researchers from University at Buffalo, New York.

in the division of respirology at St. Michael's Hospital in Toronto, Canada, he noted that the study didn't look at why menthol cigarettes might affect health differently than regular cigarettes—but he has some ideas.

Why Menthols Are More Dangerous

We do know that menthol stimulates cold receptors in the upper airway (which is why menthol feels so cool and soothing) and that when these receptors are active, people tend to hold in each breath longer than they otherwise would, said Dr. Vozoris. So the lungs would be exposed to a menthol cigarette's toxic chemicals longer. And, he added, the tiny hairlike structures in the airway, cilia, that are supposed to move toxins out of the lungs during exhalation actually slow down a little when exposed to menthol, and that impairs clearance.

So why were there more strokes but not more heart attacks for menthol smokers? Dr. Vozoris said that it's possible that menthol cigarettes and regular cigarettes affect different parts of the cardiovascular system in different ways or to different degrees. For instance, earlier studies have shown that the carotid arteries (the main arteries feeding the brain) tend to be stiffer (a bad thing) in people who smoke menthol cigarettes than

in people who smoke regular cigarettes...but there was no such difference seen in the coronary arteries (near the heart).

Bottom Line: Be particular about what you puff. If you must smoke, this recent study suggests, at least stay away from menthols.

The Tobacco Toxins That Harm Nonsmokers

Jonathan Winickoff, MD, MPH, pediatrician and associate professor, department of pediatrics, Harvard Medical School, Boston, and immediate past chair of the American Academy of Pediatrics Tobacco Consortium. He has drafted tobacco control policies for the American Medical Association and other organizations.

Ever step inside a hotel room and know instantly that someone recently smoked in it?

Or hop into a rental car and need to roll down the windows immediately to air out the stench of cigarettes?

Or maybe you occasionally get a "tobacco-y" whiff from the clothes or hair of a smoker who lives below you or in the condo next door.

So-called "thirdhand" smoke is the contamination that remains after a cigarette has been extinguished.

It's also dangerous, just like firsthand smoking and secondhand smoke—and here's why you need to avoid it...

Of Mice and Men

Believe it or not, the quintessential experiment proving the hazards of thirdhand smoke was published in *Cancer Research* way back in 1953. Researchers at the (then-called) Sloan-Kettering Institute of the Memorial Center for Cancer and Allied Diseases in New York collected cigarette smoke in a beaker and then gathered the residue that clung to the glass. They mixed the residue with a solvent and painted it on the backs of some mice...on other mice (the control group), they painted solvent alone. Researchers found that 59% of the mice exposed to tobacco residue developed skin lesions, and most of those mice went on to develop cancer. In contrast, none of the control mice developed skin lesions or cancer.

Now fast-forward to today. Sure, we're living in a time when smoking is banned from most public places in the US, but, unfortunately, many homes, apartment buildings, hotel rooms and cars are still heavily contaminated, we learned recently from Jonathan Winickoff, MD, MPH, a pediatrician and professor of pediatrics at Harvard Medical School in Boston and one of the country's top researchers on tobacco and health.

Some of these spaces are being smoked in still…others used to be smoked in…and all can hurt your health.

How We're Exposed

Thirdhand cigarette smoke adheres to all surfaces and remains there even after a butt is stubbed out. "It's surprisingly dangerous because it reacts with other compounds in the environment and with itself to create new tobacco-specific nitrosamines, compounds that are highly carcinogenic," said Dr. Winickoff.

This thirdhand smoke is, unfortunately, almost impossible to clean off most surfaces, though you'll have more luck with glass surfaces than with porous ones, such as wallboard. Usually, it just sticks around until someone comes into contact with it.

There are three ways that humans can come into contact with thirdhand smoke…

• **Through breathing.** The compounds can be reemitted into the air, so it's possible to inhale them into your lungs.

• **Through touch.** Compounds can enter the body through the skin—just by touching a wall or lamp or using an armrest, for example.

• **Through ingestion.** The microscopic compounds can settle on everything from dishware to food, making it possible for us to unknowingly eat them.

Health Consequences of Tobacco Toxins

People of any age can suffer various health consequences from any amount of exposure to thirdhand smoke, though children, in particular, are more likely to come into contact with the toxins and are more likely to be negatively affected by them.

Children breathe at faster rates than adults, so when thirdhand smoke is present, the little ones' respiratory exposure is much higher. Also, they tend to touch everything and move around surfaces like mops, which increases their skin exposure. Plus, they ingest twice the amount of house dust as the average adult, said Dr. Winickoff.

Since a child usually weighs less than what an adult weighs, exposure will impact a kid's body more. And because their bodies and brains are still developing, the exposure can have measurable effects. Studies have found that children exposed to thirdhand smoke have much higher blood levels of cotinine, which is a breakdown product of nicotine, compared with children who are not exposed to contaminated environments. "High cotinine levels have been associated with developmental delays and lower reading and math scores," said Dr. Winickoff. "Plus tobacco smoke exposure—it can be hard to tease out the effects of secondhand and thirdhand smoke—is now a leading cause of Sudden Infant Death Syndrome."

Smoke-Free Living

So if you or someone around you still smokes, this is obviously another good reason to quit—and another good reminder that smoking doesn't just harm the person who has the cigarette in his or her mouth.

If you're not a smoker, do everything you can to avoid thirdhand smoke. Try to live in a building that is smoke-free, because even if there is just one smoker around—even in another apartment—smoke moves freely in the air through ductwork or out one window and into another and can affect everyone. Reject a stinky-smelling hotel room or rental car, and ask the company for a replacement. And if a smoker (even one who is not smoking at the moment) steps into an elevator with you, step out of the elevator and take the next one. Is this inconvenient? Sure, but your good health is worth the extra hassle.

Detoxification for Ex-Smokers

Mark A. Stengler, NMD, naturopathic physician in private practice, La Jolla, California...adjunct associate clinical professor at the National College of Natural Medicine, Portland, Oregon...author of many books, including *The Natural Physician's Healing Therapies* and coauthor of *Prescription for Natural Cures* (both from Bottom Line Books).

Smoking is an extremely difficult habit to break. If you have recently stopped smoking, congratulations.

What you might not know: Anyone who has stopped smoking (whether recently or within the past year) needs to detoxify. Detoxification helps to improve liver function and get rid of some of the toxins, such as cadmium and arsenic, that have built up in the body. I recommend that all ex-smokers follow this detoxification program, which involves taking all of the following supplements below for four weeks. To further help detoxification of the lymphatic system, have a weekly massage or a dry or wet sauna, which is safe for everyone except pregnant women, children, frail elderly people and people with diabetes, heart or circulation

problems. *All of the supplements below are safe for everyone...*

• **Milk thistle.** This herb has been used for centuries for liver disorders and liver cleansing. Studies show that it enhances detoxification. Take 250 milligrams (mg) of a product standardized to contain 70% to 85% silymarin twice daily 30 minutes before meals.

• **Psyllium husks.** These husks of the seeds of an east Asian plant provide fiber and promote detoxification by regulating bowel movements and expelling toxins. While you may know psyllium husk as the main ingredient in Metamucil, it also is available on its own in powder or capsule form. Take 5 grams (one teaspoon) of powder twice daily mixed into eight ounces of water.

• **Pneumotrophin PMG.** This propriety blend, made by a company called Standard Process (800-558-8740, *www.standardprocess.com*), contains nutrients that support healthy lung tissue. Take one tablet three times daily before meals.

• **Omega-3 fatty acids.** To reduce lung inflammation, take either krill oil (1,000 mg daily) or a daily fish oil supplement with a combined 1,000 mg of eicosapentaenoic acid (EPA) and docosahexaenoic acid (DHA). Choose the omega-3 fatty acid that is easiest for you to take. Some people prefer krill oil because it is less likely to cause fishy burps or aftertaste.

• **Multivitamin.** Everyone should take a multivitamin as the basis of his/her supplement regimen. This helps to ensure that your body gets crucial nutrients.

ALZHEIMER'S DISEASE

More than five million people in the United States have Alzheimer's disease—and that number is expected to skyrocket to more than seven million by 2025. Alzheimer's disease has a unique impact on women. The latest research shows that nearly two-thirds of Americans with Alzheimer's are women. Women also make up 60% of the unpaid caregivers whose lives are also dramatically altered by the disease, providing billions of hours of unpaid care to help their family and friends. Fortunately for everyone, research is revealing new ways to help you keep your memory as you age.

www.alz.org/alzheimers_disease_facts_and_figures.asp

http://www.alz.org/shriverreport/overview.html

Chapter 16

ALZHEIMER'S RISKS AND WARNINGS

What Do "Senior Moments" Really Mean?

Until recently, most physicians have reassured older adults that so-called "senior moments" are usually a normal part of aging.

Now, recent research shows that complaints of subtle memory loss—for example, not remembering the name of a longtime acquaintance as easily as you might have five to 10 years earlier—may mean more than doctors once thought.

The findings: Researchers at New York University (NYU) School of Medicine have found that people who are concerned about episodes of memory loss may, in fact, be absolutely right, and they are at increased risk of developing Alzheimer's disease years later.

To learn more, we spoke with Barry Reisberg, MD, a renowned Alzheimer's researcher who led this important recent research.

When Does Alzheimer's Begin?

The warning signs of Alzheimer's disease are now well-known and include a gradual decline of memory and reasoning skills. However, the stages that precede Alzheimer's now are a great focus of investigation.

In the 1980s, I, along with my associates, first identified a condition that we termed mild cognitive impairment (MCI), which is generally characterized by measurable memory loss beyond the personal experiences of forgetfulness that can be associated with normal aging. With MCI, memory problems, such as forgetting recent events and frequently repeating yourself in conversations, usually are noticeable to family members and/or friends.

Research findings are mixed, but most evidence shows that about half of people who experience MCI go on to develop overt Alzheimer's disease within about four years.

Important research: NYU investigators have found that a condition they've termed subjective cognitive impairment may be evident up to 22 years before noticeable Alzheimer's symptoms manifest—many, many years before MCI.

What's the implication of this finding?

It means that scientists can refocus their research to try to find ways to prevent Alzheimer's by addressing it a decade or two before it surfaces—and individuals may have

Barry Reisberg, MD, leader of the Clinical Core of the Alzheimer's Disease Center of the New York University (NYU) School of Medicine and clinical director of the school's Aging and Dementia Research Center, both in New York City.

a crucial new clue that signals the importance of seriously following the lifestyle habits that promote brain health.

A New—Even Earlier—Sign

Subjective cognitive impairment is so subtle that it usually is not recognized by a patient's doctor or his/her family. In fact, the condition is generally apparent only to the individual, although he may confide in a spouse or close friend about the self-perceived problem.

Interestingly, when people with subjective cognitive impairment are tested, they continue to perform within normal ranges on mental and psychological tests.

So, how can subjective cognitive impairment be detected—and is it important to even do so?

What researchers currently know: Up to 56% of adults ages 65 and older experience subjective cognitive impairment. Its key known characteristic is that the person believes his memory is not as good as it was five to 10 years before. Specifically, a person with the condition may complain—or simply note—that he can't remember, say, names or where he has placed things as well as he did in previous years.

Compared with people who don't have subjective cognitive impairment, those who have the condition are 4.5 times more likely to develop MCI or full-blown Alzheimer's within seven years. In a recent study, more than half of people advanced to these more evident and more serious conditions after seven years.

What's more, research shows that those with subjective cognitive impairment who progress to MCI or Alzheimer's do so about 3.5 years sooner, on average, than those who didn't have subjective cognitive impairment.

Is This Just Normal Aging?

Since studies show that as many as 56% of people ages 65 and older have subjective cognitive impairment, it can be technically considered part of the normal aging process.

Advanced age is, after all, the single biggest risk for dementia.

However, there are unique psychological and physiological characteristics that accompany subjective cognitive impairment.

For example, research conducted at the NYU School of Medicine found that people with subjective cognitive impairment have increased urinary levels of the stress hormone cortisol and decreased brain activity in the memory and other brain regions, compared with people who don't have the condition. Increased cortisol levels have been shown in some studies to damage the brain.

In addition, European researchers have found that people with subjective cognitive impairment have significantly higher levels of spinal fluid markers that often accompany Alzheimer's, compared with people who don't have subjective cognitive impairment.

Three Important Questions

Here are a few of the questions that were used by the NYU researchers to help identify subjective cognitive impairment. *If you answer "yes" to one or more of the following, discuss this with your physician…*

1. Am I having trouble recalling names (especially names of people) more than I did five to 10 years ago?

2. Am I having trouble recalling where I placed things more than I did five to 10 years ago?

3. Is my ability to concentrate lacking compared with five to 10 years ago?

What You Can Do

If you suspect that you have subjective cognitive impairment or MCI, your doctor can determine whether a treatable factor—such as depression…anxiety…a thyroid disorder…a nutritional deficiency (such as too little vitamin B-12)…or medication (such as anticholinergic drugs taken for conditions including allergies or overactive bladder…and painkillers)—is causing memory loss. Chronic stress also may affect memory.

If your doctor rules out a treatable cause for your memory loss, it's crucial to adopt lifestyle habits, such as regular exercise, that promote brain health.

This includes eating a heart-healthy diet. A diet that emphasizes vegetables and fruit, lean protein and whole grains…avoids saturated and trans fats…and includes healthful fats, such as olive oil, promotes cardiovascular health and, in turn, the health of your brain.

There is no medication that is prescribed at the present time for people with subjective cognitive impairment. There are also no medications that have been approved specifically for MCI. However, medications such as *donepezil* (Aricept) or *rivastigmine* (Exelon), which are approved for the treatment of Alzheimer's symptoms, have been studied in MCI patients. But these medications have not shown sufficient benefit to win FDA approval as a treatment for MCI.

Alzheimer's: Is It "Type 3" Diabetes?

Isaac Eliaz, MD, LAc, integrative physician and medical director of the Amitabha Medical Clinic & Healing Center in Santa Rosa, California, an integrative health center specializing in chronic conditions. *DrEliaz.org*

For years, scientists from around the world have investigated various causes of Alzheimer's disease. Cardiovascular disease factors, such as hypertension, stroke and heart failure…other neurological diseases, such as Parkinson's disease…accumulated toxins and heavy metals, such as aluminum, lead and mercury…nutrient deficiencies, including vitamins B and E…infections, such as the herpes virus and the stomach bacterium H. pylori…and head injuries each have been considered at one time or another to be a possible contributor to the development of this mind-robbing disease.

However, as researchers continue to piece together the results of literally thousands of studies, one particular theory is now emerging as perhaps the most plausible and convincing of them all in explaining why some people—and not others—develop Alzheimer's disease.

A Pattern Emerges

Five million Americans are now living with Alzheimer's, and the number of cases is skyrocketing. Interestingly, so are the rates of obesity, diabetes and metabolic syndrome (a constellation of risk factors including elevated blood sugar, high blood pressure, abnormal cholesterol levels and abdominal fat).

What's the potential link? Doctors have long suspected that diabetes increases risk for Alzheimer's. The exact mechanism is not known, but many experts believe that people with diabetes are more likely to develop Alzheimer's because their bodies don't properly use blood sugar (glucose) and the blood sugar–regulating hormone insulin.

Now research shows increased dementia risk in people with high blood sugar—even if they do not have diabetes. A problem with insulin appears to be the cause. How does insulin dysfunction affect the brain? Neurons are starved of energy, and there's an increase in brain cell death, DNA damage, inflammation and the formation of plaques in the brain—a main characteristic of Alzheimer's disease.

An Alzheimer's-Fighting Regimen

Even though experimental treatments with antidiabetes drugs that improve insulin function have been shown to reduce symptoms of early Alzheimer's disease, it is my belief, as an integrative physician, that targeted nondrug therapies are preferable in preventing the brain degeneration that leads to Alzheimer's and fuels its progression. These approaches won't necessarily reverse Alzheimer's, but they may help protect your brain if you are not currently fighting this disease…or help slow the progression of early-stage Alzheimer's.

My advice includes…

• **Follow a low-glycemic (low sugar) diet.** This is essential for maintaining healthy glucose and insulin function as well as supporting brain and overall health. An effective way to maintain a low-sugar diet is to use the glycemic index (GI), a scale that ranks foods according to how quickly they raise blood sugar levels.

Here's what happens: High-GI foods (such as white rice, white potatoes and refined sugars) are rapidly digested and absorbed. As a result, these foods cause dangerous spikes in blood sugar levels.

Low-GI foods (such as green vegetables… fiber-rich foods including whole grains…and plant proteins including legumes, nuts and seeds) are digested slowly, so they gradually raise blood sugar and insulin levels. This is critical for maintaining glucose and insulin function and controlling inflammation.

Helpful: GlycemicIndex.com gives glucose ratings of common foods and recipes.

• **Consider trying brain-supporting nutrients and herbs.*** These supplements, which help promote insulin function, can be used alone or taken together for better results (dosages may be lower if supplements are combined due to the ingredients' synergistic effects)…

• Alpha-lipoic acid (ALA) is an antioxidant shown to support insulin sensitivity and protect neurons from inflammation-related damage.

Typical dosage: 500 mg to 1,000 mg per day.

• Chromium improves glucose regulation.

Typical dosage: 350 micrograms (mcg) to 700 mcg per day.

*Consult your doctor before trying these supplements, especially if you take any medications or have a chronic health condition, such as liver or kidney disease. If he/she is not well-versed in the use of these therapies, consider seeing an integrative physician. To find one near you, consult The Institute for Functional Medicine, FunctionalMedicine.org.

• Alginates from seaweed help reduce glucose spikes and crashes.

Typical dosage: 250 mg to 1,000 mg before meals.

• L-Taurine, an amino acid, helps maintain healthy glucose and lipid (blood fat) levels.

Typical dosage: 1,000 mg to 2,000 mg per day.

Kick Up Your Heels!

Regular exercise, such as walking, swimming and tennis, is known to improve insulin function and support cognitive health by increasing circulation to the brain. Dancing, however, may be the ultimate brain-protective exercise. Why might dancing be better than other brain-body coordination exercises, such as tennis? Because dancing is mainly noncompetitive, there isn't the added stress of contending with an opponent, which increases risk for temporary cognitive impairment.

Best: Aerobic dances with a social component, such as Latin, swing or ballroom, performed at least three times weekly for 90 minutes each session. (Dancing for less time also provides some brain benefits.) If you don't like dancing, brisk walking for 30 minutes a day, five days a week, is also shown to help protect the brain against dementia.

Alzheimer's May Progress Differently in Women, Men

Maria Vittoria Spampinato, MD, associate professor, radiology, Medical University of South Carolina, Charleston.

Clinton Wright, MD, MS, scientific director, Evelyn F. McKnight Brain Institute, University of Miami Miller School of Medicine, Miami.

Alzheimer's disease may look and act differently in men and women, new research suggests.

An emerging field known as gender-specific medicine has shown pronounced differences among the sexes in terms of heart disease and other conditions. These latest findings—if confirmed by further research—may have significant implications for diagnosing and treating Alzheimer's among the sexes.

When people develop Alzheimer's disease, their brains atrophy or shrink. In the study of 109 people with newly diagnosed Alzheimer's, brain scans showed that this atrophy happened earlier in women than men. Women also lost more gray matter in their brains in the year before their diagnosis. However, men seemed to have more problems with their thinking ability when diagnosed with Alzheimer's than their female counterparts did. What's more, men and women lost gray matter in different areas of their brain.

"It is commonly known that loss of volume in hippocampus coincides with cognitive decline, but this is more true in males than females," said study author Maria Vittoria Spampinato, MD, an associate professor of radiology at the Medical University of South Carolina.

The hippocampus is the part of the brain tasked with memory formation, organization and storage.

"The next step is to integrate this information on brain volume loss with other markers of Alzheimer's disease to understand if gender differences exist with other modalities or just brain volume alone," Dr. Spampinato said.

The study was presented at the annual meeting of the Radiological Society of North America.

Expert Commentary

Clinton Wright, MD, scientific director of Evelyn F. McKnight Brain Institute at the University of Miami Miller School of Medicine, said it's too soon to draw any conclusions about gender differences in Alzheimer's disease.

"Additional information would need to be provided to know if the findings are attributable to sex differences or other factors," Dr. Wright said. "In particular, it is not clear if the authors adjusted for age. If women were

older they might have had greater volume losses over the study period."

The finding that women had greater brain volume losses while men had worse mental function at the time of Alzheimer's diagnosis is also hard to explain, Dr. Wright said: "One would expect greater atrophy in those with worse cognition unless additional factors such as vascular damage explained these differences."

For more information about Alzheimer's disease risk factors, visit the Alzheimer's Association Web site *www.alz.org* (search "risk factors").

What's Slowly Killing Your Brain

Owen Carmichael, PhD, associate professor of neurology and computer science, Center for Neuroscience, University of California, Davis. His study was published in *The Lancet Neurology*.

There are lots of "young-ish" people—say, people in their 30s or 40s—who have been told by their doctors that they have borderline high blood pressure and whose reaction is basically, "Eh, whatever."

If this describes you—or a sibling or child of yours—please be aware that this youngish person with highish blood pressure is committing suicide of the brain.

That's because, as a recent study shows, even slightly high blood pressure starts eating up the brain even when a person is quite young.

There generally aren't any symptoms, and the person looks and feels fine (for now).

But here's where the mental trouble starts…

How High Blood Pressure Hurts the Brain

Most blood pressure research focuses on older people, so researchers were interested in exploring its effects on younger individuals.

In an analysis of data from the famous Framingham Heart Study, they examined the neurological effects of systolic blood pressure—the top number in blood pressure readings—on adults with an average age of 39.

What they found should be considered a wake-up call for some younger folks. Using high-tech scans (a traditional MRI and a special type of MRI called diffusion tensor imaging), Owen Carmichael, PhD, a coauthor of the study, and his colleagues found that the higher a person's blood pressure, the lower the volume of gray matter in the brain and the lesser the structural "integrity" of the white matter. So those with hypertension (a reading of 140/90 or higher) had more cognitive damage than those with prehypertension (a reading between 120/80 and 139/89)…those with prehypertension had more than those with "normal" blood pressure (a reading under 120/80)…and even those with "high-normal" blood pressure had more than those with "low-normal" blood pressure.

Gray matter is like a set of computers that perform the calculations that enable you to remember things, concentrate, follow a sequence of events, speak, see and hear, for example. When you have less gray matter, it's like having fewer computers to do those calculations, so it's harder to do those brain-related tasks mentioned above. White matter, on the other hand, is like the Internet wiring that allows the gray matter "computers" to communicate with each other and do those mental tasks efficiently. When the integrity of the white matter is compromised, it's as if your brain wiring has been frayed. So that also makes performing those brain-related tasks mentioned above more difficult.

Now, these aren't effects that you would necessarily notice in your 30s or 40s—you won't suddenly start forgetting your children's names or getting lost in your own house, said Dr. Carmichael. But if blood pressure isn't controlled, the negative effects begin—today—and then worsen with age. This can make you more susceptible to serious cognitive conditions, such as Alzheimer's disease.

Get Your Numbers Down

The great news, though, is that prehypertension (and even high-normal blood pressure) is very treatable. Making certain lifestyle changes (such as, of course, eating healthier foods and exercising more) and, as a last resort, even taking a medication (such as a thiazide diuretic, beta-blocker, angiotensin-converting enzyme inhibitor or calcium channel blocker) can lower your blood pressure and prevent any further brain damage. Is it possible to reverse damage that's already been done? Dr. Carmichael said that the answer isn't known, but hopefully future research will address it.

Once again, if your blood pressure is 140/90 or more, it's high. If it's under 120/80, it's normal. If it's between 120/80 and 139/89, you have prehypertension—which means that you don't have high blood pressure but are likely to develop it in the future. Even people with prehypertension in the study had more signs of brain damage than those with normal blood pressure—so you should take even a borderline reading such as that seriously.

Don't let your age give you a false sense of security.

Are Your Pots and Pans Making You Sick?

Diane S. Henshel, PhD, associate professor in the School of Public and Environmental Affairs at Indiana University in Bloomington. Her research centers on the effects of pollutants on health and the environment. She has won numerous awards, including a Presidential Citation from the Society of Environmental Toxicology and Chemistry.

You probably have a pan like this: a nonstick skillet buried in the depths of your pot cabinet that you haven't used in ages. Though its nonstick Teflon coating is slightly scratched, the pan still seems serviceable. But is it safe?

"Unquestionably, when they get scratched or overheated—which happens all the time—nonstick surfaces, such as Teflon, release potentially toxic chemicals," Diane S. Henshel, PhD, of the School of Public and Environmental Affairs at Indiana University, said. These chemicals then seep into our food—particularly fatty foods, including cooking oils. When we ingest them, the chemicals build up in the tissues in our bodies and stick around for years.

A primary chemical of concern used in making many nonstick cookware products is perfluorooctanoic acid (PFOA). According to the Centers for Disease Control and Prevention, in laboratory animals given large amounts, PFOA was found to affect growth, development and reproduction and to injure the liver. Other observational studies link PFOA to elevated cholesterol and thyroid disease in humans.

So why is cookware made with PFOA and other chemicals still on the market? Because there are conflicting conclusions about the relative risk of such cookware. What's more, cookware is not the only source of PFOA exposure—for instance, Teflon also is used in many other stain- and water-resistant products, such as clothing, carpets and furniture. PFOA and other Teflon breakdown products are found in soil, drinking water and ground water as well as in fish and other seafood.

Still, careful consumers are taking matters into their own hands. "I got rid of my nonstick cookware quite a while ago," Dr. Henshel said. "We're exposed to so many unavoidable toxic chemicals every day that it just makes sense to limit what we can."

For safer cooking: Dr. Henshel recommends using cookware made from stainless steel, cast iron, enamel-coated cast iron or glass. To deter sticking, simply use a bit of cooking oil or cooking spray.

Use ceramic cookware only if it has a clear or white glaze on the inside surface area that touches the food and is made in the US. Ceramics with glazes from foreign countries—especially those with a bright red glaze on the inside surface—may contain heavy metals, such as lead, known to be very toxic. These can be released, particularly when acidic liquids, such as tomato sauce or lemon juice, are heated.

As for aluminum, this metal has been linked to Alzheimer's disease and dementia, though scientific studies are contradictory. To be safe, if you choose to cook with aluminum, opt for anodized cookware—its surface is made with an aluminum compound that is harder than regular aluminum and won't easily scrape off or leach into food.

Dr. Henshel also commented on the newer-generation nonstick pans, such as those coated with PFOA-free Thermolon. She said, "So long as the surfaces are not scratched, they seem to be safe. Once the surfaces are scratched, though, the underlying metals could be released—and with products from some countries, the base metal may be primarily lead."

What You Should Know About Pesticide Dangers

David Pimentel, PhD, professor, department of entomology, systematics and ecology, Cornell University, Ithaca, New York.

It's almost 40 years after DDT was banned, and you would think that we'd now feel safe and comfortable in knowing that we are exposed to fewer toxic pesticides. Instead there's evidence that we're exposed to more.

About 70,000 different chemicals are used in the US today, making the chemical companies healthy even if we're not. Although many of these chemicals are known carcinogens, there isn't a lot of scientific research that has successfully proved a causal link to cancer—since, in addition to being expensive, this would take decades to prove…and, of course, no one will get rich from the results. Now research is emerging that links pesticides to other known health problems, so it's important to take a look at what we know—and what we don't know—about the dangers of the pesticides used in growing the foods we eat.

So Many Chemicals

Fruits and vegetables receive the highest dosage of pesticides, so they're more likely to be contaminated than other foods. For instance, conventional, non-organic growers can choose from as many as 62 different types of pesticide products to treat a crop of peaches (and each crop is typically treated with many different types)...52 for blueberries...42 for apples. And you may not realize that pesticides also have been found in meat and chicken, especially in the thighs.

We spoke with David Pimentel, PhD, a professor in the department of entomology, systematics and ecology at Cornell University about this trend. "About 70% of the foods that consumers buy have detectable levels of pesticide residues," Dr. Pimentel said.

Who Is Most at Risk?

Regarding the connection between cancer and pesticides, it is safe to say there's good reason to worry about one. Noting that more research is needed on this important topic, Dr. Pimentel said. "There is no question that pesticides can cause cancer—the question is, how many people do they affect?" He noted that people with a genetic risk for cancer are quite likely the most vulnerable.

Meanwhile, researchers continue to uncover more ways that absorbing pesticides—by eating, touching or breathing them—is bad for our health...most especially for people who are already somewhat unhealthy due to poor lifestyle or other conditions that depress their immunity. *Among the recent findings...*

• **Parkinson's disease.** It appears that exposure to pesticides may trigger Parkinsons's disease in genetically predisposed people. In a large 2006 study, researchers at Harvard School of Public Health found that participants exposed to pesticides (specifically, farmers, ranchers, fishermen and people who used pesticides in their homes or gar-

dens) had a 70% higher incidence of Parkinson's than those who weren't exposed. The latest research, reported in February 2011 and conducted by the National Institute of Environmental Health Sciences, shows that people exposed in their professions to the pesticides paraquat or rotenone developed Parkinson's approximately 2.5 times more often than people who were not exposed. Both pesticides cause cellular damage. Paraquat, in particular, is an extremely toxic substance originally developed as an herbicide.

• **Dementia.** A study that collected data between 1997 and 2003 from French vineyard workers who spent at least two decades applying pesticides to plants or working in buildings where pesticides were housed showed that these workers scored low on a test of memory and recall. Researchers speculate that the changes demonstrated in the mental functioning of these people indicate that they may eventually develop a neurodegenerative disease, such as Alzheimer's.

• **Infertility.** In a 2008 review of studies on pesticide exposure, epidemiologists showed a decline in the semen quality and quantity of farm workers, which impaired male fertility by 40%. "Infertility, especially in men, is increasing in proportion to greater exposure to pesticides," said Dr. Pimentel.

Kids Are Vulnerable

For children, there is bad news and good news. First of all, the problem of pesticide exposure is amplified compared with adults. "Kids are growing," noted Dr. Pimentel. "In relation to body weight, they eat more than adults." One study found that the urine of children eating a variety of conventional foods contained markers for organophosphates, a lethal group of pesticides used to disable the nervous system of pests that is, not incidentally, used to make the deadly nerve gas saran. However, the study also found that when the children's diets were switched to only organic foods, the chemicals disappeared from their bodies within 36 hours.

What to Do

You may take some comfort—briefly—in knowing that, by Dr. Pimentel's reckoning, newer pesticides are used at 1/1,000 of the amount as had been the case with DDT. But don't be fooled by this simplistic comparison—ounce for ounce or pound for pound, "These newer materials are far more toxic, not just to pests but also to humans."

Washing and peeling helps only if a chemical is on the outside of a fruit or vegetable, Dr. Pimentel noted—but the sad fact is that some of these toxins are taken up by the plant as it grows, meaning that the pesticides end up inside the flesh of the produce and therefore cannot be removed even with careful washing and peeling.

Foods least likely to have pesticide residue after washing include onions, avocados, corn, pineapples, mangoes, asparagus, sweet peas, kiwi, cabbage, eggplant, papaya, watermelon, broccoli, tomatoes and sweet potatoes. Some of these foods have thick skins that protect the food, while others face fewer threats from pests and so are sprayed less.

Avoiding the most contaminated types of fruits and vegetables or buying their organic counterparts reduces your pesticide exposure by 80%. The following foods, when grown conventionally, contain the most pesticide residue even after washing and/or peeling—celery, peaches, strawberries, apples, blueberries, nectarines, bell peppers, spinach, kale, cherries, potatoes, grapes, carrots.

Bottom line: Choose carefully, buy organic when possible and be sure to wash fruits and vegetables thoroughly to be certain they'll keep you healthy, not make you sick.

Loneliness Raises Alzheimer's Risk

A recent finding revealed that older adults who feel lonely are twice as likely to develop Alzheimer's disease as people who do not.

Self-defense: If loneliness is accompanied by symptoms of depression, consult a psychologist or psychiatrist.

Best: Maintain connections with others to safeguard your mental health.

Robert S. Wilson, PhD, researcher, Rush Alzheimer's Disease Center, Rush University Medical Center, Chicago, and leader of a study of 823 people, published in *Archives of General Psychiatry*.

Warning Sign of Alzheimer's Disease

Difficulty identifying odors may be a sign of Alzheimer's. According to a recent study, older people with mild difficulty recognizing scents, such as cinnamon and lemon, are 50% more likely to develop cognitive impairment within five years, compared with people whose odor recognition is intact. This impairment often precedes the development of Alzheimer's.

Robert S. Wilson, PhD, department of neuropsychology, Rush Alzheimer's Disease Center, Rush University Medical Center, Chicago, and author of a study of 589 people, ages 55 to 100, published in *Archives of General Psychiatry*.

Inability to Spot Lies May Warn of Dementia

Katherine P. Rankin, PhD, neuropsychologist and associate professor of neurology at the University of California, San Francisco, Memory and Aging Center and coauthor of a study presented at a meeting of the American Academy of Neurology.

Does someone you love seem increasingly gullible? Don't be too quick to dismiss this as a normal sign of aging. *Here's why...*

A recent study included 175 people ages 45 to 88, more than half of whom were in the early stages of some type of neurodegenerative disease that causes certain parts of the brain to deteriorate. Participants watched videos of two people talking. In addition to truthful statements, the video dialogue included sarcasm and lies, plus verbal and nonverbal clues to help participants pinpoint the false or insincere statements. Participants then answered yes/no questions about the video…and researchers compared their scores with results of MRI scans that measured the volume of different brain regions.

Results: Cognitively healthy people easily picked out the lies and sarcasm in the video, as did most participants with certain neurodegenerative diseases, including Alzheimer's. However, participants whose brain scans showed degeneration of the frontal and temporal lobes, a condition called frontotemporal dementia—which is as common as Alzheimer's disease among people under age 65—found it very difficult to distinguish factual statements from untruthful or sarcastic ones.

Bottom line: Increasing inability to recognize deception or sarcasm merits a consultation with a neurologist, especially if accompanied by other possible symptoms of frontotemporal dementia, such as severe changes in behavior and/or personality—yet often these are mistaken for signs of depression, a midlife crisis or normal aging. Early diagnosis of frontotemporal dementia may maximize treatment options and help protect patients vulnerable to being scammed due to their blind trust.

Falling Could Mean Alzheimer's

There's an early sign of Alzheimer's that often is ignored…Frequent falls.

Recent finding: Older people with preclinical Alzheimer's, as measured by brain scans that showed signs of amyloid plaques, are twice as likely to fall as people without preclinical Alzheimer's.

What to do: Everyone over age 65 should evaluate his/her fall risk. If you have had a fall, or a loved one has fallen, consult a physician.

Susan Stark, PhD, assistant professor, program of occupational therapy and department of neurology, Washington University in St. Louis, and lead author of a study of 125 adults, presented at the Alzheimer's Association's annual International Conference in Paris, France.

Eye Scan for Alzheimer's?

Is there an eye scan to diagnose Alzheimer's disease?

Not exactly. There is a retinal scan in development, but it is not yet available to the public.

Recent study: Researchers performed noninvasive retinal and brain scans on 136 adults (average age 73), some healthy and others with Alzheimer's disease, to measure correlations between blood vessel thickness at the back of the eye and beta-amyloid deposits in the brain—a marker of preclinical Alzheimer's disease.

Result: Those with Alzheimer's or preclinical signs of the disease in the brain had thinner retinal veins.

Theory: Alzheimer's disease affects blood vessels in the brain and may also affect blood vessels in the back of the eyes, which are easier to scan.

Although there are many people who have beta-amyloid deposits but do not have symptoms of Alzheimer's disease, studies suggest that people with the deposits often develop cognitive symptoms in 10 to 15 years. If you are concerned about Alzheimer's disease, ask your doctor about receiving a medical and neurological exam.

Shaun Frost, researcher, Commonwealth Scientific and Industrial Research Organisation, Perth, Australia.

B Vitamins May Reduce Alzheimer's Risk

Andrew L. Rubman, ND, founder and director of Southbury Clinic for Traditional Medicines, Southbury, Connecticut. *www.Naturopath.org*

While finding a cure for Alzheimer's disease remains an elusive goal for scientists, at least some progress is being made in figuring out ways to prevent it—and here's a promising installment on that quest. It's a recent study that connects some important dots in the search for how and why Alzheimer's disease develops and offers a practical and easy strategy that apparently helps slow cognitive decline.

Sixteen percent of people over age 70 suffer from mild cognitive impairment and half of them go on to develop Alzheimer's. Recent research demonstrates that daily vitamin B supplements may be helpful in slowing the process, warding off the encroaching confusion and memory loss that presage development of Alzheimer's disease in aging individuals.

Why B Vitamins Are Crucial

Earlier research had shown that vitamin B deficiency is a very common problem, especially in the elderly, and it's also known that a B vitamin deficiency (specifically B-6, B-12 and folate) is associated with elevated levels of homocysteine (an amino acid associated with increased risk of cardiovascular disease when blood levels are too high). This can lead to inflammation and fibrin development in the linings of the arteries that feed the brain, which in turn leads to degenerative changes, including memory loss and poor concentration. The question was, would supplementing with B vitamins reduce homocysteine levels and help protect against—or at least slow down—cognitive decline?

The study: At the University of Oxford in the UK, investigators examined the impact of vitamin B supplements on 168 individuals over age 70 who were experiencing mild cognitive impairment. In a randomized, double-blind controlled trial, 85 participants took a daily B vitamin combo (folic acid, B-12 and B-6) and 83 were given a placebo. All underwent MRI scans of the brain at the start of the study and again after two years. Researchers found that brain atrophy was 53% lower in people who took B vitamins as compared with those who took a placebo. Brain atrophy is when the brain shrinks and becomes progressively more dysfunctional, which correlates with worse cognitive scores and greater cognitive impairment.

This research was published in the journal *PLoS ONE*.

Vitamin B Strategy

Daily Health News contributing medical editor and naturopath Andrew L. Rubman, ND, explained that high stress and poor diet—both common here in the US—are known to deplete the body of B vitamins, with the result being that nearly all adults could benefit from supplementation. In addition to protecting cognitive health, B vitamins are important for a number of reasons—they have an effect on mood, energy, digestion and the health of skin, hair and nails. Dr. Rubman explained that older folks tend to be the most deficient because they often take multiple medications, which the body processes in the liver with the aid of vitamin B, further depleting supplies. In these seniors, a simple, safe strategy targeting homocysteine with B vitamins may slow the rate of brain atrophy and cognitive impairment.

In his practice, Dr. Rubman frequently prescribes B vitamins for older adults. He said that a typical prescription would be one 25-mg multi-B two to three times daily (this contains a broad range of the community of B vitamins, many of which are provided at 25 mg per dose) along with one 5-milligram sublingual B-12 tablet once a day. B vitamins are quite safe. It is best to take these in several doses throughout the day because most B vitamins are water-soluble and don't remain in the body longer than 15 hours or so.

Half of Alzheimer's Cases Could Be Prevented with Lifestyle Changes

According to a recent finding, many of the biggest risk factors for Alzheimer's disease are modifiable—lack of physical activity, depression, smoking, midlife hypertension, midlife obesity and diabetes. Changing or eliminating these risks could potentially prevent 2.9 million Alzheimer's cases in the US.

Deborah Barnes, PhD, MPH, associate professor of psychiatry, University of California, San Francisco, and leader of a comprehensive review published online in *The Lancet Neurology.*

Dementia-Proof?

High levels of the inflammation marker C-reactive protein (CRP) have been linked to dementia. Now, a recent study shows that among the very old (age 75 and older), those with high CRP levels are more likely to retain their memories. More research is needed to explain this finding.

Neurology

Warning: A Cold Sore Could Cause Alzheimer's

Mark A. Stengler, NMD, licensed naturopathic medical doctor in private practice, Stengler Center for Integrative Medicine, Encinitas, California…adjunct associate clinical professor at the National College of Natural Medicine, Portland, Oregon…author of many books, including *The Natural Physician's Healing Therapies* and coauthor of *Prescription for Natural Cures* (both from Bottom Line Books).

After years of research, scientists are finding that there might be a simple way to prevent Alzheimer's disease. Unbelievable? Researchers have been trying to understand the cause and progression of Alzheimer's for decades—and it would be incredible if doctors actually could do something to slow the progression of this debilitating disease.

There's growing evidence that Alzheimer's may be caused by the herpes simplex virus 1 (HSV1), the same virus that causes fever blisters or cold sores on the face and mouth. (It is not believed to be caused by the other herpes simplex virus—HSV2, genital herpes, which is transmitted sexually.) HSV1 attacks the immune system, particularly the peripheral nervous system. Once it has attacked, it never leaves the body but lies dormant and occasionally reactivates, causing a flare-up of blisters or enlarged lymph nodes, especially when set off by a trigger, such as stress or fatigue.

Research shows that HSV1 also can infect the brain—and that flare-ups of HSV1 in the brain may be a primary cause of the brain damage associated with Alzheimer's. This means that it may be possible to take steps to stave off Alzheimer's by suppressing HSV1. To learn more about preventing Alzheimer's, our editors turned to David Perlmutter, MD, an integrative neurologist and a pioneer in brain health.

According to Dr. Perlmutter, the HSV1 research, which is ongoing, is so compelling that in recent years, he has been employing the new HSV1 theory with his patients who are at risk for Alzheimer's—including those with parents who had the disease and those who have had a decline in cognitive function themselves. *Here's what he has to say…*

The Herpes Connection

For a long time, most Alzheimer's researchers focused their attention on a sticky protein or plaque, beta-amyloid, in the brains of patients with Alzheimer's. There seemed to be a correlation between the amount of this protein and the amount of cognitive impairment. The thinking was that if you could get rid of this protein, you could get rid of the disease.

But in a study published in *PLoS One,* Harvard researchers and other colleagues demonstrated that beta-amyloid could have a protective role, functioning in the immune system as an antimicrobial that attacks and destroys bacteria and viruses in the brain.

Studies focusing on HSV1 and Alzheimer's have been going on for nearly three decades. But new discoveries about genetics and genetic predispositions are inspiring researchers to clarify the link between the virus and Alzheimer's.

While it isn't known how many people with Alzheimer's have HSV1, Dr. Perlmutter believes that most people are HSV1-positive. This doesn't mean that everyone who is HSV1-positive will get Alzheimer's—it means that people who have a genetic susceptibility to Alzheimer's who also have HSV1 (that periodically reactivates causing symptoms such as fever blisters) might be more at risk for the disease. In 2008, Ruth Itzhaki, PhD, from the University of Manchester in England, estimated that 90% of adults have an HSV1 infection in areas of the brain affected by Alzheimer's.

In 2009, Dr. Itzhaki published a study in *Journal of Pathology* showing that in Alzheimer's patients, more than 70% of the HSV1 virus's DNA was located inside beta-amyloid plaques. It appears as though plaque is used by the immune system to keep the virus in check.

While HSV1 infection of the brain may be latent much of the time, stress and other triggers, combined with a genetic susceptibility to Alzheimer's, might cause it to flare up (just as it does with HSV1-related cold sores and fever blisters), leading to inflammation in the brain.

Testing for the Virus

When my patients have a family history of Alzheimer's (for example, a parent with the disease), I recommend that they get a blood test to determine if they have active HSV1. Patients who do not have a family history of the disease but want to know if they have active HSV1 also are encouraged to get tested.

Dr. Perlmutter and I use a standard viral test. We test for two antibodies produced when the body fights an infection—immunoglobulin

G (IgG) and immunoglobulin M (IgM). There are no rules about the way these tests work—IgM is produced more quickly following an infection, but this varies by person. Specific IgG antibodies can indicate the HSV1 virus, but the time this takes to be detectable varies. So a test for both antibodies is given—and the following regimen is recommended if either antibody is high.

The Protocol

Dr. Perlmutter reports that many of his patients who have Alzheimer's and follow the protocol show no further signs of cognitive decline and actually regain some cognitive function. Since Alzheimer's is such a devastating illness—and the protocol uses largely safe and natural remedies—I think it's wise for patients with cognitive decline and/or a family history of the disease to take these steps to suppress the virus.

The protocol includes the following supplements and one prescribed medication. All the supplements are available at health-food stores and online. They are safe for everyone.

•**Lysine.** This essential amino acid has been shown in studies to prevent outbreaks of cold sores caused by HSV1. It also seems to prevent outbreaks of HSV1-related inflammation in the brain. Lysine works by blocking the activity of arginine, another amino acid that HSV1 needs in order to reproduce.

Dose: 500 milligrams (mg), three times a day.

•**Vitamin D.** This vitamin has been found to prevent HSV1 activity—not by killing HSV1 but by rendering it dormant. Patients need to have their vitamin D blood levels tested regularly to ensure that they have blood levels of between 70 ng/mL and 80 ng/mL. Your doctor will tell you how much you need daily.

•**Curcumin.** The active ingredient in turmeric, this spice gives curry its color and much of its flavor. It inhibits HSV1 activity.

Dose: 200 mg to 400 mg of turmeric extract containing 95% curcuminoids daily.

Heart Disease Risk Linked to Mental Decline

Evaluating an individual's risk for cardiovascular disease by taking into account age, blood pressure, smoking, diabetes and cholesterol is a better indicator of the likelihood of mental decline later in life than the standard dementia risk test, which looks at age, education, blood pressure, body mass index and other factors.

Study of 7,800 people by researchers at French National Institute of Health and Medical Research, Paris, published in *Neurology*.

• **Antiviral treatment.** Dr. Perlmutter recommends that patients whose blood tests show active infection with HSV1 take a daily 500-mg dose of the antiviral drug *valacyclovir* (Valtrex), commonly used to prevent HSV1 from spreading. This medication, which is available by doctor's prescription only, does not produce harmful side effects and can be taken for long periods of time. Dr. Perlmutter recommends that it be used on an ongoing basis, similar to the way other drugs (such as blood thinners) are prescribed.

Unlike Dr. Perlmutter, before prescribing Valtrex, I first provide patients with other antiviral treatments, such as intravenous (IV) vitamin C, IV and oral glutathione (a powerful antioxidant) and astragalus, which increases the body's resistance to stress and disease. I do recommend Valtrex to patients whose antibody levels are not decreased by the natural therapies. If you are interested in this protocol, speak to a holistic doctor about it.

Since HSV1 stays in the body permanently once a person is infected, our thinking now is that people who want to prevent Alzheimer's need to continue this protocol for the rest of their lives. To check that the therapy is reducing HSV1, patients' antibody levels are retested annually.

Maternal Genes Raise Alzheimer's Risk

People whose mothers had Alzheimer's may be at higher risk for the disease than people whose fathers had it.

Recent finding: Adult children of women who had Alzheimer's showed reductions in sugar utilization in the brain—glucose (sugar) was available, but the brain wasn't using it properly. Decreased sugar utilization is common in Alzheimer's patients.

Theory: Maternally inherited genes may alter brain metabolism. Identifying individuals at risk may enable earlier intervention.

Lisa Mosconi, PhD, research assistant professor of psychiatry, New York University School of Medicine, New York City, and leader of a study of 49 people, published online in *Proceedings of the National Academy of Sciences*.

Chapter 17

STOP MEMORY LOSS

Cognitive Decline Prevention: Where We Stand Now

Memory loss is such a frightening and frustrating aspect of aging that, of course, we want to do what we can to keep our minds sharp. So it was a devastating disappointment to many people when a recent comprehensive analysis of studies concluded that there is simply not enough scientific evidence to support many of the strategies commonly recommended for preventing cognitive decline.

The big questions: How could the results of this analysis be so contradictory to those of numerous earlier studies? And what—if anything—can and should we do now to protect our minds?

Before we tackle those questions, let's first look at a recent analysis. An independent government panel reviewed the results from 165 scientific papers published in the last 25 years and concluded in *Annals of Internal Medicine* (AIM) that "the current literature does not provide adequate evidence to make recommendations for interventions" aimed at preventing cognitive decline. *Reasons for this conclusion…*

•**Genetic factors appear to affect susceptibility to cognitive decline**—and, of course, we can't change our genes.

•**Research on strategies to prevent cognitive decline is in a state of relative infancy.** There are numerous small studies with nonrigorous study designs—but few large-scale, long-term observational studies or randomized clinical trials. With many small studies of varying designs, it's not uncommon to get inconsistent findings and thus be unable to reach a definitive conclusion. In this regard, the panel's overall findings actually are not so surprising.

Still: A closer examination of the AIM report reveals some strategies that may indeed help.

Factors tentatively linked to a lower risk for cognitive decline include…

•**Avoiding certain medical conditions,** such as diabetes…depression or depressive symptoms…and metabolic syndrome—a

---

JoAnn E. Manson, MD, DrPH, professor of medicine and women's health at Harvard Medical School and chief of the division of preventive medicine at Brigham and Women's Hospital, both in Boston. Dr. Manson is author, with Shari Bassuk, ScD, of *Hot Flashes, Hormones & Your Health* (McGraw-Hill).

cluster of symptoms that increase risk for cardiovascular disease, including abdominal obesity, high triglycerides, high blood pressure, high blood sugar and low HDL (good) cholesterol.

•**Not smoking.** People who never smoked or quit smoking appear to be 30% less likely to experience cognitive decline than current smokers.

•**Engaging in cognitively stimulating activities,** such as reading, crossword puzzles and the card game bridge.

•**Regular physical activity,** such as walking, biking and gardening.

•**A Mediterranean diet that emphasizes fruits,** vegetables, fish and whole grains and that limits unhealthy fats…a high intake of vegetables in particular…and a high intake of marine omega-3 fatty acids, which are found in fish and fish-oil supplements. (To learn about participating in a nationwide ongoing study of marine omega-3 fatty acids being conducted by our research group at Harvard Medical School and Brigham and Women's Hospital in Boston, see *www.Vital Study.org*).

My recommendation: Although these strategies have not yet been proven to prevent cognitive decline, it seems likely that many, if not all, of them will ultimately be shown to do so. Why? A significant amount of cognitive decline is related to underlying vascular disease (diseased arteries supplying the brain or heart). There is conclusive evidence that a healthy lifestyle that includes most of the above strategies can prevent a large proportion of cases of stroke and heart disease, as well as vascular risk factors, such as diabetes and high blood pressure. This vascular protection would be expected to translate into reduced cognitive risk as well. Therefore, I'm hedging my bets and still recommending— and personally practicing—these strategies for prevention not only of vascular disease but also of cognitive decline.

What appears not to help prevent cognitive decline…

The AIM report noted that, although laboratory studies and some observational stud-ies suggest cognitive benefit for the following interventions, they have not shown benefit in available randomized trials. So, although the factors below may have other health benefits (as well as risks, in some cases), cognitive protection does not appear to be among the benefits of the following…

•**Supplements of vitamin C…vitamin E…beta-carotene…multivitamins…or the hormone DHEA.** Most of these supplements also have failed to protect against cardiovascular disease (or cancer) in large randomized trials.

•**Menopausal hormone therapy**—at least if started at age 65 or older. (We just don't know yet whether hormone therapy helps reduce dementia risk when started closer to menopause, because in most randomized trials, the women who used hormone therapy generally were older.)

•**Nonsteroidal anti-inflammatory drugs** (aspirin, *ibuprofen*)…cholesterol-lowering statins…or blood pressure-lowering medications (the quality of available data is particularly low for this last intervention).

•**Having an active social life** and/or emotional support from friends and family.

There's just too little data to say…

The panel found too little evidence to hazard a guess whether the following factors increase, decrease or have no effect on cognitive function…

•**Changes in caloric intake…or dietary fat intake.**

•**Supplements of ginkgo biloba.**

•**Having sleep apnea.**

•**The presence of trace metals in the body…or toxic environmental exposures.**

Bottom line: What should women make of this information? My opinion is that there is no harm and much to be gained in terms of prevention of other health problems (including diabetes, heart disease, stroke, depression and physical disability) by adhering to a healthful diet…maintaining an active, involved lifestyle…and controlling blood pressure and cholesterol levels as needed. As more rigorous studies are conducted, hopefully we will find that our efforts have also kept cognitive decline at bay.

The Ultimate Alzheimer's-Fighting Diet

Marwan Sabbagh, MD, a neurologist and director of Banner Sun Health Research Institute in Sun City, Arizona. He is associate director of the Arizona Alzheimer's Disease Core Center, a clinical instructor in the Banner Family Medicine Geriatrics Fellowship Program in Scottsdale, Arizona. He is author, with professional chef Beau MacMillan, of *The Alzheimer's Prevention Cookbook* (Ten Speed).

Can you really prevent Alzheimer's disease by eating certain foods? Research is not yet definitive, but there is mounting evidence that certain foods can indeed reduce dementia risk or delay the onset of symptoms.

Recent finding: In a recent analysis published in *Annals of Neurology,* researchers who reviewed the diets of more than 2,000 older adults discovered that those who ate ample amounts of fatty fish and certain vegetables, such as leafy greens, were about 40% less likely to develop Alzheimer's or some other type of dementia than those who ate less of those brain-healthy foods.

The sooner you start eating a brain-healthy diet, the better—Alzheimer's is believed to develop over decades. But even if you're an older adult, I firmly believe that eating the foods described in this article is one of the best ways to improve your odds of staying mentally sharp.

The "Orac" Powerhouses

Alzheimer's disease seems to be caused, in part, by oxidative stress—the disease-causing cellular process triggered by unstable molecules known as free radicals. One way to decrease oxidative stress is to eat antioxidant-rich foods.

In laboratory studies, animals that have been genetically engineered to develop Alzheimer's disease show lower rates of cognitive decline when they consume more antioxidants. It is likely that humans get the same benefits.

For overall health, researchers recommend a daily diet that includes 3,000 to 5,000 oxygen radical absorbance capacity (ORAC) units (a measure of antioxidant activity). *Where to start…*

•**Load up on the right kind of vegetables.** The Chicago Health and Aging Project, a study of aging and dementia that involved more than 6,000 participants, found that those who ate two to four servings of leafy green, yellow or cruciferous vegetables daily were significantly less likely to suffer from cognitive declines than those who ate less.

Best: Kale is an ORAC powerhouse with 1,770 units per one-and-a-half cup serving. Spinach has 1,260 units. In general, the darker-colored vegetables—such as Brussels sprouts, broccoli and acorn squash—have the most antioxidants. You should have at least three servings each day.

Important: Many of the nutrients and antioxidants contained in vegetables are destroyed by high-heat cooking (such as boiling and lengthy steaming). Therefore, I recommend lightly sautéing vegetables in a little olive oil. The oil provides additional antioxidants and improves the body's absorption of fat-soluble antioxidants, such as beta-carotene.

•**Use more spices.** Believe it or not, spices are the most concentrated sources of antioxidants in the kitchen. In fact, just one teaspoon of cinnamon has more antioxidants than a serving of vegetables.

Another very high antioxidant spice is turmeric, which gets a lot of attention for its brain-protective effects.

Important fact: In India, where curries and other dishes seasoned with turmeric are eaten almost every day, the rate of Alzheimer's disease is among the lowest in the world. However, other high-antioxidant spices, such as cloves, oregano, thyme and rosemary, are also worth adding to your diet. Although there's no definitive research showing how much of these spices you need to consume for brain health, it's reasonable to add as much as your taste buds permit in as many dishes as possible.

•**Be choosy about the fruit you eat.** Fruit consumption, in general, does not appear to lower the incidence of cognitive decline or Alzheimer's disease. That's probably because most fruits have a much lower concentration of antioxidants than vegetables.

Blueberries are a well-known exception to this rule. But there are other antioxidant powerhouse fruits, such as cherries and acai fruit (a slightly tart berry), that are often overlooked. So for an excellent antioxidant boost, have one cup of any type of fresh or frozen berries (including raspberries and blackberries).

Helpful: Juice (with no added sugar) is a good way to include more berry antioxidants in your diet. Pomegranate, blueberry, grape and acai juices are all high in brain-protective polyphenols. Orange and pineapple juices are high in vitamin C, but don't seem to protect against Alzheimer's—the high sugar levels of these juices aren't offset by enough benefits to justify drinking them.

My approach: I drink a six-ounce glass of unsweetened pomegranate juice every day. That's because studies suggest that pomegranate juice, in particular, reduces levels of beta-amyloid, the protein that accumulates in the brains of Alzheimer's patients. Apple and cherry juices also have been shown to reduce beta-amyloid levels. Grape juice is another good choice. Along with red wine, it contains resveratrol, a compound believed to break down the amyloid protein.

•**Don't forget tea.** Tea is possibly the most effective beverage for brain health. A study that looked at more than 1,000 elderly Japanese participants found that those who drank two cups of green tea daily had far lower rates of cognitive decline than those who drank three or fewer cups a week.

Green tea has epigallocatechin-3-gallate (EGCG), an antioxidant that seems to be particularly effective for neurodegenerative diseases, including Alzheimer's. If you don't like

green tea, drink black tea—it also contains significant levels of EGCG—or coffee. Both lower risk for Alzheimer's to a somewhat lesser extent than green tea.

•**Put fatty fish on your menu.** By now, most people have gotten the message that eating fish is good for your brain. But not all types have this effect. Lean fish, such as cod, flounder, halibut, sole and haddock, are not the best choices.

That's because it's the high levels of omega-3 fatty acids in cold-water fish (such as herring, mackerel and sardines) that offer brain protection. These healthful fats are so beneficial that you should buy the fattiest fish you can find.

Herring, mackerel and sardines are the fattiest. Salmon, another fatty fish, is also an excellent source of docosahexaenoic acid (DHA). Brain cells require DHA, a type of omega-3, to maintain their integrity—a breakdown of these cells is the hallmark of Alzheimer's disease.

Important: I advise patients to eat a three-ounce (or larger) serving of fatty fish at least three times a week—just lightly sauté the fish in olive oil, bake or broil.

At the same time, I suggest decreasing one's intake of saturated fat and processed foods (which tend to be high in soybean oil and other unhealthy fats, including omega-6s).

People who do this can achieve the recommended ratio of one part omega-3s for every three parts of omega-6s—optimal for preventing Alzheimer's and other forms of dementia.

Brain-Boosting Smoothie

Green tea offers a nice taste contrast to pomegranate juice. Matcha (finely milled green tea available at health-food stores) has a high concentration of antioxidants, and yogurt adds texture as well as protein—an important breakfast nutrient.

Combine in a blender until smooth…

1 cup plain Greek yogurt (it has less sodium and more protein than regular yogurt)

1 ripe banana, peeled and chopped

¼ cup honey
¼ cup pomegranate juice
2 teaspoons matcha
1 cup ice cubes

Foods That Fight Memory Loss

Rhoda Au, PhD, associate professor of neurology, Boston University School of Medicine, and director of neuropsychology, Framingham Heart Study.

There's a new way to potentially prevent Alzheimer's—a disease that we know frustratingly little about—and it's not some exotic, expensive or potentially dangerous drug. It's actually an affordable, natural component that's found in everyday foods. For the first time, there's a human study that confirms an association between dietary choline, an amino acid found in eggs and some other foods, and better cognitive performance. The study, from Boston University School of Medicine, appeared in the *American Journal of Clinical Nutrition*.

Brain Booster

Researchers investigated the dietary habits of 744 women and 647 men ranging from 36 to 83 years of age. None had dementia when the study started. In the early 1990s and then again between 1998 and 2001, participants filled out a questionnaire about their diets—they were asked how often they had eaten particular foods in the past year. After the second questionnaire was given, the researchers performed neuropsychological tests to evaluate the participants' cognitive skills, including verbal memory (remembering a story) and visual memory (remembering images). They also did MRI brain scans to see if there were any tell-tale lesions in the white matter areas called *white-matter hyperintensities* (WMH). WMH in the brain is considered a marker of vascular disease and is strongly associated with cognitive impairments that precede Alzheimer's disease.

The results: First, this study demonstrated that people who were currently eating the most choline performed better on tests of verbal and visual memory, compared with those who currently had the lowest choline intake. Researchers also found that those who had eaten the highest amounts of choline years earlier (as demonstrated by the first questionnaire) were more likely to have little or no WMH. In other words, eating lots of choline may make your memory sharper, and it also may reduce the risk for damage to the brain and even Alzheimer's disease.

How the Nutrient Protects Your Noggin

To learn more, we spoke with study coauthor Rhoda Au, PhD, associate professor of neurology at Boston University. Dr. Au emphasized that this is an observational study, so it doesn't prove cause and effect, but it does show a link between choline and memory. Why? Choline's crucial contribution to cognition, said Dr. Au, may be as a building block for a neurotransmitter called acetylcholine, which is known to help transmit information between neurons faster.

Diet "Dos"

How much choline do you need each day? The recommendation from the Institute of Medicine for men is a daily intake of 550 mg and for women, 425 mg. *The richest food sources are…*

- **3.5 ounces of beef liver—430 mg**
- **One large egg—126 mg**
- **3.5 ounces of salmon—91 mg**
- **3.5 ounces (just under one-half cup) of broccoli, Brussels sprouts, cauliflower or navy beans—approximately 40 mg.**

Other sources of choline include cod, almonds, tofu, milk and peanut butter.

Supplements of choline are available, but high doses (more than 3,500 mg per day for adults over age 18, according to Institute of Medicine) can cause symptoms like vomiting and excessive sweating. So if you want to take a supplement, talk to your doctor first—discuss how much you eat in your diet already so you can figure out whether (and what amount of) a supplement is necessary.

What's so exciting about this research is that while most studies concerning dementia are performed with people who already show signs of it, this study set out to investigate what people can do that might prevent dementia—and the choline connection seems promising. It's so easy to get more choline in our diets—it's in our refrigerators right now!

5 Surprising Ways to Prevent Alzheimer's

Marwan Sabbagh, MD, director of Banner Sun Health Research Institute, Sun City, Arizona. He is research professor of neurology at University of Arizona College of Medicine and associate director of the Arizona Alzheimer's Disease Center, both in Phoenix. He is author of *The Alzheimer's Prevention Cookbook: 100 Recipes to Boost Brain Health* (Ten Speed). *www.MarwanSabbaghMD.com*

Every 68 seconds, another American develops Alzheimer's disease, the fatal brain disease that steals memory and personality. It's the fifth-leading cause of death among people age 65 and older.

You can lower your likelihood of getting Alzheimer's disease by reducing controllable and well-known risk factors (see last paragraph on page 315). *But recent scientific research reveals that there are also little-known "secret" risk factors that you can address...*

Copper in Tap Water

A scientific paper published in *Journal of Trace Elements in Medicine and Biology* theorizes that inorganic copper found in nutritional supplements and in drinking water is an important factor in today's Alzheimer's epidemic.

Science has established that amyloid-beta plaques—inflammation-causing cellular debris found in the brains of people with Alzheimer's—contain high levels of copper.

Animal research shows that small amounts of inorganic copper in drinking water worsen Alzheimer's. Studies on people have linked the combination of copper and a high-fat diet to memory loss and mental decline. It may be that copper sparks amyloid-beta plaques to generate more oxidation and inflammation, further injuring brain cells.

What to do: There is plenty of copper in our diets—no one needs additional copper from a multivitamin/mineral supplement. Look for a supplement with no copper or a minimal amount (500 micrograms).

I also recommend filtering water. Water-filter pitchers, such as ones by Brita, can reduce the presence of copper. I installed a reverse-osmosis water filter in my home a few years ago when the evidence for the role of copper in Alzheimer's became compelling.

Vitamin D Deficiency

Mounting evidence shows that a low blood level of vitamin D may increase Alzheimer's risk.

A 2013 study in *Journal of Alzheimer's Disease* analyzed 10 studies exploring the link between vitamin D and Alzheimer's. Researchers found that low blood levels of vitamin D were linked to a 40% increased risk for Alzheimer's.

The researchers from UCLA, also writing in *Journal of Alzheimer's Disease*, theorize that vitamin D may protect the brain by reducing amyloid-beta and inflammation.

What to do: The best way to make sure that your blood level of vitamin D is protective is to ask your doctor to test it—and then, if needed, to help you correct your level to greater than 60 nanograms per milliliter (ng/mL). That correction may require 1,000 IU to 2,000 IU of vitamin D daily...or another individualized supplementation strategy.

Important: When your level is tested, make sure that it is the 25-hydroxyvitamin D, or 25(OH)D, test and not the 1.25-dihydroxyvitamin D test. The latter test does not accurately measure blood levels of vitamin D but is sometimes incorrectly ordered.

Also, ask for your exact numerical results. Levels above 30 ng/mL are considered "normal," but in my view, the 60 ng/mL level is the minimum that is protective.

Hormone Replacement Therapy After Menopause

Research shows that women who start hormone-replacement therapy (HRT) within five years of entering menopause and use hormones for 10 or more year might reduce the risk for Alzheimer's by 30%. But a more recent 11-year study of 1,768 women, published in *Neurology,* shows that those who started a combination of estrogen-progestin therapy five years or more after the onset of menopause had a 93% higher risk for Alzheimer's.

What to do: If you are thinking about initiating hormone replacement therapy five years or more after the onset of menopause, talk to your doctor about the possible benefits and risks.

A Concussion

A study published in *Neurology* in 2012 showed that NFL football players had nearly four times higher risk for Alzheimer's than the general population—no doubt from repeated brain injuries incurred while playing football.

What most people don't realize: Your risk of developing Alzheimer's is doubled if you've ever had a serious concussion that resulted in loss of consciousness—this newer evidence shows that it is crucially important to prevent head injuries of any kind throughout your life.

What to do: Fall-proof your home, with commonsense measures such as adequate lighting, eliminating or securing throw rugs and keeping stairways clear. Wear shoes with firm soles and low heels, which also helps prevent falls.

If you've ever had a concussion, it's important to implement the full range of Alzheimer's-prevention strategies in this article.

Not Having a Purpose in Life

In a seven-year study published in *Archives of General Psychiatry*, researchers at the Rush Alzheimer's Disease Center in Chicago found that people who had a "purpose in life" were 2.4 times less likely to develop Alzheimer's.

What to do: The researchers found that the people who agreed with the following statements were less likely to develop Alzheimer's and mild cognitive impairment—"I feel good when I think of what I have done in the past and what I hope to do in the future" and "I have a sense of direction and purpose in life."

If you cannot genuinely agree with the above statements, there are things you can do to change that—in fact, you even can change the way you feel about your past. It takes a bit of resolve…some action…and perhaps help from a qualified mental health counselor.

One way to start: Think about and make a list of some activities that would make your life more meaningful. Ask yourself, *Am I doing these?*…and then write down small, realistic goals that will involve you more in those activities, such as volunteering one hour every week at a local hospital or signing up for a class at your community college next semester.

Controllable Risk Factors…

The following steps are crucial in the fight against Alzheimer's disease…

- **Lose weight if you're overweight.**
- **Control high blood pressure.**
- **Exercise regularly.**
- **Engage in activities that challenge your mind.**
- **Eat a diet rich in colorful fruits and vegetables and low in saturated fat,** such as the Mediterranean diet.
- **Take a daily supplement containing 2,000 milligrams of omega-3 fatty acids.**

The Ultimate Brainpower Workout—Reduce Your Risk for Alzheimer's by 50%

John J. Ratey, MD, an associate clinical professor of psychiatry at Harvard Medical School and a psychiatrist at the Beth Israel-Deaconess Massachusetts Mental Health Center, both in Boston. He is author, with Eric Hagerman, of *Spark: The Revolutionary New Science of Exercise and the Brain* (Little, Brown). *www.SparkingLife.org*

We have known for a long time that exercise helps keep our bodies fit.

Now: More and more evidence shows that exercise also promotes brain fitness. For example, a study recently published in *Archives of Neurology* showed that moderate-intensity exercise reduced the odds of developing mild cognitive impairment, which often precedes Alzheimer's disease, by 30% to 40% in the 1,324 study participants (median age 80).

But what type of exercise does the best job of strengthening the brain, and how much is needed for optimal effect?

What you need to know...

The Aging Brain

After age 40, we lose about 5% of our brain cells (neurons) per decade—a process that often accelerates in those who are age 70 and older.

Since the average person has hundreds of billions of neurons, his/her cognitive reserves—that is, the brain's healthy cells that help compensate for damage by recruiting other brain areas to assist with tasks—may be sufficient to maintain mental agility...but not always.

The risk: Millions of Americans who are middle-aged and older start to "slip" in their mental capacities. Even if they have no signs of dementia, it may be harder for them to remember words, names or people than it once was. Or they may struggle to learn new information or take longer to think through problems and find solutions.

Why does this gradual mental decline affect some people much more than others?

Age-related loss of neurons, which affects all of us as we grow older, is just one factor. There's also a decline in dopamine, a neurotransmitter that controls motivation and motor function. This decline interferes with the electrical signals in the brain that allow the remaining neurons to communicate, which is necessary for memory, speech and other key brain functions.

Stronger Body, Bigger Brain

Scientists now know that the brain has plasticity, the ability to form new neurons and connections between neurons. This process can increase the brain's ability to take in information, process it and remember it.

What few people realize: Researchers have now identified a molecule—brain-derived neurotrophic factor (BDNF)—that's largely responsible for plasticity, and its levels increase dramatically with exercise. In animal studies at the University of California, Irvine, mice that exercised regularly were found to have BDNF levels that were about four times higher than those in sedentary mice. Many researchers think that humans show a similar increase.

The BDNF molecule could explain, in part, why people who exercise tend to have less memory loss, are less prone to anxiety and depression, and have up to a 50% lower risk of developing Alzheimer's disease or other forms of dementia than those who are sedentary.

Best exercises for the brain...

The Aerobic Formula

For overall fitness, the Centers for Disease Control and Prevention recommends doing some form of aerobic exercise, such as walking, for 30 minutes at least five days a week. But that's not enough for brain fitness.

Walking at an easy pace might increase your heart rate to about 50% of its maximum.

But this has little effect on the brain. For optimal brain benefits, you need to exercise hard enough so that your heart is pumping at 70% to 75% of its maximum rate.* Many treadmills have built-in heart-rate monitors, and heart-rate monitors that you wear are available at most pharmacies.

Good brands of heart-rate monitors: Garmin, Polar and Timex.

Important finding: One study published in *Archives of Neurology* found that people who walked or jogged on a treadmill for 35 minutes at a moderate intensity had improvements in cognitive flexibility (the ability to think flexibly and creatively, rather than merely repeating information) after just one session.

My advice: Exercise at a moderate intensity for 45 minutes to an hour, six days a week.

Remember, a moderate-intensity aerobic workout means elevating your heart rate to 70% to 75% of its maximum capacity. At this rate, you will most likely break a sweat and/or have difficulty carrying on a conversation. You can achieve this by jogging, bicycling, swimming or walking briskly—and then pushing yourself harder when the exercise starts to feel easy.

Example: Once you're comfortable walking for 45 minutes to an hour at the pace described above, increase the intensity by walking faster, swinging your arms or holding hand weights.

If a moderate intensity is too much for you, exercising at 60% of your maximum heart rate has also been shown to offer some improvement in cognitive health.

Cross Training

To add variety to your aerobic exercise regimen, try some form of cross training. It combines different forms of exercise to target various parts of the body. Circuit training, in

*To calculate your maximum heart rate, subtract your age from 220. The goal is to exercise at an intensity that raises your pulse to 70% to 75% of your maximum heart rate. The average 65-year-old man, for example, will need to raise his heart rate to about 108 to 116 beats per minute.

Did You Know...

Spouses of people with dementia are six times more likely to develop the illness? Increased risk may be caused by the stress associated with caring for a loved one struggling with dementia. Shared environmental factors such as diet also may be responsible.

Maria C. Norton, PhD, associate professor, department of family, consumer and human development, Utah State University, Logan, and leader of a study of 1,221 couples, published in *Journal of the American Geriatrics Society*.

which you move quickly from one exercise machine to the next without pausing, is one form of cross training. Another is swimming followed by fast walking.

Cross training is useful because it generally results in a prolonged elevation in heart rate, the critical factor for generating BDNF. Cross training is desirable because it challenges not only your aerobic capacity and strength but also calls upon parts of the brain that govern coordination, planning, etc.

My advice: Whenever possible, incorporate some form of cross training into your regular workouts. In addition, balance exercises are a good way to round out your regimen. Try to work balance exercises, such as tai chi or even any fast-paced form of dancing, into your schedule once or twice a week. These exercises are especially good because they increase your heart rate and require you to think about what you're doing.

Bonus: The social interaction that occurs in tai chi or dance classes and other group activities increases serotonin, a neurotransmitter that reduces anxiety and depression, both of which can impair cognitive functions.

The Power of Mood Workouts

Research shows that the hippocampus (the brain's memory center) is 15% smaller in depressed individuals than in those without depression. Exercise may be one of the most effective ways to reverse depression—perhaps because it influences the same neurochemicals that are affected by antidepressants.

My advice: If you suffer from depression, be sure to follow the exercise guidelines described above. This may allow you to reduce or even eliminate antidepressant medication.

Don't Forget Mental Workouts

Many different studies have shown that higher levels of education are associated with a decreased risk for dementia. But it doesn't matter where you went to school—or even if you went to school. The key factor is continued learning.

Like physical activity, mental workouts increase the number of connections between neurons that enhance memory and cognitive functions.

Perform mental workouts as often as possible.

Good choices: Try vocabulary quizzes, read books on subject matters you're not already familiar with or do any activity that requires you to push yourself intellectually.

Walk Your Way to a Sharp Mind

Cyrus Raji, MD, PhD, physician-scientist at the University of Pittsburgh and coauthor of a study on walking and cognitive decline.

We all want to know what steps we can take to protect memory and thinking skills as we age. Now data from an ongoing study suggests that one effective strategy is, quite literally, to take steps—in other words, to walk.

Background: Mild cognitive impairment refers to problems with thought processes, language, memory and judgment that are worse than typical age-related changes. More

Olive Oil Helps Your Memory

Saturated fat, such as that found in meat and cheese, contributes to declines in memory and cognition—but monounsaturated fat, like that in olive oil, seems to protect the brain.

Recent study: Women over age 65 who ate the most saturated fat were up to 65% more likely to experience cognitive decline over time than those who ate the least. Women who ate the most monounsaturated fat were 44% less likely to decline in verbal-memory scores and 48% less likely to decline in overall cognition.

Olivia I. Okereke, MD, associate psychiatrist, Brigham and Women's Hospital, Boston, and leader of a study of 6,183 women, published in *Annals of Neurology*.

severe is Alzheimer's disease, a progressive and irreversible disease that destroys memory and cognitive skills. About half of people diagnosed with mild cognitive impairment eventually develop Alzheimer's.

Recent research: Participants included 426 seniors. At the start of the study, 299 of the seniors were healthy, 83 had mild cognitive impairment and 44 had Alzheimer's. Researchers monitored how far participants walked each week...did 3-D MRI scans to measure changes in brain volume (decreases indicate that brain cells have shrunk or died)...and analyzed results of exams that track cognitive decline over time.

Findings after 10 years: To maintain brain volume and slow down cognitive decline, healthy seniors needed to walk an average of about six miles per week...those who had already had cognitive impairment needed to walk about five miles per week.

Bottom line: Walking cannot cure Alzheimer's disease, but it can improve the brain's resistance to this devastating condition. So start taking those steps today!

A Drug That Slows Alzheimer's Progression

The experimental medicine *solanezumab* improved cognitive skills among patients with mild Alzheimer's disease by 34%. The drug is still in late-stage testing. Solanezumab is one of several experimental medicines designed to remove the "sticky" protein beta-amyloid from the brain. Beta-amyloid is believed to have a toxic effect on brain function.

Study by researchers at Baylor College of Medicine, Houston, and the Alzheimer's Disease Cooperative Study, which reported the results of solanezumab testing on 2,052 patients at a recent meeting of the American Neurological Association in Boston.

The Spice That Could Keep Alzheimer's Away

Muralidhar Hegde, PhD, research scientist, and Sankar Mitra, PhD, professor of biochemistry and molecular biology, University of Texas Medical Branch, Galveston, Texas.

A recent study says that a common kitchen spice may help sweep something called cellular metal toxicity from the brain—specifically excessive amounts of iron and copper, which have been linked to diseases such as Alzheimer's and Parkinson's.

The common spice is turmeric and it contains the brain-boosting phytochemical called curcumin. The intriguing study comes from the University of Texas Medical Branch in Galveston—it was published in *Journal of Biological Chemistry*. We've been learning for years that this phytochemical can prevent and treat many diseases, such as certain cancers, but this is the first study to suggest that curcumin is also beneficial to the brain.

Sweeping Away Metals

Lead study author Muralidhar Hegde, PhD, and senior author Sankar Mitra, PhD, noted that our bodies naturally contain trace amounts of certain metals, including copper and iron. In small amounts, these metals are not only harmless but essential for good health. But some people's brain cells—for reasons that scientists don't yet completely understand—start accumulating large amounts of copper or iron, which can wreak havoc.

If you have a large amount of iron and copper in your brain cells, the extra "free" metals overwhelm the proteins that are supposed to store them and start causing two major problems. First, they initiate chemical reactions that lead to DNA damage. And then, to make matters worse, Dr. Hegde and colleagues found, they also interfere with DNA repair enzymes that attempt to fix the damage. Since too much unrepaired DNA damage can lead to neurodegenerative disorders, that's one scary situation.

The Wonder Spice

But it's not all doom and gloom. The researchers tested several chemicals called metal chelators and natural dietary and/or plant components in petri dishes to see if any of the substances would help keep iron and copper stored so they wouldn't interfere with the DNA repair enzymes. All the substances tested worked to some extent, but there was one that worked better than all the rest—curcumin. "Curcumin appeared to stop the metals from blocking the DNA repair by more than 90% to 95%—so it essentially reversed the damage to the genetic material," said Dr. Hegde.

A natural remedy that may help stave off Alzheimer's disease is exciting to think about—but, said Dr. Hegde, it's important to keep the nature of this particular finding in context. Animal testing is in order to confirm that curcumin is an effective treatment and to know exactly how much curcumin belongs in the ideal dose, then researchers can move on to human studies.

In the meantime, since what we are talking about is just a common spice, what can't hurt—and might greatly help—is to consume greater quantities of curcumin in foods like Indian and Asian dishes.

Coconut Oil May Fight Alzheimer's

Coconut oil may fight Alzheimer's disease and other cognitive disorders.

Theory: A brain compromised by Alzheimer's does not use glucose efficiently. Coconut oil helps the brain compensate for its reduced ability to use glucose as fuel. Several studies have shown promising results, but more research is needed. In the meantime, substituting several tablespoons of coconut oil for other vegetable oils in cooking and salads cannot hurt.

Preferred brand: Source Naturals, *www. SourceNaturals.com*.

Andrew L. Rubman, ND, founder and director of Southbury Clinic for Traditional Medicines, Southbury, Connecticut. *www.Naturopath.org*

Having a Purpose in Life Prevents Dementia

Patricia A. Boyle, PhD, neuropsychologist, Rush Alzheimer's Disease Center, and associate professor, department of behavioral sciences, Rush University Medical Center, both in Chicago. Her study was published in *Archives of General Psychiatry*.

You already know that staying physically and mentally active may help stave off dementia, but researchers have found yet another protective trick—having a purpose in life.

Now, this doesn't mean having a goal that has a definite end point, such as telling yourself that you'll run a marathon or write a novel.

For brain protection, having a purpose in life is a little bit different.

What are some examples of "purposes," and how can you figure out what yours is if you don't already have one?

Warding Off Brain Fog

The good news is that figuring out your life's purpose is not that hard to do. *First, here's what the study found…*

Researchers analyzed 246 senior citizens who received annual cognitive testing for about 10 years. Each was asked questions to determine whether he or she had a strong purpose in life. When participants died, they underwent brain autopsies.

What the researchers found was that in participants who had a lot of plaques and tangles in their brains—abnormal structures in and around the brain's nerve cells that are hallmarks of Alzheimer's disease—the rate of cognitive decline had been about 30% slower for people who had a strong purpose in life compared with those who had had a weaker purpose or no purpose at all.

Here's what these findings could mean: The stronger your purpose in life, the less likely you'll suffer cognitive decline as you age, even if your brain is affected by Alzheimer's signs.

Of course, it could be the other way around—it could be that some people have a biological problem that makes them less able to cope with brain plaques and tangles and, also, less able to feel that their lives have purpose.

Go for It Anyway

When we spoke with lead study author Patricia A. Boyle, PhD, a neuropsychologist in the Alzheimer's Disease Center at Rush University Medical Center in Chicago, she acknowledged that her study doesn't prove whether purposefulness helps our brains work better or is simply a side effect of a brain that is already working better. Maybe research will determine that one day. But on the other hand, since having a sense of purpose seems to make people happier, she said, why not cultivate one?

Based on her work with the study subjects, Dr. Boyle defines a life purpose as "the sense that one's life has meaning and direction—that one is intentional and motivated to engage in activities that one finds important and fulfilling." In other words, it's what gets you out of bed each day and makes you feel that life is worth living.

A purpose doesn't have to be ambitious or complicated. In fact, many purposes are simple, said Dr. Boyle. It just can't have a definite end point—it has to last throughout your life. For example, some purposes include spending time every day with loved ones…helping other people (for example through long-term volunteer work)…learning something new every day…or passing down a certain set of knowledge or skills to a younger generation. If you love running marathons or writing novels, as mentioned earlier, make sure that your goal is to continue pursuing those goals through life—and not just run one marathon or write one novel.

It's not so much what your purpose is, Dr. Boyle said—what's critical is how it makes you feel. If it stirs you up inside and makes you feel passionate, energetic and excited, then you've found it!

Omega-3s Boost Brain Power

According to a recent finding, people with low blood levels of omega-3 fatty acids had smaller brain volumes and performed more poorly on tests of visual memory, abstract memory and executive function than people with high levels. Omega-3s are found in fatty fish and can be taken as supplements.

Study of 1,575 dementia-free people, average age 67, by researchers at University of California, Los Angeles, published in *Neurology*.

Brain Stimulation for Alzheimer's

Ten Alzheimer's patients received a placebo or repetitive transcranial magnetic

Hormone Replacement Therapy (HRT) May Reduce Alzheimer's Risk

Recent finding: Women who take hormones within five years of menopause have a 30% lower risk for Alzheimer's, compared with women who never take them. The issue of HRT remains complex and controversial—discuss your personal situation with your doctor.

Study of 1,768 women by researchers at Johns Hopkins Bloomberg School of Public Health, Baltimore, published in *Neurology*.

stimulation (rTMS), which applies magnetic pulses to the brain at high frequencies.

Result: The rTMS group improved sentence-comprehension test scores by 11%, while the placebo group showed no change. Benefits lasted for up to eight weeks.

If a loved one has Alzheimer's: Ask the patient's doctor about rTMS—it is available at several US hospitals and research centers.

Maria Cotelli, PhD, researcher, Centro San Giovanni di Dio Fatebenefratelli, Brescia, Italy

Learn Another Language for a Better Brain

When researchers examined clinical records of 211 adults diagnosed with probable Alzheimer's disease, those who spoke multiple languages over their lifetimes showed initial Alzheimer's symptoms an average of five years later than those who spoke one language.

Theory: Bilingual people build concentration skills by focusing on the language they are speaking while minimizing interference from a second language.

If you are bilingual: It's not enough to hear or read a second language—contact libraries, universities and cultural centers to find groups that converse. If you are not bilingual, learning a second language can help promote brain health.

Fergus Craik, PhD, senior scientist, The Rotman Research Institute, Toronto, Canada.

Nicotine for the Brain?

A study of nonsmokers with mild cognitive impairment found that nicotine patches restored 46% of normal, long-term memory within six months.

Theory: Nicotine stimulates brain receptors involved in thinking and memory.

Neurology

Help for Severe Alzheimer's

The drug *donepezil*—already prescribed for mild-to-moderate-stage Alzheimer's symptoms—preserves cognitive function in late-stage alzheimer's patients as well.

Sleep Well

Poor sleep is linked to Alzheimer's disease. People who wake up frequently (more than five times in an hour) or who are awake for more than 15% of the time that they are in bed are significantly more likely than better sleepers to show physiological changes associated with early Alzheimer's disease.

Not yet known: Whether it is poor sleep that causes the brain changes—or vice versa.

Yo-El Ju, MD, assistant professor of neurology and a sleep medicine specialist at Washington University School of Medicine, St. Louis, and leader of a study presented at the American Academy of Neurology's 2012 annual meeting.

Recent finding: 63% of patients who took donepezil exhibited stable or improved memory, language, attention and recognition of their own names. The donepezil users also showed slower declines in overall social functioning than the placebo users.

Sandra E. Black, MD, professor of neurology, Sunnybrook Health Sciences Centre, University of Toronto, canada, and leader of a study of 343 people, published in *Neurology*.

Memory Loss May Soon Be Reversible

Amy Arnsten, PhD, professor of neurobiology and psychology at Yale School of Medicine, New Haven, Connecticut. Dr. Arnsten is a member of Yale's Kavli Institute of Neuroscience, a group that focuses on innovative approaches to study of the human brain.

If you can't remember where you put your glasses or the last name of the couple that you've just been introduced to, be sure to remember this one word—*guanfacine*. It's the name of a drug, currently used to treat high blood pressure, attention deficit hyperactivity disorder (ADHD) and anxiety, that might be able to reverse a major type of short-term memory loss in older people, according to a recent study. That's right—reverse memory loss. Even if an elderly person's ability to remember has deteriorated over 15 or 20 years, doctors may soon be able to prescribe guanfacine to restore the memory to the way it was during young adulthood. Now, we're not talking about memory loss due to Alzheimer's disease or other forms of dementia—we're talking about the loss of working memory, which occurs in nearly everyone, sometimes starting as early as age 50 and almost certainly after the mid-60s.

We spoke with Amy Arnsten, PhD, the study's lead researcher and a professor of neurobiology and psychology at Yale University School of Medicine in New Haven, Connecticut, to find out how this drug works.

Unlocking Secrets of Memory

Prior studies have shown that the faster neurons fire, the better the working memory. What Dr. Arnsten and her colleagues explored is how aging affects the firing of the neurons—and whether guanfacine might help speed up the firing.

For the study, she gathered six rhesus monkeys of three different age groups. Two were "young adults," two were "middle-aged" and two were "aged." The monkeys played a game that required them to remember the locations of objects on computer screens. During the game, a tiny electrode that had been painlessly inserted into each monkey's prefrontal cortex allowed researchers to monitor their brain function. Compared with the young adult monkeys, the neurons in the middle-aged and aged monkeys fired more slowly.

Earlier tests done by Dr. Arnsten's lab had shown that neurons in the prefrontal cortex of humans and other animals fire more slowly when there's a buildup there of a substance called cyclic adenosine monophosphate (cAMP). So in this study, researchers injected the monkeys with guanfacine, which is known to inhibit the production of cAMP in the prefrontal cortex. Afterward, neuron firing doubled, on average, in both the middle-aged and aged monkeys, compared with the firing speed of their neurons when they weren't given the guanfacine injection. These results appeared in *Nature*.

From Monkeys to Humans

The question remains: Would guanfacine have the same effect on humans? Dr. Arnsten said that she and her colleagues are optimistic because the prefrontal cortex functions similarly in both species. In fact, researchers at Yale have already begun clinical trials on the effect of guanfacine on the working memory of people age 75 or older (who don't suffer from dementia or Alzheimer's). Results of these tests are expected in the near future.

Meanwhile, there's the question of whether guanfacine could or should be prescribed now, off-label, for memory loss. Dr. Arnsten thinks that it's too early to try this—because it hasn't yet been proven to reduce memory loss in humans.

For the Alzheimer's Caregiver...Finally... There's a Way to Connect with a Loved One Who Has Dementia

Gerontologist Tom Brenner, MA, cofounder, with his wife, Karen Brenner, MA, of Brenner Pathways, a consulting and educational company in Chicago that specializes in the Montessori Method for Positive Dementia Care, *www.BrennerPathways.org*. He and his wife are also coauthors of *You Say Goodbye and We Say Hello: The Montessori Method for Positive Dementia Care* (Brenner Pathways).

Henry had been diagnosed with early-onset Alzheimer's and was quiet and withdrawn. When he was younger, he had collected vintage cars, so his caregiver gave him some old hubcaps and polish. After 30 minutes of polishing, Henry began talking with a great deal of emotion about his time as a soldier. Perhaps the process of polishing the hubcaps reminded him of polishing his boots, and an important memory was triggered. This activity enabled Henry and his caregiver to connect, even if only for a short time.

One of the most heartbreaking and frustrating aspects of caring for a loved one with dementia is the loss of meaningful interaction.

But there's good news on this front: The Montessori Method for Positive Dementia Care, a nondrug approach (often used in combination with medication), is now being used by some caregivers in home-care settings and nursing homes with dramatic results.

Through basic Montessori principles (see next page), this method offers ways to be in the moment with a dementia patient and possibly have a deep connection. Patients become more secure, confident and calm. And caregivers are less likely to get frustrated and burn out.

Recent research: In a study involving nine residential facilities in Melbourne, Australia, dementia patients were two times more actively engaged when participating in Montessori-based activities than when they were not doing these activities.

Background: Developed more than 100 years ago as a method of teaching "unreachable" children with learning disabilities, the Montessori approach encourages the use of all five senses to stimulate different areas of the brain and the use of "muscle memory"* to develop small-muscle coordination and promote confidence. The Montessori method also advocates an environment that meets the specific physical and emotional needs of those using it.

Montessori classrooms for children are uncluttered but homey and filled with natural light and materials to promote use of the senses. Students are free to move about and engage in activities that appeal most to them. This sets the stage for focused and calm activity. Research has shown that Montessori pupils learn to excel at problem solving, adapting to change and social skills—all areas that are difficult for adults with dementia.

Key Montessori tenets and how they can help dementia patients...

•**Emphasis on environment.** The surroundings of the dementia patient should be familiar and comforting and designed to foster as much independence as possible. For example, the layout of a facility, or your home if a loved one is living with you, should be uncomplicated so there is less potential for confusion. Visual cues, such as large-print labeling indicating what can be found in drawers, are also very helpful. Clutter should be minimized, but the use of natural elements—such as plants, pictures of nature,

---

*Sometimes called procedural memory, this involves physical movements fixed into memory through repetition (think of riding a bike or playing a musical instrument).

Best Way to Fight Memory Loss

The combination of computer use and exercise is better than mental or physical activity alone. The exact reason is not yet known, but it may be that physical activity improves blood flow to the brain and therefore delivers more nutrients...while mental activity works at the molecular level to boost synaptic activities.

Yonas E. Geda, MD, MSc, a neuropsychiatrist at Mayo Clinic, Scottsdale, Arizona, and leader of a study of 926 people, ages 70 to 93, published in *Mayo Clinic Proceedings.*

---

natural lighting, etc.—can induce a feeling of calm.

•**Muscle memory stimulation.** While the mind of a dementia patient might be faltering, the muscles often "remember" how to do an activity that was done repetitively and enjoyably in the past. The key is to discover a patient's unique strengths, passions and interests—not only tapping muscle memory but strong emotions as well. Focusing on a physical task and having success helps dementia patients feel more secure and confident and less angry and agitated.

A caregiver might take a former golfer to the driving range to jump-start his/her muscle memory. Or a long-retired handyman might be given a toolbox with a tape measure, paintbrushes and a level so that he can tinker.

These activities also build muscle coordination and can simply make life more pleasant and enriching for a dementia patient.

•**Sharing stories.** This is one of the most effective tools for helping dementia sufferers stay connected. Moments when patients share their stories, even if the time is fleeting, can enable the patient and caregiver to feel a deep connection, boosting the patient's sense of security.

To encourage a patient to share a story: A caregiver might give him a meaningful object to hold—something important from the patient's life or an object from nature. This simple act can help spark a memory and get the patient talking.

• **Art therapy.** Painting, singing and playing an instrument can provide patients new avenues of self-expression and strengthen their spirits. These activities also can give patients the opportunity to engage their senses.

Good activity: Flower arranging. Patients are encouraged to feel and smell the flowers, cut stems and pour water. This exercise calls on small motor skills, essential for independence and range of motion. Key areas of the brain are also exercised when deciding how to arrange the flowers.

• **The Knobbed Cylinder.** This classic Montessori tool—a long wooden block with 10 different-sized holes in which the user places matching cylinders—builds focus and small-muscle coordination. Dementia patients might be asked to fill only two holes—the point is for the patient to feel success and build confidence through this activity.

• **Finish a phrase.** Old sayings may never leave our minds. With this technique, the caregiver holds up the first half of a statement on a piece of paper ("The whole nine...") and asks the patient to finish the saying ("...yards"). It's astonishing to see dementia sufferers suddenly become very vocal and involved.

Benefits for the caregivers: The Montessori method gives the caregiver more tools to care for a dementia patient. It encourages the caregiver to use his imagination and allows him to act more like a guide than a director. Plus, patients are less agitated and aggressive, so they are easier to be with. All this helps minimize caregiver burnout and frustration.

Try out a few of these exercises with your loved one. To find a facility that offers this specific approach, you'll need to ask the director of the center you are considering.

How to Cope with Behavior Problems

Victor A. Molinari, PhD, a psychologist and professor in the department of aging and mental health disparities at Florida Mental Health Institute of the University of South Florida in Tampa. He is coeditor with Sheila LoboPrabhu, MD, and James Lomax, MD, of *Supporting the Caregiver in Dementia* (Johns Hopkins University Press).

Alzheimer's disease robs its victims not only of memories and mental skills, but also of the ability to control their behavior. This leaves family caregivers struggling to cope with their loved ones' behavioral problems—and even can provoke regrettable behavior from frustrated caregivers themselves. *Why this happens...*

• **Nine out of 10 Alzheimer's disease patients display behavioral and psychological symptoms,** such as yelling, restlessness and/or delusions, at some point. Often family members are on the receiving end of verbal or physical aggression. For caregivers who are constantly giving of themselves, this can be very upsetting.

• **Spending an average of 100 hours a week taking care of a loved one** leaves caregivers with no time to exercise or see friends. Isolation is one reason why depression is more common among caregivers than noncaregivers.

• **Family caregivers often deplete their own finances to handle their loved ones' needs.** Caregivers with full-time jobs miss more than three weeks of work per year, on average...20% quit their jobs. The financial burden is extremely stressful.

As the strain mounts, many caregivers cannot help lashing out.

Recent study: 52% of people caring for a relative with dementia admit to screaming at, swearing at or threatening their loved ones. Caregivers then feel guilty—which adds to their stress. *What helps...*

Working With the Doctor

The more effectively you can communicate with your loved one's doctor, the more likely the patient is to receive treatment that minimizes behavioral difficulties. *Ask the doctor about…*

•**Cholinesterase inhibitors.** These prescription drugs, such as *donepezil* (Aricept) and *rivastigmine* (Exelon), generally are used to treat cognitive symptoms of Alzheimer's.

Recent finding: These drugs also reduce behavioral and psychological symptoms, such as aggression, wandering and paranoia.

How: Alzheimer's patients have depleted levels of acetylcholine, a brain chemical that helps with cognition, memory and judgment. By raising acetylcholine, cholinesterase inhibitors promote communication between nerve cells, stabilizing or even improving symptoms. If your loved one experiences digestive upset with one drug, consider trying a different one.

•**Sleep disorders.** Up to 80% of Alzheimer's patients have sleep apnea (frequent halts in breathing during sleep). Apnea reduces oxygen in the brain, impairs cognition and causes sleep deprivation—all of which can negatively impact behavior.

Promising: Patients showed cognitive improvement after three weeks of continuous positive airway pressure (CPAP) treatment. The CPAP machine provides pressurized air via a face mask worn during sleep.

Handling Problem Behaviors

Practical strategies help reduce negative behaviors. *Here's how to deal with your loved ones…*

•**Agitation.** Alzheimer's patients often get upset, act restless or pace around. Keep a log to help you identify circumstances that provoke these reactions, then develop a plan to work around such triggers.

Example: If your loved one gets upset when you try to bathe him in the morning, try it in the afternoon instead. Once you find a routine that is comfortable for your loved one, stick with it. Isolation and understimulation also can provoke agitation, so try to keep your loved one active and engaged during the day—for instance, by listening to music or going for a walk together.

•**Aggression.** Shouting, shoving and hitting can be signs of frustration or pain.

To avoid triggers: Protect your loved one from overstimulation (from clutter or noise)…confusion (from being given too many instructions)…and physical discomfort (from medication side effects or an unnoticed injury).

Soothing: Try to maintain a calm and reassuring demeanor, refrain from arguing or lecturing—and don't take your loved one's behavior personally.

•**Wandering.** Place a large, solid-colored, dark, rubber-backed mat in front of each door to the outside. Your loved one probably won't remember if you say not to go past that point—but mats act as visual deterrents, discouraging an Alzheimer's patient from leaving home unattended.

Also: Install sliding bolts high enough on each door that a person must reach up to unlock them (but not so high as to impede the family's departure in an emergency, such as a fire). Chances are that a person with advanced Alzheimer's will not figure out how to open them.

Useful tool: The Alzheimer's Association Comfort Zone program includes a GPS-like service that alerts you (via telephone or the Internet) to your loved one's location.

Information: 877-259-4850, *www.alz.org/ ComfortZone.*

•**Nighttime restlessness.** Many Alzheimer's patients suffer disturbances in circadian rhythms that affect sleep cycles and alertness. Keep the house brightly lit between 7 pm and 9 pm each evening…then help your loved one get ready for bed, following a consistent routine. This helps normalize his/her body clock, improving sleep and decreasing nocturnal disturbances.

Finding Support

Compared with caregivers who get little support from others, those who get the most support keep their loved ones at home longer...feel healthier...and find caregiving more rewarding. *Best...*

• **Ask family and friends for help.** Be specific. Instead of saying, "Can you help me out sometime?" say, "Can you watch Mom for three hours on Monday?" Having even a few hours off a week helps significantly.

• **Contact support organizations.** The Alzheimer's Association (800-272-3900, *www.alz.org*) offers a toll-free helpline, guidance on financial and legal matters, online message boards, information on local support groups and more.

Also helpful: Alzheimer's Disease Education and Referral Center (800-438-4380, *www.nia.nih.gov/Alzheimers*).

• **Consider professional aid.** Your local Alzheimer's Association office can connect you with geriatric health professionals, meal-delivery programs, adult day-care centers and respite-care providers (who come to your home so you can have time off).

• **Recognize the rewards.** Many family caregivers report that they receive significant emotional benefits from taking care of their loved ones. You can, too, if you allow yourself to take pride in your ability to help and to find joy in your deepened sense of devotion.

How to Stay Connected to a Loved One with Alzheimer's

Marjory Abrams, chief content officer, Bottom Line newsletters (Boardroom Inc., 281 Tresser Blvd., Stamford, Connecticut 06901), with Nancy Pearce, author of *Inside Alzheimer's* (Forrason Press).

The news that a friend or relative has Alzheimer's disease is not only devastating—it also can be intimidating.

Most people don't quite know what to say or do when they are with the person. Yet there are specific ways you can stay close with the loved one and contribute to his/her ongoing comfort and serenity, says medical social worker Nancy Pearce, author of *Inside Alzheimer's: How to Hear and Honor Connections with a Person Who Has Dementia* (*http://dev.forrasonpress.com/*). She offers the following guidelines, which work whether the person was recently diagnosed or is now quite impaired...

• **Decide to connect.** Before every visit, think about what might be getting in the way of interacting with this person. Often it's our innermost feelings, such as, This is just so sad or This is too hard. Such thinking distracts us from being truly present.

• **Another obstacle to connection is how you communicate nonverbally.** A person with dementia still can feel your tensions, distractions or apathy because these are broadcast through your stance and voice. Before you go into the room, take a moment and breathe deeply to release tension.

• **Let go of rigid thinking, and think about what is best for the person.** Here's an example—Pearce once worked with a 92-year-old man who every day anxiously asked for his mother—and every time was told that she had died. Each day, he grieved anew. His caregivers meant well, but their concern with accuracy actually was cruel. When his caregivers realized what really was behind the request—the need to feel taken care of—they were able to make the patient's life much more peaceful. For example, when he wanted his mother to do something for him, his caregivers let him know that she could not be there at that time, but that they would help him instead.

• **Open your heart and enter the person's world,** rather than getting caught up in the nuts and bolts of the disease by asking about symptoms and so on. Pearce knew a man with dementia whose longtime golf buddy picked him up every week to play. When the man could no longer hit the ball, his friend found other things for him to do at the golf course—drive the cart or clean the balls—so they still could happily share their mutual interest. There was another woman whose beloved grandmother had Alzheimer's, and as a result, the grandmother often was angry. After much trial and error, the woman learned that what opened both their hearts was to watch old movies together.

• **Embrace silence.** When it comes to talking, less can be more, especially for people who may be frustrated about losing their ability to speak and comprehend. You don't have to fill every silence with conversation.

• **Express gratitude.** No matter how advanced the disease, notice and thank the person for all the little things you appreciate about being with him. You might simply thank him for allowing you the time spent together.

With Dementia, a Little Humor Goes a Long Way

Peter Spitzer, MB BS, Churchill Fellow, a physician in private practice, and medical director and cofounder of the Humour Foundation, Australia.

Humor therapy has long been practiced with children in hospitals. To see whether it could also help dementia patients, staff at The Humour Foundation in Australia trained health-care workers in humor therapy and then sent them to three dozen nursing homes in and around the city of Sydney to treat several hundred residents. All the residents had dementia, some had agitation and some were taking antipsychotic meds. The workers performed humor therapy for two hours a week for 12 weeks, usually one-on-one with a patient.

To learn more about what the health-care staffers did and how effective the therapy was, we contacted one of the lead investigators, Peter Spitzer, MD, medical director and cofounder of the Humour Foundation.

Mainstream humor—like the kind that dementia patients see on TV sitcoms and talk shows—doesn't really connect with them, said Dr. Spitzer, so health-care workers had to "find the key that would open the door to the patients' humor." During each session, the workers would wear red clown noses and attempt to engage patients by using mime, music, massage, touch, stories and magic tricks. In many cases, they would ask a simple question like, "Which way is the bathroom?"…and then, after the patient gave the correct answer, the worker would play the fool and purposefully walk in the wrong direction. This might elicit a laugh—but there was another positive effect, too. For patients who have already lost so much independence, this type of humorous play can give them a brief but uplifting sense of personal power and control, said Dr. Spitzer.

The study didn't just make patients smile—its results made the researchers smile. Immediately after 12 weeks of humor therapy—and even six months after treatment ended—frequency of overall patient agitation as measured by standard psychological surveys was down by 20%, on average, compared with measurements taken at the beginning of the study. Since the patient population included some people who were already being treated for agitation with antipsychotic meds, the results are promising—especially because they seem to last, which is remarkable. "These findings suggest that humor therapy may be as effective as antipsychotic drugs in reducing agitation—while providing more happiness and no dangerous side effects," said Dr. Spitzer. Controlled studies that compare antipsychotic medications to humor therapy need to be done in the future.

Make a Patient Laugh

Right now, one of the few organizations in the US providing humor therapy for seniors in nursing homes is Big Apple Circus's Vaudeville Caravan in Chicago and Montrose, New York. Dr. Spitzer suspects that as more "psychosocial" research is done with dementia patients, more resources will become available. Dr. Spitzer added that humor therapy could be effective in a residential setting, too. So if you're caring for a dementia patient at home who has agitation, Dr. Spitzer said to try goofy humor to play and ease symptoms—even if you don't have formal training—so you can bring a smile to your loved one's face.

Brain-Power Boost for Dementia Patients

Bob Woods, MSc, professor of clinical psychology of the elderly and codirector of the Dementia Services Development Centre Wales at Bangor University in Bangor, Wales, and lead author of a study on dementia published in *Cochrane Database of Systemic Reviews*.

Mastering a new language, learning to play a musical instrument and other such complex mental tasks may help keep our brains sharp as we age—and may even provide some protection against dementia. But what about less challenging activities, such as putting together puzzles, tending to plants or chatting about the past? Such pursuits are pleasurable, sure...but can they protect brain power for those who need help most—people who already have dementia?

Researchers from the UK decided to find out by pooling the results of 15 randomized controlled trials involving a total of 718 patients with mild-to-moderate dementia. Patients in the various studies' cognitive stimulation groups participated in a wide range of activities that aimed to stimulate thinking and memory generally. Examples included discussing past and present events, playing word games, doing jigsaw puzzles, listening to music, baking and indoor gardening. Typically these were done as group activities involving trained staff plus a handful of dementia patients, though in some cases family caregivers provided the cognitive stimulation to their relatives on a one-to-one basis. Activities averaged 45 minutes, three times per week...and continued for anywhere from one month to two years.

Findings: Patients who participated in the cognitive stimulation activities reported improved quality of life and well-being...were found to communicate and interact with others better than they had previously...and their scores on tests of memory and thinking improved, too. The beneficial effects were seen not only at the end of treatment, but also during the study follow-up periods, which ranged from one to three months.

Brain gain: If a loved one has mild-to-moderate dementia, make a point of initiating stimulating discussions and involving the person in interesting group activities.

Protect yourself, too: Even for people who don't have dementia, lack of cognitive stimulation appears to hasten mental decline over the years—so pull out the jigsaw puzzles and Scrabble board and invite a few friends over for some brain-building fun.

PHYSICAL INJURY

It's hard to imagine falls being as serious as diseases like cancer and heart disease, but the reality is that one-third of people over 65 fall each year. Those falls can result in everything from minor injuries like cuts and sprains to serious problems such as hip fractures and head trauma. The good news is that you can prevent most of these injuries by getting your eyes checked, making your home safer and doing exercises that improve balance. Keep reading for more ways to prevent falls.

Chapter 18

SECRETS TO STAYING STEADY ON YOUR FEET

The Injury-Prone Time of the Month

When we women talk about "that time of the month," we're usually referring to our periods, with the accompanying physical hassles and emotional upheavals. But there is another time in the menstrual cycle that should be on our radar—ovulation. We're not talking about getting pregnant (though fertility generally does peak at this time as the ovary releases a mature egg). Instead, we want to caution you about an increased risk for injury, particularly during exercise.

Reason: Around the time of ovulation, the increases in levels of hormones such as estrogen and relaxin that allow the egg to pop through the ovarian capsule also cause a loosening and stretching of ligaments and tendons. These are the same hormones that, late in pregnancy, help loosen a woman's pelvic ligaments in preparation for childbirth.

"Women who participate in intense exercise in the days around ovulation are at heightened risk for tearing any area where connective tissue may be aggressively stretched by a movement or an impact during sports," explained Andrew L. Rubman, ND, medical director of the Southbury Clinic for Traditional Medicines in Southbury, Connecticut. Vulnerable areas include the shoulders, knees, ankles and back.

A woman typically ovulates mid-cycle. The first day of your period is considered day one, so if your cycle lasts 28 days, ovulation is likely to occur around day 14—though it could happen earlier or later. Dr. Rubman noted that the peak injury-prone time lasts from a day before until a day after ovulation.

Self-defense: There's no need to avoid exercise entirely during this time, Dr. Rubman said, but you should take added precautions against injury. *Here's how…*

• **Be extra-sure to warm up before working out…**and to cool down and stretch afterward.

• **For weight lifting, use somewhat lighter weights than usual.** You can make up for this by increasing the number of repetitions.

• **Avoid sports that involve sudden angular movements that would challenge tendons and ligaments,** such as tennis and basketball—or at least try not to play full-out.

Andrew L. Rubman, ND, is founder and medical director of the Southbury Clinic for Traditional Medicines in Southbury, Connecticut. *www.Southbury Clinic.com*

• **Focus on gentle stretching and low-impact activities such as bicycling, swimming and walking.**

Not Sure When You're Ovulating?

Watch for these signs: Lower abdominal discomfort or an ache in the general area of your ovaries (a sensation called mittelschmerz)…and/or vaginal secretions that increase in amount and that change from just wet to tacky and slippery (similar in look and feel to uncooked egg whites). If you still can't tell, take your temperature with a basal thermometer first thing every morning before getting out of bed—temperature rises slightly during ovulation. Charting your daily temperature for a few months will familiarize you with the rhythms of your cycle.

Don't Get Hurt When Working Out at Home

Barbara Bushman, PhD, professor in the department of kinesiology at Missouri State University in Springfield, a fellow of the American College of Sports Medicine (ACSM) and editor of *ACSM's Complete Guide to Fitness and Health* (Human Kinetics).

Exercising in the comfort of your own home is convenient and can save a bundle in gym fees over time. But there's a potential downside, too, and it has to do with safety—because unlike at a good gym, at home there's no professional trainer correcting your improper technique or making sure damaged equipment gets repaired. When it comes to treadmills, multistation home-gym machines and stationary bikes, the risks can be substantial.

We spoke with Barbara Bushman, PhD, a professor in the department of kinesiology at Missouri State University, to discuss strategies that can keep you safe when you're using major home exercise equipment. (For safety tips when using simple home exercise equipment, such as hand weights, resistance bands, balance boards and fitness balls, see page 335.) *What you need to know about using a…*

• **Treadmill.** The treadmill causes more injuries than any other type of exercise equipment, according to the Consumer Product Safety Commission.

• If your treadmill has a safety cord that clips to your clothing, be sure to use it (and if your unit does not have this feature, consider upgrading to one that does). At one end of the cord is a key that plugs into the treadmill. If you lose your footing and fall, the cord disengages from the machine, shutting off the treadmill automatically. Without this safety feature, you could wind up having your face sandpapered by the treadmill's moving belt.

• Familiarize yourself with your treadmill's speed and grade options. Incorrectly manipulating the controls could cause the treadmill to speed up or raise its incline when you were expecting to go slower or lower, Dr. Bushman warned—and that could send you flying.

• Use caution when placing towels, magazines, water bottles or other objects on the console at the front of the treadmill. An object that drops onto the treadmill could wind up underfoot, causing you to trip.

• **Multistation Home-Gym Machine.** These combination units are designed to provide a full-body workout—which means they have many moving parts that can cause injury if the equipment is improperly assembled or maintained.

• It is worth paying extra to have a professional set up your unit, Dr. Bushman said. If you're buying a new multistation, ask the store manager whether professional assembly is included in the purchase price—and confirm that the job won't be done by an untrained deliveryman. For help putting together a used unit or to make sure that yours has been assembled correctly, check with a local store that sells similar equipment.

• Even with all the nuts and bolts in the right places, inattention can lead to accidents—so stay alert and keep hands and

Got Hurt? What's Sending Us to the ER

The leading causes of nonfatal injuries treated in US hospital emergency departments…

#1…Falls

#2…Unintentionally being struck by or against an object

#3…Overexertion

#4…Being inside a motor vehicle that's involved in an accident

#5…Cuts

Centers for Disease Control and Prevention

Even Simple Home Exercise Equipment Can Be Tricky When It Comes to Safety

Barbara Bushman, PhD, is a professor in the department of health, physical education and recreation at Missouri State University in Springfield, a fellow of the American College of Sports Medicine (ACSM) and editor of *ACSM's Complete Guide to Fitness & Health* (Human Kinetics).

Exercising at home is convenient and economical. Yet even with simple equipment, such as weights, resistance bands, balance boards and balls, there's a risk for injury if appropriate safety precautions are not taken. At a good gym, professional trainers are on hand to help, and equipment is regularly checked for damage—but at home, you're on your own. That's why we contacted Barbara Bushman, PhD, a professor in the department of health, physical education and recreation at Missouri State University, to discuss safety measures for home exercisers.

Here's how to stay safe when using…

Hand weights or barbells with weight plates…

•**Wear weight-lifting gloves to help you maintain your grip**—otherwise a barbell or dumbbell can easily slip out of sweaty hands.

•**Always wear shoes to help protect your feet in case you do drop a weight.**

•**If you have a weight bench, check regularly to assure that all nuts and bolts are tight**—these can loosen over time and make the bench unstable, Dr. Bushman cautioned.

•**Never try to lift more weight than you can comfortably handle unless another person is right there to spot you.**

Elastic resistance bands or tubes…

•**These are economical, portable and versatile alternatives to weights,** but they do wear out—so before each use, check for

other body parts well clear of the multistation's moving weight stacks, leverage arms, pulleys and cables.

•Examine your unit's pulleys, connections and other moving parts at least once a month for signs of wear, including fraying or other damage. Follow the manufacturer's directions for lubricating and tightening the unit's components and replacing worn parts promptly.

•**Stationary Bicycle.** These are relatively safe, but you'll still want to exercise caution.

•Avoid wearing pants that flare at the ankle—depending on your bike's style, the fabric could get trapped in the spinning mechanism and wrench your leg. The same goes for untied or unnecessarily long shoelaces.

•A seat that is too low puts strain on your knees.

Best: Adjust the seat height so that there's a slight bend in the knee when your foot is at the far reach of the pedal stroke.

•A new study in *The Journal of Sexual Medicine* found that using a bike on which the handlebars were positioned lower than the saddle was linked with decreased genital sensation in women.

Best: To lessen the pressure, raise your handlebars higher than your seat. Dr. Bushman also suggested using a cushioned seat cover or wearing padded shorts to increase comfort—so you'll be eager to get back on your bike when it's time to work out again.

tiny tears. If you spot a rip or weak area, it's time to replace your band or tube.

•**If the equipment has a handle (as many tubes do),** be sure the elastic tubing is properly secured in the handle.

•**Avoid abruptly letting go of the band or tube while it is stretched**—otherwise, it may snap back and hit you. This can be particularly serious if it hits you in the eye.

•**When anchoring the band or tube to another object,** choose something stationary, such as a door hinge. Do not anchor to a lightweight piece of furniture or a doorknob—if the furniture suddenly moves or the door flies open, you could lose your balance and fall.

Balance boards…

•**Typically a flat board atop an inflated base shaped like an upside-down dome**, these also are called wobble boards because they challenge your balance—so the primary safety concern is to prevent falls.

Best: Do your workout next to a bar or other stable surface (choose one with no sharp edges) that you can grab if you start to lose your balance.

•**Opt for a balance board with a textured top surface rather than a smooth one.** This helps keep feet from slipping.

•**Master simple stationary exercises** (such as just standing on the balance board) before challenging yourself with exercises involving movement or the addition of hand weights.

Inflatable fitness balls…

•**If a ball explodes while you're sitting or lying on it,** the sudden fall to the floor could leave you with an injury to the back, neck, head or other area. That's why Dr. Bushman recommended paying a few extra dollars for a ball labeled "burst-resistant," which is designed to deflate relatively slowly if punctured.

•**Also check the product label for inflation instructions.** Overinflating may cause the ball to pop while you're pumping it up, potentially hurling pieces of plastic into your eye.

•**If possible, do your ball workout on a floor that is carpeted or padded with rubber tile** so you won't land as hard in the event of a sudden fall.

•**Be sure the floor is free of sharp objects…**stay away from furniture…and keep pets out of the area.

For added safety: No matter what type of equipment you choose, if you are not familiar with it, Dr. Bushman suggested taking a few lessons from a qualified fitness professional…or buying a how-to DVD featuring a credentialed instructor, not a celebrity.

How to Choose the Right Athletic Shoe

Vahan Agbabian, clinical instructor and rehabilitation specialist, MedSport sports medicine program, University of Michigan Health System, Ann Arbor.

When you work out or play a sport, your shoes affect your performance—and your risk for injury.

Key: Choose sport-specific footwear.

Examples: Tennis shoes have side support and flexible soles for fast changes in direction…running shoes give maximum shock absorption…walking shoes need low heels that bevel inward so feet roll easily through the stride. *Also…*

•**Learn your foot type.** Ask a podiatrist or athletic trainer…or visit a shoe store that offers computerized foot-type analysis.

Wide feet: A too-narrow shoe leads to shin splints, so if even wide-size women's shoes feel tight, try men's shoes.

High arches: Look for a shoe with a thick, shock-absorbent heel, such as a gel heel or air bladder.

For feet that roll inward: You need a deep heel cup and wide mid-foot base.

For feet that roll outward: Choose a somewhat rigid shoe.

• **Check a shoe's flexibility by bending and twisting it.** It's too flexible (and thus can lead to ankle sprains) if it bends at mid-sole instead of the ball…flattens at the heel cup…or wraps like a towel when twisted. A shoe that's hard to bend or twist is too rigid (except for cycling) and may cause shin splints.

• **Know when to purchase a new pair.** Wear and tear affect a shoe's ability to support and protect. Replace sports shoes after they've taken about 500 miles' worth of steps. If you're a walker or runner, that's easy to calculate. Otherwise, replace shoes when treads and heels are visibly worn.

Car Most Likely to Have Crash Injuries

Toyota Yaris has the most injury claims. Personal-injury claims were filed 28.5 times for every 1,000 insured Yaris vehicles for model years 2009 through 2011 (most recent data available). The second-highest claims rate was for the Suzuki SX4, with 26.6 claims per 1,000 insured vehicles. The Yaris was among the 2012 top safety picks by the Insurance Institute for Highway Safety—but its small size makes its occupants more vulnerable in crashes with larger vehicles.

Lowest rate of injury claims: Porsche 911, with 4.5 per 1,000 vehicles.

Other vehicles with low claims rates (through 2011): Chevrolet Corvette and Silverado, Jeep Grand Cherokee, Lexus LX 570.

Highway Loss Data Institute, Arlington, Virginia. *www.IIHS.org*

Drugs That Increase the Risk for Car Crashes

Hui-Ju Tsai, MPH, PhD, associate investigator, division of biostatistics and bioinformatics, Institute of Population Health Sciences, National Health Research Institutes, Taiwan. She is lead author of a study published in *British Journal of Pharmacology*.

It's been known that taking antianxiety medications called benzodiazepines (such as Xanax, Ativan and Klonopin) raise your odds of getting into a car accident while driving.

But a group of researchers wanted to find out whether other types of drugs that fall into this psychotropic category (including antidepressants, sleeping pills and antipsychotics) are risky for drivers, too.

And what they discovered may make many people hesitant to get behind the wheel.

If you are among the millions of people taking any of these drugs, then you'll definitely want to know whether or not you're at increased risk…

Which Drugs Were Studied?

Researchers looked at two groups of data on people age 18 or over. One group was made up of people who had a record of being in a car accident (as a driver, not a passenger) at some point over a recent 10-year span, and the other group comprised people of similar ages who had no record of being in a car accident (as a driver, not a passenger) over the same 10-year span. (The researchers couldn't be sure that the accident was the driver's fault—there was no way to tell, based on the data. And determining blame in accidents is sometimes subjective.) *Then researchers analyzed who in the accident group had taken any of the following drugs within one month of the accident…*

• **Antipsychotics**
  • Thorazine (chlorpromaxine)
  • Depixol (flupentixol)
  • Loxitane (loxapine)
  • Zyprexa (olanzapine)

- Seroquel (quetiapine)
- Risperdal (risperidone)
- **Antidepressants**
  - SSRIs (selective serotonin reuptake inhibitors):
    - Prozac (fluoxetine)
    - Paxil (paroxetine)
    - Zoloft (sertraline)
    - Celexa (citalopram)
    - Lexapro (escitalopram)
  - Tricyclic antidepressants:
    - Trofanil (imipramine)
    - Elavil (amitriptyline)
  - "Others":
    - Wellbutrin (bupropion)
    - Effexor (venlafaxine)
    - Cymbalta (duloxetine)
- **Benzodiazepines**
  - Hypnotics:
    - Halcion (triazolam)
    - Dalmane (flurazepam)
  - Anxiolytics:
    - Xanax (alprazolam)
    - Klonopin (clonazepam)
    - Valium (diazepam)
    - Ativan (lorazepam)
- **"Z-drugs" or sleeping pills**
  - Ambien (zolpidem)
  - Sonata (zaleplon)

Then researchers compared people of the same age and gender in both groups to see whether those who had taken any of the drugs mentioned above were more likely to have been in car accidents.

Impaired Driving Skills

We contacted study author Hui-Ju Tsai, MPH, PhD, to learn more about the results. She and her colleagues found that only two categories of drugs—antipsychotic drugs and "other" antidepressants—were not associated with a higher risk of having a car accident while every other category was.

It is, of course, possible that the underlying medical conditions that caused people to take the drugs—depression, anxiety and insomnia—contributed to the car accidents.

Future research will need to address that. But there is some evidence that the drugs themselves may have played a role.

Dr. Tsai noted that many psychotropic drugs impair cognitive and psychomotor abilities—and of course, cognitive and psychomotor abilities are crucial for driving. While on these drugs, you might feel more drowsy or more confused, and your reflexes might be slower. All of these things may negatively impact your judgment and coordination.

Dr. Tsai isn't exactly sure why antipsychotic drugs and "other" antidepressants weren't shown to be associated with car crashes. It could be due to the smaller number of subjects taking these drugs in the study…or it could be that people on these particular drugs drive less often…or it could be that these drugs impair cognitive and psychomotor abilities less than the other drugs mentioned above.

Protect Yourself on the Road

If you take any of the types of drugs listed above that were associated with having car accidents, here's some advice from Dr. Tsai…

For those who take the medication in the morning, ask your doctor whether you can take it at night instead. The effects of many psychotropic drugs are strongest after you first take them, and since people tend to drive most in the daytime, this simple switch might help.

Ask your physician if you can take a lower dosage of the drug or possibly be weaned off the drug altogether. Perhaps you can use a natural treatment or make a lifestyle change instead.

If you have to stay on the drug and there is someone else who can drive you places (such as a spouse, sibling, child or friend), see if it's possible to become a passenger for at least the time being.

People who must drive: Stay extra alert while you're on the road, drive slowly and, of course, wear your seatbelt. And be sure not to drive if you are tired or upset.

Biggest Road Risk for Seniors Isn't Driving

Jonathan J. Rolison, PhD, a psychology lecturer at Queen's University, Belfast, Ireland. His study was published in *Journal of the American Geriatrics Society.*

Let's say you were asked this question: Are senior citizens at greatest risk of dying from a car-related injury while walking, riding in the passenger seat of a car or driving?

Your guess most likely would be driving. It's just part of being human—as we age, our eyesight and reflexes (and maybe even our mental focus) all diminish…and those are all vital for something as risky and difficult as driving.

Well, a recent study conducted in Britain found that seniors are actually in most danger while walking.

How can that be possible? *Here's the explanation…*

Pedestrian Perils

A research team lead by Jonathan J. Rolison, PhD, analyzed all fatal injuries reported by police in Britain between 1989 and 2009 that were classified as "road traffic fatalities." Meanwhile, the UK National Travel Survey had estimated the number of excursions—whether as a driver, passenger or pedestrian—made each year by individuals age 21 and up. When the researchers combined these two sets of data, they were able to calculate the risk that an individual would be fatally injured for each excursion. *Here's what they found…*

When it came to both driver and passenger fatality rates, people age 70 and older had a higher rate than people who were considered "middle-aged" (between 30 and 69). But the rate of the older set was about equal to that of the youngest set—people between ages 21 and 29.

When it came to the pedestrian fatality rate, however, seniors were far more likely to die than people in any other age group—and they were far more likely to die as pedestrians than while driving or sitting in a passenger seat.

"In other words, seniors shouldn't just be cautious about driving and riding in passenger seats in cars—they should also be cautious while walking," said Dr. Rolison. "Walking is riskier than they might think."

Safeguarding Seniors

Anyone who is elderly should be extra careful while walking on or near roads. Seniors typically walk more slowly than younger individuals, and they more often misjudge the speed of approaching vehicles—often due to declining hearing and/or sight. "These things compromise their ability to safely cross streets," said Dr. Rolison. And because they are usually more frail and susceptible to injury than younger people, they should cross streets only at designated crossing areas, ideally when no cars are in sight. It's best for them to choose crossing areas that have timers if their neighborhood has any, because those will ensure that seniors have a particular amount of time to safely cross.

Why Seniors Fall

Stephen Robinovitch, PhD, professor, kinesiology and engineering science, Simon Fraser University, British Columbia, Canada. His study was published in *The Lancet.*

You've probably already heard that falling is the most frequent cause of injury among people age 65 and older.

But here's a question to ponder…

Why do most seniors fall?

You might think that most falls are due to tripping or slipping, but a recent study, where actual falls were caught on video tape, points to a different, more surprising cause.

It's something that most of us do every day without even thinking—and it's something that can be easily avoided.

Falls Caught on Video

In the first study of its kind, Canadian researchers set up shop at two long-term-care facilities for the elderly that had video cameras installed in common areas (dining rooms, lounges, hallways, etc). Whenever an elderly resident fell on camera, researchers analyzed the video footage to determine what caused the fall. Here are the problems that caused the falls and the percentage of falls that each problem caused…

- **Unknown cause:** 2%
- **Slipping:** 3%
- **Bumps or hits:** 11%
- **Loss of support:** 11%
- **Collapse:** 11%
- **Trips or stumbles:** 21%
- **Incorrect weight-shifting** (more on this below): 41%!

So something the researchers called "incorrect weight-shifting" was, unexpectedly, the top cause of falls. Now, what does that mean exactly? Incorrect weight-shifting is when you abruptly change your center of gravity so that the bulk of your weight isn't aligned between your feet—it's thrown off to one side, which can cause your body to tilt off balance. This is different from tripping, for example (when your balance is thrown off by some external object)—this problem is internal or self-induced, due to the way you move around.

Guard Against Tumbles

You can fall at any age, of course, but the rate of falls during normal daily activities increases with age, said lead study author Stephen Robinovitch, PhD. So the older you get, the more careful you need to be. And age isn't the only risk factor—certain conditions also can play a role, such as vision impairment, cognitive problems and reduced muscle strength, to name just a few.

To help protect yourself (or a loved one) from taking a spill, focus on the number-one form of prevention, according to this study—try not to shift your center of gravity outside the base of support provided by your feet while moving around. *Here are some tips from Dr. Robinovitch, which may help you avoid doing exactly that…*

- **When standing: Keep your body weight evenly distributed between your feet**—don't lean too far sideways or on the heels or balls of your feet.
- **When walking: Avoid abrupt turns**—turn slowly, with your whole body at once (don't swivel your head and torso around without moving your lower half, too, for instance).
- **When reaching: Instead of grasping for high items that are near the limit of your reach** (such as the door of a kitchen cabinet that's above the refrigerator) and causing your body to lurch awkwardly, use a wide, low step stool or call someone taller to help.
- **When bending: If you've dropped, say, your car keys,** instead of leaning down with your upper body while keeping your legs straight (which causes your center of gravity to shift forward), lower yourself by bending your knees and moving into a squatting position.

Is the Way You Walk Giving You a Warning?

Mary Harward, MD, a geriatrician in private practice in Orange, California. She specializes in the diagnosis and treatment of gait disorders and other diseases affecting older adults. She is editor of *Medical Secrets* (fifth edition, Mosby Elsevier).

Have you surprised yourself recently with a stumble or a fall? If you blamed it on your shoes…your eyesight…or an obstacle, such as a throw rug, you may not be getting at the root cause of why you stumbled or fell. The fact is, the real reason many people fall (and sometimes die from it) is the way that they walk.

A problem that goes undetected: Most people who have treatable abnormalities in their gait (the way in which a person walks) never even discuss it with their doctors.

Here's why: When you go to the doctor, odds are that you are taken to an exam room and asked to "have a seat" until the doctor arrives. The problem is, you'll probably stay seated during the entire visit, and your doctor may miss a symptom—a dangerous gait—that's just as important as abnormal x-rays or blood tests.

Take It Seriously

It's never normal to shuffle, be off-balance or have an unusual posture. A gait disorder always means that something—or, in most cases, a combination of factors—is awry.

Problems with gait affect about 15% of adults age 60 and older and more than 80% of those age 85 and older. Gait disorders, which interfere with stability and balance, are not only among the most common causes of falls and subsequent hospitalizations, but also can be one of the first health problems that eventually leads to nursing home care.

My advice: Doctors should ask every patient if he/she has fallen in the last year. In addition, if you're age 65 or older, you should ask your doctor to check your gait at least once a year.

What's Behind It?

Patients often assume that problems with one's gait are due to neurological disorders, such as Parkinson's disease or multiple sclerosis (MS). With Parkinson's disease, patients also experience a resting tremor or shaking of one hand, muscle rigidity and slow movements, while MS typically is accompanied by vision problems, dizziness and trouble speaking. *But there are other possible causes of gait problems…*

- **Arthritis.** Gait problems are common in patients with arthritis, particularly osteoarthritis of the knee or hip. If you have knee or hip pain, you may favor that side and use other muscles to compensate. This throws off your posture and body mechanics, which may cause you to limp or take tentative steps.

Helpful: Ask your doctor if it's appropriate to see a physical therapist for advice on exercises to strengthen the muscles around the arthritic joint—this will help you walk normally and with less pain.

- **Pain control is also very important.** Apart from making you more comfortable, it will help you do the exercises that you need for a better gait. If you don't get adequate relief from over-the-counter pain relievers, talk to your doctor about stronger forms of pain control. Stretching, massage, heating pads, cold packs and/or acupuncture are helpful to some people.

- **Back problems.** A gait problem often is due to a painful back. Patients with lumbar stenosis, for example, will frequently experience nerve pressure from damaged vertebrae in the spine, affecting their ability to walk. Patients with sciatica (nerve pain that often accompanies lower-back problems) will have difficulty walking or standing. Suspect nerve problems if you have back or leg pain that gets worse when you walk or stand for more than a few minutes and gets better when you're off your feet. See your doctor for treatment advice.

- **Balance disorders.** If you sometimes feel as though you're about to fall (even when you're not), see a doctor right away. Problems with balance—often accompanied by dizziness, spinning sensations, etc.—are a major cause of falls. Potential causes include ear infections, inner-ear disorders, neuropathy (nerve damage) and circulatory problems.

Also: Ask your doctor to test your vitamin B-12 level. Older adults often have low levels of intrinsic factor, a protein that's needed for B-12 absorption. It's also common for vegetarians to be deficient in this vitamin because meat is a major source of B-12. Low B-12 can make you feel light-headed, cause numbness and/or tingling in the feet and make it difficult to walk.

Similar foot and leg symptoms are caused by diabetic neuropathy, nerve damage that may occur in patients with poorly managed (or undiagnosed) diabetes. Bunions and other foot conditions also can contribute to gait disorders.

● **Drug side effects.** It's not surprising that sedating medications such as *diazepam* (Valium) can increase fall risk. What many people don't realize is that nonsedating medications also can be an issue.

Example: Medications that lower blood pressure, such as diuretics, can cause orthostatic hypotension, a sudden drop in blood pressure that can make you dizzy or lightheaded. Some blood pressure drugs also decrease magnesium, which can cause leg weakness or cramps. Your doctor might advise changing medications. Alcohol or drugs that lower blood sugar or affect mood or sleep also can change one's gait.

Important: Be especially careful after eating. Studies have shown that dizziness and gait problems tend to get worse about 30 minutes after meals—blood travels to the digestive tract after meals, sometimes lowering blood pressure.

● **Reduced brain circulation.** Gait disorders are often the first sign of infarcts, areas of brain damage caused by impaired circulation. Infarcts occur in patients who have had a stroke or other problems that affect blood vessels in the brain, such as hypertension or high cholesterol.

A patient who has multiple infarcts might walk very slowly…take short steps…stand with his feet wider apart than usual…and/or hesitate when starting to walk or have trouble slowing momentum when stopping.

How's Your Gait?

If you've noticed changes in the ways in which you move, see your doctor for an evaluation. *He/she will give you tests that may include…*

● **The timed get-up-and-go test.** This measures the time it takes you to get up from a chair (without using your hands to push off from the armrests), walk 10 feet, turn around and walk back to the chair. You should be able to complete the sequence safely in 14 seconds or less. If it takes longer than 20 seconds, your gait is seriously impaired.

How to Fall Down Without Getting Hurt

Hal Needham, who appeared as a stuntman in more than 4,000 television episodes and more than 300 feature films. He is author of *Stuntman! My Car-Crashing, Plane-Jumping, Bone-Breaking, Death-Defying Hollywood Life* (Little, Brown).

When we fall, our natural instinct is to reach out for the ground with our hands. Unfortunately, that only increases our odds of injury—our hands, wrists and arms are full of small bones that are easily broken. Instead, when you realize you are falling…

1. Buckle your knees. This can in essence lower the height that your upper body falls by as much as a foot or two, significantly reducing the impact when you hit the ground. In a forward fall, it might result in bruised knees, but that's better than a broken bone in the upper body.

Helpful: In a backward fall, tuck your head into your chest as you buckle your knees—try to turn yourself into a ball.

2. Throw one arm across your chest whether you're falling forward or backward. Do this with enough force that it turns your body to one side. It doesn't matter which arm you use.

3. Rotate the rest of your body in the direction that you threw your arm, increasing your spin. If you can rotate enough, you

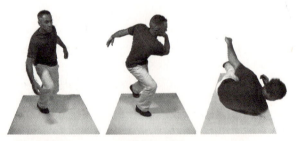

Model demonstrates falling technique.

can come down mainly on your backside, a well-padded part of the body unlikely to experience a serious injury.

Trouble is, while stuntmen know exactly when and where they're going to fall, real-world falls usually take people by surprise. It can be difficult to overcome instinct and put this falling strategy into action in the split second before hitting the ground.

Practice can help. If you have access to a thick gym mat and you don't have health issues that make it risky, try out this falling technique until it feels natural.

Falls—Beware of the Hidden Causes

Rosanne M. Leipzig, MD, PhD, vice chair for education and Gerald and Mary Ellen Ritter Professor of Geriatrics in the Brookdale Department of Geriatrics and Adult Development at Mount Sinai School of Medicine in New York City.

Anyone can trip and be thrown momentarily off balance. But can you regain your balance—or do you go down? Anything that makes an initial misstep more likely or interferes with a person's ability to self-correct increases the risk for falls. And many such factors become more common with age. *For example…*

•**Muscle weakness.** If you stumble, it requires coordinated actions of your feet, ankles, knees and hips to prevent a fall. Muscle weakness in any of those areas impairs this ability. That's why physical inactivity is a common—though often unrecognized—cause of falls.

Exercise helps slow the loss of muscle mass that occurs with aging. Stair-climbing is an excellent way to strengthen critical thigh muscles.

Also helpful: Leg extensions—while sitting in a chair, raise your lower leg until it is in line with the thigh. Repeat 10 times and switch legs. Perform this exercise three times a day.

•**Impaired nerve function.** The nervous system plays a part in sensing loss of balance early and guiding the self-correction process. Blunted nerve function in the feet often is due to peripheral neuropathy, which can be caused by diabetes, vitamin B-12 deficiency or low thyroid levels (hypothyroidism).

•**Thinning bones.** Bone mass declines with age. If the thinning process goes far enough, osteoporosis can develop—in both women and men—and those dangerously fragile bones are liable to fracture. Osteoporosis can worsen the consequences of a fall, but in some cases, weakened bones are the cause, rather than the effect.

Here's what happens: As bones lose density, the body's center of gravity shifts forward, causing an older person to lean progressively forward. Balance becomes more precarious, so a slip is more likely to become a fall. Small fractures of the vertebrae caused by osteoporosis accentuate the forward shift.

•**Low vitamin D levels.** An analysis of five studies published in *The Journal of the American Medical Association* found a more than 20% reduction in falls in healthy older people who took vitamin D supplements, compared with those who didn't.

Researchers theorize that vitamin D may have an effect on muscle that helps reduce falls. Although the Daily Value (the FDA's reference guideline for daily nutrient intake) for vitamin D is 400 international units (IU), most studies have found that daily doses of 700 IU to 800 IU are needed to prevent falls and fractures.

Vitamin D deficiency is more common than previously believed—it's often due to a lack of regular sun exposure and/or a low intake of foods containing or fortified with vitamin D. If either of these factors applies to you, ask your doctor to check your blood level of vitamin D.

Vision and Hearing Loss

"Silent" vision problems, such as cataracts and glaucoma that have not yet caused difficulties in reading or other activities, can increase a person's risk for falls. Subtle vision changes, such as a decline in the ability to see contrasts in color or light and dark, can be missed as well. This makes tripping over curbs and on stairs or escalators more of a danger.

Correcting nearsightedness or farsightedness with glasses will help but initially can be risky. It takes time to adjust to new glasses—particularly when they have multifocal (bifocal, trifocal or variable) lenses. An Australian study found that in the period just after patients got new glasses, they were more likely to fall.

Even hearing loss may be linked to increased falls—possibly because some hearing problems reflect damage to the eighth cranial nerve, which also controls the inner-ear system that maintains balance. Maintaining and regaining balance is key to preventing falls.

Dangerous Medications

Any drug that causes sedation can impair alertness, slow reaction time and disable the coordinated interplay of nerves and muscles that protects against falls. Some medications lower blood pressure when you stand up—these can cause weakness and light-headedness that can lead to a fall.

Among the most common culprits: Some antidepressants and anti-anxiety drugs… medications taken for enlarged prostate… painkillers, such as codeine and *oxycodone* (OxyContin)…and pills for high blood pressure.

Important: The more medications you take, the higher your risk of falling.

Hidden menace: Over-the-counter (OTC) drugs. For example, older OTC antihistamines that can have sedating effects, such as *diphenhydramine* (Benadryl), should not be used by older adults, who may experience confusion when taking such drugs. First try a nonsedating antihistamine, such as *loratadine* (Claritin).

Try Another Way to Sleep

Sleeping pills can cause more risks than benefits.

Recent finding: Researchers analyzed studies involving 2,417 people who took either a placebo or a prescription sleep aid, such as *zolpidem* (Ambien), or over-the-counter medication, such as *diphenhydramine* (Benadryl), for five or more consecutive nights.

Result: People who took sedatives were more than twice as likely to report daytime fatigue, headache, dizziness, nausea and falls as they were to gain a better quality of sleep.

If you have trouble sleeping: Ask your doctor about nondrug strategies, such as cognitive behavioral therapy and/or exercise.

Nathan Herrmann, MD, head, division of geriatric psychiatry, Sunnybrook Health Sciences Centre, University of Toronto, Canada.

Sleep Problems

Lack of sleep can increase fall risk by impairing alertness and slowing reaction time. However, sleeping pills aren't the solution—their effects often linger, dulling the senses and slowing reaction time. Even newer sleep medications, such as *zolpidem* (Ambien), which are designed to be shorter acting, keep working longer in older people, possibly contributing to falls.

Anything that gets you out of bed in the middle of the night—such as an urgent need to urinate—also increases your fall risk. Keep a clear path to the bathroom, use night-lights and keep a cane or walker easily accessible, if necessary.

Undiagnosed Illness

Falls also can be a harbinger of a new health problem, such as pneumonia, a urinary tract infection, heart attack or heart failure. In some cases, weakness that can lead to a fall is more evident than the usual symptoms for these illnesses.

Small Changes That Help

The exact cause of a fall is often impossible to pin down and may actually be due to several subtle factors working together—such as a slight loss of sensation in the feet, mild sedation due to medication and minor difficulty with balance.

Fortunately, safety is cumulative, too. Slight adjustments can be lifesaving. For example, avoid shoes that don't fit snugly or have slippery soles...instead, wear sneakers or walking shoes. In addition, get rid of any throw rugs...make sure that lighting is adequate and handrails are available where needed...and don't be vain about using a cane or walker if it helps you move about safely.

Are Your Bone-Building Drugs Bad for You?

Harris H. McIlwain, MD, founder of the Tampa Medical Group and an adjunct professor at the University of South Florida College of Public Health, both in Tampa. Dr. McIlwain is coauthor of *Reversing Osteopenia* (Henry Holt) and *The Osteoporosis Cure* (Avon).

A 65-year-old woman recently fell in her bathroom and fractured three vertebrae. If she had been taking medication to strengthen her thinning bones, might her injuries have been less severe? Maybe. But given the growing evidence of bone-building drugs' side effects—including increased risk for certain fractures and even jawbone death—such drugs might actually have done her more harm than good. Her plight draws attention to how important it is for women to keep abreast of the latest research on osteoporosis treatment. We spoke with Harris H. McIlwain, MD, coauthor of *Reversing Osteopenia* and *The Osteoporosis Cure. Here's what all women need to know about bone-building meds...*

When bone-building medications known as bisphosphonates were introduced more than 20 years ago, they were hailed as near-miracle drugs for people with thinning bones.

Studies showed that these drugs—first, *alendronate* (Fosamax) and later, *risedronate* (Actonel), *ibandronate* (Boniva) and *zoledronic acid* (Reclast)—significantly reduced the incidence of hip and spine fractures in people with osteoporosis and osteopenia (bone loss that is less severe than osteoporosis).

Now: Despite the established benefits of bisphosphonates, the medications are increasingly coming under fire for having potentially serious side effects. For example, studies have shown that the drugs may increase risk for various conditions, such as breakage of the femur (thigh bone)...osteonecrosis (death of bone tissue) in the jaw...and even esophageal cancer. Two FDA advisory panels recently wrote in a report that, due to the potential risks associated with long-term use of bisphosphonates, bisphosphonate therapy could be safely discontinued in some cases—but did not specify when or for how long to discontinue the drug.

Studies on the safety of bisphosphonates are ongoing. Thus far, the research is mixed on the benefits of taking the drug for more than five years. For example, research has shown that women who took Fosamax for another five years (for a total of 10 years) had the same rate of femur fractures as those who took a placebo. The risk for spine fracture, however, was higher in the group taking a placebo.

Finding the Best Treatment

The decision to take bisphosphonates (or any medication) requires balancing benefits against risks. People at high risk for fractures should not stop taking these medications but instead work with their doctors to determine the duration of treatment. This includes people who have had previous fractures or a family history of fractures...and those with rheumatoid arthritis, which can increase bone loss. Other high-risk individuals include those who take the corticosteroid prednisone for a chronic condition...women who weigh under 127 pounds...people who lead a sedentary lifestyle (weight-bearing exercise strengthens bones)…and smokers (their risk for bone loss is twice that of a nonsmoker).

Women and men who have a high risk for fracture but who have other health concerns may want to talk to their doctors about taking a nonbisphosphonate bone-strengthening medication. *Examples…*

•*Denosumab* **(Prolia),** a monoclonal antibody that reduces the body's bone-breakdown mechanism. If you have gastro-esophageal reflux disease, this drug, which is delivered via an injection, may help you avoid the gastrointestinal side effects common with bisphosphonates. However, in a few rare cases, osteonecrosis of the jaw has been reported.

•*Teriparatide* **(Forteo),** a type of para-thyroid hormone that builds bone. This injectable drug increases bone thickness, so if you have a history of periodontal disease, you may be better off with this drug.

How Bones Age

Bones are living tissue in a constant state of flux. Children and teenagers generally produce more bone than they lose until they reach peak bone mass in their mid-20s. By the time women and men reach their early 30s, the amount of bone loss is about the same as the amount that is created.

After that, as estrogen levels start to decline in women, the rate of bone loss slowly begins to exceed the amount that is built. During menopause, when estrogen levels decline even more sharply, bone loss accelerates markedly.

In fact, according to the National Osteoporosis Foundation, women can lose as much as 20% of their bone mass in the first five to seven years of menopause. Men in their 50s do not rapidly lose bone mass the way women do after menopause, but by age 65, men and women lose bone mass at the same rate.

Keys to Better Bone Health

Women at low risk for fracture but who have osteopenia are the best candidates for discontinuing (or not starting) bisphosphonates, but they should talk to their health-care providers first to discuss benefits versus risks and continue having regular bone mineral density tests. *They should also talk to their doctors about the following steps to promote bone health…*

•**Eat a diet rich in calcium.** Calcium is the main mineral in bone. Low-fat dairy foods, such as skim milk, yogurt and cheese, are excellent sources of calcium. If you don't like dairy or are unable to tolerate it, try eating leafy greens, tofu, almonds and salmon. Aim to get 1,200 mg to 1,500 mg of calcium a day through a combination of diet and supplements.

Note: Also talk to your doctor about magnesium. Adequate levels of this mineral are needed for optimal calcium absorption.

•**Get your vitamin D through a combination of diet and supplements.** Fortified milk, salmon and cod-liver oil are good dietary sources of vitamin D. Talk to your doctor about getting a blood test to measure your vitamin D level (nearly half of people with osteoporosis have low vitamin D levels)… and about taking 1,000 international units (IU) of vitamin D a day to maintain a vitamin D blood level of 32 ng/mL or higher.

•**Don't forget vitamin K.** It helps the bones absorb calcium. Aim for 65 micrograms (mcg) to 80 mcg a day. Good sources include leafy greens, broccoli, beef liver and soybean oil. Vitamin K is also available in supplement form.

•**Do 30 minutes of weight-bearing exercise every day,** such as walking, hiking, yoga, tai chi or jogging, to stimulate the body to produce new bone. If it's been awhile since you exercised, start slowly and work your way up to a half hour a day.

•**Add back exercises.** Back exercises typically involve strengthening the abdominal (core) muscles, which support the spine.

•**Ask your doctor about strontium.** Strontium is a natural element that is prescribed in Europe for osteoporosis. It works by slowing bone resorption and increasing bone production. Strontium supplements are available at health-food stores. Ask your doctor what dosage of strontium would be best for you.

Fight Osteoporosis the Natural Way

Mark A. Stengler, NMD, licensed naturopathic medical doctor. He is founder and medical director of the Stengler Center for Integrative Medicine, Encinitas, California, and associate clinical professor at the National College of Natural Medicine, Portland, Oregon. He is author of *The Natural Physician's Healing Therapies* (Bottom Line Books).

Misconceptions abound when it comes to osteoporosis, a dreaded disease marked by porous, brittle bones and hunched backs. Most people think of osteoporosis as a women's disease, but it's more than that. While 8 million American women have been diagnosed with osteoporosis, more than 2 million men also are affected by it.

Osteoporosis: A Silent Problem

Osteoporosis can develop because, starting at about age 35, our bone cells do not make new bone as fast as it is broken down. Our bones become more frail and fracture more easily. Fractures, especially of the hip, spine and wrist, are more likely to occur, even without trauma. Osteoporosis has no symptoms until a bone is fractured. Many people go for decades without a diagnosis of osteoporosis—until they fall and an x-ray reveals porous bones.

Bone density can be measured with a dual-energy x-ray absorptiometry (DEXA) scan, but many people don't get this test. I recommend a baseline DEXA scan by age 50, and if results are normal, follow-ups every three to five years.

The most worrisome risk for a person with osteoporosis is a hip fracture. According to the National Osteoporosis Foundation (*www.nof.org*), an average of 24% of hip-fracture patients age 50 or older die in the year following their fractures, often as a result of long-term immobilization that leads to blood clots or infection. Six months after a hip fracture, only 15% of patients can walk unaided across a room.

Virtually every person with osteoporosis who has come to my clinic is confused about the best way to promote bone health. Conventional doctors typically prescribe osteoporosis medication, such as *alendronate* (Fosamax) and *ibandronate* (Boniva). However, these drugs can cause side effects, such as digestive upset and blood clots, and they don't address the underlying nutritional deficiencies that promote bone loss.

The natural protocol I recommend includes a healthful diet (rich in vegetables, fruit and fish and low in refined-sugar products and red meat)…weight-bearing exercise (such as walking and stair-climbing)…and good hormone balance (deficiencies of some hormones, such as testosterone, accelerate bone loss). I also suggest certain bone-protecting supplements.

Caution: People with kidney disease should not take supplements without consulting a doctor. With kidney disease, the kidneys cannot process high doses of nutrients.

My recommendations for women and men: To help prevent osteoporosis, take the first three supplements listed below. If you have osteoporosis or osteopenia (mild bone loss that can be diagnosed with a DEXA scan), take the first three supplements listed and as many of the others as you're willing to try, in the dosages recommended…

Super Trio Prevents and Treats Osteoporosis

• **Calcium is the most prevalent mineral in bone tissue.** Taking supplements helps prevent a deficiency. Most studies have found that calcium slows bone loss but does not increase bone density when used alone. Women with osteoporosis should take 500 mg of calcium twice daily with meals. It should be a well-absorbed form, such as citrate, citrate-malate, amino acid chelate or hydroxyapatite. To boost absorption, take no more than 500 mg per dose. Calcium carbonate, which is widely used, is not well-absorbed. For osteoporosis prevention, men and women, as well as boys and girls starting at age 13, should take 500 mg daily.

Calcium supplementation for men with osteoporosis is more complicated. Some recent research has identified a link between high calcium intake (from dairy products) and increased prostate cancer risk. A meta-analysis in the *Journal of the National Cancer Institute* that reviewed 12 studies on this association concluded, "High intake of dairy products and calcium may be associated with an increased risk for prostate cancer, although the increase appears to be small." A recent study found that calcium intake exceeding 1,500 mg a day (from food and supplements) may be associated with a higher risk of advanced, and potentially fatal, prostate cancer. The saturated fat in dairy products may raise prostate cancer risk.

Until there is more definitive information, I recommend that men who have osteoporosis, regardless of whether they have eliminated calcium-rich foods from their diets, take no more than a 500-mg calcium supplement daily. Men with prostate cancer should consult their doctors before using calcium supplements.

• **Vitamin D promotes absorption of calcium.** Deficiencies of this vitamin are more common in Americans over age 50 than in younger adults. Sun exposure prompts the body to produce vitamin D, and the kidneys help convert it to its active form. As we age, our skin cannot synthesize vitamin D as effectively from sunlight, and our kidneys become less efficient. People with darker skin, those with digestive problems (due to malabsorption conditions, such as Crohn's disease) and those with limited exposure to sunlight are also at greater risk for vitamin D deficiency. Preliminary studies indicate that an inadequate intake of vitamin D is associated with an increased risk of fractures.

Hearing Loss Increases Risk for Falls

Researchers tested the hearing of 2,017 adults (ages 40 to 69) and asked them about recent falls.

Finding: Those with even mild hearing loss were three times more likely to have fallen within the previous year than those with normal hearing. Each 10-decibel loss of hearing raised risk of falling 1.4-fold.

Theory: Hearing loss may overwork the brain, leaving fewer resources to maintain gait and balance.

Frank R. Lin, MD, PhD, assistant professor of otolaryngology and epidemiology, The Johns Hopkins University, Baltimore.

For the prevention of osteoporosis, I recommend 600 IU to 800 IU of vitamin D daily. People with osteoporosis should take 800 IU to 1,200 IU daily. Vitamin D is fat soluble, meaning it is better absorbed when taken with meals (containing small amounts of fat).

For many patients with low vitamin D levels, I recommend 2,000 IU of vitamin D daily. To ensure that vitamin D levels are optimal, I monitor blood levels once or twice a year. Overdosing can lead to heart arrhythmia, loss of appetite, nausea and other ill effects.

• **Magnesium, an important constituent of bone crystals, is crucial for the proper metabolism of calcium.** A deficiency of magnesium impairs bone-building cells known as osteoblasts. Like calcium, magnesium requires vitamin D for absorption.

Researchers at Tel Aviv University in Israel looked at the effect of magnesium supplementation on bone density in 31 postmenopausal women with osteoporosis. This two-year, open, controlled trial (both the researchers and patients knew who was receiving the placebo or the supplement) involved giving the participants 250 mg to 750 mg of magnesium daily for six months and 250 mg for another 18 months. Twenty-two patients (71%) experienced a 1% to 8% increase in bone density. The mean bone density of all treated patients increased significantly after one year and remained at that level after two years. Among an additional 23 postmenopausal women not receiving magnesium, mean bone density decreased significantly.

For osteoporosis prevention, take 400 mg to 500 mg of magnesium daily…for osteoporosis, take 500 mg to 750 mg daily. In both cases, take in divided doses.

If You Have Bone-Loss Disease

•**Vitamin K has received attention in recent years for its role in treating osteoporosis.** It activates osteocalcin, a bone protein that regulates calcium metabolism in the bones and helps calcium bind to the tissues that make up the bone. It also has been shown to inhibit inflammatory chemicals that cause bone breakdown.

Studies have shown that low vitamin K intake and blood levels are associated with reduced bone density and fractures in people who have osteoporosis. A recent meta-analysis published in the American Medical Association's *Archives of Internal Medicine* found that vitamin K supplements were associated with a consistent reduction in all types of fractures. Leafy, green vegetables, such as spinach, kale, collard greens and broccoli, are the best sources of vitamin K, yet many people do not consume these vitamin K–rich foods on a regular basis.

High-dose vitamin K (above 2 mg) should be used only under the supervision of a doctor, because excess vitamin K may increase blood clotting. Vitamin K supplements should not be used by people who take blood-thinning medication, such as warfarin (Coumadin) or heparin, or by pregnant women or nursing mothers.

I typically recommend 2 mg to 10 mg daily of vitamin K for people who have osteoporosis to help increase their bone density.

•**Essential fatty acids (EFAs) have been shown to improve bone density in older women** and are believed also to promote bone health in men. Many researchers theorize that osteoporosis develops because of chronic inflammation of bone tissue (due to stress, toxins, poor diet and infection). EFAs, especially those found in fish oil, reduce inflammation. Some studies show that EFAs also improve calcium absorption. I recommend that people with osteoporosis take fish oil daily (containing about 480 mg of EPA and 320 mg of DHA), along with 3,000 mg of evening primrose oil, which contains inflammation-fighting gamma-linolenic acid (GLA). Because EFAs have a blood-thinning effect, check with your doctor if you are taking a blood thinner.

•**Strontium is a mineral that doesn't get much attention,** because it is not regarded as essential for the human body. However, 99% of the total amount of strontium found in the body is located in the teeth and bones. Supplemental strontium is not the radioactive type that you may have heard about in relation to nuclear facilities. Strontium is a valuable mineral for people with osteoporosis, and I often recommend it.

A clinical trial in *The New England Journal of Medicine* found that strontium prevents vertebral fractures and increases bone density. The most common supplemental forms are strontium chloride and strontium citrate. I suggest a supplement that contains 680 mg of elemental strontium daily (similar to the dose used in most studies).

Because calcium inhibits strontium absorption, strontium should be taken at least four hours before or after calcium is taken. Strontium should not be taken by pregnant women and nursing mothers. It is not available at most health-food stores, but you can buy it from Vitacost (800-381-0759, *www.vitacost.com*).

•**Soy, as a supplement and/or food, has been shown in several studies to improve bone density.** Soy contains isoflavones, estrogen-like constituents that support bone mass and relieve menopausal symptoms in women. Women and men with osteoporosis or osteopenia should take 125 mg of soy isoflavones daily in soy protein powder or supplement form and consume three to five servings of soy foods weekly. (One serving equals one-half cup of tofu...one-half cup of soy beans...or one cup of soy milk.)

Caution: Soy supplements are not well studied in women who have had breast cancer, so they should avoid supplements and nonfermented soy products.

• **Vitamin C is required for the production of the protein collagen, a component of bone tissue.** I recommend that people with osteoporosis take 1,000 mg twice daily. Reduce the dosage if loose stools develop.

Silicon is a trace mineral required for bone formation. I recommend 2 mg to 5 mg daily.

Best Osteoporosis Formulas

These products contain all the vitamins and minerals described in this article, in the therapeutic doses used for osteoporosis treatment...

• **BoneUp by Jarrow.** To find an online retailer, call 310-204-6936 or go to *www.jarrow.com.*

• **OsteoPrime by Enzymatic Therapy.** To find a retailer, call 800-783-2286 or go to *www.enzymatictherapy.com.*

• **Pro Bone by Ortho Molecular Products is available from health-care professionals,** including naturopaths, holistic MDs, chiropractors, nutritionists and acupuncturists. If you cannot locate a health-care professional in your area who sells the formula, it is available from my clinic at 858-450-7120, *http://markstengler.com.*

Fix Your Feet to Prevent Falls

Hylton Menz, PhD, deputy director of the Musculoskeletal Research Center at La Trobe University in Victoria, Australia. He is author of the textbook *Foot Problems in Older People: Assessment and Management* (Churchill Livingstone).

Each year, about one in every three people over age 65 suffers a fall, a mishap that is far more dangerous than most people realize.

Important new research: In a 20-year study of nearly 5,600 women ages 70 and older, breaking a hip doubled the risk for death in the following year. Men who suffer a broken hip after a fall are also at increased risk for an untimely death.

Most people know the standard recommendations to reduce their risk for falls—get medical attention for balance and vision problems...improve the lighting in and around their homes...and eliminate loose carpets, cords and other obstacles.

What often gets overlooked: Painful feet...foot deformities such as bunions... weak foot and ankle muscles...and improper footwear also can significantly increase one's risk for falls.

Recent scientific evidence: In a 2011 study in the *British Medical Journal,* a comprehensive program of foot care reduced falls by one-third among a group of older people with assorted foot problems.

Get a Firm Foundation

With age, the muscles that support our ankles and feet often become weak—a common problem that contributes to foot pain and reduced activity levels. Structural abnormalities in the feet, such as bunions and hammertoes, undermine stability. And conditions that blunt sensations in the feet, such as nerve damage commonly caused by diabetes, may impair the ability of one's feet to react quickly and adjust to potentially hazardous conditions.

Basic Fall-Prevention Workout

Stretching and strengthening exercises can reduce foot pain—and lower your risk for falls. Basic exercises to perform daily...

To increase your ankles' range of motion: Sit in a chair with one knee extended. Rotate your foot in a clockwise, then counterclockwise direction. Repeat 10 times with each foot, in each direction.

To strengthen your toe muscles: Place small stones or marbles on the floor in front of you. While seated, pick up the stones with your bare toes and place them in a box, one by one. Pick up 20 stones with each foot, then repeat.

To stretch your calf muscles: Stand about two feet from a wall, then lean into it with one leg slightly bent at the knee about three inches in front of the other. Then reverse the position of your feet and lean forward to stretch the muscles of the other calf. Hold the stretch for 20 seconds, three times for each leg.

Proper Footwear

The right shoes are essential for everyone, but especially those with problem feet.

Most women know to avoid high heels, which make it more difficult to maintain balance. But many people opt for flimsy slip-on footwear, such as flip-flops, which may be comfortable but often become loose or come off the foot altogether, creating a balance hazard. It's far better to wear shoes that fasten to your feet with laces, Velcro or buckled straps.

Surprising fact: Most people assume that thick, cushiony soles, such as those found on most sneakers, help prevent falls because they tend to provide good support for your feet. But thinner, harder soles, such as those on some walking shoes, are safer because thin-soled shoes allow your feet to feel the sensations that help you maintain balance. A trade-off between comfort and safety may be necessary—you may have to wear less cushiony shoes that optimize balance.

Also, be sure that your shoes are the right size. Your feet may slide around in shoes that are too loose, while tight footwear won't allow your toes to respond to variations in the ground to help maintain stability while walking.

Remember: Shoe size often changes with age, as feet swell and spread. So have your feet measured every time you buy shoes.

Slightly more falls occur indoors than outdoors, and the proportion increases with age. Therefore, even when you're at home, proper footwear is crucial.

Important recent finding: When researchers at Harvard's Institute for Aging Re-

search followed a group of older adults for more than two years, they found that more than half of those who fell indoors were barefoot, in their stocking feet or wearing slippers. These injuries tended to be more serious than those of people who were wearing shoes when they fell.

Best to wear at home: Sturdy, thin-soled shoes that have more structural integrity than the average slipper.

Do You Need Orthotics?

Many adults over age 65 could benefit from wearing orthotics—inserts that fit inside the shoe—to help prevent falls by providing additional support.

Properly made orthotics may improve the way your feet move as you walk, distribute your weight more broadly to reduce pressure on sensitive spots and help convey sensory information to your feet, all of which may lessen the risk for falls.

If you have structural foot problems due to diabetes or rheumatoid arthritis, you may need customized orthotics from a podiatrist.

Typical cost: About $400. Insurance coverage varies. But over-the-counter versions (made with firm material, not just a soft cushion) may work as well if your feet are relatively normal and your foot pain is fairly mild. Good brands include Vasyli and Langer. Usually, you will be able to transfer orthotics between shoes.

Most people find that full-length orthotics are less likely to slip inside the shoe than the half-length variety. Full-length orthotics also may feel more comfortable, especially if you have corns or calluses under the toes or on the ball of your foot.

Getting Help

If you have foot problems, seek care from a podiatrist or other health professional—and be sure to mention any concerns about falling. Also ask for exercises, in addition to the ones described here, to address your specific foot issues.

Fall-Proof Your Life

Mary Tinetti, MD, director of the Program on Aging and the Claude D. Pepper Older Americans Independence Center at the Yale School of Medicine in New Haven, Connecticut. She is professor of epidemiology and investigative medicine and the Gladys Phillips Crofoot Professor of Medicine (geriatrics), also at the Yale School of Medicine.

Every year in the US, about one-third of people age 65 and older fall, with 1.6 million treated in emergency rooms and 12,800 killed. But falling is not an inevitable result of aging.

Falling is associated with impairments (such as from stroke, gait or vision problems, or dementia) that are more common with age. But risk for falling is also increased by poor balance and muscle strength and by side effects of certain drugs, especially those prescribed for sleep and depression.

Training That Works

Balance training and strength training are often underutilized ways to prevent falls.

With some types of balance training, you move continuously while simultaneously "perturbing" your center of gravity—that is, you intentionally become off-balance during movement, and your body learns how to respond, building your sense of balance. Do not try this on your own. Balance training is taught by physical therapists at many rehabilitation centers.

Another type of balance training is tai chi. This meditative martial art combines gentle, flowing movements with breathing and improves balance with moves that shift weight and increase awareness of body alignment. Teachers don't have to be licensed, so look for one with at least five years' experience.

Surprising: Dancing is a form of balance training. Any type will do, including ballroom, polka or salsa. Take lessons—and go out dancing!

In strength training, you build lean muscle mass by using your body weight (in squats, push-ups and ab crunches), free weights or elastic bands, all of which provide resistance to muscular effort. Stronger muscles and good balance often make the difference between a stumble and a fall.

You can safely learn strength training at a health club with a certified instructor who can correct your form and modify moves as needed. To do these exercises at home, use a book or DVD by a certified instructor, but check with your doctor first.

Caution: If you've had two or more falls in the past year, or feel unsteady on your feet, see a doctor for a referral to a physical therapist, who can create a safe balance- and strength-training program for you.

Risky Medications

Several types of widely prescribed drugs have been linked to an increased risk for falls, including....

•**Sleep medications,** such as the new generation of drugs heavily advertised on TV, including *eszopiclone* (Lunesta) and *zolpidem* (Ambien).

•**Antidepressants,** including selective serotonin reuptake inhibitors, such as *citalopram* (Celexa)...selective serotonin-norepinephrine reuptake inhibitors, such as *duloxetine* (Cymbalta)...and tricyclic antidepressants, such as *amitriptyline* (Elavil).

•**Benzodiazepines (antianxiety medications),** such as *alprazolam* (Xanax).

•**Anticonvulsants,** such as *pregabalin* (Lyrica), a class of drugs that is prescribed not only for epilepsy but also for chronic pain problems, such as from nerve damage.

•**Atypical antipsychotics,** such as *quetiapine* (Seroquel), which are used to treat bipolar disorder...schizophrenia...and psychotic episodes (such as hallucinations) in people with dementia.

•**Blood pressure medications,** including diuretics, such as *furosemide* (Lasix)...and calcium channel blockers, such as *nifedipine* (Procardia).

Important: Taking five or more medications also is linked to an increased risk for falls.

Low Blood Pressure

Side effects of several medications (including drugs for Parkinson's disease, diuretics and heart drugs such as beta-blockers) may increase the risk of falling by causing postural hypotension (blood pressure drops when you stand up from lying down or sitting). Not enough blood flows to the heart to keep you alert and stable, and the body's normal mechanism to counteract this fails.

What to do: Ask your doctor to test you if you have symptoms, including feeling light-headed or dizzy after standing. He/she will have you lie flat for five minutes, and then check your blood pressure immediately when you stand up. You will remain standing and have your pressure checked one or two minutes later. If systolic (top number) blood pressure drops at least 20 mmHg from lying to standing, you have postural hypotension.

If this is the case, ask about reducing your dosage of hypertensive, antidepressive and/or antipsychotic medications—the three drug types most likely to cause this condition.

Also: Drink more water—at least eight eight-ounce glasses a day. Dehydration can cause postural hypotension and is common among older people, who have a decreased sense of thirst.

Helpful: When you wake up in the morning, take your time getting out of bed. Sit on the edge of the bed for a few minutes while gently kicking forward with your lower legs and pumping your arms. This will move more blood to your heart and brain. Then stand up while holding on to a nearby stable object, such as a bedside table.

Vitamin D

Vitamin D promotes good muscle strength, so people with low blood levels of vitamin D may be at increased risk for falls. If your level is below 30 ng/mL, ask your doctor about taking a daily vitamin D supplement.

"Fall-Proof" Your Home

To prevent falls at home…

Careful on Weekends

Patients who suffer head injuries on the weekends are 14% more likely to die than those hurt during the week. This "weekend effect" is probably due to reduced weekend hospital staffing.

Johns Hopkins Medicine

• **Maintain bright lighting throughout the house.**

• **Eliminate throw rugs that could cause you to trip or slip,** or use strong double-sided tape to secure them.

• **Have handrails mounted on both sides of stairs** (the most common spot for falls)… and clearly mark the bottom stair with a contrasting color, such as a light-color paint on dark wood.

For more information: Go to the CDC's Web site, *www.cdc.gov*, and type "Home Fall Prevention Checklist" in the search field.

Natural Ways to Feel Much Better After a Fall…

Jamison Starbuck, ND, naturopathic physician in family practice and a guest lecturer at the University of Montana, both in Missoula. She is past president of the American Association of Naturopathic Physicians and a contributing editor to *The Alternative Advisor: The Complete Guide to Natural Therapies and Alternative Treatments* (Time Life).

Ever since I took that fall, I haven't felt quite right." This is a refrain that I hear from a surprising number of my patients. We tend to think of falls as affecting only older adults and causing primarily physical injuries. But neither is true. People of all ages fall, and the aftereffects can be harmful in a variety of ways.

My theory is that unexpected falls destabilize the nervous system. Even if you aren't badly hurt, these falls are scary. Our inner protective mechanisms become hypervigilant—our muscles become tense and we hold ourselves more rigidly. We also struggle with a lingering sense of unease and begin to mistrust our ability to safely do everyday activities. When a patient falls, I perform a thorough exam to rule out a concussion and possibly order an x-ray to check for fractures. I also treat the patient's nervous system. In addition to the use of ice to treat an injury for the first 48 hours, followed by heat and painkillers, if needed, I've found that natural medicine can help people avoid lasting problems from falls. *My favorite approaches...**

• **Use natural remedies.** Arnica is a well-known homeopathic remedy that is used topically for physical trauma. Arnica lotion, for example, can be applied to bruises or sprains several times a day until they are healed. Along with arnica, I recommend using homeopathic Aconite, a remedy that is excellent in treating the fright that follows sudden, violent accidents. Aconite is best taken within 48 hours of a fall. I typically recommend one dose (two pellets of Aconite 30C) taken under the tongue. If 24 hours after taking Aconite you remain anxious or scared about your fall, repeat the same dose once a day for up to a week.

• **Try nervine herbs.** Chamomile, valerian and hops are plant medicines that calm the nervous system and help the body recover from a fall by promoting rest and muscle relaxation. Take these herbs alone or in combination in tea or tincture form.

Typical dose for a single herb or mixture: **Drink 10 ounces of tea three times a day or take 60 drops of tincture in one ounce of water three times a day for up to two weeks.**

• **Get plenty of rest.** Soaking in a warm bath with Epsom salts relaxes muscles and helps you get a good night's sleep. Until you

*Check with your doctor first if you have a chronic condition or take medication.

have fully recovered from the fall, it also helps to take 150 mg of magnesium citrate (the form most easily absorbed) twice daily. This mineral promotes relaxation.

• **Consider bodywork.** Soon after a fall, consider getting full-body massage or acupressure treatment several times. These therapies not only promote circulation and healing, but also help people regain trust in their bodies after a scary event.

Caution: If you hit your head, are bleeding significantly or suspect a fracture from a fall, get to a hospital emergency department. If you experience headache, vision changes, dizziness, confusion, nausea, vomiting or a balance problem (even days after the fall), you may have a head injury and must seek immediate medical help.

Bed Rails Can Be Deadly

During the last nine years, 150 patients (mostly older, frail and in nursing homes) were reported to have died after their heads or chests became trapped in hospital bed rails—about 36,000 more required emergency room treatment for their injuries. The FDA issued public safety warnings about adult bed rails in 1995, but manufacturers weren't required to put safety labels on their products.

Alternative: A mattress with raised edges.

Steven Miles, MD, professor of medicine and bioethics, University of Minnesota Medical School, Minneapolis.

Stress Could Trigger Falls

In a new study, about one-third of nearly 5,000 men over age 65 who had experienced at least one stressful event, such as the death of a loved one or serious financial problems, fell significantly more often within the following year than those who didn't have a life shock.

Possible reason: Stress may trigger negative neurohormonal responses, which could affect balance and vision.

If you have had a life shock within the past year: Talk to your doctor about ways to reduce your risk for falls.

Howard Fink, MD, MPH, staff physician, Minneapolis VA Medical Center.

Taking Multiple Medicines Causes Falls Among All Ages

Falling has been viewed as an issue for older adults—but a new study finds that young and middle-aged adults who took at least two medicines were 2.5 times as likely to have fall-related injuries as those who took fewer medications.

Drugs most associated with falling: Blood pressure and lipid-lowering medicines, including statins.

Study of 687 people by University of Auckland School of Population Health, New Zealand, published in *Injury Prevention*.

Sleeping Pills Dangerous for Hospital Patients

The fall rate in hospital patients given the sleep medication *zolpidem* (Ambien) was more than four times higher than in patients who didn't take the drug. Zolpidem posed greater susceptibility for falls than other risk factors, such as age or cognitive impairment, regardless of the dose.

If you're having trouble sleeping in the hospital: Ask that nighttime interruptions and noise be kept to a minimum and/or bring earplugs.

Timothy I. Morgenthaler, MD, professor of medicine, Center for Sleep Medicine, Mayo Clinic, Rochester, Minnesota.

DIABETES

Diabetes is a difficult disease for anyone, but it can be especially challenging for women. Not only can diabetes show up during pregnancy (called gestational diabetes), it can also create other problems unique to women. For example, elevated blood glucose levels can trigger yeast infections, birth control pills can elevate blood sugar levels, and the hormonal changes that occur during menopause can send blood glucose levels out of control. Here's the help women need to conquer diabetes.

http://www.diabetes.org/living-with-diabetes/treatment-and-care/women/women-and-diabetes-frequently-asked-questions-faq.html

Chapter 19

BEST WAYS TO CONTROL— EVEN CURE—DIABETES

The Best Way to Prevent Diabetes—No Drugs Needed

If your doctor ever tells you (or has already told you) that you have prediabetes, you'd be wise to consider it a serious red flag. It means that your blood sugar level is higher than normal—though not yet quite high enough to be classified as diabetes—because your pancreas isn't making enough insulin and/or your cells have become resistant to the action of insulin.

A whopping 35% of American adults now have prediabetes. Nearly one-third of them will go on to develop full-blown diabetes, with all its attendant risks for cardiovascular problems, kidney failure, nerve damage, blindness, amputation and death.

That's why researchers have been working hard to figure out the best way to keep prediabetes from progressing to diabetes. And according to an encouraging recent study, one particular approach involving some fairly quick action has emerged as the winner—slashing prediabetic patients' risk for diabetes by an impressive 85%…without relying on drugs.

New Look at the Numbers

The recent study draws on data from the national Diabetes Prevention Program, the largest diabetes prevention study in the US, which began back in 1996. The program included 3,041 adults who had prediabetes and were at least somewhat overweight.

Participants were randomly divided into three groups. One group was given a twice-daily oral placebo and general lifestyle modification recommendations about the importance of healthful eating, losing weight and exercising. A second group was given twice-daily oral *metformin* (a drug that prevents the liver from producing too much glucose) and those same lifestyle recommendations. The third group was enrolled in an intensive lifestyle-modification program, with the goal of losing at least 7% of their body weight and exercising at moderate intensity for at least 150 minutes each week.

The original analysis of the data, done after 3.2 years, showed that intensive lifestyle modification reduced diabetes risk by 58%

Nisa M. Maruthur, MD, assistant professor of medicine, The Johns Hopkins School of Medicine and the Welch Center for Prevention, Epidemiology, and Clinical Research, both in Baltimore. Her study was published in *Journal of General Internal Medicine.*

and metformin use reduced diabetes risk by 31%, as compared with the placebo group.

Updated analysis: Researchers wanted to know whether those odds could be improved even further, so they did a new analysis, this time looking specifically at what happened in the first six months after prediabetes patients began treatment and then following up for 10 years. What they found…

• **At the six-month mark, almost everyone (92%) in the intensive lifestyle-modification group had lost weight…**while more than 25% in the metformin group (and nearly 50% in the placebo group) had gained weight. The average percentage of body weight lost in each group was 7.2% in the lifestyle group…2.4% in the metformin group…and 0.4% in the placebo group. Ten years later, most of those in the lifestyle group had maintained their substantial weight loss—quite an accomplishment, given how common it is for lost pounds to be regained.

• **In the intensive lifestyle-modification group, those who lost 10% or more of their body weight in the first six months reduced their diabetes risk by an impressive 85%.** But even those who fell short of the 7% weight-loss goal benefited. For instance, those who lost 5% to 6.9% of their body weight reduced their risk by 54%…and those who lost just 3% to 4.9% reduced their risk by 38%.

If you have prediabetes: Don't assume that diabetes is an inevitable part of your future…and don't assume that you necessarily have to take drugs. By taking action now, you can greatly reduce your risk of developing this deadly disease. So talk with your doctor about joining a program designed to help people with prediabetes adopt healthful dietary and exercise habits that will promote safe, speedy and permanent weight loss. Ask your doctor or health insurer for a referral… or go to *http://www.ymca.net/diabetes-pre vention/* to find a YMCA Diabetes Prevention Program near you. For more information on a drug-free prevention and diabetes cure program, see "The 30-Day Diabetes Cure" on page 379.

What Causes Diabetes? Add Stress to the List

Masuma Novak, PhD, researcher, department of molecular and clinical medicine, Sahlgrenska Academy, University of Gothenburg, Sweden. Her study was published in *Diabetic Medicine*.

When you think about ways to prevent diabetes, you probably don't think about stress. But as it turns out, a particular type of stress can increase the odds of developing type 2 diabetes quite significantly.

The news comes from a long-term study conducted in Sweden that began back in 1970. Participants included about 7,000 men who, at the time, were 47 to 56 years old and free of any history of diabetes, heart disease or stroke. These men completed questionnaires that asked, among other things, about their stress levels. Stress was defined as "feeling tense, irritable or filled with anxiety, or having sleeping difficulties as a result of conditions at work or at home." Nearly 16% of the men reported that they had been feeling "permanent" stress, meaning that it had been ongoing for one to five years or more.

Fast-forward 35 years: By searching through national death records and hospital discharge reports, the researchers determined that, over the following three-and-a-half decades, 899 of the study participants were di-

Curcumin Stops Diabetes from Progressing

Recent finding: When given a curcumin extract (1.5 grams daily) for nine months, study participants at risk for diabetes did not develop the disease. Among a similar group given a placebo, 16.4% developed the disease. Curcumin is the main compound in turmeric, a spice in curry powders and mustards.

Study of 240 people by researchers at Srinakharinwirot University, Bangkok, Thailand, published in *Tufts University Health & Nutrition Letter.*

agnosed at some point with type 2 diabetes. Next, the researchers analyzed the data, adjusting for other factors that influence diabetes risk, such as physical activity level, body mass index, high blood pressure and age.

Findings: Men who had reported feeling ongoing stress at the start of the study had a 45% higher probability of developing diabetes, compared with men who had not had ongoing stress. Interestingly, there was hardly any difference in diabetes risk between the men who had reported periodic stress and those who had reported little or no stress.

The Stress Connection

There are several reasons why stress could contribute to diabetes risk. One is that increased levels of the hormone cortisol, which the body produces in response to stress, may prevent insulin from efficiently removing glucose from the blood. Another is that cortisol may promote the development of belly fat, which is a known risk factor for diabetes. Also, when we're under stress, our bodies produce cytokines, which are proteins that promote inflammation—and evidence suggests that inflammation caused by cytokines is closely involved in the development of type 2 diabetes.

Does ongoing stress also increase diabetes risk in women? Further research is needed to answer that question, but the mechanisms described above are likely to apply to women as well.

Self-defense: Of course, it's not easy to completely eliminate stress from your work or home life (in fact, it's hard to imagine that there are people in the world who experience no stress at all). Still, there are many helpful steps you can take to keep stress from becoming the kind of permanent, endless presence that seems to have given those unfortunate Swedes diabetes. Exercise is known to relieve stress…certain nutrients can reduce stress…and meditation helps, too, by limiting stress-induced inflammation and restoring cortisol levels to more normal levels. What if you still feel stressed much of the time despite your best efforts to reduce stress? Be es-

pecially sure to reduce your other risk factors for diabetes by eating a healthful diet, staying physically active and keeping your weight and blood pressure under control.

Magnesium-Rich Foods Fight Type 2 Diabetes

Magnesium is needed for the hormone insulin to deliver glucose to cells. A magnesium deficiency leads to high blood glucose levels, which may contribute to insulin resistance—a sign of type 2 diabetes.

Self-defense: Eat more magnesium-rich whole grains, nuts, legumes and green leafy vegetables to reach the recommended dietary allowance of 320 milligrams (mg) for women and 420 mg for men.

Examples: One-quarter cup of wheat bran contains 89 mg of magnesium…one ounce of dry-roasted almonds contains 80 mg…one-half cup of cooked frozen spinach, 78 mg…one ounce of dry-roasted cashews, 74 mg…three-quarters cup of bran flakes cereal, 64 mg…one cup of instant fortified oatmeal, prepared with water, 61 mg.

Environmental Nutrition. *www.EnvironmentalNutrition.com*

Eat Walnuts… Prevent Diabetes

Frank Hu, MD, PhD, professor of medicine, Harvard School of Medicine and Channing Division of Network Medicine, Brigham and Women's Hospital, and professor of nutrition and epidemiology, Harvard School of Public Health, all in Boston. His study was published in *Journal of Nutrition.*

We've been losing the fight against diabetes—the prevalence of this deadly disease has increased by more than 175% since 1980.

Good news: There's an easy and economical way to help guard against type 2 diabetes. Just eat a particular type of nut—the walnut.

The news comes from a huge Harvard study that looked at data on nearly 138,000 women. Every two years, participants answered detailed questions about their health and lifestyle. Every four years, they completed lengthy questionnaires about their diets, indicating how often they consumed each of more than 130 foods, with answers ranging from "never or less than once per month" to "six or more times per day." At the start of the study, none of the women had diabetes… by the end of the 10-year follow-up, nearly 6,000 had developed the disease.

The researchers performed a careful analysis that adjusted for age, body mass index, family history of diabetes, smoking, menopausal status and other factors that affect diabetes risk. They also adjusted for consumption of various unhealthful foods (such as sugar-sweetened drinks and processed meats) and healthful foods (whole grains, fish, fruits, vegetables and various types of nuts).

What they found: Women who ate two or more ounces of walnuts per week, on average, had a 24% lower risk for type 2 diabetes…those who ate just one ounce of walnuts per week had a 13% lower risk.

Other types of nuts conferred some benefits, but mainly through weight control, the researchers said. The walnut, however, has a number of properties that make it a winner in the fight against diabetes. For one thing, of all the common tree nuts, walnuts are highest in polyunsaturated fats, containing 47% of these fats by weight—and there is good evidence that polyunsaturated fats have favorable effects on how the body uses insulin. Walnuts also are the richest of all nuts in a particular type of healthful polyunsaturated fat called alpha linolenic acid. What's more, walnuts are high in fiber and plant protein and have been shown to decrease total cholesterol and LDL "bad" cholesterol. These nuts also are loaded with vitamin E and polyphenols that have antioxidant properties.

Bonus: Even though walnuts (like other nuts) are high in calories, they don't seem to cause weight gain in a balanced diet—perhaps because they are so filling and satisfying.

Do men get similar protection against diabetes from eating walnuts? Research will have to prove it, but odds are good that they would.

Going nuts: The best part is that walnuts aren't some specialty product you have to go out of your way to buy, and you don't have to drown yourself in walnuts to get the benefits. Two ounces is only 28 walnut halves per week…that's just four halves per day.

Walnuts are a great snack to have on the road or at work because they don't need to be refrigerated (though if you're going to store them for a while, putting them in the fridge or freezer will keep them fresher longer). While this new study did not look at whether the participants ate their walnuts raw, roasted or otherwise cooked, you can certainly use them in cooking if you like because heat won't significantly affect their health benefits. To increase your intake, try adding chopped walnuts to cereal, salad, rice or soup…stirring ground walnuts into a smoothie or yogurt…and spreading walnut butter on celery sticks or apple slices.

Antidepressants Can Increase Diabetes Risk

In a recent study, people at high risk for type 2 diabetes who did not take diabetes medications were two to three times more likely to develop diabetes if they were taking antidepressants than similar people who were not taking antidepressants. If you are taking an antidepressant and are at risk for diabetes—for example, because you are overweight or have a family history of diabetes—talk to your doctor.

Richard Rubin, PhD, coinvestigator, Diabetes Prevention Program Research Group, Baltimore.

Does Whole Milk Help Prevent Diabetes?

Dariush Mozaffarian, MD, DrPH, codirector of the cardiovascular epidemiology program and an associate professor in the division of cardiovascular medicine at Brigham and Women's Hospital, Harvard Medical School and Harvard School of Public Health, all in Boston.

We're often told to forgo whole milk, cheese and yogurt in favor of low-fat or skim—but recent research suggests that the higher-fat dairy foods may provide significant protection against diabetes.

Background: Dairy products naturally contain a fatty acid called trans-palmitoleic acid. The higher the dairy fat content, the more trans-palmitoleic acid. People who consume whole-fat dairy foods tend to have higher blood levels of trans-palmitoleic acid.

New study: In 1992, researchers took blood samples from 3,736 adults, then followed the participants for 14 years.

Results: Compared with people whose blood levels of trans-palmitoleic acid were lowest, those whose blood levels were highest were 62% less likely to develop diabetes...and they also had more healthful levels of cholesterol, triglycerides, insulin and C-reactive protein (a marker of inflammation) and slightly less body fat.

Theory: Trans-palmitoleic acid affects metabolism in beneficial ways.

This is a very exciting finding, given the current epidemic of diabetes. However, it is possible that people with low trans-palmitoleic acid were generally consuming foods that were less healthful and that this accounted for their greater diabetes risk. In any event, more research is needed before experts would start suggesting that people routinely choose whole-milk dairy products over low-fat or skim. In the meantime, ask your doctor for guidelines on dairy consumption, especially if you've been told that you're at risk for diabetes.

No Two Diabetes Patients Are the Same

Ildiko Lingvay, MD, MPH, an assistant professor in the departments of internal medicine and clinical science and a practicing endocrinologist at The University of Texas Southwestern Medical Center in Dallas. Dr. Lingvay is an internationally recognized researcher who has authored several dozen articles related to type 2 diabetes, obesity and metabolic syndrome.

Chances are you know one or more people who have type 2 diabetes, or perhaps you have been diagnosed with the condition yourself.

The number of Americans with diabetes is truly staggering—a new case is diagnosed every 17 seconds. And, of course, the consequences of uncontrolled diabetes are dire, including increased risk for heart attack and other cardiovascular problems...blindness... leg amputation...kidney failure...and, ultimately, premature death.

To help meet this enormous challenge, medical research has been stepped up.

Now: American researchers have joined forces with their European counterparts to devise new strategies to diagnose and manage diabetes more effectively than ever before.

What you need to know...

Easier Diagnosis

In the US, about 26 million people have diabetes. This includes roughly 19 million who have been diagnosed and an estimated seven million who are undiagnosed. Experts hope that a change in the diagnostic process will lead to more widespread testing and fewer undiagnosed cases.

Until recently, diabetes was typically diagnosed using one of two standard tests—a blood test that requires an overnight fast to measure blood glucose levels...and an oral glucose tolerance test, which involves drinking a high-sugar mixture and then having blood drawn 30 minutes, one hour and two hours later to show how long it takes blood glucose levels to return to normal.

The problem: Both of these tests are inconvenient for the patient, and they measure blood glucose levels only at the time of the test. Many people never get tested because they don't like the idea of having to fast overnight or wait hours to complete a test.

New approach: More widespread use of the A1C test. For decades, the A1C test, which provides a person's average blood glucose levels over a period of two to three months, has been used to monitor how well people with diabetes were controlling their disease. However, it wasn't deemed a reliable tool for diagnosis.

Now, after major improvements that have standardized the measurements from laboratory to laboratory, the A1C test is considered a practical and convenient diagnostic option.

The A1C requires no fasting or special preparation, so it's the perfect "no excuses" test. A1C tests analyzed by accredited labs (such as LabCorp and Quest Diagnostics) meet the latest standardization criteria.

New Treatment Guidelines

Recently, the American Diabetes Association and the European Association for the Study of Diabetes collaborated on recommendations for best treatment practices for type 2 diabetes. The most significant change in the new guidelines is the concept of individualized treatment.

The problem: In the past, diabetes care was based on a one-size-fits-all strategy—with few exceptions, everyone with the condition got basically the same treatment.

New approach: The recently released guidelines acknowledge that there are multiple treatment options for each patient and that the best treatment for one patient may be different from what another patient requires.

This is important because diabetes affects an enormously wide range of people. For example, diabetes can strike a thin 77-year-old woman or a 300-pound teenage boy, and their treatment needs and goals will be as different as their characteristics.

After reviewing a patient's medical history and individual lifestyle, the doctor and patient consider treatment options together and decide on the best fit. *Factors that are more explicitly spelled out in the new guidelines include…*

• **Other medical conditions and medications.** If diabetes treatments interact badly with a patient's current medications, it may cause one of the medications to become ineffective…amplify the effects of the drugs…or cause allergic reactions or serious, even life-threatening side effects. This is especially true for people being treated for kidney disease or heart problems, as many diabetes medications may exacerbate those health issues.

• **Lifestyle and daily schedule.** Diabetes management is easier for people who have predictable schedules. For example, a full-time worker who regularly wakes up at 7 am, eats breakfast, takes a lunch hour and is home for dinner will have simpler treatment needs than a college student who sleeps past noon, eats cold pizza for breakfast, then pulls an all-nighter.

If a physician gives standard insulin recommendations to someone who has an unusual eating and sleeping schedule, it is easy to have blood sugar drop too low—a dangerous condition called hypoglycemia. That's why it is important that patients share as many details of their lives as possible, even if the information seems irrelevant.

Better Treatment Strategies

Until recently, diabetes has been treated with a stepwise approach—starting with conservative treatment, adding medication later only when needed. This sounds good, except that new treatments are incorporated only after previous treatments fail and blood glucose rises.

The problem: Depending on scheduled doctor visits, blood sugar may remain elevated for months or even years before anyone catches the change.

New approach: Research suggests that if physicians intervene more intensively at the beginning, they have the potential to stop the progression of diabetes. With this in mind, treatment aims to decrease the rate at which the body loses insulin-producing ability...and prevent diabetes complications by not allowing blood sugar to exceed safe levels.

Under this new scenario, doctors hit diabetes full force with the patient's individualized treatment plan (including lifestyle changes and medication), instead of with graduated, step-up treatments.

What the new guidelines mean for anyone diagnosed with diabetes: If your current diabetes treatment plan does not address the points described in this article, see your doctor. Your treatment may need to be more customized.

Study Examines Link Between Breast Cancer and Diabetes

Diabetologia, news release

Postmenopausal breast cancer survivors are at increased risk for developing diabetes and should be screened for the disease more closely, a new study suggests.

The Study

Researchers analyzed data from 1996 to 2008 from the province of Ontario, Canada, to determine the incidence of diabetes among nearly 25,000 breast cancer survivors ages 55 or older and nearly 125,000 age-matched women without breast cancer.

During a median follow-up of more than five years, nearly 10% of all the women in the study developed diabetes. Compared to those who had not had breast cancer, the risk of diabetes among breast cancer survivors was 7% higher two years after cancer diagnosis and 21% higher 10 years after cancer diagnosis, the investigators found.

The risk of diabetes, however, decreased over time among breast cancer survivors who had undergone chemotherapy. Their risk compared to women without breast cancer was 24% higher in the first two years after cancer diagnosis and 8% higher 10 years after cancer diagnosis, according to the study, which was published in the journal *Diabetologia*.

Possible Explanations

"It is possible that chemotherapy treatment may bring out diabetes earlier in susceptible women," said study author Lorraine Lipscombe, MD, director, Centre of Integrated Diabetes Care of Women's College Hospital and Women's College Research Institute in Toronto. "Increased weight gain has been noted [after receiving] chemotherapy for breast cancer, which may be a factor in the increased risk of diabetes in women receiving treatment."

"Estrogen suppression as a result of chemotherapy may also promote diabetes," Dr. Lipscombe added. "However, this may have been less of a factor in this study where most women were already postmenopausal."

The study authors suggested that there may be other factors involved for women who received chemotherapy, including glucocorticoid drugs, which are used to treat nausea in patients receiving chemo and are known to cause spikes in blood sugar. In addition, breast cancer patients undergoing chemotherapy are monitored more closely and thus are more likely to have diabetes detected, they noted.

The researchers said it is unclear why diabetes risk increased over time among breast cancer survivors who did not receive chemotherapy.

"There is, however, evidence of an association between diabetes and cancer, which may be due to risk factors common to both conditions," Dr. Lipscombe said. "One such risk factor is insulin resistance, which predisposes to both diabetes and many types of cancer—initially insulin resistance is associated with high insulin levels and there is evidence that high circulating insulin may increase the risk of cancer."

"However, diabetes only occurs many years later when insulin levels start to decline," she said. "Therefore, it is possible that cancer risk occurs much earlier than diabetes in insulin-resistant individuals, when insulin levels are high."

Advice

Overall, the "findings support a need for closer monitoring of diabetes among breast cancer survivors," Dr. Lipscombe concluded.

The American Cancer Society outlines what happens after breast cancer treatment. Visit *www.cancer.gov* and search "after breast cancer treatment."

Some Moisturizers and Soaps May Raise Diabetes Risk

Phthalates are chemicals found in some personal-care products such as moisturizers, nail polishes, soaps, hair sprays and perfumes.

Recent finding: Women who had the highest concentrations of certain phthalates in their bodies had twice the risk for diabetes, compared with women who had the lowest levels of those chemicals. Phthalates also are found in adhesives, electronics, toys and other products. They are known to disrupt the body's endocrine system, which may cause a change in insulin resistance that leads to diabetes.

Study of urinary concentrations of phthalates in 2,350 women, ages 20 to 80 years old, by researchers at Brigham and Women's Hospital, Boston, published online in *Environmental Health Perspectives*.

The Alarming Omission That Puts Moms and Babies at Risk

Jon M. Nakamoto, MD, PhD, laboratory medical director for Quest Diagnostics and an associate professor of pediatrics and endocrinology at the University of California, San Diego. He is coauthor, with other Quest Diagnostics medical experts, of a study on gestational and postpartum diabetes screening published in *Obstetrics & Gynecology*.

There's a vitally important screening test that expectant and new moms need to protect their babies' health and their own. So it's shocking to learn from a new study just how often this test is omitted. We're talking about screening for diabetes during and after pregnancy. *What women must know…*

• **Gestational diabetes develops when a pregnant woman's blood sugar is too high** and her body cannot make and use all the insulin it needs. Based on updated diagnostic criteria, the American Diabetes Association now estimates that this condition affects 18% of pregnancies—a far higher percentage than previously believed.

Risks: Unless diagnosed and controlled, gestational diabetes increases the mother's risk for high blood pressure and triples the likelihood that a cesarean delivery will be needed…it also doubles the baby's risk for serious injury at birth, quadruples the odds of being admitted to the neonatal intensive care unit, and increases the child's risk for obesity and diabetes in adulthood. For most women with gestational diabetes, the condition goes away after childbirth, but about 10% develop type 2 diabetes—a chronic and potentially deadly condition—during the postpartum period. That's why the American College of Obstetricians and Gynecologists recommends that all pregnant women get tested for gestational diabetes between the 24th and 28th week of pregnancy…and that all those diagnosed with gestational diabetes get retested six to 12 weeks after delivery.

Alarming findings: Analyzing data on 924,873 women from pregnancy through six months after delivery, researchers found that 32% were never tested for gestational diabetes...and, worse, that 81% of women who had been diagnosed with gestational diabetes, and therefore should have been screened for postpartum diabetes, did not receive the test.

Based on recent studies, the International Association of Diabetes and Pregnancy Study Groups now recommends that doctors use the 75-g oral glucose tolerance test to screen for diabetes. If you are pregnant or postpartum, discuss this with your obstetrician.

Good Dog!

Dogs can detect blood sugar drops in diabetics. Trained dogs can detect a faint odor emitted by humans as much as 20 minutes before blood sugar drops to a critical level. Such drops can cause diabetics to collapse or go into a coma if they do not receive medication immediately. A trained dog is valued at $20,000, but Dogs4Diabetics and other providers often require only $150 for people in need.

Dogs4Diabetics, Nylabone Training Center, Concord, California. *www.dogs4diabetics.com*

Say What? A Surprising Link to Hearing Loss for Women

Derek J. Handzo, DO, otolaryngology resident and Kathleen Yaremchuk, MD, chair of the department of otolaryngology–head and neck surgery at Henry Ford Hospital in Detroit.

Needing to turn up the volume on the TV or radio yet again...straining to catch a dinner companion's words in a crowded restaurant...having trouble identifying background noises. It's normal to notice an increase in such experiences as we get older.

But: A study has highlighted an important and often overlooked risk factor that can make age-related hearing loss among women much worse than usual—diabetes that was not well controlled.

Researchers reviewed the medical charts of 990 women and men who, between 2000 and 2008, had had audiograms to test their ability to hear sounds at various frequencies...participants also were scored on speech recognition. Study participants were classified by age, gender and whether they had diabetes (and, if so, how well controlled their blood glucose levels were).

Results: Among women ages 60 to 75, those whose diabetes was well controlled were able to hear about equally as well as women who did not have diabetes—but those with poorly controlled diabetes had significantly worse hearing. (For men, there was no significant difference in hearing ability between those with and without diabetes, no matter how well controlled the disease was, though this finding could have been influenced by the fact that men generally had worse hearing than women regardless of health status.)

Now hear this: Diabetes also increases the risk for heart disease, vision loss, kidney dysfunction, nerve problems and other serious ailments...so this new study gives women with diabetes yet one more important motivation for keeping blood glucose levels well under control with diet, exercise and/or medication.

If you have not been diagnosed with diabetes: If your hearing seems to be worsening, ask your doctor to check for diabetes—particularly if you have other possible warning signs, such as frequent urination, unusual thirst, slow wound healing, blurred vision and/or numbness in the hands and feet.

Your Eyes Can Reveal Early Warning Signs of Diabetes

Emily Y. Chew, MD, medical officer and deputy director in the division of epidemiology and clinical applications at the National Eye Institute, part of the National Institutes of Health, Bethesda, Maryland.

The eyes may be the windows to the soul, but they also are the windows to the body. Via the eyes, doctors can view internal structures, including nerves and blood vessels. What they learn can provide important clues about your whole body—and your current and future health.

Regular eye exams are obviously important for visual health. But they also can detect conditions that you might not know you have—and that your primary care doctor might have missed.

Clues, such as damaged blood vessels, may be overlooked by your primary care doctor. And damaged blood vessels could indicate diabetes.

Patients with diabetes have a high risk for diabetic retinopathy, a diabetic eye disease in which blood vessels in the retina are damaged, causing vision loss and blindness. During an eye exam, your doctor will look for microaneurysms, areas where blood vessels are swollen or leaking, a sign of diabetic retinopathy. Your doctor also might notice the growth of new, abnormal blood vessels, which could indicate advanced diabetes and diabetic retinopathy.

Most diabetics get regular eye exams because they know about the risk for eye damage. But in some cases, patients who don't know that they have diabetes—or who have it but aren't controlling their blood sugar—first learn there's a problem during a routine eye exam.

Is It Riskier to Be a Thin Diabetic?

Mercedes R. Carnethon, PhD, associate professor of preventive medicine, associate chair for faculty development and mentoring, department of preventive medicine, Feinberg School of Medicine, Northwestern University, Chicago. Her study was published in *The Journal of the American Medical Association.*

It's well-known that obesity raises the risk for type 2 diabetes, but roughly 11% of people with the disease have a "normal" body mass index between 18.5 and 24.9.

They are what you might call "thin people with diabetes."

If you're one of them, you might assume that you're at lower risk for serious complications from your diabetes—but a new study actually shows the opposite.

It has found that people with type 2 diabetes who are not overweight have a higher risk for death from any cause, compared with overweight or obese people with type 2 diabetes.

How much greater was the risk?

And how can that be? We spoke with the researchers to find out…

Puzzling Paradox

In the study, scientists analyzed data that followed a total of 2,625 people from the time of their type 2 diabetes diagnoses for anywhere from seven to 28 years (or their death).

It showed that people who were of normal weight at the time of diagnosis had more than twice the risk of dying from any cause as people who were overweight or obese at the time of diagnosis, and this held true even after adjusting for factors such as age, smoking and blood pressure.

That finding seemed backward, so we spoke with lead author Mercedes Carnethon, PhD, to learn more.

The Skinny On Risk

Dr. Carnethon said that there are several possible explanations for why normal-weight people with diabetes might die sooner than overweight people with diabetes, including…

• **Loss of lean muscle.** As people age, some drop pounds because they lose muscle and bone—not fat. That's a problem, though, because fat isn't as sensitive to insulin as muscle is, so the higher your fat-to-muscle ratio, the less your body is able to use circulating glucose for energy. In other words, it's possible that a person with a "normal" weight who has a high fat-to-muscle ratio could have a higher risk for death than a person who is classified as "overweight" and has a lower fat-to-muscle ratio.

• **Other illnesses.** Diabetes is generally an obesity-related disorder, so having diabetes and a normal weight might reflect another underlying illness—and that underlying illness might be what raises the risk for death. The researchers did exclude participants who died within two years of developing diabetes, but they were not able to account for other diseases participants may have had, such as cancer.

• **Less aggressive treatment.** It's possible that leaner people with diabetes are screened less frequently and/or less carefully…or that they are undertreated once their diabetes is diagnosed, because doctors may mistakenly perceive them to be at lower risk for complications and death compared with overweight people with diabetes.

It's Not an Excuse to Eat Fried Foods

So if you are of normal weight and have type 2 diabetes, what can you do to help prolong your life? Certainly, the results of this study do not suggest that you should just gobble food to gain weight. But there are a few things that you can do, Dr. Carnethon explained…

1. Talk to your physician about it. Make sure that your doctor fully appreciates that even though you are not overweight or obese, your diabetes still represents a risk to your well-being and you should be evaluated and treated no less aggressively than your overweight counterparts. In fact, show him or her

this article about death rates if you need to! And ask: "Do we fully understand the reason I got diabetes…and are we doing everything possible to treat that underlying cause?"

2. Make yourself strong. Exercise of any kind will help improve your blood sugar control, but strength training, in particular, is a great way to lose fat and increase muscle.

By following these two simple tips, you'll have a better chance of living a long, healthy life!

Psoriasis Sufferers: Keep an Eye on Blood Sugar!

Joel M. Gelfand, MD, associate professor of dermatology and epidemiology at Perelman School of Medicine, University of Pennsylvania, Philadelphia. He was senior author of a study published in *Archives of Dermatology*.

If you have psoriasis—as millions of Americans do—the scaly, itchy patches of skin on your scalp and/or other body parts aren't the only health problems to be concerned about.

We're not talking about the well-known increased risks, such as the risks for heart attack, stroke, arthritis and certain cancers.

There's yet another disease to add to the already long list.

A recent study found that people with psoriasis are at increased risk for also developing type 2 diabetes—even if they don't have any of the risk factors that are common to both diseases, such as obesity. And the more severe the psoriasis, the greater the risk of type 2 diabetes.

How much extra risk do you have? In the study, people with mild psoriasis had an 11% greater risk of developing type 2 diabetes, compared with those who did not have psoriasis…and people with moderate-to-severe psoriasis had a 46% higher risk.

The Common Thread: Inflammation

To find out more about why having a skin disease might increase the risk for type 2 diabetes, we spoke with senior study author Joel M. Gelfand, MD.

"Both diseases are caused by chronic inflammation," Dr. Gelfand noted, "and we think that the same inflammation that causes psoriasis also prevents the body from responding to insulin as well as it should, which is what leads to type 2 diabetes."

A Two-Part To-Do List

So if you have psoriasis, what does this mean for you?

First of all: Dr. Gelfand said that it's important to get regular blood sugar screenings to test for type 2 diabetes, since the earlier you find out that you have diabetes, the easier it is to keep it in check. "If you have psoriasis, I recommend beginning blood sugar screenings at age 18 and then getting checked at least every three years after that—depending on your particular health conditions and what your doctor advises," he said. For many people, blood sugar is checked as part of their annual physical.

"Think of your psoriasis as a window into what's happening in your body," he continued. "Those rashes on your skin aren't necessarily just exterior problems—they may be a sign of other metabolic issues that are happening in the interior of your bloodstream."

Second of all: In the meantime, do everything you can to help prevent (or at least delay) type 2 diabetes from developing. That means—you guessed it—following a healthy diet, exercising regularly and losing excess weight, Dr. Gelfand said.

He also stressed that these recommendations are especially important for people with psoriasis who are 40 or older because the risk of developing diabetes increases with age.

We also asked Dr. Gelfand whether reducing psoriasis symptoms might lower your risk of type 2 diabetes. "There is some evidence that it might help, so it's worth a shot, but scientists don't yet know," he said.

One Food That Diabetics Really, Really Need

David Jenkins, MD, PhD, DSc, professor, department of nutritional science, and Canada Research Chair in Nutrition and Metabolism, University of Toronto, Canada. He also is director of the Risk Factor Modification Centre, St. Michael's Hospital, Toronto, and lead author of a study on legumes and diabetes control published in *Archives of Internal Medicine*.

A humble everyday food is amazingly good at helping to control diabetes and prevent the complications of this deadly disease—yet many diabetes patients ban it from their diets.

We're talking about legumes—beans, chickpeas, lentils—which truly are close to magical when it comes to their health effects, particularly for folks with type 2 diabetes.

So if you're among the "bean holdouts," we're hoping to convince you to give beans and other legumes a place of honor in your daily diet.

Your life could depend on it! *Here's why...*

Beans and Your Blood Sugar

For diabetes patients, keeping blood sugar levels as close to normal as possible is crucial...but controlling those fluctuating levels can be a real challenge. Many patients take antihyperglycemic drugs for this purpose, yet diet remains a major factor in diabetes management.

A lot of people with diabetes focus on high-fiber foods such as whole grains to help avoid problems like heart disease. And fiber does help (though the exact mechanism is unknown). But now a new Canadian study shows that beans and other legumes do the job even better.

The secret behind legumes' awesome power lies in their low glycemic index (GI) status. The GI is a scale from 0 to 100 that ranks foods based on their immediate effects on blood glucose levels. The lower its GI, the less of a blood sugar spike a particular food causes.

Beans Best the Competition

The study included 121 men and women with type 2 diabetes. Participants were divided into two groups and assigned to follow one of two healthful diets that were fairly equal in total calories, fat, protein and carbohydrates consumed.

As part of their diet, the first group was told to consume about 190 grams (two half-cup servings) of beans or other legumes each day. The second group's diet included an equal amount of whole grains, such as whole-wheat cereals and breads and brown rice. Each group also avoided the alternate food—in other words, the bean group avoided whole grains and the whole-grain group avoided beans.

After three months: The whole-grain group did benefit from their diet—but the bean-eaters benefited even more. *Specifically…*

• **Hemoglobin A1C values**—indicated by a blood test that measures average blood glucose levels for the previous three-month period—dropped significantly more in the legume group than in the whole-grain group.

Using an equation that calculates risk for coronary heart disease (CHD), researchers found that the legume group's CHD risk score fell from 10.7 to 9.6. This was largely the result of the legume eaters' decrease in systolic blood pressure (the top number of a blood pressure reading) from 122 to 118. In contrast, in the whole-grain group, neither the CHD risk score nor blood pressure decreased significantly.

Also: In the legume group, the average weight loss and waist-size reduction slightly exceeded those of the high-fiber group.

Give a High-Five for Low GI

When we spoke with the study's lead author, David Jenkins, MD, PhD, DSc, he said that his team purposely chose study participants who already had reasonably good diets. "We wanted to see how people doing well could make further improvements," he explained.

And in fact, both the legume group and the high-fiber group did improve. On the hemoglobin A1C test, for instance, both groups got their levels down below 7.0—a benchmark that often allows patients to eventually decrease their diabetes medication.

Still, the legumes came out ahead for several reasons. Unlike whole grains, beans are a very good source of protein—and protein does not cause blood sugar to fluctuate the way carbs can. Beans also provide plentiful potassium, which may reduce blood pressure by counteracting the effects of sodium. But the primary factor in beans' favor, Dr. Jenkins said, is that they are among the lowest-GI foods because their complex carbohydrates are digested slowly.

Who Should Give A Hill of Beans

Legumes are particularly good for diabetes patients, but just about everyone can benefit from better blood sugar control. Are you hesitant because you don't care for the taste or texture? There are many types of beans and other legumes to choose from—so keep experimenting until you find some you enjoy!

It's easy to incorporate one cup of these potent orbs into your daily diet since they are so versatile.

Tasty suggestions: Add white beans to vegetable soups and meat stews…use black or kidney beans plus tofu as the basis for chili…top salads with edamame (boiled green soy beans)…serve lentils as a side dish or salad…enjoy the many varieties of hummus, made from chickpeas…or purée any type of bean to make dip, adding what tastes good to you—olive oil, pepper and/or other spices you love.

And don't worry about gas. Despite the "musical" reputation of beans, the study participants registered few complaints in this department. However, if you are concerned about bloating or flatulence, Dr. Jenkins advised starting with just one-half cup per day and increasing gradually over several weeks to give your digestive system time to adjust.

Red Wine and Diabetes

Is it safe to drink red wine if you have diabetes—or even recommended?

Red wine in moderation usually is not harmful to people with diabetes and may benefit them by decreasing stress and lessening feelings of deprivation. *But talk to your doctor…*

If you take insulin: Alcohol lowers blood sugar, so you may need less insulin.

Also: Eat when you drink to buffer the alcohol's effect.

If you take the drug metformin (Glucophage): The combination of metformin and alcohol can increase the risk for a serious condition called lactic acidosis.

Anne Peters, MD, professor of medicine, University of Southern California, and director of the USC Westside Center for Diabetes, both in Beverly Hills. She is author of *Conquering Diabetes* (Penguin).

The One-Day Sugar Challenge

Miriam Nelson, PhD, director of the John Hancock Research Center on Physical Activity, Nutrition, and Obesity Prevention and a professor of nutrition at the Friedman School of Nutrition Science and Policy, both at Tufts University in Boston. She also is the author or coauthor of many books, including *Strong Women Stay Young* (Bantam) and *The Social Network Diet* (FastPencil Premiere).

Sparkling prettily in the sun, that bowlful of sugar on your kitchen table probably looks harmless enough…and a spoonful certainly makes your bitter coffee taste better. Yet in a recent article published in *Nature*, researchers from the University of California, San Francisco, said that sugar was so dangerous that it ought to be controlled the way alcohol and tobacco are!

That's a wake-up call for folks who know that it would be wise to cut back on sugar but could use some help getting started. Well, here is that help—the One-Day No-Added-Sugars Challenge from Miriam Nelson, PhD, a professor of nutrition at Tufts University and coauthor of *The Social Network Diet*. We spoke with Dr. Nelson for details on the challenge, which I'll share in a moment. *First, some background…*

Dr. Nelson said that human beings are genetically programmed to like sweet foods—we're born that way. However, worldwide sugar consumption has tripled in the last 50 years, bringing with it a host of health problems. These developments have nothing to do with our normal affinity for naturally sweet foods, such as fruit…and not much to do with the bit of sugar we stir into our coffee. Rather, the overconsumption crisis is primarily due to the ubiquity of added sugars that manufacturers put into today's processed foods. In addition to obviously sweet treats (packaged cookies, candies, soda, sugary breakfast cereals), we unwittingly consume copious added sugars snuck into nonsweet products such as bottled salad dressings, condiments, pasta sauces, crackers, cereals and sliced bread.

Freaky fact: The average American woman takes in about 24 teaspoons of added sugars every day (and the average man takes in even more).

The dangers: You know that sugar contributes to obesity and increases the odds for insulin resistance and type 2 diabetes. But you may not realize that excessive sugar consumption also has been linked to increased risk for high blood pressure and high triglycerides…osteoporosis…liver disease…gout…hormonal disruptions…impaired cognitive function…impaired immunity…and various types of cancer. Plus, sugar can trigger cravings for even more sugar, creating an escalating cycle of harm.

The solution: Dr. Nelson's challenge is straightforward—for just one day, give up all added sugars. This means forgoing the spoonful you might normally use to sweeten your coffee or cereal, but more importantly, it means becoming attuned to all the unexpected places added sugars lurk. "When you do this, you see the 'stealth sugar' that has come into our food supply," Dr. Nelson said. "When I did my own challenge, I realized that there were very simple substitutions—like choosing naturally sweet balsamic vinegar for my salad rather than French dressing, which has 11 grams of added sugar per serving." By avoiding added sugars, Dr. Nelson said, you can reduce your calorie count by nearly 400 in a single day!

Manufacturers use oodles of sneaky synonyms to fool unwary consumers. So check the ingredients and avoid not only items that list sugar, but also anything that contains corn syrup…dextrose…fructose…fruit juice concentrate…glucose…honey…lactose…malt syrup… maltodextrin…maltose…maple syrup…molasses…rice syrup…sucrose…tagatose…treacle…or trehalose. (Note that whole fruits, vegetables and milk provide naturally occurring sugars, which are fine to eat during your challenge.)

Why do this for just one day rather than vowing to give up added sugars all the time? Because this challenge doesn't require a major commitment—and diet-wise, most people can do almost anything for a single day. "This is a mind-jogger. Once you're more aware of where all the added sugars come from, it's easier to make a few permanent shifts in your diet. For instance, you'll still be getting some sugar, but maybe only half as much," Dr. Nelson explained. That level of improvement can bring significant health benefits. And it's likely to curb your sugar cravings to boot—which will help you cut back even further in the future.

Sugar Alternatives If You Need to Watch Your Blood Sugar

Suzanne Havala Hobbs, DrPH, a licensed, registered dietitian and clinical associate professor in the departments of health policy and management in the Gillings School of Global Public Health, University of North Carolina at Chapel Hill. She is author of *Living Vegetarian for Dummies* and *Living Dairy-Free for Dummies* (both from Wiley).

Do you need to watch your sugar intake, but love to bake? *Best nonsugar alternatives for baking…*

Sugar adds sweetness and flavor to quick breads, cookies, cakes, muffins and other baked goods, but it also affects texture, moistness and color. In some recipes, you can reduce the amount of sugar by 25% with good results. In other recipes, you can't replace or reduce the sugar at all.

You sometimes can compensate for the loss of sweetness by adding extra vanilla, almond flavoring, cinnamon, nutmeg or even bits of fruit such as raisins, diced apples, dried cherries or mashed, ripe banana, which come with fiber and nutrients in exchange for the small number of added calories.

Sugar substitutes such as *aspartame* (Equal) and *sucralose* (Splenda) aren't ideal for baking because their sweetening power is degraded by heat and they don't contribute to the texture or color of baked goods. Sugar substitutes that incorporate sugar, such as Equal Sugar Lite and Splenda Sugar Blend, make for better baking.

Alert for Diabetes Patients

Warning: There have been reports of insulin-delivery pumps and glucose-monitoring devices being potentially damaged after passing through full-body or x-ray scanners used by airport security.

If you use one of these devices for diabetes care: Get a letter from your doctor that will allow you to bypass the scanners and be hand-screened instead.

H. Peter Chase, MD, clinical director, Barbara Davis Center for Childhood Diabetes, University of Colorado, Aurora.

How Full Fat Helps Diabetes

Dariush Mozaffarian, MD, DrPH, associate professor, department of medicine, Brigham and Women's Hospital and Harvard Medical School, department of epidemiology, Harvard School of Public Health, Boston.

After all these years a follower of health news can't help but notice that certain basic nutritional truths keep reasserting themselves. For instance, it seems blatantly obvious that we could save lots of money researching the root causes of chronic illness by saying simply this—always eat in moderation, and choose foods that are as close to their natural states as possible.

As the latest example, some research says people who consume whole-fat dairy products—as opposed to their processed, lower-fat versions—have a 60% lower incidence of diabetes! This flies in the face of what experts have been advising for decades—that everyone but babies and toddlers should choose milk, cheese, yogurt and other dairy products with the lowest possible fat content, because the saturated fat that's prominent in dairy products is bad for your health.

Fat Is Beautiful?

Now, in a study from Harvard published in *Annals of Internal Medicine,* a team of researchers has found that people with the highest circulating levels of a type of fatty acid that is found only in whole-fat dairy are one-third as likely to get diabetes as those with the lowest circulating levels. Higher levels of the fatty acid—called trans-palmitoleic acid—were also associated with lower body mass index (BMI)…smaller waist circumference…lower triglycerides (potentially harmful blood fats)…higher levels of HDL "good" cholesterol…less insulin resistance…and lower levels of C-reactive protein, a marker for general inflammation.

How the study was done: At the study's start, researchers began with baseline measurements of glucose, insulin, inflammatory markers, circulating fatty acids and blood lipids (such as triglycerides and cholesterol) from stored 1992 blood samples of 3,736 participants in the National Heart, Lung, and Blood Institute-funded Cardiovascular Health Study. Those data were compared with the same participants' dietary records and recorded health outcomes (including the incidence of diabetes) over the following 10 years. During this period, 304 new cases of diabetes were recorded. When the participants were grouped according to their circulating levels of trans-palmitoleic acid, the researchers discovered that those with higher levels had the lowest rates of diabetes.

You May Have Type 2 Diabetes and Not Even Know It

With type 1 diabetes, the pancreas produces little or no insulin, a hormone needed to convert sugar into fuel for cells. This soon leads to excessive thirst and hunger, frequent urination, weight loss, lethargy and blurry vision. However, the more common type 2 diabetes—in which the body's cells do not use insulin properly—often causes no symptoms in the early stages. You could have the disease for five years or more before developing telltale signs, including those above plus slow-healing sores, frequent vaginal and/or bladder infections, and patches of dark, thickened skin.

Best: Talk to your doctor about diabetes risk factors—high cholesterol, high blood pressure, excess weight, history of gestational diabetes, family history of diabetes or being of African American, Native American, Latino, Pacific Islander or Asian descent.

Steven V. Edelman, MD, professor of medicine at University of California, San Diego, Veterans Affairs Medical Center, and founder and director of the not-for-profit education organization Taking Control of Your Diabetes, both in San Diego. *www.tcoyd.org*

How Much Dairy?

We spoke with the study's lead researcher, Dariush Mozaffarian, MD, DrPH, associate professor of epidemiology at Harvard School of Public Health, who said that other studies have suggested a similar phenomenon with dairy consumption, but that his is the first to have used objective chemical markers in the blood to determine the relationship between this specific fatty acid and the onset of diabetes. The participants with the highest levels averaged about two servings of whole-fat dairy foods a day.

This is not a license to indulge yourself in a daily serving of strawberry shortcake with extra whipped cream or a giant ice cream from Cold Stone Creamery…but you might want to consider switching from skim milk to whole milk with your morning cereal and selecting full-fat yogurt over low-fat or nonfat. The difference in calories isn't great—and you may be getting some real metabolic and cardiovascular benefits.

Recent Diabetes Diagnosis? You May Be at Risk for This Cancer

Babette S. Saltzman, PhD, research assistant at Seattle Children's Hospital and leader of a study conducted while at the Fred Hutchinson Cancer Research Center in Seattle.

If you recently learned that you have diabetes, the last thing you want to hear about is yet another potential health problem—in this case, an increased risk for cancer of the endometrium (uterine lining). But knowledge is power, so please take note of a study in the *American Journal of Epidemiology.*

Researchers analyzed data on 3,082 women ages 45 to 74. Compared with women who did not have diabetes, those who did have diabetes had a 30% higher risk for endometrial cancer if their diabetes had been diagnosed five or more years earlier…and a more than twofold higher risk for endometrial cancer if their diabetes had been diagnosed less than five years earlier.

Theory: Like other hormones (such as estrogen), insulin can influence endometrial cancer risk…and in the prediabetic or early diabetic stages, hyperinsulinemia (elevated blood level of insulin) often has not yet been adequately controlled.

Diabetes patients: The more recently your diabetes was diagnosed, the more important it is to speak with your doctor about strategies that can lower endometrial cancer risk—including many of the same strategies associated with good cardiovascular and overall health.

Helpful: Losing excess weight (obesity is a known risk factor for endometrial cancer)…exercising regularly…and eating a diet low in saturated fats and high in fruits and vegetables. If you are premenopausal, also ask your doctor about birth control pills—according to the National Cancer Institute, endometrial cancer risk decreases by about 50% after five years of oral contraceptive use.

Up all Night? Watch Out for Diabetes

Frank B. Hu, MD, PhD, MPH, professor of nutrition and epidemiology at Harvard School of Public Health and a professor of medicine at Harvard Medical School, both in Boston. He also is coauthor of a study on shift work and diabetes published in *PLoS Medicine.*

Working a rotating shift that includes both nights and days is tough on many levels, as you've probably heard from sleep-deprived friends who do it. Now a recent study reveals yet another concern with this increasingly common type of work schedule—an elevated risk of developing type 2 diabetes.

Researchers combed the data on 177,184 US women who participated in the Nurses' Health Study, analyzing age, weight, diet, exercise habits and work schedules...and tracking who got diabetes during the two-decade study period. For the study, a rotating night shift was defined as working three or more nights per month in addition to working some days and evenings in that same month.

Results: Compared with women who did not work rotating night shifts, those who worked such shifts for three to nine years were 20% more likely to develop diabetes. The risk for diabetes rose 40% when rotating night shifts were worked for 10 to 19 years... risk rose 58% with 20 or more years of such work.

Explanation: Rotating shift work disrupts the body's circadian rhythm, elevating blood glucose and insulin levels as well as increasing blood pressure and reducing sleep efficiency.

Self-defense for rotating night-shift workers: Diabetes can be deadly, so be sure that your doctor is aware of your work schedule. Discuss an appropriate schedule for screening for diabetes. And immediately alert your doctor if you develop any possible warning signs of the disease (excessive thirst, increased urination, blurred vision). Also, remember that lifestyle changes—adopting a healthy diet, getting regular exercise, losing excess weight—go a long way in guarding against the development of diabetes.

The Sleep Cure for Blood Sugar Balance

Michelle M. Perfect, PhD, assistant professor, school psychology, University of Arizona, Tucson.

I f you (or someone in your family) has diabetes and you do your best to manage your blood sugar levels throughout the day, yet your levels often are still curiously high, a recent study has shed light on why that might be the case.

Getting poor-quality sleep at night may be secretly sabotaging your blood sugar—even when you're doing everything right!

And this is a recipe for diaster. So spoke with study author Michelle Perfect, PhD, an assistant professor of psychology, disability and psychoeducational studies at The University of Arizona in Tucson to find out more.

A Chicken-and-Egg Conundrum

This study was done on kids with type 1 diabetes, but as you'll see later, this news about sleeping applies to all types of diabetics of all ages.

The study: Fifty children ages 10 to 16 with type 1 diabetes were compared with a matching number of similarly aged kids without the condition. Participants underwent a home-based sleep study for five nights, wearing equipment that measured their blood sugar, sleep stage (one of four stages ranging from light to heavy), speed of breathing and heart rate. Parents and children also answered questions about topics such as mood level and amount of daytime sleepiness. School records were obtained to analyze grades. And the kids and their parents were told to administer insulin as they normally would.

The findings, which appeared in the January 2012 issue of *Sleep*, were intriguing. Children in the control group (no diabetes) spent 19% of their sleep time in deep sleep, while children with diabetes spent only 15% of their sleep time in deep sleep. Sleep apnea—a serious condition that causes dangerous pauses in breathing during sleep and awakenings during the night and that heightens risk for heart attack and stroke—was experienced by about one-third of the children with diabetes. Compared with the control group, the diabetics were more likely to have high blood sugar, which was expected, said Dr. Perfect, since very few kids achieve perfect glucose control. But interestingly, the diabetic kids with sleep apnea had much higher blood sugar levels compared with diabetic kids who did not have sleep apnea.

So that raises the question—does poor-quality sleep cause blood sugar irregularities, or do these sugar fluctuations lead to troubled sleep? It could be either or both, said Dr. Perfect, who didn't set out to answer that question and said that more research needs to be done to figure out the answer. There are theories supporting both angles. For example, prior studies from other research teams established that not getting enough deep sleep causes the brain to release less of a chemical that helps stabilize blood glucose levels. But on the other hand, Dr. Perfect said that if you have diabetes, you may sometimes need to get up in the middle of the night to check your blood sugar, so having diabetes may also cause more sleep disturbances, though that wasn't specifically analyzed in this study. It's also possible that poor blood glucose control—such as not administering enough insulin at the proper times—could lead to sleep problems.

Tips for Solid Shut-Eye

When asked whether these findings might apply to adults with type 1 diabetes and anyone with type 2 diabetes, Dr. Perfect said that her findings support what other studies on type 2 diabetics and sleep have found—the better your sleep, the better your blood sugar control. So people of any age with diabetes should pay close attention to how well they're sleeping and should ask their family members to keep an ear out for lots of snoring or gasping while sleeping—a sign of sleep apnea, which is dangerous and would require immediate attention from a doctor.

Dr. Perfect advises diabetics of all ages to ask themselves the following questions…

•**Most of the time, do I feel refreshed when I wake up?**

•**Am I easily awoken during the night?**

If the answer to these questions is "no" and then "yes," then Dr. Perfect advises that you talk to your doctor, because it may mean that you're not getting enough deep sleep. There isn't any quick trick that can make you sleep deeply throughout the night, but you can be more diligent about ensuring good

sleep habits—including minimizing light and noise in the bedroom…abstaining from caffeine and stimulating activities such as exercising or Web surfing near bedtime…and keeping your bedroom a little cooler than the rest of the house. Quality sleep is important for everyone—and, it seems, even more so if you have diabetes.

Got Diabetes? The Extra Help You Need

Joel Zonszein, MD, CDE, FACE, FACP, professor of clinical medicine, Albert Einstein College of Medicine, director, Clinical Diabetes Center, Montefiore Medical Center, New York City.

If you've been diagnosed with type 2 diabetes, you may think that you have a good handle on keeping your blood sugar under control…and maybe you do…but you probably don't. Research has shown that only 16% of people with type 2 diabetes properly carry out the recommended "self-care behaviors," such as eating healthy foods, staying active, taking medications and monitoring blood sugar. A recent study has found that diabetics who get regular individual instruction from a nurse or dietitian do much better and feel much better.

Getting Face Time

To learn more about how much of an impact one-on-one instruction can have, we called Joel Zonszein, MD, director of the clinical diabetes program at Montefiore Medical Center in New York City. He took a close look at the new research, which was conducted in Minneapolis and Albuquerque, New Mexico, and was published in *Archives of Internal Medicine*.

Participants included 623 patients (men and women, average age 62) who had had type 2 diabetes for 12 years, on average. Researchers considered only patients who had taken a type of blood test called the A1C, which measures the average blood sugar levels within the previous two to three months, and selected only those whose A1C scores were above 7%—that's higher than what is considered healthy, so it indicated that, like the vast majority of diabetics, these people were poorly managing their condition. These patients were then split into three groups—one group received individual education, another received group education and another received no education.

After seven months, the researchers asked participants to take the A1C test again. *And here's what they discovered…*

• **It was basically "no contest" when comparing the results from group to group.** The no-education group lowered its A1C score by 24% (perhaps because they knew that they were being studied)…those who received group education, by 27%…and individual-education participants lowered their A1C scores by a whopping 51%.

• **The proportion of participants who got their scores into a healthy range (under 7%) was highest among those who were individually educated—21% of those participants achieved this fantastic result.** Meanwhile, only 13% of the no-education group and 14% of the group-education group got into the healthy range.

• **What's even better is that the individual education didn't take up much time at all**—it consisted of exactly three one-hour sessions with a certified diabetes educator (either a nurse or a dietitian) about one month apart. Three short visits! The educators focused on topics that included all the healthy behaviors mentioned above (eating right, staying active, taking medications and monitoring) along with problem solving (for instance, if a patient doesn't take a pill, maybe it's because he doesn't understand why he needs it and what it does)…healthy coping (such as if a patient is frustrated, instead of grabbing a bag of chips, he's taught to go for a walk or listen to calming music)…and setting personalized, action-oriented goals (for example, scheduling an eye exam once a year to prevent diabetic complications such as retinal detachment or blindness).

Why It Works So Well

Dr. Zonszein stressed one word—accountability. Having to face someone regularly and acknowledge mistakes that you may be making is a powerful motivator—apparently more powerful than just the idea of being healthy, he said. "It's also about empowerment—teaching diabetics to be in charge of the disease rather than letting the disease control them," he added. And there's another, slightly darker side to all this—doctors aren't typically trained to give appropriate diabetes education, and they aren't reimbursed for the time they spend educating patients about it, as Dr. Zonszein noted. So in too many cases, after an initial diagnosis and a hastily written prescription, patients are essentially sent out into the cold to muddle through on their own—not a shining example of great health care.

So, what can you do for you? In Dr. Zonszein's opinion, the best diabetes education programs are hospital-based with certification from the American Diabetes Association (ADA), since these are regularly evaluated to ensure that they meet high standards. To find one in your area, check the ADA's site, *www. Diabetes.org*. Call the programs in your area and ask them specifically if they offer one-on-one instruction, what it costs and whether it is covered by insurance. Dr. Zonszein suggests trying one-on-one counseling for at least three months. At the very least, don't assume that you already know all that you need to know about managing your diabetes—ask your doctor for diabetes brochures and visit reputable Web sites such as *www.Diabetes. org* for the latest information and advice. And then make a point to discuss the info with your doctor at your next appointment. (Don't expect him or her to bring it up.)

Though one-on-one counseling might make you feel embarrassed or might seem like a nuisance, it's clear that the more you know about your disease and the more accountable you are about taking care of yourself, the better you will manage it…it's just human nature…so get the help!

30-Day Diabetes Cure— You May Even Be Able to Throw Away Your Meds!

Stefan Ripich, ND, a naturopathic physician based in Santa Fe, New Mexico. He practiced for 10 years at the Palo Alto Veterans Administration Medical Center and established the first holistic clinic in the VA system. He is coauthor, with Jim Healthy, of *The 30-Day Diabetes Cure* (Bottom Line Books).

In the US, a new case of diabetes is diagnosed every 30 seconds. And many of those people will be given drugs to treat the disease.

You can control high blood sugar with medications, but they aren't a cure and they can have side effects. They also are expensive, costing $400 or more a month for many patients.

Much better: Dietary remedies that have been proven to reduce blood sugar, improve the effects of insulin (a hormone produced by the pancreas that controls blood sugar), promote weight loss and, in many cases, eliminate the need for medications. A UCLA study found that 50% of patients with type 2 diabetes (the most common form) were able to reverse it in three weeks with dietary changes and exercise.

How you can do it, too…

• **Eliminate all HFCS.** A 2010 Princeton study found that rats given water sweetened with high-fructose corn syrup (HFCS) gained more weight than rats that drank water sweetened with plain sugar, even though their calorie intake was exactly the same.

Reasons: The calories from HFCS fail to trigger leptin, the hormone that tells your body when to quit eating. Also, HFCS is more likely than natural sugar to be converted to fat…and being overweight is the main risk factor for diabetes.

What to do: Read food labels carefully. HFCS is the main sweetener in soft drinks and many processed foods, including baked goods such as cookies and cakes.

• **Don't drink diet soda.** If you give up HFCS-laden soft drinks, don't switch to diet soda. Diet sodas actually cause weight gain by boosting insulin production, leading to excessively high insulin in your blood that triggers greater fat accumulation and even more cravings for sugar.

A study published in *Diabetes Care* found that drinking diet soda every day increased the risk for type 2 diabetes by as much as 67%.

If you crave sweet bubbly beverages, pour one inch of pure fruit juice into a glass and then top it off with carbonated water.

• **Eat barley.** I advise patients to eat foods that are as close to their natural state as possible—whole-grain cereals and breads, brown rice, etc. These "slow carbohydrates" contain fiber and other substances that prevent the spikes in glucose and insulin that lead to diabetes.

Best choice: Barley. Researchers at the Creighton Diabetes Center in Omaha compared the effects of two breakfasts—one consisting of oatmeal (one of the best slow carbohydrates) and the other consisting of an even slower breakfast cereal made from barley. Participants who ate barley had a postmeal rise in blood sugar that was significantly lower than participants who ate the oatmeal breakfast.

You can eat cooked barley as a side dish…sprinkle it on salads…or mix it into tuna, chicken, tofu or lentil salad.

• **Season with cinnamon.** About one-quarter teaspoon of cinnamon daily reduces blood sugar, improves insulin sensitivity and reduces inflammation in the arteries—important for reducing the risk for heart disease, the leading cause of death in diabetics.

Research published in *Diabetes Care* found that people with type 2 diabetes who ate at least one-quarter teaspoon of cinnamon daily reduced fasting blood sugar levels by up to 29%. They also had up to a 30% reduction in triglycerides (a blood fat) and up to a 27% drop in LDL (bad) cholesterol.

• **Eat protein at breakfast.** Protein at breakfast stabilizes blood sugar and makes people feel satisfied, which means that you'll consume fewer calories overall. Lean protein includes eggs, chicken and fish.

• **Eat more meat (the good kind).** We've all been told that a diet high in meat (and therefore saturated fat) is inherently unhealthy. Not true. Other things being equal, people who eat more saturated fat actually tend to weigh less and have smaller waist measurements than similar adults who eat less.

The real danger is from processed meats, such as bacon, hot dogs and many cold cuts. These foods have more calories per serving than natural meats. They're higher in sodium. They have a lower percentage of heart-healthy omega-3 fatty acids and other beneficial fats that lower inflammation.

A large study that looked at data from 70,000 women found that those who ate processed meats with every meal were 52% more likely to develop diabetes than those who ate healthier meats and other foods.

I advise people to look for grass-fed beef. It's lower in calories and fat than industrialized grain-fed factory feedlot beef and higher in omega-3s.

• **Snack on nuts.** Healthful snacking between meals keeps blood sugar stable throughout the day. Nuts are the perfect snack because they're high in fiber (which reduces abrupt increases in glucose and insulin) and protein (for appetite control). They also are good sources of important nutrients and antioxidants.

A Harvard study of 83,000 women found that those who frequently ate almonds, pecans or other nuts were 27% less likely to develop diabetes than those who rarely ate nuts. A small handful every day is enough.

Caution: "Roasted" nuts usually are a bad choice because they often are deep-fried in coconut oil. They also have added salt and/or sugar. "Dry-roasted nuts" have not been fried in fat but usually have salt and sugar.

If you like roasted nuts, it's best to buy organically grown raw nuts and lightly toast them in a dry fry pan over very low heat (or in your oven).

• **Supplement with vitamin D.** In theory, we can get all the vitamin D that we need from sunshine—our bodies make it after the sun hits our skin. But about 90% of Americans don't get adequate amounts—either because they deliberately avoid sun exposure or because they live in climates without much sun.

A Finnish study found that participants with high levels of vitamin D were 40% less likely to develop diabetes than those with lower amounts. Vitamin D appears to improve insulin sensitivity and reduce the risk for diabetes-related complications, including heart disease.

Recommended: Take 1,000 international units (IU) to 2,000 IU of vitamin D-3 daily.

• **Remember to exercise.** It's just as important as a healthy diet for preventing and reversing diabetes. The Diabetes Prevention Program (a major multicenter clinical research study) found that people who walked as little as 17 minutes a day, on average, were 58% less likely to develop diabetes.

Walking for 30 minutes most days of the week is optimal.

Some Diabetes Drugs Are Linked to Vision Loss

Macular edema—swelling in the central retina that can lead to blindness—is more common among patients taking Actos or Avandia. But the medicines, known as thiazolidinediones, generally have more benefits than risks, and the risk for macular edema is small. Patients taking the medications should have more frequent eye examinations to detect early signs of the condition.

Joel Zonszein, MD, FACE, FACP, a certified diabetes educator, professor of clinical medicine and director of the Clinical Diabetes Center, University Hospital of the Albert Einstein College of Medicine, Montefiore Medical Center, Bronx, New York.

Weight Loss Surgery Can Help Diabetes

According to recent research, weight-loss surgery treats type 2 diabetes better than standard therapy.

Diabetes went into remission in 73% of obese diabetes patients who had laparoscopic adjustable gastric-banding surgery (in which an adjustable band is surgically placed around the stomach, limiting the amount of food that can be eaten)—compared with 13% given conventional treatment, including drugs and counseling on exercise and weight loss. Surgical patients lost 20.7% of body weight, compared with 1.7% of body weight for patients given conventional treatment. More research is needed, but many doctors expect surgery for diabetes patients to become common within a few years.

John Dixon, PhD, obesity researcher, Monash University Medical School, Melbourne, Australia, and leader of a study published in *The Journal of the American Medical Association*.

Which Exercises Are Best If You Have Diabetes?

John P. Porcari, PhD, program director of the Clinical Exercise Physiology (CEP) program at the University of Wisconsin–La Crosse.

Exercise can lower blood sugar almost as well as medication. Recent guidelines for people with diabetes recommend 150 minutes of moderate to strenuous aerobic exercise weekly,* in addition to three strength-training sessions that work all the major muscle groups—increasing muscle mass is believed to be a particularly effective way of controlling blood sugar.

*Always talk to your doctor before starting a new exercise program. If you have a chronic illness, it may be useful to consult a physical therapist for advice on exercise dos and don'ts for your particular situation.

All aerobic exercises are beneficial, but those that use both your upper- and lower-body muscles are best because they help deliver blood glucose to muscle cells throughout your body—try an elliptical machine, the Schwinn Airdyne (a stationary bike that adds arm movements) or NuStep (a recumbent stepper that incorporates arm movements). If you walk, use poles to involve your arms. Try to do some type of exercise every day—this helps ensure its blood sugar–lowering benefits.

If you use insulin on a regular schedule: Exercise at the same time each day, if possible, to help maintain even, predictable blood sugar levels. Insulin should typically be used 60 to 90 minutes after your workout—check with your doctor or diabetes educator.

To prevent excessive drops in blood sugar: Eat something before or just after exercise and adjust your insulin dose on the days you work out. Talk to your doctor for specific advice.

How Women with Diabetes Should Exercise

Jane Yardley, PhD, postdoctoral fellow, Human and Environmental Physiology Research Unit, University of Ottawa, Ontario, Canada. The study was published in *Diabetes Care*.

If you have type 1 diabetes (the kind where your body can't produce insulin), then you know that regular exercise is essential because it helps keep blood sugar under control and reduces the chance of complications such as high blood pressure and high cholesterol.

But when you exercise, which do you do first—cardio/aerobic…or strength training?

That may sound like a silly question, but a new study suggests that the order in which you do your exercises can make a big difference in terms of how well you control your blood sugar.

Using the Proper Fuel

To understand the recent research, keep in mind that the human body can use either glucose or fats as fuel—and, of course, for people with diabetes, the level of glucose in the blood tends to be out of whack.

Now, in previous studies, it's been shown that in healthy people (who do not have diabetes), performing strength training immediately before aerobic exercise increases the body's use of fats—not glucose—as fuel. And insulin, which is key to the proper maintenance of blood glucose, plays a less important role when fats are being used as fuel. Therefore, researchers were curious to find out whether exercising in this particular order might better protect individuals with diabetes from hypoglycemia (low blood sugar).

Let's Get Moving

We spoke with the study's lead author, Jane Yardley, PhD, a postdoctoral fellow in the human and environmental physiology research unit at the University of Ottawa in Ontario, Canada. The research involved 12 men and women (average age 32) with type 1 diabetes who already lifted weights and ran at least three times a week. For the study, each participant completed two exercise sessions held at least five days apart. In one session, each subject ran on a treadmill for 45 minutes and then lifted weights for 45 minutes. In the other session, the sequence was reversed.

Both sessions were held at the same time of day and the participants ate the same foods the day before, the day of and the day after they exercised. Whenever a participant's glucose dropped too close to a hypoglycemic level during exercise, the exercise was interrupted and the participant was given a carbohydrate supplement to bring glucose back up. The participants were set up with continuous glucose monitoring starting the day before their exercise sessions and ending the following day.

Results: Those who performed strength training first were less likely to reach the hypoglycemic danger zone. In fact, 43% more glucose supplementation was needed when running came first.

Plus, the blood sugar benefits of strength training first lasted through the night. Researchers found that nighttime episodes of hypoglycemia were, on average, shorter (48 minutes rather than 105 minutes) and less severe following an exercise session that began with strength training.

Lift Before You Run

Why might strength training first have such a positive effect on blood sugar? Dr. Yardley said that more growth hormone is secreted during anaerobic exercise (such as strength training), and growth hormone might increase the use of fats as fuel, rather than glucose.

Another possibility: Performing strength training first can cause lactate to circulate in the blood. Some lactate could be converted to glucose, so blood sugar wouldn't drop as quickly.

So should all people with type 1 diabetes strength train before doing cardio? Dr. Yardley recommends it, though she did point out one limitation to the study, which is that the participants were fit, and fit people may use glucose differently than people who aren't in such good shape. But whether you're fit or unfit, it wouldn't hurt to strength train first, said Dr. Yardley. Even if you can't handle 45 minutes of each type of exercise, it's not the total time that matters—it's the order.

We asked Dr. Yardley whether this advice would also hold true for type 2 diabetics. She explained that most type 2 diabetics are not insulin-dependent, so hypoglycemia isn't as big a risk. Therefore, the order in which they do those exercises isn't likely as critical.

Statins and Diabetes

Statins raise diabetes risk in postmenopausal women.

According to a recent finding, postmenopausal women who took cholesterol-lower-

One in Three US Adults Could Have Diabetes by 2050

Currently one in nine people has the disease. The predicted increase in cases is attributable to aging of the population, obesity, sedentary lifestyle, people with diabetes living longer and an increase in the population of minority groups that are at higher risk for type 2 diabetes.

Ann Albright, PhD, RD, director, Division of Diabetes Translation, Centers for Disease Control and Prevention, Atlanta. *www.cdc.gov*

ing statin drugs had a 48% higher likelihood of developing type 2 diabetes than women who did not take statins. Statins lower risk for cardiovascular disease in people who already are at risk for cardiovascular disease.

Caution: Talk to your doctor about the risks and benefits. Do not stop taking statins on your own.

Yunsheng Ma, MD, PhD, epidemiologist and associate professor of medicine, University of Massachusetts Medical School, Worcester, and leader of a study of 153,840 postmenopausal women, published in *Archives of Internal Medicine.*

Say Good-Bye to Your Diabetes Medication

Mark A. Stengler, NMD, licensed naturopathic medical doctor in private practice, Stengler Center for Integrative Medicine, Encinitas, California...adjunct associate clinical professor at the National College of Natural Medicine, Portland, Oregon...author of many books, including *The Natural Physician's Healing Therapies* and coauthor of *Prescription for Natural Cures* (both from Bottom Line Books).

Some of my patients who have type 2 diabetes are able to keep the disease under control with diet, exercise and supple-

ments. Lucky them! But for other diabetes patients, that's not enough and they must take pharmaceutical medications.

I'm happy to report that there is another natural treatment option for diabetes patients who currently take pharmaceutical medications. Research has found that a plant extract called berberine can control diabetes as well as, or better than, common medications such as *metformin* (Glucophage) and *rosiglitazone* (Avandia). And it does this with no side effects—and without damaging the liver, as some medications do. *Here's how berberine can help people with diabetes...*

• **A naturally occurring chemical compound, berberine is found in the roots and stems of several plants,** including Hydrastis canadensis (goldenseal), Coptis chinensis (coptis or goldthread) and Berberis aquifolium (Oregon grape). Long used as a remedy in Chinese and Ayurvedic medicines, berberine is known for its antimicrobial properties and as a treatment for bacterial and fungal infections. Several decades ago, berberine was used to treat diarrhea in patients in China. That was when doctors noticed that the blood sugar levels of diabetes patients were lower after taking the herbal extract—and berberine began to be investigated for this purpose.

• **Over the past 20 years, there has been much research on berberine and its effectiveness in treating diabetes.** In 2008, Chinese researchers published a study in *Metabolism* in which adults with newly diagnosed type 2 diabetes were given 500 milligrams (mg) of either berberine or the drug metformin three times a day for three months. Researchers found that berberine did as good a job as metformin at regulating glucose metabolism, as indicated by hemoglobin A1C (a measure of blood glucose over several weeks)...fasting blood glucose...blood sugar after eating...and level of insulin after eating. Berberine even reduced the amount of insulin needed to turn glucose into energy by 45%! In addition, those taking berberine had noticeably lower trigylceride and total cholesterol levels than those taking metformin.

• **In another 2008 study published in** ***Journal of Clinical Endocrinology*** **and** ***Metabolism,*** researchers found that type 2 diabetes patients who were given berberine had significant reductions in fasting and postmeal blood glucose, hemoglobin A1C, triglycerides, total cholesterol and LDL (bad) cholesterol—and also lost an average of five pounds, to boot, during the three-month study period.

In a 2010 study in *Metabolism*, Chinese researchers compared people with type 2 diabetes who took either 1,000 mg daily of berberine or daily doses of metformin or rosiglitazone. After two months, berberine had lowered subjects' fasting blood glucose levels by an average of about 30%, an improvement over the rosiglitazone group and almost as much as people in the metformin group. Berberine also reduced subjects' hemoglobin A1C by 18%—equal to rosiglitazone and, again, almost as good as metformin. In addition, berberine lowered serum insulin levels by 28.2% (indicating increased insulin sensitivity)…lowered triglycerides by 17.5%…and actually improved liver enzyme levels. Pharmaceutical medications, on the other hand, have the potential to harm the liver.

These were remarkable findings. Here was a botanical that was holding up to scientific scrutiny—and performing as well as, or better than, some drugs that patients had been taking for diabetes for years.

How Berberine Works In the Body

Berberine helps to lower blood glucose in several ways. One of its primary mechanisms involves stimulating the activity of the genes responsible for manufacturing and activating insulin receptors, which are critical for controlling blood glucose.

Berberine also has an effect on blood sugar regulation through activation of incretins, gastrointestinal hormones that affect the amount of insulin released by the body after eating.

How Berberine Can Help

I recommend berberine to my patients with newly diagnosed type 2 diabetes to reduce their blood sugar and prevent them from needing pharmaceutical drugs. When a diet, exercise and supplement program (including supplements such as chromium) is already helping a diabetes patient, I don't recommend that he/she switch to berberine.

Some patients are able to take berberine—and make dietary changes—and stop taking diabetes drugs altogether. People with severe diabetes can use berberine in conjunction with medication—and this combination treatment allows for fewer side effects and better blood sugar control. I don't recommend berberine for prediabetes unless diet and exercise are not effective. Berberine is sold in health-food stores and online in tablet and capsule form. The dosage I typically recommend for all diabetes patients is 500 mg twice daily.

For patients with diabetes who want to use berberine, I recommend talking to your doctor about taking this supplement. It's also important for every patient with diabetes to participate in a comprehensive diet and exercise program.

Note that berberine helps patients with type 2 diabetes, not type 1 diabetes (in which the body does not produce enough insulin).

The Body Part That's Aging Fastest If You Have Diabetes

Hongha Vu, MD, clinical gastroenterology fellow, Washington University, St. Louis.

People with type 2 diabetes have a lot of balls to keep in the air, medically speaking.

They need to, of course, keep their blood sugar in check, get regular eye screenings and monitor their feet, which often can suffer from nerve damage.

Now recent research may add another item to that already-long checklist.

It suggests that people with type 2 diabetes should start getting colonoscopies earlier and, perhaps, get them more frequently.

Here's why...

Type 2 Diabetics Have "Older" Colons

Researchers from Washington University in St. Louis reviewed colonoscopy records of male and female patients over a six-year span, comparing the incidence of precancerous polyps in three groups—those ages 40 to 49 with type 2 diabetes...those ages 40 to 49 without type 2 diabetes...and those ages 50 to 59 without type 2 diabetes.

Their first finding was expected, since age increases the risk for precancerous polyps. Nondiabetics in their 50s had a much higher rate of precancerous polyps (32%) than nondiabetics in their 40s (14%).

But their second finding was alarming. Diabetics in their 40s had nearly the same rate of precancerous polyps (30%) as nondiabetics in their 50s (again, 32%). And this was after individual cancer risk factors—such as gender, race, obesity, smoking, high cholesterol and alcohol use—were taken into account.

"It's almost as if the colons of diabetics are 10 years older," said study author Hongha Vu, MD, a clinical gastroenterology fellow at the university. It's believed that the culprit is a high level of insulin in type 2 diabetics, since insulin is thought to promote cell growth in the colon, she said.

Should Screening Guidelines Change?

Current guidelines from the American Cancer Society (ACS) suggest that colorectal cancer screenings should begin at age 50 for people at average risk for colon cancer. ACS advises those at high risk (anyone with inflammatory bowel disease, a personal history of colorectal cancer or a family history of colorectal cancer) to get screened even earlier (the age varies by risk factor). In addition, the site for the American College of Gastroenterology says, "Recent evidence suggests that African-Americans should begin screening earlier at the age of 45."

What about people with type 2 diabetes? The American Diabetes Association, while acknowledging that type 2 diabetes is linked with a higher risk for colorectal and other cancers, urges diabetics to reduce lifestyle-related cancer risk factors but doesn't deviate from the "begin screening at age 50" recommendation for those at average risk.

Dr. Vu, however, is hoping that her research—and future studies that replicate it—will change that. Her study suggests that type 2 diabetics should consider getting their first colorectal cancer screening earlier than age 50.

In her view, doctors should be open to discussing the idea of earlier colorectal cancer screenings with diabetic patients based on their overall risk factors, and it might help to bring a copy of this article with you if you want to broach the idea with your physician. Unfortunately, if you're a type 2 diabetic who wants to get a colorectal cancer screening before the age of 50 but you're considered to be at "average risk," according to the current guidelines, it's unlikely that insurance will cover it, said Dr. Vu, and a colonoscopy can cost around $1,200 or more. If more research confirms Dr. Vu's findings and screening guidelines change, colonoscopies are more likely to be covered in the future.

If you're a type 2 diabetic who is over the age of 50 and you've already started getting colorectal cancer screenings, Dr. Vu said that there is no data yet on whether or not more frequent screenings are necessary, but if you're concerned, talk to your doctor. ***Also:*** This increased risk for colorectal cancer does not apply to people of any age with type 1 diabetes, said Dr. Vu, because type 1 is caused by a lack of insulin.

What Your Doctor May Not Tell You About Your Diabetes

Frederic J. Vagnini, MD, a cardiovascular surgeon and director of the Heart, Diabetes & Weight Loss Centers of New York in Lake Success. His clinical interests include heart disease, diabetes, weight loss and nutrition. Dr. Vagnini is author, with Lawrence D. Chilnick, of *The Weight Loss Plan for Beating Diabetes* (Fair Winds).

For most of the 19 million Americans diagnosed with type 2 diabetes, the main goal of treatment is simply to control their glucose (blood sugar) levels with diet, exercise and sometimes medication.

But there's much more that should be done to help prevent serious complications, which can shorten the life expectancy of a person with diabetes—by about 7.5 years in men and 8.2 years in women.

Sobering statistics: About 80% of people with diabetes die from cardiovascular complications, such as a heart attack. About half the patients with poor glucose control will eventually suffer from nerve damage (neuropathy). Another 20% to 30% may experience retinopathy or other eye disorders.

Whether or not you're taking medication for diabetes, virtually all of these complications can be avoided—and, in some cases, reversed—with natural approaches.

Important: Be sure to speak to your doctor before following any of the steps in this article—some may affect diabetes drugs and other types of medication.

Best ways for people with diabetes to avoid complications…

Controlling Inflammation

People with diabetes typically have elevated levels of C-reactive protein, a blood protein that indicates chronic low-level inflammation, the underlying cause of most cardiovascular, eye and nerve disorders. Inflammation also exacerbates arthritis, which is more common in diabetics than in those without the disease. *Effective options…*

•**Stop eating wheat.** Many people with diabetes are allergic or sensitive to gluten, a protein found naturally in wheat, barley and rye—and sometimes in other grains, such as oats, because they become "cross-contaminated" during processing. Even trace amounts of gluten can stimulate the production of cytokines, substances that increase inflammation. (See below to self-test for gluten sensitivity.)

Besides increasing inflammation in these patients, exposure to gluten may lead to fatigue and joint problems. Gluten may also impair digestion in these people, making it harder to lose weight—a serious problem because excess body fat increases inflammation even more.

Important: Read food labels. Besides avoiding obvious sources of gluten such as wheat bread and wheat pasta, look for terms such as "amino peptide complex," "filler flour," "hydrolyzed protein" and "vegetable starch"—these indicate that gluten is or may be found in the product. Gluten is also present in unexpected sources, such as soy sauce, malt and graham flour, as well as thousands of nonfood products, including some medications. To determine if a medication contains gluten, call the drug manufacturer.

•**Give up dairy.** Oftentimes people who are sensitive to gluten also have problems digesting casein, a dairy protein.

To test for a gluten or dairy sensitivity: Eliminate each food type one at a time for several weeks. If you notice an improvement in energy, or a reduction in joint pain or digestion problems, you're probably sensitive to one or both. To make sure, reintroduce dairy and/or gluten foods one at a time to see if your symptoms return.

Important: Foods that are labeled "lactose-free" or "dairy-free" are not necessarily casein-free. Foods that are both gluten-free and casein-free can be found online at *www.TraderJoes.com* or *www.wholefoods.com*.

To keep it simple: Remember that all un-processed meats, vegetables and fruits are gluten-free and dairy-free.

•**Supplement with omega-3 fatty acids.** The American Diabetes Association recommends a diet high in these fatty acids because of their ability to reduce inflammation and other diabetes complications. Unfortunately, many people find it difficult to eat enough omega-3–rich foods, such as salmon, mackerel and herring—two six-ounce servings a week are recommended—so supplements often are a good choice.

My advice: Take a daily supplement with at least 1,500 mg of eicosapentaenoic acid (EPA), the component in fish oil that helps reduce the inflammation that contributes to diabetes-related complications. If you're allergic to fish, you can use an omega-3 supplement derived from algae.

Omega-3 fatty acids, also found in flaxseed and walnuts, have the additional benefit of helping to lower triglycerides, blood fats that have been linked to atherosclerosis and cardiovascular disease.

Fight Arterial Calcification

The Rotterdam Heart Study, which looked at the dietary histories of more than 4,800 patients, found that those with low blood levels of vitamin K2 were 57% more likely to develop heart disease, due in part to an increase in calcium in the arteries. Paradoxically, these patients had lower bone levels of calcium, which increases the risk for fractures.

Because diabetic patients have an extremely high risk for heart disease, I routinely recommend a daily supplement (45 mcg) of vitamin K2. You can also get more of this nutrient by eating such foods as liver, eggs and certain cheeses.

Caution: Because there are different forms of vitamin K—some of which interfere with the effects of *warfarin* (Coumadin) and other blood thinners—always speak to your doctor before taking any vitamin K supplement.

Overcome Fatigue

Both inflammation and elevated blood sugar increase fatigue, making it one of the most common symptoms of diabetes. *Helpful…*

•**Coenzyme Q10 (CoQ10) increases the body's production of adenosine triphosphate (ATP),** a molecule that enhances the performance of mitochondria, the energy-producing components of cells. CoQ10 is also an antioxidant that reduces inflammation. Typical dose: 100 mg to 200 mg, twice daily.

•**Magnesium is involved in glucose and insulin reactions** and is typically lower than normal in people with diabetes who experience fatigue. Patients who eat a healthy diet, including magnesium-rich foods such as nuts and oatmeal, and supplement with magnesium often report an increase in energy. They also show improvements in blood pressure and cardiac performance. Talk to your doctor about the appropriate dosage of a magnesium supplement—especially if you have kidney disease or heart disease, both of which can be worsened by too much magnesium.

All forms of supplemental magnesium can be used, but magnesium citrate causes diarrhea in some people. If this happens to you, take a different form, such as magnesium taurate or magnesium glycinate.

Avoid Diabetic Neuropathy

Excess blood sugar can damage the tiny blood vessels that carry blood and nutrients to nerves in the fingers, legs and/or feet, causing neuropathy. Neuropathy can eventually lead to tissue damage that requires amputation. *What to try…*

•**Alpha-lipoic acid makes the cells more sensitive to insulin and can relieve symptoms of diabetic neuropathy.** Typical dose: 600 mg to 1,200 mg daily for people with diabetes who have neuropathy. To help prevent neuropathy, 100 mg to 300 mg daily is the typical dose.

•**B-complex supplement may help prevent neuropathy or reduce symptoms in patients who already have it.** *Typical dose:* Two B-100 complex supplements daily for people with diabetes who have neuropathy...one B-100 complex daily to help prevent neuropathy.

Prevent Eye Damage

High blood sugar can cause diabetic retinopathy, which can lead to blindness. It can also increase eye pressure and lead to glaucoma.

Self-defense: Eat more fresh fruits and vegetables. These foods contain antioxidants such as lutein, zeaxanthin and vitamin C, which strengthen eye capillaries, fight free radicals and reduce the risk for blindness. Frozen fruits and vegetables also can be used.

Best choice: Blueberries or bilberries—both contain anthocyanins, antioxidants that help prevent eye damage and appear to improve glucose levels.

Treatment for Diabetic Neuropathy

Up to 70% of diabetes patients have some form of neuropathy. The most common is peripheral neuropathy, in which nerves in the feet, legs, arms and/or hands are damaged. Symptoms include numbness that results in a reduced ability to feel pain. The first step in treating diabetic neuropathy is to bring blood glucose (sugar) levels within the normal range—high levels can injure nerve fibers throughout the body. Blood sugar levels should be 90 mg/dL to 130 mg/dL before meals and less than 180 mg/dL two hours after meals. Consistently keeping blood sugar within this target range can help delay progression of diabetic neuropathy and may improve existing symptoms. If you keep your blood sugar under control but continue to experience pain in your legs, feet, arms or hands, you may want to ask his doctor about taking *pregabalin* (Lyrica), an anticonvulsant drug that has been approved by the FDA to treat pain associated with diabetic neuropathy.

Larry Deeb, MD, president for medicine and science, American Diabetes Association, Tallahassee, Florida.

Natural Remedy for Neuropathy

People with peripheral neuropathy, damage to the nerves in the extremities, often experience pain and numbness in their hands and/or feet. Studies show that the nutrient acetyl-l-carnitine (ALC) can increase and repair nerve fibers. Although not studied for hereditary peripheral neuropathy, I have seen ALC reduce the symptoms of other types of neuropathy. I recommend 1,000 mg of ALC three times daily between meals. Acupuncture also can help to reduce your symptoms. A holistic doctor can provide you with other natural therapies, such as injectable or intravenous vitamin B-1, which can help the neurological system.

Mark A. Stengler, NMD, licensed naturopathic medical doctor in private practice, Stengler Center for Integrative Medicine, Encinitas, California...adjunct associate clinical professor at the National College of Natural Medicine, Portland, Oregon...author of many books, including *The Natural Physician's Healing Therapies* and coauthor of *Prescription for Natural Cures* (both from Bottom Line Books).

Nausea from Diabetes? Electrical "Acupressure" to the Rescue

Jiande Chen, PhD, professor of medicine and director, Clinical Physiology Laboratory, University of Texas Medical Branch, Galveston. His study was presented at the American College of Gastroenterology's 77th Annual Scientific Meeting.

About 10% to 15% of diabetes patients develop a digestive complication called gastroparesis, in which food takes too long to leave the stomach—and the symptoms are nasty. But help may be on the horizon, a new study shows. The secret weapon is a small electrical device that a patient simply straps onto his or her wrist or leg.

Background: Gastroparesis develops when high blood glucose levels cause chemical changes, damaging the vagus nerve. This nerve controls the muscles that move food through the digestive tract. Gastroparesis symptoms include nausea, vomiting, heartburn, bloating, abdominal pain, stomach spasms and an uncomfortable feeling of abdominal fullness. What's more, the condition can worsen diabetes by making blood sugar control more difficult. Medication often fails to relieve the problem. Some patients, unable to keep any food down, wind up needing feeding tubes that go straight to their intestines.

The study: Researchers developed a watch-sized microstimulator, a device that delivers a short, painless burst of electrical stimulation. Diabetes patients with gastroparesis were asked to wear the device on their wrists or legs for two hours after lunch and for two hours after dinner, continuing daily for eight weeks. For four of those weeks, the device was positioned to make contact with specific acupressure points associated with nausea relief. (The acupoints were PC6, on the inner wrist about two-and-a-half finger widths up from the wrist crease...and ST36, on the front of the leg about four finger widths below the kneecap, just outside the shinbone.) For the other four weeks, the device was positioned slightly differently so that it did not contact the acupoints, thus delivering a sham treatment.

Throughout the study, researchers monitored patients' symptoms and conducted electrogastrogram (EGG) tests, recording the electrical signals that control muscle contractions and nerve activity of the stomach.

Results: Electrical stimulation of the acupressure points, on average, reduced patients' nausea by 30%...vomiting by 40%...retching by 31%...bloating by 21%...and abdominal fullness by 21%. The treatment also improved muscle and nerve function in the stomach, as shown on the EGG. The sham treatment produced no improvement in symptoms or EGG results. No side effects from electrical stimulation were reported.

These are very promising results, especially since the treatment is noninvasive, risk-free and can be used at home—but there are some caveats. For one thing, this was a small study with just 26 participants, and though it was presented at a recent meeting of the American College of Gastroenterology, it has not yet been published in a peer-reviewed journal. Also, the device used in the study isn't available to the public yet. Though further studies are need, researchers hope that the microstimulator treatment will be available by prescription within a year or two.

In the meantime: There is another approach that, in theory, might be helpful for patients with diabetes-induced gastroparesis. Talk to a licensed acupuncturist about having professional acupressure stimulation of the same acupoints used in the study...or consider electroacupuncture, which is similar to traditional acupuncture except that an electrical current makes the needle stimulation stronger and steadier. To find a licensed acupuncturist in your area, visit the American Association of Acupuncture and Oriental Medicine Web site at *http://www.aaaom online.org/.*

PNEUMONIA
AND INFLUENZA

Believe it or not, the eighth leading cause of death in America is pneumonia and flu, with pneumonia claiming the most lives. People over the age of 65 are more susceptible to these diseases. Therefore it is not only critical to be aware of the signs and symptoms, but also to know all the steps you can take to boost your immunity and prevent these diseases right now.

http://www.lung.org/lung-disease/influenza/in-depth-resources/pneumonia-fact-sheet.html

Chapter 20

EVERYTHING YOU NEED TO KNOW ABOUT PNEUMONIA

The Nutrient That Beats Pneumonia

Pneumonia is the eighth leading cause of death in the US. Sadly, antibiotics alone often aren't enough to save the lives of pneumonia patients when their immune systems are so weak.

The good news is that adding a nutrient "booster" to the antibiotics has been shown to prevent more pneumonia deaths, according to a recent study.

The best part is that this nutrient is both cheap and easy to find.

One Mighty Mineral

The study took place in a developing country, Uganda, and it looked only at kids under five years old, but the researchers said that its findings apply to people of all ages all over the world—even those in developed countries. Researchers looked at 352 male and female children between six months old and five years old who were suffering from severe pneumonia. In addition to getting the prescribed antibiotics, half of the children received a daily supplement pill that contained the current Ugandan Recommended Daily Allowance (RDA) of zinc (10 milligrams per day for children under one year old and 20 milligrams per day for older children) and the other half received a daily placebo pill. (The US RDA is slightly lower.) Before starting treatment, the average level of zinc in the blood of all the children was measured and found to be below the normal range.

Findings: Children receiving zinc supplements were much less likely to die from the pneumonia. Within seven days, about 4% of the children receiving zinc died, while 12% of the children receiving the placebo died. (Remember, all received the same antibiotic treatment.) Researchers followed the children for only seven days, because due to past research they suspected that a child who survived pneumonia would likely have recovered by the seventh day of treatment. But they did not track how many (if any) children died after seven days.

According to one of the study authors, James Tumwine, MBChB, MMed, PhD, a professor of pediatrics and child health at the School of Medicine at Makerere University in Uganda, zinc increased survival because

James Tumwine MBChB, M.Med, PhD, professor of pediatrics and child health, School of Medicine, Makerere University, Kampala, Uganda, whose study was published in *BMC Medicine*.

the children were deficient in zinc and the added zinc may have helped boost their immune systems. For example, zinc increases the function of T-cells (types of white blood cells), as well as the hormone thymulin, both of which help increase immunity.

Cheap and Easy to Find

If you think that the only people who are deficient in zinc are those in developing countries or are young children, think again. For example, the ongoing National Health and Nutrition Examination Survey has found that about 35% to 45% of Americans age 60 or older aren't getting as much zinc as they should. And vegetarians also are at risk for zinc deficiency—not only because they do not consume the foods that are high in zinc (such as oysters and meat), but also because two staples of their diets, legumes and whole grains, contain phytates which inhibit zinc absorption.

Many people do not know whether they're zinc deficient. And you can have a healthy level for years and then it can suddenly drop once an infection such as pneumonia develops, said Dr. Tumwine, so asking a doctor to check your level at your annual checkup doesn't necessarily do any good.

If you get pneumonia, ask your doctor whether taking a daily zinc supplement or getting more of it through foods including red meat, poultry, oysters, nuts and zinc-fortified cereals may boost recovery. The RDA for zinc in the US for adults is 11 milligrams (mg) per day for men over age 19 and 8 mg per day for women over age 19. *For kids, it varies…*

• **7 months to 3 years old:** 3 mg

• **4 to 8 years old:** 5 mg

• **9 to 13 years old:** 8 mg

• **14 to 18 years old:** males, 11 mg; females, 9 mg

• **19 and older:** males, 11 mg; females, 8 mg

Fortunately, zinc is a mineral that's cheap and widely available. The cost of a zinc supplement is just pennies per tablet, and you can find zinc wherever nutritional supplements are sold.

How Not to Get Pneumonia—Proven Ways to Avoid This Deadly Illness

Neil Schachter, MD, professor of medicine at Mount Sinai School of Medicine and the medical director of respiratory care at Mount Sinai Hospital, both in New York City. He is author of *Life and Breath: The Breakthrough Guide to the Latest Strategies for Fighting Asthma and Other Respiratory Problems—At Any Age* (Broadway).

Most people tend to worry about pneumonia during the winter months, but it can strike at any time of year.

Recent development: For reasons that are not yet understood, older men have been found to be 30% more likely than older women to die from community-acquired pneumonia—a type of pneumonia that develops in people who have had little or no contact with hospitals or other medical settings where the illness is often contracted. Even though everyone should take precautions to avoid this potentially life-threatening illness, older men should be especially vigilant.

What you need to know to protect yourself—and loved ones…

What Is Pneumonia?

Pneumonia is inflammation of the lungs due to infection—usually bacterial or viral. Of the estimated four million Americans who contract pneumonia each year, 1.2 million are hospitalized and 55,000 die. Pneumonia is the fifth-leading cause of death among Americans over age 65.

Symptoms include cough, chills, fever, fatigue and trouble breathing.

Caution: Since an older adult's normal body temperature is often below 98.6°, he/she may not seem to have a fever.

Pneumonia Avoidance Made Easy

In addition to not smoking (smoking increases risk for all respiratory illnesses), getting the seasonal flu vaccine has long been a cornerstone of pneumonia prevention. Because flu weakens the immune system and damages the airways, the illness makes it easier for bacteria and viruses to multiply and turn into pneumonia. The flu vaccine is recommended for anyone over age 50 and for people of any age with pneumonia risk factors, such as asthma, heart disease or any other chronic illness. (If you didn't get a seasonal flu vaccine this winter, it's even more crucial for you to follow the advice below.)

Important steps—besides getting vaccinated for the seasonal flu—that help guard against pneumonia…

1. Get a pneumonia vaccination. A vaccine against pneumococcal pneumonia, which is caused by Streptococcus pneumoniae (the most common cause of bacterial pneumonia), is available for adults and lasts for five years. The vaccine helps prevent pneumococcal pneumonia's most serious complications, such as bacteremia (infection in the bloodstream) and septicemia (infection throughout the body).

Important finding: A recent report shows that a significant number of adults—more than 30% of older adults in most parts of the US—have not received the pneumococcal pneumonia vaccine.

My advice: Get this vaccine if you're over age 65 or you are any age and have pneumonia risk factors, such as diabetes…chronic obstructive pulmonary disease (COPD) or other chronic lung or heart problems…or you are on immunosuppressive medical therapy, including chemotherapy or inhaled corticosteroids.

Bonus: Recent research indicates that the pneumonia vaccine also reduces heart attack risk among people with cardiovascular risk factors—possibly by preventing arterial inflammation that can accompany pneumonia.

2. Get measles and chicken pox vaccinations, if needed. Both of these diseases can lead to pneumonia. If you didn't have chicken pox or the measles and weren't vaccinated against them as a child, get vaccinated now.

3. Wash your hands frequently. Even though most bacterial pneumonia results from germs in our own bodies—for example, on our teeth or tonsils or in our sinuses—pneumonia-causing bacteria and viruses (including those that cause the flu) can be passed among people. Frequent hand-washing with soap or alcohol-based cleansers helps minimize disease transmission.

4. If you do get the flu, discuss antiviral medication with your doctor. A review of the medical records of 70,000 patients age 60 and older found that taking *oseltamivir* (Tamiflu) decreased the incidence of pneumonia in older Americans by 59%.

5. Drink alcohol only in moderation. Alcohol depresses the cough and sneeze reflexes, making it easier for microbes to enter the lower respiratory tract. It also impairs the function of white blood cells, which are responsible for destroying bacteria in the lungs. Men should not exceed one drink daily…women should limit their alcohol consumption to three drinks weekly.

6. Brush and floss—and treat gum disease and sinus infections promptly. Gum and sinus infections increase the amount of bacteria inhaled into the airways. Good oral hygiene and treatment of such infections are key preventive measures, especially for people with impaired immunity or other risk factors that increase susceptibility to pneumonia. Be sure to brush at least twice daily, floss once daily and get a dental checkup at least every six months.

7. Use caution with inhaled corticosteroids. Treatments such as chemotherapy and *prednisone* are known to suppress the immune system, thus increasing pneumonia risk. Now, studies show that extended use (24 weeks or more) of inhaled corticosteroids for COPD increases pneumonia risk by 50%. Among people age 65 and older, this figure jumps to almost 75%. However, the benefits of using an inhaled corticosteroid often outweigh the pneumonia risk. Monitor yourself closely with your physician's help.

8. Treat GERD, but follow your doctor's advice about medication. Gastroesophageal reflux disease (GERD), in which stomach contents chronically wash back up the esophagus, boosts pneumonia risk by increasing the bacteria inhaled into the airways. However, treating GERD with acid-suppressing proton-pump inhibitor (PPI) drugs, such as *lansoprazole* (Prevacid) or *esomeprazole* (Nexium), also raises pneumonia risk by encouraging bacterial growth in the stomach.

Recent finding: While PPIs increase risk for community-acquired pneumonia only slightly, they appear to be a major factor in hospital-acquired pneumonia, which strikes up to 1% of all hospital patients in the US and kills 18% of its victims (in part because more virulent bacteria are present in hospitals).

One recent study estimates that PPIs and other acid blockers, such as H2-receptor antagonists—for example, *cimetidine* (Tagamet) and *ranitidine* (Zantac)—may cause some 30,000 pneumonia-related deaths each year. The study also found that many patients were routinely given PPIs and other acid blockers despite not really needing them.

If you need to take one of these GERD drugs (even in an over-the-counter product) for more than two weeks, consult your doctor.

Natural Ways to Prevent Pneumonia

Jamison Starbuck, ND, naturopathic physician in family practice in Missoula, Montana.

Even though many people think of pneumonia as a wintertime illness, it can strike during any season of the year. It can be caused by one of many different types of bacteria, viruses, fungi—or even an injury, such as exposure to chemical fumes (from a chlorine spill, for example). People who are at greatest risk for pneumonia are older adults and newborns, smokers, heavy drinkers, people with pre-existing lung disease or compromised immune systems, or anyone who is bedridden or has limited mobility (which increases risk for buildup of mucus in the lungs). Fortunately, you can take steps to protect yourself. *My secrets to avoiding pneumonia…*

• **Consider getting a pneumonia vaccination.** Discuss the vaccine with your doctor if you are age 65 or older—or at any age if you have congestive heart failure, a compromised immune system, liver or lung disease or diabetes, or if you are a smoker or heavy drinker. The vaccine can help prevent a common type of pneumonia caused by the Streptococcus pneumoniae bacterium.

• **Take vitamin A daily.** Vitamin A deficiency can cause drying of the respiratory-tract lining and a reduction in cilia, the hairlike tissues that move mucus and debris out of the lungs. Both changes make the lungs vulnerable to infection and inflammation. A total daily dose of 10,000 international units (IU) of vitamin A can help keep your lungs healthy.

Caution: Vitamin A is toxic when consumed in high doses over long periods of time. Consult your doctor before taking more than 10,000 IU of vitamin A daily. If you have liver disease or are pregnant, do not take supplemental vitamin A. In addition, some research suggests that smokers should not take vitamin A supplements.

• **Get more vitamin C daily.** The results of studies on the immune-enhancing effects of vitamin C have been mixed. However, I'm convinced—based on my clinical experience—that a daily dose of vitamin C does, in fact, help the immune system resist disease and is essential to combating the immune-draining effects of stress, a chief cause of illness.

Recommended: A daily total of 1,000 mg of vitamin C.

• **Treat upper respiratory infections (URIs) promptly and effectively.** Quite often, pneumonia develops from the spread

Test for Pneumonia in Minutes

Results from current tests for "walking pneumonia" can take days. A new experimental test measures spectral signatures from laser light bouncing off a specimen from a throat swab. Results are available in 10 minutes.

PLoS ONE

of inflammation caused by a viral infection, such as bronchitis.

Advice: Rest (forgo your usual activities, including going to work)…and hydrate (drink 68 ounces of water daily). For a cold or bronchitis, I recommend drinking a tincture made from extracts of the powerful antiviral botanical medicines elder, echinacea, eyebright and licorice—15 drops of each in one ounce of water, 15 minutes before or after meals, every four waking hours for several days.

Caution: Omit licorice if you have high blood pressure or heart disease—the herb may affect blood pressure or cause heart problems.

• **Don't delay a doctor visit if you suspect pneumonia.** Typical symptoms include a cough, fever, shortness of breath and fatigue. An early diagnosis increases your chance of a good outcome.

Can't Catch Your Breath? Is It Pneumonia?

Len Horovitz, MD, an internist and pulmonary specialist at Lenox Hill Hospital and director of Carnegie Medical PC, a private practice, both in New York City.

Perhaps climbing a flight or two of stairs has never really affected your breathing—until now. Or maybe you notice that it's harder to breathe even when you're simply watching television. What's going on?

You might wonder whether you are developing a common lung problem such as asthma or chronic obstructive pulmonary disease (COPD)—especially if you're over age 40…you have a history of allergies…are a current or former smoker…or have been exposed for long periods to secondhand smoke, heavy dust or chemical fumes.

But don't be too quick to make assumptions. There's a chance that your lungs have nothing to do with your shortness of breath.

Even a slight cold or the flu can take your breath away, but don't assume that a cold or the flu is all you have.

Many people who think they have a cold actually have pneumonia, a lung infection that kills about 50,000 Americans every year.

Walking pneumonia, the term for mild cases, usually clears up on its own within a week to 10 days.

More serious cases of pneumonia, however, often require hospitalization and treatment with antibiotics. Serious cases of pneumonia usually are caused by bacteria rather than viruses.

Red flags: Fever, cough, discolored or bloody mucus, chest pain and chills—especially when accompanied by shortness of breath—warrant a visit to your doctor right away.

Also important: Get vaccinated for pneumonia if you're age 65 or older…or if you have pneumonia risk factors such as smoking or a history of heart/lung disease, diabetes or liver disease.

Acute bronchitis, inflammation of the main air passages to the lungs, is less serious than pneumonia but also can cause shortness of breath. Check with your doctor.

Pneumonia Patients at Risk for Cardiac Arrest

Researchers examined data on 5,367 pneumonia patients (average age 68) who had cardiac arrest while in the hospital. Many of these cardiac arrests were unexpected—almost 40% occurred outside of the intensive care unit, and most patients were not receiving mechanical ventilation or blood pressure–boosting medications.

Theory: Patients with pneumonia may be susceptible to abrupt physical deterioration due to the illness.

If a loved one is hospitalized with pneumonia: Speak to the doctor about careful monitoring of the patient's respiratory and cardiac status.

Gordon Carr, MD, pulmonary and critical care fellow, The University of Chicago Medical Center.

Chronic Pneumonia

If you or a loved one is frequently hospitalized with pneumonia, you need to determine the cause of the recurrences. There could be an underlying condition, such as chronic obstructive pulmonary disease, bronchiectasis, congestive heart failure, asthma, a swallowing disorder or diabetes. Treating these conditions may help you (or your loved one) avoid repeated bouts of pneumonia. Also, smoking and excessive alcohol use partially paralyze the airway's cilia, tiny hairlike projections that sweep out bacteria and viruses. Stress and excess weight can significantly lower immunity.

Pneumonia is a very serious and potentially fatal illness. It needs to be treated with antibiotics, bronchodilators and, if necessary, oxygen until the lungs are strong enough to function optimally on their own.

Each bout of pneumonia can reduce lung function. Eventually, these repeated infections will make daily activities difficult and leave you short of breath. To help reduce pneumonia risk, ask your doctor about a pneumonia vaccination.

Neil Schachter, MD, professor of pulmonary, critical care and sleep medicine, Mount Sinai School of Medicine, New York City.

Common Drugs Linked to Fatal Pneumonia

An analysis of nearly 35,000 health records found that patients regularly using benzodiazepines, such as *diazepam* (Valium) or *temazepam* (Restoril), prescribed as sedatives or sleep aids, had a 54% higher-than-normal risk for pneumonia.

If you need a sedative or sleep aid: Ask your doctor about alternatives, including nondrug treatment.

Robert Sanders, MD, PhD, senior clinical research associate, Wellcome Department of Imaging Neuroscience, Institute of Cognitive Neuroscience, University College London.

Pneumonia Scare After Heart Surgery

John Puskas, MD, MSc, professor of surgery at Emory University and chief of cardiac surgery at Emory University Hospital Midtown in Atlanta.

We all know that heart surgery is a serious procedure, and that just like any other surgery, there is always a risk for major infection.

But recently, a group of researchers were shocked when their study showed that the kind of major infection most frequently associated with heart surgery wasn't at all what they expected (an infection at the site of the incision)—it was pneumonia.

And even more surprisingly, this dangerous condition often either didn't occur or wasn't diagnosed while the patient was still in the hospital during the post-op stay. The researchers had hypothesized that any such dangerous condition would be evident during this critical period. Instead, it was usually diagnosed about two full weeks after the operation!

Dangerous Post-Op Infections

The objective of the study was to find out what types of major infections occur after heart surgery and when they occur. So researchers collected clinical records of 5,185 male and female heart surgery patients with an average age of 64 at 10 medical centers—nine in the US and one in Canada—over the course of eight months. The surgeries included coronary artery bypass and aortic valve and/or mitral valve procedures.

First major finding: Researchers discovered that about 5% of heart surgery patients contracted major infections. And at the top of the list was not an infection at the site of the surgical incision, as the researchers had expected.

Pneumonia, a lung infection, was the most common infection. It was followed by clostridium difficile colitis (an infection in the colon that can cause diarrhea, abdominal cramps and sometimes fever, nausea, weight loss and dehydration)...bloodstream infection...infection at the site of the surgical incisions...and, lastly, mediastinitis (the infection and inflammation of the area between the lungs).

You probably already know that pneumonia and these other types of infections can cause weeks and sometimes even months of discomfort, serious complications or even death.

John Puskas, MD, MSc, a coauthor of the study and the head of cardiac surgery at Emory University Hospital in Atlanta, said that he's not entirely sure why pneumonia came out on top, but he has some theories. For one thing, after a heart operation, breathing is often uncomfortable, which causes recovering patients to take shallow breaths. As a result, the lungs are not well-aerated, and bacteria that would normally be exhaled with deep breaths are left inside to multiply. Moreover, heart disease itself can cause fluid to build up in the lungs. Another potential conduit for infection is the breathing tube that's inserted into the lungs during surgery.

We asked Dr. Puskas whether these infections implied hospital error, such as using unsterile instruments or other supplies. He said that the study uncovered no evidence of that and that these serious post-op infections most likely occur because patients have low-level, preexisting infections before surgery... or because their immune systems are too weak to fight off bacteria that are naturally present in the air, in their lungs or on their skin after surgery. Dr. Puskas added that the risks for infection during a heart operation can be reduced by appropriate safety procedures, but they can't be eliminated.

Why Were the Infections Delayed?

The second major finding of the study was equally important—Only half of the infections were diagnosed during patients' post-op hospital stays of five to seven days. The other half were diagnosed much later—about 14 days after the surgery, on average.

This is worrisome, because patients may assume that once they're home, they're healthy, so there's no need to look out for symptoms of infection. It's also concerning, said Dr. Puskas, because patients at home are not prompted by nurses and respiratory therapists to walk around, breathe deeply and clear mucus from their lungs, which can help prevent and treat infection. And they won't get immediate care if they need it.

Dr. Puskas said that this time frame might illustrate how long it takes some infections to appear. And sometimes, he added, the reason for the delay is that diagnosis itself can be a lengthy process that can require multiple visits over the course of a few days or weeks.

What You Must Do

Dr. Puskas said that it's important for heart surgery patients to be on the lookout for symptoms of infection after the surgery—even after they return home feeling fine. Be especially alert for symptoms of pneumonia, which may include chills, fever, cough, shortness of breath, a sharp chest pain when you inhale, headache or pain anywhere in your body, said Dr. Puskas. Call your doctor immediately if you experience any of these. And be diligent about following your doctor's post-op advice—walk around regularly, cough to clear mucus from your lungs, and breathe deeply.

Down the Wrong Hatch—Aspiration Can Lead to Pneumonia

Ali I. Musani, MD, director of the Interventional Pulmonology Program at National Jewish Health, a teaching affiliate of the University of Colorado Denver, and an associate professor of medicine and pediatrics at the University of Colorado Denver School of Medicine.

We all know that pneumonia can develop after a person has been exposed to certain germs. But there's another form of pneumonia that is far lesser known but that can also be deadly. It usually results when food being swallowed goes into the trachea (windpipe) instead of the esophagus (food pipe). Then, the food (or liquid, mucus or foreign substance) is aspirated—inhaled into the lungs.

Aspiration pneumonia occurs most often in adults age 65 and older. Like other types of pneumonia, it can cause symptoms such as a wracking cough (often accompanied by green or yellow foul-smelling phlegm)…fever…shortness of breath…wheezing…chest pain…and/or difficulty breathing.

Up to 15% of so-called community-acquired pneumonia is caused by aspiration, according to research in the *New England Journal of Medicine*. Also, the fatality rate for hospital-acquired pneumonia from aspiration can reach 25%.

Another danger: If a person aspirates a large object (or a mouthful of food), it can obstruct a major airway even if it makes it past the opening at the back of the throat. This may interfere with breathing and even cause a lung to collapse.

Is There a Harmful Disease Lurking in Your Car?

Legionnaire's disease risk: Using water instead of windshield wiper fluid.

Recent finding: Drivers who did not add windshield wiper fluid to the water in their car reservoirs had an increased risk for Legionnaire's disease, a rare disease that can result in severe pneumonia.

Theory: When the water in the reservoir is sprayed on the windshield, the bacteria can come through the car vents and enter the lungs of the driver and passengers, causing infection. Adding windshield wiper fluid kills infection-causing bacteria and decreases risk.

Anders Wallensten, MD, PhD, epidemiologist, Swedish Institute for Infectious Disease Control, Stockholm, Sweden, and coauthor of a study of 142 people, published in *European Journal of Epidemiology*.

Who Is at Risk?

It's fairly common for food and liquid to be aspirated, but lung specialists and emergency teams have found everything from dentures and tooth fillings to thumbtacks and batteries in patients' lungs. These are typically spotted and removed using a bronchoscope viewing instrument and "grabber" device or, in rare cases, with surgery.

What most people don't realize, however, is that material from their own bodies, particularly stomach contents, can be aspirated and can be equally dangerous.

Nearly half of healthy adults aspirate small amounts of contents from the stomach while they sleep. Most never experience symptoms because the amount of aspirated material is small and the body's defenses (such as coughing) are strong enough to remove the material.

The aspiration of larger amounts of material is much more dangerous. It's among the most feared complications of anesthesia—and the reason that patients are usually asked to fast for at least six to eight hours before having deep sedation.

Patients in intensive care units (ICUs) have a high risk for aspiration. So do those who have suffered a stroke or have dementia or a neuromuscular disorder, such as Parkinson's disease. Anything that impairs consciousness or muscular control, including the use of sedatives or heavy alcohol consumption, increases the risk.

In healthy adults, aspiration may occur with certain types of foods, such as popcorn or peanuts, because people tend to toss these to the back of the mouth.

Common scenario: A man is popping food into his mouth without thinking about it, while reclining (increasing his risk for aspiration) in his favorite chair and watching TV. He's also not chewing thoroughly. Suddenly, he may cough or choke and possibly aspirate pieces of food.

Dangerous Inflammation

Patients who aspirate food, foreign objects, or vomit or other secretions can develop lung irritation and inflammation without infection. Damage to the lungs can impair the normal exchange of oxygen and carbon dioxide. If the object/material isn't removed quickly, some patients may experience irreversible destruction of lung tissue.

Possible tip-offs that something has been aspirated include repeat pneumonia in the same area of the lung despite having taken antibiotics, a history of choking or, in older adults, possibly even missing dentures.

I once had a patient who aspirated a pill (in this case, an iron supplement). The supplement lodged in the lung for months and released corrosive chemicals that destroyed the surrounding lung tissue and caused large amounts of scar tissue.

Easy Ways to Stay Safe

Be careful while eating and drinking. Nearly everyone occasionally aspirates a small amount of food.

Red flag: If you frequently choke during meals, you are probably eating too quickly and/or have developed bad swallowing habits that need to be corrected. *For example, you may need to…*

• **Stop talking while you eat.** Talking while you chew is risky in two ways. You're not paying attention to the act of chewing and swallowing, and you are more likely to take a deep breath at the wrong time and suck particles of food into the airways.

• **Position a straw at the side of your mouth if you use a straw when drinking.** Using a straw in this way reduces the risk that a jet of liquid will go straight to the back of the throat and then into the airways.

• **Use a thickening agent in beverages and runny foods if you have a neuromuscular disease,** such as Parkinson's disease, or some other condition that makes it difficult to swallow.

Thin liquids are more likely to cause aspiration because they move so quickly through the mouth and throat. Products, including Resource ThickenUp Instant Food Thickener and Thick-It Instant Food Thickener, are available in pharmacies.

• **Lower your chin slightly when swallowing.** This slows the passage of foods/liquids down the throat.

• **Don't eat within two hours of bedtime.** You're more likely to aspirate stomach contents during sleep if you've recently had a meal.

Helpful: You can use wood blocks underneath the head of your bed to raise it by two to four inches. The force of gravity makes it harder for stomach contents to move "upstream."

In hospital patients, one of the best ways to prevent aspiration is to elevate the head of the bed to 30° to 45°. Since we started doing this in ICUs around the country, the incidence of aspiration has been significantly reduced.

Important: If you have difficulty swallowing and think that you may have aspiration, see your doctor, who can direct you to a swallowing specialist (usually a gastroenterologist), if needed.

Chapter 21

INFLUENZA—EXPERTS' FLU-FIGHTING SECRETS

Flu-Fighting Facts That May Surprise You

The flu is an illness that you hear so much about year after year that it's easy to assume you know all there is to know about it. That's a mistake. Widely held assumptions about the flu often are wrong—and dangerous. By learning the facts, you can help yourself and loved ones from being among the estimated 36,000 Americans who will die this year due to pneumonia and other flu-related complications. *Common misconceptions…*

Misconception #1. **People who have the flu are contagious only when they have symptoms.** Actually, most people with the flu are able to spread the illness beginning about a day before showing any symptoms and up to seven days after symptoms begin.

And you don't even have to be in very close proximity. The influenza virus can spread to a person six feet away—mainly when the sick person sneezes, coughs or even talks. Of course, you can also become contaminated if you touch your eyes, nose or mouth after coming in contact with an object, such as an elevator button, handrail or doorknob, that harbors a flu virus. These viruses can live up to eight hours on such objects.

Helpful: Wash your hands or use hand sanitizer several times a day—and always after you've been out in public or in contact with someone who has the flu.

Also: If you get the flu and have a fever, stay home until your fever has been gone for at least 24 hours without the use of fever-reducing medication.

Misconception #2. **If you're not running a fever, you don't have the flu.** Flu symptoms aren't always predictable. A fever is common with the illness, but it doesn't occur in everyone. Typical flu symptoms include body aches, extreme fatigue and a dry cough. However, some flu patients may also experience sneezing, a stuffy nose and sore throat—symptoms that usually occur with the common cold. In rare cases, flu patients even suffer vomiting and diarrhea. Although flu symptoms vary, a hallmark of the illness is that it comes on quickly and makes you feel quite sick.

Misconception #3. **If you think you have the flu, you should go right to bed**

William Schaffner, MD, a professor of preventive medicine and infectious diseases at Vanderbilt University Medical Center in Nashville.

until you feel better. Getting plenty of rest is important for flu recovery, but if you suspect that you have the flu and are in the high-risk category for flu complications (for example, you are over age 65, pregnant or have a chronic health condition such as asthma or heart disease), you should also alert your doctor right away.*

He/she may recommend a rapid flu test (using a nose or throat swab) that can diagnose the flu in about 30 minutes. If the result is positive, you may be prescribed the antiviral medication *oseltamivir* (Tamiflu). *Key:* This drug works best when started within 48 hours of getting sick.

Important: Adults produce much less of the flu virus and for a shorter time than children. If the rapid flu test is negative, it doesn't necessarily mean that you don't have the flu, and your doctor may want to treat you anyway.

If you're generally healthy and get a mild case of the flu, you may simply want to get a lot of rest and drink plenty of fluids. To control symptoms, you can use over-the-counter drugs—cough medicine or *acetaminophen* (Tylenol) or a nonsteroidal anti-inflammatory drug such as *naproxen* (Aleve) for fever, if necessary.

Misconception #4. **The flu vaccine must be given early in the season to be effective.** You will certainly have protection for a greater part of the flu season if you get vaccinated early on, but it's still worth getting the vaccine even as late as January if the flu is still circulating. But don't wait! It takes about two weeks for the vaccine to trigger the development of antibodies and confer maximum protection.

Misconception #5. **All flu vaccines offer the same level of protection.** Again, not true. Traditional flu vaccines, known as *trivalent* vaccines, protect against three types of viruses—two strains of Type A (which cause the most severe illness) and one Type B strain.

For the entire list of CDC flu recommendations, go to CDC.gov/flu.

New option for upcoming flu seasons: Manufacturers have introduced *quadrivalent* vaccines, which add a second type of B strain to the mix. It is more likely than older vaccines to protect against the variety of virus strains that circulate each year.

Ask your doctor—or the pharmacist where you get your shot—if the new version is available. The extra protection is worth it. The "quad" vaccine will probably become standard in the next few years. For the 2013/2014 seaon, however, it was in short supply because manufacturers hadn't fully changed their operations.

Important: If the quad vaccine is not available in your area, don't skip your vaccination.

Misconception #6. **People who are allergic to eggs can't get a flu vaccination.** A new vaccine, Flublok, doesn't use eggs in

Too Healthy to Get the Flu? Think Again!

Many people believe that if they're basically healthy, they won't benefit from flu vaccination and that only high-risk individuals need the vaccine. That's absolutely false. Perhaps you've dodged this bullet in past flu seasons, but that doesn't mean you will this year or in any future year. While it's true that people in high-risk groups are more likely to develop potentially deadly complications (such as pneumonia, dehydration and even heart attacks) from the flu, many perfectly healthy people contract the flu each year, and some of those cases turn out to be devastating. Even people without symptoms can spread the flu: Younger adults (in their 20s and 30s) can get the flu but have no symptoms and pass it on to others, including those in high-risk categories. If younger adults get vaccinated, it helps cut down on the spread of the virus.

William Schaffner, MD

production—as do traditional vaccines that culture flu viruses in eggs. Instead, it's made with recombinant DNA technology in which insect viruses are used to produce a protein found in flu viruses. The vaccine is FDA-approved for adults ages 18 to 49 (the ages of people in a study that was performed). It is just as effective as egg-based vaccines.

Misconception #7. The flu vaccine doesn't work very well. The CDC recently reported that the flu vaccine was about 56% effective at overall prevention and about 27% effective in adults age 65 or older.

The immune system gets less robust with age. It produces fewer antibodies in response to vaccines. To help older adults, manufacturers have recently introduced a higher-dose vaccine that research has shown to be about 24% more effective than older vaccines.

Important: These percentages may seem low but represent *complete prevention* in people who respond to the vaccine. Even though the flu vaccine isn't effective for everyone, it's better than no protection. The vaccine also makes the flu milder in people who do get it and reduces deadly complications such as pneumonia.

If you are age 65 or older, your doctor or pharmacist will probably recommend the Fluzone High-Dose vaccine.

Note: A small percentage of people will have arm soreness and/or a headache.

Misconception #8. All flu shots contain mercury. Questionable research that once claimed that the mercury-containing preservative *thimerosal* caused autism in children has been completely debunked. Even though there's no credible evidence of harm caused by thimerosal, some people refuse to get a flu shot because they are still concerned about the preservative and assume that all flu shots contain it. If you would rather avoid thimerosal, ask your doctor for a single-dose flu vaccine (the preservative is used only in multi-dose vials that provide vaccine for multiple injections). The FluMist nasal spray also doesn't contain thimerosal.

Top Naturopath's Cold and Flu Protection Plan

Mark A. Stengler, NMD, naturopathic medical doctor and leading authority on the practice of alternative and integrated medicine. Dr. Stengler is author of the *Health Revelations* newsletter, author of *The Natural Physician's Healing Therapies* (Bottom Line Books), founder and medical director of the Stengler Center for Integrative Medicine in Encinitas, California, and adjunct associate clinical professor at the National College of Natural Medicine in Portland, Oregon. *http://MarkStengler.com*

Every year, I advise my patients to protect themselves against colds and flu. The best defense against these illnesses is a strong immune system. *Here's how to protect yourself this winter…*

My Flu-Prevention Protocol

I don't recommend the flu vaccine for healthy people, although I do suggest that some people consider getting the flu vaccine (see below). Instead, I recommend a powerful protocol for flu prevention that my patients, my family and I all follow. Begin this protocol in October—and continue it through April. (All of these products can be found at health-food stores and online.)

The protocol includes…

• **Influenzinum.** I have recommended this homeopathic remedy on its own for more than 15 years. The manufacturers of Influenzinum reformulate it annually based on the flu viruses expected to predominate that year. One French survey found that 90% of 453 people who took Influenzinum did not get the flu.

Dosage: Follow label instructions. Adults and children (age six and older) should take one dose (three pellets of a 9C potency) dissolved under the tongue once weekly for six weeks, beginning at the start of flu season. (For infants starting as young as one day old, crush one pellet and place on the tongue.) Influenzinum is available at health-food stores and online. It is made by several manufacturers including Boiron.

•**Vitamin D.** Many studies show an association between low levels of vitamin D and respiratory tract infections. A study published in *The American Journal of Clinical Nutrition* found that only 10% of school-age children who took vitamin D got the flu, compared with 18% who took a placebo.

Dosage: Adults and children age 13 and older should take 2,000 international units (IU) daily, then increase to 5,000 IU during peak flu months (January through March). This is higher than the dose I typically recommend, which is 1,000 IU to 2,000 IU, but these higher doses of vitamin D are safe. Infants and children up to age 12 should take 1,000 IU daily, then increase to 2,000 IU during peak flu months, though for infants, check with a pediatrician before increasing the dose to 2,000 IU.

•**N-acetylcysteine (NAC).** This antioxidant helps prevent flu and reduces severity of symptoms if infection occurs. A landmark Italian study found that only 25% of older people who were injected with flu virus after taking NAC for six months experienced flu symptoms, versus 79% who took a placebo.

Dosage: Adults and children age 13 and older should take 1,000 milligrams (mg) daily. Children ages six to 12 can take 500 mg daily. At the first sign of flu symptoms, increase to 4,000 mg daily for adults and 1,500 mg daily for children, and continue until symptoms subside. Higher doses, such as 4,000 mg, may cause digestive upset. Reduce the dose if needed.

Natural Cold Remedies

•**Colds can be hard to distinguish from flu.** Colds come on slowly with symptoms affecting the chest, neck and head. Flu comes on quickly with more intense symptoms, including bodywide aches and pains, high fever and often digestive complaints.

Even if you follow my immune-boosting flu-prevention protocol, there's always a small chance that you will catch a cold. Take one or both of the herbal remedies below at the first sign of a cold until symptoms are

---

Vitamin D Reduces Risk for Colds and Flu

Healthy adults with high blood levels of vitamin D in fall and winter were less likely to develop viral respiratory infections than those with low levels of vitamin D.

Best: Take 2,000 international units (IU) to 4,000 IU of vitamin D daily. The amount depends on body weight, where you live, skin tone and the season—talk to your doctor.

James R. Sabetta, MD, associate clinical professor of medicine, Yale University, New Haven, Connecticut, and coauthor of a study of 198 people, published in *PloS One.*

---

gone. There are no side effects, except as noted—and you can safely take more than one of these remedies at the same time. For dosing information for adults and children, follow label instructions.

•**Pelargonium sidoides.** The focus of more than 20 clinical studies, this South African plant has been found to be effective in relieving cold symptoms, sinusitis, sore throat and bronchitis. It is available in many forms, including syrup, lozenge and chewable tablet.

Brand to try: Nature's Way Umcka Cold-Care or Umcka Cold+Flu (*www.NaturesWay. com*).

COLD–FX. This remedy contains Panax ginseng extract, which is used in Chinese medicine to increase energy. Studies show that COLD-FX can strengthen the immune system to beat the common cold. A study published in the *Canadian Medical Association Journal* found that healthy adults who took COLD-FX had 25% fewer colds per person than those in the placebo group. COLD-FX is available online and at health-food stores.

Get the Flu Vaccine?

I have concerns about flu vaccines—mainly because we don't know the long-term impact of using them. However, the flu vaccine (mercury-free is best) should be considered by those who are over age 65...suffer from chronic pulmonary or cardiovascular disease...have a weakened immune system from a chronic disease such as cancer...and by women who are pregnant. Contrary to the recommendations of mainstream medicine, healthy caregivers do not need to get the vaccine.

6 No-Fuss Germ-Fighting Secrets

Philip M. Tierno, Jr., PhD, director of clinical microbiology and immunology at New York University Langone Medical Center and a member of the faculty at New York University School of Medicine, both in New York City. He is author of *The Secret Lives of Germs* (Atria).

During the fall and winter, we're all on high alert to avoid germs that cause colds and flu. But there are other microbes—some quite dangerous—that we should also protect ourselves from all year long.

The majority of people know that methicillin-resistant Staphylococcus aureus (MRSA), an antibiotic-resistant organism that often affects hospital patients, is now infecting more and more people in community settings, such as health clubs, assisted-living facilities and other public places.

What you may not know: There's been a significant increase in the prevalence of MRSA in the noses of healthy adults and children, according to research published in *The New England Journal of Medicine*. Since anyone can harbor MRSA without getting sick, this means that an infected person could unknowingly spread the dangerous bacterium by sneezing into his/her hand before touching a doorknob, for example, or other surface.

Know Where the Germs Hide

Most people know that hand-washing with warm water and plain soap for at least 20 seconds is a highly effective germ-control strategy. However, there are some little-known secrets that you also should be aware of to help protect yourself—and your family—from germs that cause colds or the flu or infection with MRSA or other dangerous bacteria...

SECRET 1: **Opt for sanitizer wipes instead of gel.** Alcohol-based gels are effective, but sanitizer wipes (with 62% ethyl alcohol) are better because the friction caused by wipes helps remove bacteria and skin debris containing dead skin cells that can harbor infectious agents.

My advice: Keep sanitizer wipes in your bag or a shirt pocket, and use them whenever you've been out in public and can't get to a bathroom to wash your hands.

If you do use gel: Apply a dollop about the size of a quarter. Using less won't completely cover the hands.

Whether you're using a gel or wipe, use the product for at least 20 seconds. It takes this long to completely cover the hands, rub between fingers, etc. Let the sanitizing agent dry, do not wipe it off, and be sure to apply it under the fingernails, too.

SECRET 2: **Use triclosan in certain situations.** If you or someone in the family is sick with a communicable illness such as the flu, a cold, stomach virus or any infection that can be transmitted, wash your hands with a soap that contains triclosan. It's an antimicrobial agent that kills both bacteria and viruses.

Important: Some researchers worry that soaps with triclosan might increase antibiotic resistance. This does not occur when people use products such as Dial Complete liquid soap, which has a ratio of about 4:1 of surfactant (a detergent-like agent) to triclosan.

My advice: To help protect against bacteria and viruses when you or someone in your home is ill, use Dial Complete liquid soap.

SECRET 3: **Bring your own reading material to the doctor's office.** Cold and flu viruses can survive up to 48 hours on the pages of magazines—longer if the reader has left behind smudges of hand cream or make-up, which can help some organisms survive.

My advice: Bring your own magazine or book to read. If you do read one of the doctor's magazines, do not moisten your finger in your mouth when turning the pages—and keep your hands away from your eyes, nose and mouth until you've had a chance to wash your hands.

SECRET 4: **Air-dry bath towels.** Most people, after using a bath or hand towel, fold it over and hang it neatly on a towel rod. This is the worst thing you can do because it traps moisture and makes it possible for germs to thrive.

A few staph bacteria deposited on a damp towel will increase to about 100,000 in four hours. Some organisms can live for several hours to days on a damp towel.

Danger: Suppose you have a cut on your skin, then wipe yourself with a staph-infected towel. Because of the bacterial "bloom," you'll be exposing the cut to very high concentrations of staph bacteria.

My advice: To avoid doing multiple loads of laundry, completely air-dry towels between uses by hanging them in such a way that air can reach every part of the surface. If you follow this practice, it's fine to wash towels just once or twice a week. If someone in your home has a communicable illness, he/she should use a personal towel and keep it separate from other towels.

SECRET 5: **Keep your toothbrush upright.** Like bathroom towels, a toothbrush that stays moist can accumulate enormous quantities of bacteria and cold and flu viruses in just a few hours.

My advice: Don't lay your brush down to store it—stand it up with the bristles at the top so that it will dry completely between uses. Also close the toilet lid before you flush. The flushing action in some toilets can spray invisible water droplets—which contain fecal and other disease-causing organisms—up to 20 feet. An exposed toothbrush is an easy target.

Also helpful: Sanitize your toothbrush by submerging the bristles in a germ-killing mouthwash for about five minutes. Do this several times a week or with each use if you are ill.

SECRET 6: **Use hotter water.** Everyone wants to save money on utility bills, but some people do this by turning down the thermostat on the water heater.

The risk: Undergarments and bath towels can harbor enormous amounts of dangerous organisms, including the hepatitis A virus (transmitted primarily via human stool) and bacteria such as staph and Escherichia coli. Washing clothes in cool or warm water will remove some of these germs, but it won't kill them. Hot water is needed to kill these organisms as well as cold and flu viruses.

My advice: Make sure the water temperature in your washing machine is at least 150° F by checking it with a candy thermometer. This is hot enough to kill microbes. If your washer doesn't have a heating cycle that uses water this hot, raise the hot-water setting on your water tank—just be careful of scalding from tap water.

Helpful: Wash underwear separately so that any surviving organisms won't be transferred to other clothes.

Also: Use bleach on whites—it kills microbes.

The Best Way to Stay Away From the Flu

Dena Schanzer, MSc, PStat, researcher, senior statistical analyst, Public Health Agency of Canada, Ottawa, Ontario, Canada.

Little kids sure can be cute, but when they're all sneezy and drippy, who can blame us for not wanting to get too close—imagine the germs! And when flu season hits, the thought of being sidelined with a hacking cough, fever and chills is enough to make us want to step back just a bit further from those sweet little faces. Hold on though—it turns out that small children may be getting a bad rap when it comes to spreading the flu. Dena Schanzer, MSc, PStat, a senior statistical analyst with the Public Health Agency in Ontario, Canada, published research recently in the *American Journal of Epidemiology* that suggests that, in fact, teenagers and young adults may be the real drivers of seasonal and pandemic flu outbreaks…not young children.

Curious, we called Schanzer, who said that she had looked at data from influenza lab tests compiled by the Canadian government between 1995 and 2006. She and her colleagues found that seasonal flu peaked in two of the groups studied, those ages 10 to 19 and those 20 to 29, one week earlier than it did in kids under 10 and older adults. During the much-buzzed-about H1N1 flu pandemic in 2009, cases involving that strain peaked in preteens and teens four days before it did in younger and older groups. And teens ages 15 to 19 were the one group most often associated with the earliest infections (including seasonal flu, swine flu and H1N1).

Schanzer and her team said they could only speculate why these groups would be the Typhoid Marys of the flu, but it's pretty clear that the social habits of teens and young adults—who tend to frequently gather at malls, parties, concerts and other communal events—makes them particularly vulnerable to the flu virus. These age groups have mobility on their side as well, she surmised—they have fewer responsibilities to tie them down than older people and, unlike little kids, they can move around at will in cars and by public transportation—no mom or dad needed!

The results agree, she said, with a prior study of social contacts that showed that high school students and young adults are likely to be the "transmission backbone" for the next pandemic because of the nature of their social networks. So despite the "high attack rate" (susceptibility to infection) of younger school-aged children between five and nine years old, these kids aren't in the lead group

spreading the flu. There's no question that if exposed, they have the greater potential to catch it, but they're not the main culprits when it comes to passing it on.

Schanzer would like to see this study design repeated in other countries to see if age patterns are similar. Her instincts tell her that they will be—and that the findings of this study should be considered in the age-specific recommendations for vaccination—in other words, if we want to reduce the spread of flu throughout every age group, the most effective place to focus would be with our preteens, teens and young adults.

Rev Up Your Immunity

Michael T. Murray, ND, one of the country's best-known naturopathic physicians. He serves on the Board of Regents of Bastyr University in Seattle and has written more than 30 books, including *The Encyclopedia of Natural Medicine* (Atria) with coauthor Joseph Pizzorno, ND. *www.DoctorMurray.com*

Colds are potentially more dangerous than most people realize. That's because they often weaken an already compromised immune system, making the sufferer more vulnerable to the flu and pneumonia.

A nutritional deficiency is the most common cause of depressed immunity, but even people who make a point to eat a well-balanced diet often fall short when it comes to getting enough key nutrients. For this reason, many Americans turn to dietary supplements for extra protection.

But which ones really work?

For answers, we spoke to Michael T. Murray, ND, a leading naturopathic physician who has spent more than 30 years compiling a database of more than 60,000 scientific articles on the effectiveness of natural medicines, including supplements.

Here are some of the most effective supplements for preventing and treating colds and related upper-respiratory ailments. Start with the first supplement and add others (all are available at health-food stores), based on specific symptoms…*

• **Mixed antioxidants.** When it comes to fortifying your body to fight off colds, it's wise to start with a high-potency multisupplement. I recommend one that combines zinc, selenium, beta-carotene (or other carotenes) and vitamins C and E. This antioxidant mix helps prevent oxidative damage to the thymus gland—a robust thymus is needed to produce T lymphocytes, a type of white blood cell that recognizes and attacks viruses and other infectious agents.

Typical daily dose: 20 mg to 30 mg zinc… 200 micrograms (mcg) selenium…25,000 international units (IU) beta-carotene…500 mg vitamin C…and 200 IU vitamin E. You'll find roughly these amounts in any high-potency multisupplement. Many people take a multisupplement year-round.

• **Astragalus.** Few Americans know about this herb, although it's a standard treatment in Traditional Chinese Medicine (TCM). It is getting more attention these days because scientists have learned that it contains polysaccharide fraction F3 and other substances that stimulate different parts of the immune system.

Test-tube and animal studies have found that astragalus has potent antiviral effects—important for preventing colds and the flu. In one study, 115 patients who took the herb for eight weeks showed significant improvement in their counts of infection-fighting white blood cells.

Typical daily dose: 100 mg to 150 mg of powdered extract combined with any liquid, three times daily, whenever you have a cold or the flu or throughout the winter months if your immunity is low (for example, due to extra stress).

Caution: If you have rheumatoid arthritis or some other autoimmune disease, use astragalus only under a doctor's supervision—

*Consult your doctor before trying these supplements—especially if you have a chronic medical condition and/or take medication. Some of these remedies may interact with medication. Most supplements need to be taken for at least six weeks to reach their full effect.

the increase in immune activity could worsen your autoimmune symptoms.

• **South African geranium.** Also known as umckaloabo, this herbal remedy is commonly used for bronchitis, an upper-respiratory infection that often follows colds, particularly in winter.

In a study of 205 patients with bronchitis, those taking it had reduced bronchitis-related symptoms, such as a cough and shortness of breath. Other studies have shown similar effects.

Although doctors who specialize in herbal medicine typically recommend this supplement for patients who have been diagnosed with bronchitis or sinusitis, I advise taking it if you have a cold because it reduces symptoms and helps prevent a secondary bronchial infection.

Typical daily dose: 20 mg, three times daily, until the symptoms subside.

• **Beta-glucan.** This class of compounds is found in baker's yeast, medicinal mushrooms (such as maitake) and a variety of grains. Supplemental forms have been shown to stimulate the activity of immune cells. They also stimulate immune signaling proteins, which help the body fight viral infections.

In a study of 54 firefighters (who are susceptible to colds because of frequent exposure to smoke and other fumes), those who took a beta-glucan supplement had 23% fewer upper-respiratory infections compared with those who took a placebo.

Typical daily dose: 250 mg to 500 mg daily. This dose is effective for treatment of viral infections as well as prevention (for example, when you feel a cold coming on). I recommend Wellmune WGP (it contains a substance derived from yeast that has been shown to strengthen immune cells) or Maitake Gold beta-glucan supplements—the research is more solid with these than with other products.

• **Echinacea.** This herb has been the subject of more than 900 studies. A few years ago, researchers reported that it was not effective for colds—probably because these scientists were using products that had insufficient amounts of active compounds. In my experience, echinacea is very effective both for prevention and treatment.

Example: One study, involving 120 patients who had just started to experience cold symptoms, found that only 40% of those taking echinacea went on to develop a full-fledged cold compared with 60% of those not taking the herb. When patients in the echinacea group did get sick, their symptoms started to improve after four days versus eight days in those taking placebos.

Typical daily dose: One-half to one teaspoon of liquid extract, which can be added to a glass of water or taken straight, three times daily, when you have a cold or feel one coming on. Buy a product that is made from the fresh aerial portion of the plant. This information will be printed on the label. You will receive a higher concentration of active compounds. People who have allergies to plants in the daisy family (which includes ragweed) should not take echinacea.

Add a Dose of Stress Relief

It's important to remember that virtually everyone is more likely to get sick during times of stress.

Reasons: Stress increases blood levels of adrenal hormones, which suppress the immune system. In addition, stress triggers the release of cytokines and other substances that decrease the activity of white blood cells and inhibit the formation of new ones.

What to do: In addition to getting regular exercise and sleeping at least seven hours a night, make a habit of doing activities that improve your mood. Deep breathing, meditation or simply having a good time with friends will all help you stay healthier.

Ditch the Sugar!

If you want to stay healthy this winter, cut way back on sugar. This is important because the simple sugars in sweets and sweet beverages (including fruit juices) diminish the ability of lymphocytes to fight off viruses. When you consume sugar, the immune system weakens

Better Flu Recovery

Researchers divided 154 healthy adults (age 50 and older) into three groups—one that was trained to meditate daily for 45 minutes, one that exercised daily for 45 minutes and a control group that did neither.

Result: During a single flu season, the meditation and exercise groups had similarly fewer acute respiratory infections than the control group, but the meditation group's symptoms were far less severe than those of the other two groups.

Theory: Daily meditation reduces stress, which may protect against infection.

Bruce Barrett, MD, associate professor of family medicine, University of Wisconsin School of Medicine and Public Health, Madison.

within just 30 minutes—and it remains in a depressed state for more than five hours.

It's not clear why sugar has such serious effects on immunity. It's possible that elevated blood sugar prevents vitamin C from attaching to and entering white blood cells, which makes the immune system less effective.

My advice: Have no more (and preferably less) than 15 g to 20 g of sugar in any three-hour period. Sugar-content information is, of course, found on food labels. A four-ounce glass of fruit juice, for example, will have about 12 g of sugar.

Eat When Fighting the Flu Despite the Old Adage "Starve a Fever"

Even if you are not hungry, eat a normal number of calories if possible. The flu comes in new strains every year, so the body must make new antibodies. To do that, it requires fuel to produce natural killer cells. Eating fewer calories slows recovery. Eat fresh fruits and vegetables—they help create an alkaline environment in which viruses cannot survive.

Caution: Limit sweets while you are ill—sugar feeds viruses.

Study by researchers at Michigan State University, East Lansing, published in *The Journal of Nutrition*.

Hydrotherapy for Flu Aches

Thomas A. Kruzel, ND, a naturopathic physician at the Rockwood Natural Medicine Clinic in Scottsdale, Arizona. He is author of *The Homeopathic Emergency Guide: A Quick Reference Guide to Accurate Homeopathic Care* (North Atlantic). *www.Rockwood NaturalMedicine.com*

One way to know that you have the flu rather than a cold is the presence of severe muscle aches. *Ibuprofen* and aspirin can help with the aches, but they also reduce fever—and fever is one of the body's healing mechanisms.

Better: Home hydrotherapy. Before you go to bed, soak a cotton T-shirt in cool water. Wring it out as much as possible and put it on. Then put a dry shirt over that. It may feel uncomfortable for a minute after you put on the damp shirt, but this therapy is very effective. Or you can try damp socks instead. Either way, your body responds by raising your body temperature between one-half and one degree. This increases immune activity and reduces muscle aches. *Caution:* This technique is not advisable for anyone in a frail state, especially the elderly.

Also helpful: Homeopathic Nux Vomica, Gelsemium or Eupatorium. See a homeopathic physician at the first signs of flu—the remedies work best when they're taken within 48 hours of the first symptoms.

Protect Your Pet From the Flu

Flu sufferers may make their pets sick. Certain strains of influenza, including the pandemic H1N1 strain, are known to pass from animals to humans, but now it's being reported that the transmission of such viruses also can occur in reverse. One dog and 13 cats appear to have been infected with this virus by humans. The animals developed similar symptoms, such as labored breathing and, in some cases, even stopped eating and died.

Pet owners: Follow your doctor's advice about flu prevention, and make sure that your pet gets veterinary care if it develops flulike symptoms.

Christiane Löhr, DVM, associate professor of anatomic pathology, Oregon State University, College of Veterinary Medicine, Corvallis.

Vitamin D Reduces Risk for Colds and Flu

Healthy adults with high blood levels of vitamin D in fall and winter were less likely to develop viral respiratory infections than those with low levels of vitamin D.

Best: Take 2,000 international units (IU) to 4,000 IU of vitamin D daily. The amount depends on body weight, where you live, skin tone and the season—talk to your doctor.

James R. Sabetta, MD, associate clinical professor of medicine, Yale University, New Haven, Connecticut, and coauthor of a study of 198 people, published in *PloS One*.

KIDNEY DISEASE

This dangerous condition is on the rise in the US, affecting more than 10% of the population, most of whom don't even know they have it. And the two biggest risk factors for chronic kidney disease are having diabetes or high blood pressure (conditions that are also epidemic in this country). In this chapter, you'll discover the signs, symptoms and best ways to take care of your kidneys.

Chapter 22

HOW TO SPOT AND STOP KIDNEY DISEASE

Hidden Dangers of Kidney Disease

When Charlotte, a 66-year-old retired schoolteacher from New Jersey, was recently screened for kidney disease, she assumed that she was in good health. She had no symptoms, worked out four times a week and had no family history of kidney problems. When test results showed that she had kidney failure (that is, her kidneys were no longer able to perform normal functions, including the removal of waste products), Charlotte was shocked but relieved that she could begin treatment immediately to help prevent further damage to her kidneys. *What you need to know…*

Hidden Dangers of CKD

When your kidneys function properly, they remove excess fluid, waste and minerals from the body. The kidneys manufacture hormones that produce red blood cells, strengthen bones and regulate blood pressure. When the kidneys fail—a condition sometimes known as end-stage renal disease—you're at increased risk for complications such as anemia, weak bones and nerve damage.

What you may not know: Because chronic kidney disease (CKD)—gradual loss of kidney function—can damage blood vessels and organs, including the heart, it also increases the risk for heart and blood vessel disease.

Troubling trend: CKD is on the rise—due in large part to the surge in risk factors for CKD, such as high blood pressure (hypertension) and diabetes, according to a study in the *Journal of the American Medical Association.* In fact, CKD now affects 26 million Americans—roughly 13% of all American adults, according to the National Kidney Foundation.

Important finding: Impaired kidney function in older adults also accelerates memory problems, according to a recent study published in *Neurology.*

Are You at Risk?

CKD is often a silent condition, especially in the early stages. One study found that only

Joseph Vassalotti, MD, associate clinical professor of medicine at the Mount Sinai School of Medicine and chief medical officer of the National Kidney Foundation, *www.kidney.org,* both in New York City.

12% of men and 6% of women with CKD had been diagnosed with the disorder.

Latest development: Researchers have linked diets high in sodium and artificially sweetened beverages to declines in kidney function.

If kidney failure goes undetected, it usually progresses, causing uremia, a group of symptoms that result from impurities in the blood that accumulate because of the kidneys' inability to excrete waste and water. *Symptoms of kidney failure (or CKD) include…*

• **Foamy urine** (resembling the foam on the surface of eggs as they are scrambled).

• **Swelling of the feet or ankles or around the eyes** (due to fluid retention).

• **Difficulty concentrating and doing simple calculations,** such as counting money.

• **Fatigue and trouble sleeping.**

• **Dry, itchy skin.**

• **Frequent urination** (more often than the norm for the individual)—especially at night—or decreased urine output.

Even if you have no symptoms (such as those described earlier), you should be screened for CKD if you…

• **Are over age 60.**

• **Have cardiovascular disease, high blood pressure, diabetes or a family history of kidney disease (in a parent or sibling)**—all increase risk for CKD.

• **Have an autoimmune disease,** such as lupus, or a chronic infection, such as hepatitis B. Autoimmune diseases and certain chronic infections can cause kidney disease that is related to the body's immune response.

The Tests You Need

If you are at increased risk for CKD or have symptoms of kidney failure (as described earlier), ask your doctor for screening tests to measure…

• **Estimated glomerular filtration rate (eGFR).** This is determined with a blood test for creatinine (a by-product of normal muscle metabolism that is removed by the kidneys). The amount of creatinine indicates how well the kidneys are filtering blood. An eGFR below 60 mL per minute is considered abnormal.

• **Urinary albumin-to-creatinine ratio (UACR).** Albumin is a protein in the blood that passes through the kidneys' microscopic filtering units, known as glomeruli. When albumin is found in the urine, it means that the kidneys have been damaged and can no longer properly filter albumin—much like a coffee filter that leaks coffee grinds. A normal UACR is less than 30 mg per gram of creatinine. A reading above that level is considered high and possibly a sign of early kidney disease.

An abnormal result for either of these tests doesn't necessarily mean that you have CKD. But you should be tested again in about three months. If either of these tests still shows abnormalities at that time, you are diagnosed with CKD.

Both tests are relatively inexpensive and typically covered by health insurance—the blood tests for creatinine and albumin are $40 to $50 each.

How to Fight CKD

High blood pressure and diabetes cause two-thirds of the cases of CKD. High blood pressure is harmful to the kidneys because it increases pressure on the walls of the blood vessels, including those in the kidneys.

When blood sugar levels rise too high in people with diabetes, the kidneys and other organs often are damaged. For these reasons, one of the best ways to guard against CKD is to avoid high blood pressure and diabetes.

If you are diagnosed with CKD, it's crucial to control the root cause. For example, people with CKD and hypertension need to get their blood pressure below 130/80 mm Hg (typically through dietary changes, such as limiting sodium intake, and blood pressure–lowering medication).

People with CKD and diabetes need to get their hemoglobin A1C level—the average blood glucose level over three months—below 7% (usually through careful attention to diet and the use of diabetes medications).

If CKD progresses to end-stage renal disease, a kidney transplant or dialysis, in which machines do the job of your kidneys, is required.

Important: If you have CKD, review all your medications, vitamins and herbs with your doctor. In people with advanced kidney disease, fat-soluble vitamins (such as vitamin A) can accumulate in the body, causing vitamin toxicity. In addition, certain herbal medications, such as those containing aristolochic acid, can be toxic to the kidneys. Certain medications, including the diabetes drug *metformin* (Glucophage), and nonsteroidal anti-inflammatory drugs, such as *naproxen* (Aleve) and *ibuprofen* (Motrin), can worsen CKD.

People with CKD also should take precautions when undergoing certain medical tests. For example, dyes used as contrast agents for computed tomography (CT) scans and other procedures can weaken the kidneys. Oral sodium phosphate bowel preparations used for colonoscopies, such as Visicol, OsmoPrep and Fleet Phospho-soda, also can be harmful. If you have CKD, tell your doctor about it before undergoing radiological tests that use contrast agents or taking a sodium phosphate product prior to a colonoscopy.

Lower Risk of Kidney Disease Up to 150%

Alexander Chang, MD, a nephrology fellow in the department of nephrology and hypertension at Loyola University Medical Center in Maywood, Illinois. He is a member of the American Society of Nephrology, the National Kidney Foundation and the American Society of Hypertension.

We hear a great deal about the best dietary strategies to help prevent heart disease and diabetes. But what about kidney disease?

Recent development: For the first time, researchers have identified some of the key

Do You Have Chronic Kidney Disease?

In an effort to encourage people to undergo free screening for kidney disease, the National Kidney Foundation has designated March as Kidney Month. To find the screening location nearest you, consult the Web site for the Kidney Early Evaluation Program at *www.keeponline.org*. Nearly 26% of all people who have participated in this program have been found to have CKD, but only 2% were aware of their risk.

Joseph Vassalotti, MD

eating habits that help prevent the onset of kidney disease.

Why this is important: Kidney disease, which affects all the body's main physiological functions, significantly increases one's risk for serious medical conditions such as cardiovascular disease, including heart attack and stroke...sexual dysfunction...and bone fractures. *What you need to know...*

Kidney Damage Occurs Slowly

Like hypertension and diabetes, kidney disease can progress over decades. Patients can lose up to 75% of their kidney function without experiencing kidney disease's eventual symptoms, which include fatigue and loss of appetite, difficulty concentrating, muscle cramps, swelling in the feet and/or ankles and/or low urine output. Increased risk for heart attack and stroke begins when kidney function has declined by about 50%—further declines usually require medication, dialysis or a kidney transplant.

Losing weight if you're overweight and following very specific dietary strategies are among the best ways to prevent kidney disease—and to minimize further damage if you are one of the 26 million Americans who already have it. Obesity increases the risk for hypertension and diabetes, which are the two most common causes of kidney disease.

Key dietary approaches recently identified by researchers…

•**Drink fewer sugar-sweetened drinks.** In a recent unpublished analysis of data from a 25-year study of young adults, Loyola researchers found that those who drank just 3.5 soft drinks or other sweetened beverages, such as energy drinks or fruit drinks, per week were 150% more likely to develop kidney disease than those who didn't drink them.

It's possible that the sweet beverages' high concentration of fructose, in particular (in refined sugar and high-fructose corn syrup) is responsible for the increased risk.

My advice: In general, Americans consume too much sugar. Switch to diet soft drinks.

Even better: Choose unsweetened beverages, such as water with a lemon slice.

•**Get less animal protein.** In our analysis, people who ate an average of more than 1.5 servings a day of red meat or processed meat were 139% more likely to develop kidney disease than those who ate less than that. In patients with kidney disease, reducing overall protein intake lessens stress on the kidneys and can delay disease progression and the need for dialysis.

My advice: If you have kidney disease, consider working with a nutritionist to find healthful ways to limit daily protein to 40 g to 50 g. Fish (salmon, herring, mackerel and sardines) and lean meats provide high-quality protein with less saturated fat than you would get from typical red meat. Some research suggests vegetarian diets are especially beneficial for people with kidney disease.

For prevention: Include the most healthful protein sources. For example, beans and whole grains provide not only high-quality protein but also antioxidants, vitamins and minerals.

•**Consume much less salt.** For many people, a high-salt diet is a main cause of high blood pressure—a leading risk factor for kidney disease.

My advice: Even though some recent research raises questions about universal sodium restrictions, most health organizations recommend limiting daily sodium intake to 2,300 mg.

For some people with hypertension, reducing salt to 1,500 mg daily can lower systolic (top number) and diastolic (bottom number) pressure by about 11 points. That's comparable to the reduction that typically occurs with the use of antihypertensive medications.

•**Drink low-fat milk.** A study published in the *American Journal of Clinical Nutrition* that looked at 2,245 participants found that those who consumed the most low-fat milk, along with other low-fat dairy products, reduced their risk of developing hypertension by about 7%. Keeping one's blood pressure under control also contributes to healthy kidneys.

It's possible that the proteins and minerals (such as calcium) in dairy foods are responsible. Even though full-fat dairy contains the same minerals and proteins, the higher level of saturated fat may offset the benefits.

My advice: Check the USDA's Web site, *www.choosemyplate.gov,* for general guidelines regarding daily intake of low-fat or nonfat dairy.

•**Limit phosphorus intake.** The RDA for phosphorus in adults is 700 mg daily. However, the average adult consumes about twice as much because phosphorus is found in nearly every food—and it's added to processed foods to preserve colors and improve taste and/or texture.

Healthy adults excrete excess phosphorus. But in those with impaired kidney function, phosphorus can accumulate and cause conditions such as hyperphosphatemia, a buildup of this naturally occurring element that can lead to accelerated bone loss.

My advice: If you have kidney disease, ask your doctor if you need to lower your phosphorus levels—and work with a nutritionist to find the best ways to stay within healthy limits. It's wise for everyone to stay away from processed foods. In general, foods that are high in protein, such as meats, are also high in phosphorus. So are cola soft drinks, starchy vegetables and hard cheeses.

Important: To avoid high-phosphorus processed foods, look for "phos" on food labels. High-phosphorus additives include phosphoric acid, calcium phosphate and monopotassium phosphate.

For more information on kidney disease, consult the National Kidney Foundation's Web site, *www.kidney.org.*

Key Facts About the Kidneys

The kidneys are fist-sized organs that remove waste (about two quarts) from the approximately 200 quarts of blood that are processed daily. Each kidney contains about one million filtering units—tiny, delicate networks of blood vessels and tubes that are easily damaged by diabetes, high blood pressure and other chronic diseases.

Is It Just a Bladder Infection...or Are Your Kidneys in Danger?

Mildred Lam, MD, is an associate professor at Case Western Reserve University School of Medicine and an attending physician in the division of nephrology at MetroHealth Medical Center, both in Cleveland. She specializes in the care of patients with acute and chronic kidney disease.

A barely there bladder infection can turn into a kidney infection that can result in serious, or even fatal, complications. *How to stop a bladder infection from getting worse...*

According to kidney specialist Mildred Lam, MD, of Case Western Reserve University School of Medicine, in most cases of urinary tract infection (UTI), bacteria get into the urethra (the tube that carries urine out of the body), travel into the bladder and multi-

ply. Called a bladder infection or cystitis, this generally is easily treated with antibiotics.

But sometimes the bacteria travel farther and invade the kidney itself, causing a kidney infection. Possible consequences of this type of UTI include temporary or permanent kidney failure...chronic kidney disease...and potentially life-threatening septicemia if bacteria enter the bloodstream.

Women are more vulnerable to UTIs than men because in women, the urethra and bacteria-laden anus are closer together...and the urethra is shorter, so bacteria don't have to travel as far to reach the bladder and kidneys. *Other risk factors...*

•**Being postmenopausal**—accompanying hormonal changes can diminish muscle tone in the urinary tract, making it easier for bacteria to invade.

•**Sexual activity,** especially with a new partner—perhaps because, over time, a woman develops antibodies to her partner's bacteria.

•**Diabetes**—sugar in the urine promotes bacterial growth.

•**Kidney stones**—these provide a place for bacteria to grow and also impede the flow of urine (and therefore bacteria) out of the body.

•**Congenital defects that let urine travel upward from the bladder to the kidney**—normally urine only travels downward from kidney to bladder.

Because a kidney infection can quickly become serious, Dr. Lam urges women to be on the lookout for symptoms. *Call your doctor today if you notice...*

•**Discomfort or burning pain when urinating.**

•**Frequent urge to urinate** (even if little comes out).

•**Cloudy or blood-tinged urine.**

•**Low-grade fever.**

•**Mild to moderate pain in the middle of the lower back.**

These symptoms suggest a bladder infection. A urine test can confirm the diagnosis.

Remember: Prompt treatment—typically a three-to-five-day course of oral antibiotics—helps keep a bladder infection from moving to the kidneys. If you need a pain reliever, your doctor may recommend *acetaminophen* (Tylenol). "High-dose aspirin, *ibuprofen* and *naproxen* carry a small risk for kidney failure," Dr. Lam cautioned.

• **Severe pain in the "flank" area of the back,** at the lower edge of the ribs on the left or right side.

• **Chills and/or fever above 102°.**

• **Nausea and vomiting.**

These symptoms suggest a kidney infection. "To minimize the risk for permanent kidney damage, high-dose IV antibiotics are needed to quickly achieve high antibiotic levels in both the blood and the urine," Dr. Lam said. You may be given IV fluids if dehydrated or very nauseated. Once fever subsides and you can take fluids and medication by mouth, you'll switch to oral antibiotics, taking these for 10 to 14 days to eradicate the bacteria.

Dr. Lam's bladder and kidney infection prevention strategies…

• **Don't hold your urine too long**—going when you need to go helps flush bacteria out of the bladder.

• **Always wipe from front to back after using the toilet.**

• **Drinking cranberry juice or taking cranberry supplements may help**—cranberries contain a compound that makes it difficult for bacteria to cling to the bladder walls.

• **Stay hydrated.**

• **Urinate before and after intercourse.**

If you are especially prone to UTIs (getting more than two in a six-month period), ask your doctor about taking a single dose of an antibiotic immediately after intercourse.

Better Kidney Disease Test

Researchers stored blood samples from 2,300 adults with healthy kidneys for 10 years, then tested the samples for six biomarkers.

Results: Levels of three of the biomarkers, when considered together, identified people at high risk for chronic kidney disease.

Theory: Screening for these biomarkers (homocysteine, aldosterone and B-type natriuretic peptides), along with known risk factors (such as diabetes and high blood pressure), could identify 7% more adults at risk for the disease. Early detection can help prevent full-blown kidney disease.

Caroline Fox, MD, assistant clinical professor of medicine, Harvard Medical School, Boston.

Backache…or Bad Kidney?

When your back hurts, how can you tell if it's due to an injury or a kidney infection?

If you feel pain only when you move, it is most likely a back injury. Back pain often occurs from strained muscles and ligaments when you work around your house or in your garden, for example, participate in sports or suffer a sudden jolt, such as from a car accident. A kidney infection, on the other hand, may cause fever, pain when you urinate, shaking, chills, blood in your urine and deep back pain that hurts with or without movement. If you have any of these symptoms, contact your doctor immediately. If you have an infection, antibiotics are typically prescribed.

Leslie Spry, MD, kidney specialist, Lincoln Nephrology and Hypertension, Lincoln, Nebraska.

Are Swollen Ankles a Serious Problem? It May Mean Kidney Disease

Leo Galland, MD, director of the Foundation for Integrated Medicine in New York City...founder of Pilladvised.com, an online resource for learning about medications, supplements and food...and author of *Power Healing: Use the New Integrated Medicine to Cure Yourself* (Random House). *www.mdheal.org*

Dismissing ankle swelling as inconsequential can sometimes be a big mistake, according to Leo Galland, MD, a practicing physician, author and director of the Foundation for Integrated Medicine in New York City. It could be a sign of kidney disease. *Here are the warning signs to watch for...and what to do to protect yourself...*

The kidneys' job includes removing waste and excess fluids from the blood, maintaining the proper balance of salt and minerals in the blood, and helping regulate blood pressure. When kidney function is impaired, fluids build up in the body.

Watch for swelling that...

• **Affects both ankles.**

• **Gradually worsens.**

• **Also affects the hands, face and/or abdomen.**

Accompanied by...

• **Increased or decreased urination.**

• **Urine that is darker or foamier than usual.**

• **Itchy skin.**

• **A metallic or ammonia-like taste in the mouth.**

What to do: Immediately alert your doctor—untreated kidney disease can lead to irreversible kidney failure.

Preeclampsia May Forewarn Future Kidney Problems

Bjørn Egil Vikse, MD, PhD, doctor and researcher, renal research group, Haukeland University Hospital, Bergen, Norway.

If you had preeclampsia during a pregnancy your risk for kidney failure later in life may be elevated. Results of a Norwegian study recently published in *The New England Journal of Medicine* indicate that a history of preeclampsia is associated with nearly a five times greater likelihood of end-stage renal disease later in life. Specifically, the study found greater risk of kidney disease severe enough to require dialysis or a kidney transplant.

Preeclampsia, which occurs during about 5% of pregnancies, is characterized by high blood pressure, swelling of the hands, face, feet or entire body, and the presence of protein in the urine during the second half of the pregnancy. Doctors at Haukeland University Hospital in Bergen, Norway, identified a few years ago that women who had preeclampsia during their first pregnancy were more likely to later need a kidney biopsy than women whose pregnancies were free of this complication.

Recent research by the same team goes further, confirming that the association between preeclampsia and later kidney failure is "strong," according to Bjørn Egil Vikse, MD, PhD, a renal researcher and lead author of the study. "In Norway we are fortunate to have access to large databases of health information on virtually everyone born in the country since 1967," he said. Linking the Medical Births Registry of Norway with the Norwegian Renal Registry showed that women who gave birth to their first child in that country between 1967 and 1991 and who had also had preeclampsia during that pregnancy were more likely to have developed end stage renal disease later in life, on average 17 years afterward, he said.

Prolonged Sitting Linked to Kidney Disease

In a recent finding, women who sat a total of eight hours or more daily were about 30% more likely to develop chronic kidney disease than women who sat for three hours or less. Men who spent the most hours sitting had 19% increased risk.

Thomas Yates, PhD, senior lecturer at University of Leicester, Leicester, England, and lead researcher on a study of 6,379 people, published in *American Journal of Kidney Diseases*.

Other Risk Factors

An elevated risk of kidney failure was found in women who experienced preeclampsia with more than one pregnancy, as well as among women who had delivered prematurely or given birth to a low-birth-weight child, even if there was no preeclampsia. The registry does not contain information on such factors as whether the mothers at greater risk were also obese, smokers or had a history of high blood pressure, Dr. Vikse said, so those factors were not part of the study.

Dr. Vikse and his colleagues emphasize that the overall risk of end-stage renal disease for a woman who had preeclampsia is very small, around 0.5%. But, because of the seriousness of kidney disease, he recommends that all women who have had preeclampsia, especially those who have given birth to a premature child (before the 37th week) or a baby with a low birth weight (less than 5.5 pounds) discuss these aspects of their health history with their physician and have regular cardiovascular examinations, since heart disease is also linked to preeclampsia and kidney disease. Though there is not yet information on how to prevent the problem, catching kidney disease in the early stages is far better than later on when much more damage will have occurred.

Mammogram May Help Detect Kidney Disease

When 71 women with advanced kidney disease had routine mammograms, the images from 63% of them showed signs of calcification in breast artery tissue. This is a marker of vascular disease, which is common in people with kidney disease. By comparison, only 17% of a matched group of women without kidney disease showed calcification.

When having a mammogram: Ask the radiologist to look for breast tissue calcification. If spotted, talk to your doctor about screening for undetected vascular disease and kidney disease.

W. Charles O'Neill, MD, professor of medicine, Emory University School of Medicine, Atlanta.

Dialysis: New Ways to Get Better Results

Joel Neugarten, MD, professor of medicine at Albert Einstein College of Medicine of Yeshiva University and an attending nephrologist at Montefiore Medical Center, both in New York City. In addition to his clinical practice, Dr. Neugarten has conducted extensive research on the link between gender and risk for chronic kidney disease.

About one in every nine American adults will develop kidney disease in his/her lifetime (often as a result of diabetes or high blood pressure), and 1.5%, or about 400,000, are now undergoing dialysis.

Latest development: While this lifesaving treatment has been available for decades, the roughly 5,700 dialysis centers located throughout the US are now doing more and more to make the experience as pleasant as possible—providing comfortable chairs equipped with personal televisions, for example, and free Wi-Fi for Internet use.

What's most important: These "extras" are appealing to many people, but what matters most is the quality of the treatment itself. Fortunately, there are several recent discoveries that can help make dialysis more effective than ever before. *What you need to know...**

More Frequent and Longer Sessions

While three- to four-hour dialysis sessions, performed three times weekly, have long been the standard of care in the US, there's a growing body of evidence that patients may do better with more frequent and/or longer dialysis treatments.

Benefits of more frequent sessions: A 2010 study published in *The New England Journal of Medicine* found that undergoing dialysis two hours per day, six days per week, improved patients' quality of life and survival rates compared with three four-hour sessions.

Another recent study of 32,065 dialysis patients linked the two-day weekend wait that typically occurs with thrice-weekly dialysis to increased cardiac death risk.

Possible reason: Among other things, more frequent dialysis reduces fluid accumulation between treatments, which helps control blood pressure and reduces risk for ventricular hypertrophy (enlarged heart).

Benefits of longer sessions: Longer dialysis has been linked to increased "clearance rate"—a measure of toxin removal. In France, the country with the best dialysis outcomes, patients undergo three eight-hour dialysis sessions per week.

While there's no conclusive proof that increasing the duration of dialysis sessions improves long-term outcomes, several large-scale studies investigating this question are under way.

Increasing dialysis duration may improve...

*Before starting dialysis, go to the Medicare Web site, *www.Medicare.gov*, and click on "Forms, Help & Resources" and then "Find doctors, hospitals & facilities" to see how the outcomes of the center you're considering stack up against those of other centers.

- **Removal of "middle molecules"—** larger toxins, such as beta2-microglobulin, which aren't filtered out easily during standard dialysis.

- **Removal of phosphorus.** Elevated phosphorus is linked to loss of bone density and increased risk for death in patients with chronic kidney disease. For these reasons, dialysis patients are commonly prescribed phosphorus-lowering medications. With more frequent dialysis, such medications, which have side effects that may include gastrointestinal problems, may be unnecessary.

- **Cognitive function and sleep quality.** Improved cognition and sleep may be due to more efficient clearance of uremic toxins.

Maximizing Convenience

If more frequent and/or longer in-center dialysis sessions are not an option for you, the following alternative approaches are generating increasing interest for their effectiveness and convenience...

- **Nocturnal dialysis.** Undergoing dialysis at night while sleeping is appealing because it frees up daytime hours while also extending the treatment's duration. Some centers now accommodate overnight dialysis stays,

Even Seniors Can Donate a Kidney

Donation is safe for people over 70 years old. They are no more likely to die within one, five or 10 years of the procedure than healthy people of the same age who are not donors. Kidneys donated by healthy people over age 70 last as long as ones from younger deceased donors, although not as long as those from younger living donors.

Jonathan Berger, MD, department of surgery, Johns Hopkins University School of Medicine, Baltimore, and leader of a study of 219 adults over age 70 who donated kidneys, scheduled for publication in *Clinical Journal of the American Society of Nephrology.*

but it may not be covered by insurance. Nocturnal dialysis also can be done at home.

Emerging evidence links nocturnal dialysis with increased longevity and fewer hospital visits. Compared with the conventional approach, nocturnal dialysis produces a better clearance rate and reduces "urea rebound"—the rise in blood urea nitrogen (BUN), a marker for waste buildup, that can occur after a dialysis session ends.

Important research: In a 2007 study of 52 Canadian dialysis patients published in *The Journal of the American Medical Association*, half switched to nocturnal dialysis. After six months, their left heart ventricles shrank, on average, and their mineral and blood pressure levels also improved, allowing them to reduce blood pressure drugs and other medications.

• **Home dialysis works well for more frequent daytime sessions and nocturnal dialysis.** Home dialysis has been linked to improved heart function, sleeping patterns, energy levels and overall well-being—and it costs less than in-center dialysis. Most health insurers cover the cost of home dialysis.

With home dialysis, patients use portable, fully automated home-dialysis machines. The leading US device, NxStage, uses a convenient, preformulated dialysis solution that helps restore vital electrolytes that can be lost during dialysis.

Studies indicate that complications, such as cramping, occur no more often with home dialysis than in a dialysis center.

What's more, patients can typically sleep through the night without interruption while receiving home dialysis. A caregiver (a spouse or home health aide, for example) is typically trained by the dialysis center to monitor home dialysis.

Home dialysis is now used by 55% of dialysis patients in New Zealand…30% in Australia…and 20% in Canada. Only 8% of US patients use this approach, but that could change as people become more aware of its safety, convenience and cost-effectiveness. You may want to ask your doctor about home dialysis.

Strong Muscles Help Kidney Disease Patients Live Longer

Kidney disease patients on dialysis live longer—and are happier—if they have robust muscles, say researchers from Harbor-UCLA Medical Center in Los Angeles. Measuring lean muscle mass in the arm, researchers found that patients with the highest amount of lean muscle mass were 37% less likely to die during the five-year study period than those with the least amounts. Techniques such as weight training to build lean muscle mass can help kidney disease patients.

K. Kalantar-Zadeh, et al., "Mid-Arm Muscle Circumference and Quality of Life and Survival in Maintenance Hemodialysis Patients," *Clinical Journal of the American Society of Nephrology* (2010).

A Probiotic for Kidney Disease

Mark A. Stengler, NMD, licensed naturopathic medical doctor in private practice, Stengler Center for Integrative Medicine, Encinitas, California…adjunct associate clinical professor at the National College of Natural Medicine, Portland, Oregon…author of many books, including *The Natural Physician's Healing Therapies* and coauthor of *Prescription for Natural Cures* (both from Bottom Line Books)…and author of the *Bottom Line/Natural Healing* newsletter. *http://markstengler.com*

Patients with chronic kidney disease (CKD) often ask me about natural treatments that can help them. There's a probiotic product called Renadyl (formerly named Kibow Biotics) that can help kidney function. I'm a great believer in probiotics—ingesting "good" bacteria daily inhibits growth of harmful bacteria and enhances immune function. There now are probiotic combinations targeted to help specific conditions—and one of these is for compromised kidney function.

What Is Dialysis?

When a person loses 85% to 95% of his/her kidney function, dialysis is used to perform the job of healthy kidneys. In the US, hemodialysis is the most popular form. With this treatment, blood is removed from the patient's body via a needle and catheter and filtered through a dialysis machine to extract excess water and waste products. "Clean" blood is then returned to the patient's body. Treatments (usually three to four hours each) are performed three times a week, typically at outpatient centers.

Joel Neugarten, MD.

In CKD, the kidneys no longer filter toxins efficiently. As a result, toxins accumulate in the bloodstream where they can damage a wide range of organs. Renadyl contains three strains of probiotics—Streptococcus thermophilus...Lactobacillus acidophilus... and Bifidobacterium longum. These bacteria strains metabolize toxins and convert them into nontoxic substances that then are excreted by the colon. In essence, this probiotic enables the colon to remove more toxins, thus reducing the kidneys' exposure to this substance.

By lessening the kidneys' workload and reducing the buildup of toxins in the blood, probiotics offer significant benefits for people with Stage 3 or Stage 4 kidney disease, whose kidneys still are functioning to some degree. It also helps reduce strain on the kidneys for those with Stage 1 or Stage 2 kidney disease. But it won't help people who are undergoing dialysis because their kidneys have failed completely.

In a 2010 study published in *Advances in Therapy*, researchers from the company that makes the probiotic and outside researchers gave patients with Stage 3 and Stage 4 CKD three capsules (equaling 90 billion colony-forming units) daily of Renadyl. After taking the probiotic for six months, about 63% of the study participants had decreased levels of blood urea nitrogen (which means that this toxin was being eliminated), and 86% reported substantially improved quality of life, which for CKD patients means eating more of the foods they want, sleeping better and having more energy because they don't have to urinate as many times at night.

Renadyl can be purchased from Kibow Biotech (888-271-2560, *www.kibowbiotech. com*). Cost is $135 for a three-month supply. Patients with CKD should speak to a holistic doctor before taking this probiotic or any other supplement.

New Statin Side Effects

Statins are linked to cataracts and kidney failure, in addition to previously known effects on the liver and muscles. Risks are highest during the first year of use, according to a huge study of the popular cholesterol-lowering medications, which include *atorvastatin* (Lipitor), *fluvastatin* (Lescol) and *simvastatin* (Zocor).

Better news: The research suggests that statins decrease risk for esophageal cancer.

Bottom line: Discuss benefits and risks of statins with your physician.

Julia Hippisley-Cox, MD, professor of clinical epidemiology and general practice, University of Nottingham, Nottingham, United Kingdom, and coauthor of a study of 2,004,692 patients, published in *British Medical Journal* (BMJ).

Far from the Road?

A study of about 1,100 adults found that those living within about a half-mile of a major road were more likely to have impaired kidney function than those who lived farther away.

Journal of Epidemiology & Community Health

Better Kidney Monitoring

When researchers compared kidney function tests in 701 adults with type 2 diabetes and kidney disease, the albumin-to-creatinine ratio taken from a first-after-waking urine sample best predicted kidney disease progression. Doctors typically use a 24-hour collection (in which all urine excreted during that period is collected in a cup) to measure protein excretion.

If you have type 2 diabetes: Ask your doctor about monitoring your kidney function with the more convenient morning urine test.

Hiddo Lambers Heerspink, PhD, researcher, University Medical Center Groningen, the Netherlands.

Calcium Supplements Can Lead to Kidney Stones

Recent finding: Women who averaged 1,800 milligrams (mg) a day of calcium primarily from supplements were 17% more likely to develop kidney stones than women who averaged about 1,145 mg of calcium a day. But women in the study with the highest intake of calcium from food were 65% less prone to kidney stones than those with the lowest dietary calcium consumption.

Self-defense: Try to get calcium from food sources. If your intake is low, talk to your doctor about taking calcium supplements.

Robert B. Wallace, MD, professor, department of epidemiology, University of Iowa School of Public Health, Iowa City, and leader of a study of 36,282 women over seven years, published in *American Journal of Clinical Nutrition.*

Gene Linked to Kidney Stones

According to a recent laboratory finding, the claudin 14 gene, when activated by a high-salt, high-calcium or low-water diet, causes excess calcium to enter the urine—the cause of most kidney stones. This may lead to better treatments and new screenings.

EMBO Journal

Best and Worst Drinks for Preventing Kidney Stones

Pietro Manuel Ferraro, MD, physician, department of internal medicine and medical specialties, Catholic University of the Sacred Heart, Rome, Italy. His study was published in *Clinical Journal of the American Society of Nephrology.*

Mention kidney stones and everyone within earshot winces—because we've all heard how painful these stones can be. So if you want to be stone-free, you're probably following the common advice to drink lots of liquids. But instead of focusing on how much you drink, the crucial question is what you drink, a recent study reveals. Certain beverages—including some very surprising ones, such as beer!—are particularly helpful in protecting against stones, while other drinks do more harm than good.

Unfortunately, kidney stones are common, plaguing 19% of men and 9% of women in the US at least once in their lifetimes—and recurrences are quite common. Drinking plenty of water helps prevent stones from forming…but actually, there are other fluids that can be even more effective.

Drink This, Not That

Using data from three large studies, researchers followed 194,095 people, none of whom had a history of kidney stones, for more than eight years. Participants periodically completed questionnaires about their diet and overall health. During the course of the study, there were 4,462 cases of kidney stones.

Researchers adjusted for health factors (age, body mass index, diabetes, medications, blood pressure) as well as various dietary factors (including intake of meat, calcium and potassium) known to affect kidney stone risk. Then they calculated the stone risk associated with various types of beverages.

How the comparison was done: For each analysis, the effects of drinking an average of one or more servings per day were compared with drinking less than one serving per week. Because data from three different studies were used, serving sizes were not necessarily alike across the board. But in general, a serving was considered to be 12 ounces of soda or beer…eight ounces of coffee, tea, milk or fruit punch…five ounces of wine…and four to six ounces of juice. The researchers' findings were eye-opening.

Kidney stone risk boosters…

•**Sugar-sweetened noncola sodas increased kidney stone risk by 33%.**

•**Sugar-sweetened colas increased risk by 23%.**

•**Fruit punch increased risk by 18%.**

•**Diet noncola sodas (but, surprisingly, not diet colas) increased risk by 17%.**

Kidney stone risk reducers…

•**Beer reduced kidney stone risk by 41%.**

•**White wine reduced risk by 33%.**

•**Red wine reduced risk by 31%.**

•**Caffeinated coffee reduced kidney stone risk by 26%.**

•**Decaf coffee reduced risk by 16%.**

•**Orange juice reduced risk by 12%.**

•**Tea reduced risk by 11%.**

Consumption of milk and juices other than orange juice did not significantly affect the likelihood of developing kidney stones.

Theories behind the findings: Because sugar-sweetened sodas and fruit punch are associated with higher risk, researchers suspect that their high fructose concentration may increase the amount of calcium, oxalate and uric acid in the urine—and those substances contribute to kidney stone formation. So how to explain the beneficial effects of orange juice, which is also high in fructose? Perhaps orange juice's high concentration of potassium citrate offsets the fructose and favorably changes the composition of urine.

Regarding the beneficial effects of coffee and tea, it could be that their caffeine acts as a diuretic that promotes urine production and thus helps prevent stones. Tea and coffee, including decaf, also contain antioxidants that may help combat stone formation. Alcohol, too, is a diuretic, and wine and beer contain antioxidants as well—though of course, with any type of alcoholic beverage, moderation is important.

Diet to Prevent Hypertension Also Fights Kidney Stones

The DASH diet (Dietary Approaches to Stop Hypertension) is high in fruits, vegetables, nuts, whole grains and low-fat dairy products and low in sodium, sweetened beverages and processed meats.

Recent finding: In addition to having lower risk for hypertension, people who consume a DASH-style diet are 40% to 45% less likely to develop kidney stones. To learn more about the DASH diet, go to *www.nhlbi. nih.gov/health* (click on "High Blood Pressure" and "Your Guide to Lowering Your Blood Pressure with DASH" farther down the page).

Eric Taylor, MD, assistant professor, department of internal medicine, Brigham and Women's Hospital, Cambridge, Massachusetts, and leader of a study of 241,766 people, published in *Journal of the American Society of Nephrology*.

Lemonade for Kidney Stones

Roger L. Sur, MD, urologist, assistant professor of surgery and director of the University of California, San Diego (UCSD), Comprehensive Kidney Stone Center.

More than half a million Americans go to emergency rooms each year due to kidney stones, and about one in 10 Americans will suffer a kidney stone at some time in his/her life.

Simple home remedy: Drink lemonade. A study I published in *The Journal of Urology* found that patients who drank a little more than two quarts of lemonade (made with about four ounces of lemonade concentrate) daily for an average of 44 months had an increase in urinary citrate that was comparable to the increase in a group taking oral potassium citrate, which is commonly prescribed for kidney stones. More urinary citrate means a lower risk for calcium kidney stones, the most common form. Drinking water alone has not been found to raise urinary citrate levels.

If you've had kidney stones in the past, you have a 50% chance of getting one or more additional stones within five to 10 years. Drinking two quarts of lemonade daily could reduce this risk by 90%—without the expense or side effects of medication. I advise using an artificial sweetener or honey instead of refined sugar.

Other citrus juices, including orange and grapefruit juice, also contain citrate, but not as much as juice made from lemons.

Plastic Dishes May Cause Kidney Stones

Recent finding: When volunteers ate hot soup from plastic bowls made with melamine, levels of the chemical in their urine were up to 6.4 times higher than in people who ate soup from ceramic bowls.

Theory: Melamine-containing dishes release large amounts of the chemical, which has been linked to kidney stones, when used to serve high-temperature foods.

Best: Serve hot food in ceramic dishes. Check for melamine on the label when purchasing plastic dishes.

Ming-Tsang Wu, MD, ScD, professor and attending physician, Kaohsiung Medical University Hospital, Taiwan.

SEPSIS AND OTHER INFECTIOUS DISEASES

Septicemia and sepsis are extremely serious blood infections (usually bacterial), which need to be treated quickly and aggressively or they can result in death. According to recent research, infectious diseases are becoming more widespread as environmental conditions change, global travel increases and as more contagious strains become resistant to current medical treatments. Fortunately there are dozens of steps you can take to avoid getting these life-threatening infections.

http://healthyamericans.org/newsroom/releases/?releaseid=298

Chapter 23

PROTECT YOURSELF FROM KILLER INFECTIONS

Millions Die from Sepsis—How to Detect And Cure Quickly

Sepsis is the tenth-leading cause of death in the US. It doesn't have to be. **The challenge:** There isn't a single test that can diagnose sepsis. Because its symptoms can be very similar to those caused by the original infection, the diagnosis sometimes is overlooked—and even a brief delay in treatment can be deadly.

Every year, at least 750,000 Americans develop severe sepsis and about 40% of patients with severe sepsis will die from it. The death rate approaches 50% in patients who develop septic shock (a dangerous drop in blood pressure that can lead to organ failure), which can't be reversed by the administration of intravenous (IV) fluids.

Who's at Risk

Sepsis often is triggered by a bacterial infection. It also can be caused by viral or fungal infections. Pneumonia is the infection most likely to lead to sepsis.

The risk for sepsis is highest among adults age 65 and older, particularly those in the hospital who get IV lines, urinary catheters or other invasive devices. But you don't have to be elderly or seriously ill or be in a hospital to develop sepsis. About half of all cases occur in nonhospital settings. If you have any type of infection—an infected cut, a urinary tract infection, the flu—it can progress to sepsis.

Examples: Many of the 18,000 deaths that were linked to the swine flu outbreak in 2009 actually were caused by sepsis. In 2012, a New York sixth-grader cut his arm during a basketball game and got an infection. He died from sepsis three days later.

Warning Signs

For reasons that still aren't clear, some infections are accompanied by an exaggerated immune response. It's normal for the body to respond to an infection with local inflammation. In patients with sepsis, the inflammation is systemic—it spreads throughout the body and often causes a loss of fluids that leads to plummeting blood pressure and shock. It also triggers microscopic blood

Derek C. Angus, MD, MPH, the Mitchell P. Fink Endowed Chair in Critical Care Medicine and professor of critical care medicine, medicine, health policy and management, and clinical and translational science at University of Pittsburgh School of Medicine.

clots that can block circulation to the heart, kidneys and other organs.

Warning signs…

•**You're sicker than expected.** Suppose that you have a bladder infection or an infected cut. If the severity of your symptoms seems to be out of proportion to the illness, call your doctor.

Go to the emergency room if you or a loved one also has two or more of the following symptoms…

•**Rapid heartbeat.** Patients developing sepsis usually will have tachycardia, a rapid heartbeat that exceeds 90 beats/minute.

•**High or low temperature.** Both hypothermia (a body temperature below 96.8°F) and fever (above 100.4°F) can indicate sepsis.

•**Rapid breathing, or tachypnea.** Patients with sepsis may have a respiration rate of 20 breaths/minute or higher.

•**Mucus.** The common cold is unlikely to cause sepsis, but it's not impossible. Call your doctor if a cold or other respiratory infection is accompanied by foul-smelling, discolored (rather than clear) mucus. This could indicate that you have developed a more serious infection.

•**Mental confusion.** When sepsis has reached the stage that it's interfering with circulation, it often will cause mental confusion.

•**Mottled skin.** There may be blue patches on the skin. Or if you press on the skin, there might be a delay before it returns to its normal color. Both of these changes indicate that circulation is impaired—a sign of severe sepsis.

Important: When patients begin to develop signs and symptoms suggesting that vital organ function is compromised, sepsis already is an emergency. For example, altered mental status, falling blood pressure, difficulty breathing or mottled skin all suggest that the inflammatory response intended to help is now causing life-threatening harm.

What Comes Next

Sepsis always is treated in the hospital. To confirm that you have it, your doctor will do a variety of tests, including a blood pressure check and a white blood cell count. You also will need blood cultures to identify the organism that is causing the infection so that your doctor can choose the most effective treatment.

•**Treat first, diagnose later.** A study in *Critical Care Medicine* reported that the risk of dying from sepsis increases by 7.6% for every hour that passes without treatment. If your doctor suspects that you have sepsis, he/she will immediately start treatment with an antibiotic—usually a broad-spectrum antibiotic that's effective against a wide variety of organisms. Later the drug may be changed, depending on what the blood cultures show.

•**Intravenous fluids.** They often are needed to counteract the capillary leakage that causes blood pressure to drop.

•**Vasopressor treatment.** Depending on the severity of sepsis, you might be given *dopamine* or *norepinephrine*—medications that increase blood pressure and improve circulation to the heart, kidneys and other organs.

Other treatments may include supplemental oxygen, anti-inflammatory steroids and sometimes kidney dialysis.

Preventing Sepsis

There's no way to predict who will get sepsis or the type of infection that's most likely to cause it in a particular person. So don't watch and wait. If you suspect sepsis, call your doctor. *And to build up your defense against sepsis in the future…*

•**Get a pneumococcal pneumonia vaccination if you're 65 years old or older… have chronic health problems…take medications that lower immunity…or you're a smoker.** Most people should get a pneumonia vaccination every five years.

•**Get an annual flu shot.** The rate of sepsis increases by about 16% during flu season. Getting an annual flu shot—along with washing your hands several times a day—reduces your risk for sepsis.

•**Clean wounds thoroughly.** If you have a cut, scrape or burn and are taking care of it yourself, wash it several times a day with soap and water, and apply an antibacterial ointment. Call your doctor immediately if there is pus, increased or streaking redness, or if the wound feels warm.

The Truth About Steroid Shots for Back Pain

David Borenstein, MD, a clinical professor of medicine at The George Washington University Medical Center in Washington, DC, with a private practice at Arthritis and Rheumatism Associates based in Chevy Chase, Rockville and Wheaton, Maryland, and Washington, DC. The author of *Heal Your Back* (M. Evans & Company), Dr. Borenstein is also the host of *Speaking of Health with Dr. B*, a weekly radio program on WomensRadio.com. *www.ARAPC.com*

Steroid injections have long been considered a much needed pain-relieving treatment for people with sciatica and other back conditions.

Now: Many patients are thinking twice about having the injections after contaminated doses of the drug created a nationwide outbreak of meningitis that began in September 2012 and claimed more than 60 lives and sickened more than 750 people.

Possible Risks

Injected steroids are much less likely to cause side effects than oral steroids, but there are some risks…

•**Severe infection.** This occurs in only about 0.01% to 0.1% of injections. Even so, steroid injections usually are not recommended for people with compromised immunity due to diabetes or cancer treatments, for example, or those with an active infection. *Important:* To reduce contamination risk, your doctor should use a brand-name drug rather than a

drug from a compounding pharmacy (as was the case in the meningitis outbreak).

•**Bleeding.** This can occur in patients taking blood thinners or in those with underlying health problems (such as cirrhosis of the liver) that interfere with blood clotting.

•**Nerve damage.** This occurs in only about one in every 10,000 cases but could happen if the doctor accidentally jabs a nerve during the procedure. Nerve damage could result in incontinence, chronic back pain and, in rare instances, paralysis.

Meningitis Vaccine

Meningitis vaccine for kids benefits the elderly, too.

Recent finding: Since the meningitis vaccine was introduced in 2000 for children ages two months to two years, not only have meningitis cases declined by 64% among children, they also have dropped by 54% among people 65 and older.

Reason: With fewer children spreading germs, fewer adults are getting the disease.

Nancy Bennett, MD, director, Center for Community Health, University of Rochester School of Medicine and Dentistry, Rochester, New York, and coauthor of a study of data collected from 1998 to 2005, published in *The New England Journal of Medicine*.

Travel Vaccination Recommendations

Below are the vaccinations needed for popular travel destinations…

•**Brazil**—yellow fever, typhoid, rabies and hepatitis.

•**Cambodia**—Japanese encephalitis, typhoid, rabies and hepatitis.

•**Kenya**—yellow fever, meningococcal meningitis, typhoid, rabies, hepatitis and polio.

•**Peru**—yellow fever, hepatitis, typhoid and rabies.

• **Thailand**—hepatitis, Japanese encephalitis and typhoid.

More information: www.cdc.gov/travel (click on "Destinations").

Centers for Disease Control and Prevention, Atlanta.

Alert on Mosquito-Borne Illnesses, Including Dengue Fever

Roxanne Connelly, PhD, president, Florida Mosquito Control Association, associate professor of medical entomology, Institute of Food and Agricultural Sciences, University of Florida, Vero Beach.

In 2010, Florida's Key West was hit with an outbreak of dengue fever, a tropical mosquito-borne disease seldom seen in this country. In July 2013, an outbreak occurred in Marin County, Florida. Dengue fever generally isn't deadly, but it does make people very, very sick. It joins a list of other mosquito-borne illnesses in the US, some of which are far more serious, including West Nile virus, St. Louis encephalitis and LaCrosse encephalitis. All are caused by viruses transmitted to humans through mosquito bites. We spoke with Roxanne Connelly, PhD, associate professor at the University of Florida and president of the Florida Mosquito Control Association, to discuss what moms and families (who love the outdoors) need to know to protect ourselves from this array of illnesses as the buggy season kicks in…

Dengue Fever in the US

Although dengue (pronounced den-gay) is found primarily in tropical climates, there have been occasional outbreaks here in the US. Dengue is the most common virus transmitted by mosquitoes worldwide and also often the cause of fever in people who return ill from vacations in the Caribbean and Central America.

Where it occurs: Rarely in the US, outside of occasional outbreaks (recently in Florida and isolated cases reported in Texas since 1980).

When you may get sick: Four to seven days after you are bitten.

Watch out for these symptoms: Headache, high fever and muscle, bone and joint aches, nausea and vomiting. The virus usually causes mild illness—with any luck, you'll never even know that you were infected. But, because of the potential for severe aches and pains, dengue is also known as "breakbone fever." In the worst-case scenario, you may develop dengue hemorrhagic fever, which can be fatal. This is rare—occurring, for instance, when a person is infected with two different strains of the virus—and it occurs most often in children. *What to watch for:* After several days of being sick, the patient becomes irritable and sweaty, then goes into a shocklike state. Sudden bleeding (from the gums or nose) or bruising may appear. Be alert for tiny spots of blood on the skin and larger patches of blood pooled beneath.

The treatment: There are four strains of the virus. Once you have been infected with one strain, you are at risk for more serious disease if you are bitten by a mosquito carrying a different strain. Treatment is to relieve symptoms, which usually resolve on their own within a few weeks. The hemorrhagic form is a medical emergency and requires hospitalization.

West Nile Virus

The first case of West Nile virus in the US was documented in 1999, when an epidemic hit New York City. Most people who are bitten by an infective mosquito don't get sick, but if you're over age 50, your odds of getting sick are higher—and the older you are, the sicker you're likely to get. There's a mild form called West Nile fever that is usually uncomfortable at worst (only 20% of people who are infected even have symptoms), but there's also a more severe form, West Nile encephalitis or meningitis, that affects a small percentage (less than 1%). This form may result in seizures and even death.

Where it occurs: In most states in the US. See a state-by-state map at *www.cdc.gov/ ncidod/dvbid/westnile/mapsincidence/surv& control10IncidbyState.htm.*

When you may get sick: Two to 15 days after you are bitten.

Watch out for these symptoms: Fever, headache, body aches and a skin rash (characterized by large red patches with a varied surface, both raised and flat) are signs of West Nile fever, which lasts several days to weeks. The severe and potentially fatal form, West Nile encephalitis (an inflammation of the brain), strikes in one in 150 cases and causes neck stiffness, disorientation, muscle weakness, paralysis, convulsions and coma. Severe symptoms may last for months, says Dr. Connelly.

The treatment: Treatment focuses on symptom control (e.g., *acetaminophen* to lower fever and oral fluids to prevent dehydration). People with West Nile encephalitis may require hospitalization for intravenous fluids, respiratory assistance and other support.

St. Louis Encephalitis

As with West Nile, most people bitten by a mosquito carrying the virus that causes St. Louis encephalitis do not fall ill. The first known epidemic of the disease broke out in St. Louis in 1933.

Where it occurs: Don't make the mistake of thinking this is a problem only in Missouri—it occurs throughout the country, though most outbreaks have been concentrated in the southeastern and midwestern states. See a state-by-state map at www.cdc. gov/sle/technical/epi.html#casesbystate.

When you may get sick: Four to 21 days after you are bitten.

Watch out for these symptoms: Fever, headache, nausea, vomiting, dizziness and tiredness for several days to a week. Severe disease attacks the central nervous system and often involves encephalitis—which may

cause a stiff neck, disorientation, lethargy, and, very rarely, coma, convulsions, paralysis and death.

The treatment: As in the case of West Nile virus, treatment consists of supportive care to relieve symptoms. In rare cases, long-term disability or death can result. The risk for death increases with age.

How to Mount an Aggressive Anti-Mosquito Defense

Doctors do not always think to check for a mosquito-borne virus, especially when the symptoms are so similar to other illnesses such as the flu. If no major outbreak has been publicized in the news, it is a good idea to ask your doctor if your flulike symptoms could be from a mosquito-borne virus. But in the meantime, the best way to protect yourself from mosquito-borne illnesses is to take precautions to limit mosquito bites. *Here's how…*

•**Use mosquito repellent.** Choose an EPA-approved mosquito repellent, advises Dr. Connelly, one that contains DEET, picaridin or oil of lemon eucalyptus. Apply a light layer to exposed skin and clothing.

Caution: Do not use repellent near or in your eyes or mouth, under clothing or on cuts or irritated skin, and use sparingly on your ears (making sure that it does not get down inside the ears). Do not use products that combine sunscreen and repellent. Since sunscreen must be applied often and liberally, you can potentially get too much repellent—even a toxic dose. When you return indoors, wash treated skin thoroughly to avoid spreading repellent.

•**Eliminate standing water.** Mosquitoes lay their eggs in standing water. Reduce mosquito populations around your house by eliminating their breeding grounds.

Your job: Get rid of unnecessary buckets, flowerpots and other items that hold water. Change water in birdbaths once a week. Don't let rain gutters get clogged. (Many people think about their gutters only in autumn when leaves are falling, but they can become clogged any time of year.)

• **Avoid peak mosquito hours.** Steer clear of outdoor activities around dusk and dawn. If you have to go out at these times, use insect repellent (on exposed skin only) and wear repellent-treated protective clothing such as long sleeves and pants.

Don't waste your money: Gimmicks like antimosquito bracelets and necklaces that claim to have repellent qualities don't work, says Dr. Connelly. Likewise, there is no evidence that sound-emitting devices will keep you from getting bitten.

• **Repair damaged window and door screens, or install new ones.** Only tight, well-fitting screens will keep mosquitoes outside when your windows are open.

Do it yourself: For advice on how to make simple screen repairs inexpensively, visit *http://edis.ifas.ufl.edu/fy811.*

Beware—Valley Fever Is On the Rise

Clarisse Tsang, MPH, epidemiologist, Office of Infectious Disease Services, Epidemiology & Disease Control Services, Arizona Department of Health Services, Phoenix.

If you have a cough and fever that land you in the doctor's office and he/she asks if you've done any traveling lately, it's not just small talk—the information you give may help pin down your diagnosis. Doctors all over the US are now on the alert for new cases of a serious health problem affecting residents of and visitors to the southwestern US. Called "valley fever," this flulike illness is being spread by the spores of ground-dwelling fungi, which are easily stirred up and blown about by the wind. While most people exposed to the fungi don't fall ill, others get quite sick and may end up missing weeks, even months, of work or school. In less than 1% of people who get valley fever, the infection can spread from the lungs to the rest

of the body, causing meningitis (spine and brain infection) or infection in the bones and joints and can eventually lead to death (although this is rare).

According to the Directors of Health Promotion and Education in Washington, DC, an affiliate of the Association of State and Territorial Health Officials and an advocate for promoting health and preventing disease, an estimated 50,000 to 100,000 people are affected by valley fever each year. According to the Centers for Disease Control, some researchers estimate that each year the fungus infects more than 150,000 people, many of whom are sick without knowing the cause or have cases so mild they aren't detected.

Valley fever (one popular name for coccidioidomycosis) is now affecting people in Arizona, New Mexico, southern and central California, desert areas in Texas and Nevada, southern Utah, northern Mexico, and parts of Central America and southern South America. It's not contagious but according to Clarisse Tsang, MPH, an epidemiologist in the

MRSA at the Beach

You can catch MRSA anywhere—even at the beach. Methicillin-resistant Staphylococcus aureus (MRSA) is an antibiotic-resistant strain of bacteria that can cause difficult-to-treat skin and systemic infections. Staphylococcus bacteria are everywhere—many people carry them without realizing it. Beachgoers may pick up bacteria left behind in sand or water by other visitors.

Self-defense: Shower with soap after leaving the beach. Consider staying out of the water if you have an open cut or sore—these can be bacterial entry points.

Lisa Plano, MD, PhD, associate professor, departments of pediatrics and of microbiology and immunology, Miller School of Medicine, University of Miami, Florida, and leader of a study of 1,303 people, presented at a meeting of the American Association for the Advancement of Science.

Arizona Department of Health Services, it's more widespread than was initially thought.

Ms. Tsang is the lead author of a paper on valley fever that was published in the Centers for Disease Control and Prevention's *Emerging Infectious Diseases.* First documented in Argentina in 1892, the spores are spread when the ground gets stirred up—such as by farming, construction, military field training, archaeology, gardening, etc. In this study, of the 493 patients interviewed, 44% went to an emergency room and 41% were hospitalized. Ms. Tsang said that researchers found that patients are suffering with the disease longer than expected, with symptoms typically lasting about four months—far longer than the 21-day duration that was previously reported. Symptoms may include coughing, fatigue, fever, headache, joint and muscle aches, rash and/or shortness of breath.

The severe cases—in which the fungus spreads from the lungs to other parts of the body, including the skin, bones, joints or brain—affect about 1% of patients, and African-Americans, Asians and Filipinos, as well as pregnant women and people with compromised immune systems seem to be most vulnerable. Valley fever usually can be treated successfully with prescription antifungal medication (*fluconazole* and several other drugs known as "azoles"), but the diagnosis often is missed because the symptoms are common to many other illnesses.

You can learn more about this problem from the Valley Fever Center for Excellence (*www.vfce.arizona.edu*) or the Arizona Department of Health Services (*www.Valley FeverArizona.org*).

Visiting the Desert?

If you live in or will be visiting an area where valley fever is known to be a problem, you can follow these simple precautions…

• **Minimize dust exposure.** Stay indoors when it's windy, especially during a dust storm.

• **Avoid activities that mean you are breathing potentially spore-bearing soil** that has been stirred up, such as gardening. Persons who are immunocompromised should especially keep this in mind.

If you have any collection of the symptoms described above for two weeks and are not getting better…and you have visited an area where you may have been exposed to the spores…Ms. Tsang said you should ask your doctor to test you for valley fever. The simple blood or sputum test can be done at a local lab, with results usually available within one to two weeks.

How NOT to Get a Deadly Infection

Susan Kellie, MD, associate professor of medicine in the division of infectious diseases at University of New Mexico (UNM) Health Sciences Center and hospital epidemiologist for the UNM Health Sciences Center and the New Mexico Veterans Administration Healthcare Systems, Albuquerque.

The virulent strain of methicillin-resistant *Staphylococcus aureus* (MRSA) continues to cause dangerous infections in otherwise healthy adults and children.

Several years ago, MRSA made headlines when a Virginia high school student died after MRSA spread quickly through his internal organs. Local officials closed 21 schools for disinfection.

The good news is that infections are on the downslide. Looking at data from 2005, government researchers estimated that were more than 94,000 life-threatening MRSA infections in the US annually, contributing to the deaths of an estimated 19,000 Americans per year. The most recent figures from the Centers for Disease Control (CDC), reported in the September 16, 2013, issue of *JAMA Internal Medicine*, found that 30,000 fewer MRSA infections occurred in 2011 compared to 2005.

MRSA is considered a "superbug" because it's resistant to nearly all treatments, including the powerful antibiotic methicillin.

Risk Still Exists

The ordinary Staphylococcus aureus (staph) bacterium is among the most common causes of infection. Up to one-third of Americans have a relatively innocuous form of staph in the nose or on the skin. It usually causes nothing more serious than boils or a hair-follicle infection.

MRSA is a strain of this organism that is resistant to certain antibiotics and has long been a problem in hospitals. The JAMA study, conducted by researchers at the Centers for Disease Control and Prevention (CDC), found that about 85% of MRSA cases are connected with hospitals and other health-care settings—after surgery, in dialysis patients, etc.—but the more recent form of MRSA, known as USA 300, can be found in healthy Americans. *Examples…*

• **The Veterans Administration in Pittsburgh recently reported a four-fold increase** in emergency room treatments for skin and soft-tissue (tissue under the skin) infections caused by MRSA.

• **A study in *The New England Journal of Medicine*** found that nearly 60% of skin and soft-tissue infections at 11 university-affiliated emergency rooms were caused by MRSA.

• **In 2005, researchers investigated an outbreak of skin infections among the St. Louis Rams** and found that 9% of the football players had MRSA skin infections. In addition, 42% of nasal swabs taken from the players and staff members tested positive for MRSA. All carried the USA 300 form of MRSA, which was simultaneously being discovered throughout the country. This suggests rapid, widespread transmission.

• **Studies indicate that 1% of healthy Americans are colonized with MRSA**—bacteria are present but haven't caused infection. In group-living settings, such as prisons and military training camps, the colonization rate is as high as 2.5% to 3%. Among hospitalized patients, the rate of colonization is eight to 10 times higher than previously suspected.

What to Look For

MRSA—particularly the USA 300 variant—can be a serious public health threat, but while MRSA is resistant to some antibiotics, it is still vulnerable to others, such as *vancomycin*. Most patients, including those with systemic infection, can be treated successfully if they get an antibiotic promptly.

Infection with MRSA usually starts with the skin. Patients often notice what looks like a spider bite. There will be a small, swollen area with a halo of redness around it. The area will be tender…might become a larger abscess…and the middle area might turn black from tissue breakdown. Sometimes, the bacteria remain confined to the skin—but they also can burrow deep into the body, causing potentially life-threatening infections.

If you suspect that you have a staph infection, call your doctor. If he/she is not available, go to an emergency room.

Prevention

The CDC has identified five conditions, known as the 5 Cs, that increase the risk for MRSA—crowding…contact (usually skin to skin)…compromised skin…contaminated surfaces…and cleanliness (or the lack of it).

Patients in health-care settings have the highest risk, followed by those who spend time in communal settings—team locker rooms, prisons, etc. But the emergence of the community-acquired USA 300 form of MRSA means that everyone is potentially at risk.

Important steps to protect yourself…

• **Wash your hands with friction.** Most people with MRSA carry it in the nose, and people tend to touch their noses frequently. Wash your hands at least four times a day, rubbing them together briskly for at least 15 seconds and applying friction to all surfaces. Be sure to do this before meals and after touching gym equipment, shaking hands, etc. Use regular soap—antibacterial soap isn't necessary.

If you are in the hospital or another health-care setting, insist that doctors, nurses and technicians wash their hands before touching you—even if they wear gloves while doing the procedure.

• **Dry your hands with an air blower or a disposable paper towel.** Don't share towels with others, even at home.

• **Use an alcohol-based hand-cleaning gel.** Look for a product that contains at least 62% alcohol. A thorough application of the sanitizer takes only a few seconds and is a highly effective alternative to hand washing.

• **Cover wounds.** Damaged, open skin is the main pathway to infection. Wash cuts and scratches carefully...and keep them covered until they're completely healed.

• **Stay safe in gyms and locker rooms.** Wipe down sweaty equipment (barbells, exercise benches and exercise machine handles) with disinfectant before using...shower after exercise...wear flip-flops to protect your feet in the shower and locker room...and sit on your own towel, rather than on a bare bench.

• **Get vaccinated.** People who have had the flu are vulnerable to post-influenza MRSA pneumonia, which is potentially deadly. In older adults, an annual flu vaccination can reduce mortality from all causes by 50%.

• **Don't take unnecessary antibiotics.** In hospitals and nursing homes, between 20% and 30% of MRSA infections are attributed to antibiotic use. ***Reason:*** Antibiotics kill many of the normal, healthy bacteria in the body. Eradicating "good" bacteria can allow MRSA to proliferate.

Patients often ask their doctors for antibiotics when they have a cold or another viral illness—and doctors often give them to keep their patients happy. But antibiotics are useless for viral infections.

What's Really Making Us Sick

Do you know which infectious diseases you're most likely to catch—and which are surprisingly rare? *Diagnosed in the US in 2010, there were...*

1,307,893...Cases of chlamydia

309,341...Gonorrhea

54,424...Salmonellosis (an infection with Salmonella bacteria)

35,741...HIV

30,158...Lyme disease

11,182...Tuberculosis

1,773...Malaria

467...Typhoid fever

82...Toxic shock syndrome

63...Measles

2...Plague

Centers for Disease Control and Prevention

Antibiotic Creams May Increase MRSA Resistance

Over-the-counter triple-antibiotic creams and ointments, such as Medi-Quik and Neosporin, seem to be leading to the emergence of a form of methicillin-resistant Staphylococcus aureus (MRSA) that resists *bacitracin* and *neomycin*—two of the antibiotics found in the creams.

Self-defense: Washing with soap and water is all that many scrapes and cuts require. If you do use an antibiotic cream, apply only a small amount and use it for as short a time as possible.

William Schaffner, MD, professor of preventive medicine, Vanderbilt University School of Medicine, Nashville, commenting on a study by Japanese researchers, published in *Emerging Infectious Diseases.*

Infection Facts

15%…US nursing homes cited for deficiencies in infection control practices every year.

One reason: Staffing shortages can lead nurses and aides to cut corners on anti-infection measures, such as proper hand-washing.

American Journal of Infection Control

47%…Meat and poultry from US grocery stores that is contaminated with *staphylococcus aureus*, a bacterium linked to various diseases in humans, including pneumonia and heart infection. Proper cooking can kill staph bacteria.

Translational Genomics Research Institute

88%…Increase in the rate of syphilis among American women from 2004 to 2008… though the rate fell by 7% in 2009, and continued to fall from 2009 to 2012 (the most recent year for which statistics are available). Total US syphilis cases (men, women and children) in 2012: 49,903.

Centers for Disease Control and Prevention

Half of People with HCV Ignore the Essential Follow-Up RNA Test

Centers for Disease Control and Prevention's *Morbidity and Mortality Weekly Report*.

You've heard that all baby boomers need to get tested for hepatitis C, a common viral infection. But here's what is happening way too often—people get that initial screening test, but when the results come back positive, about half of those infected don't bother to take the simple yet all-important next step! This oversight can prove deadly…which is really a shame because, thanks to new therapies, hepatitis C often can be cured.

What's going on? The hepatitis C virus (HCV) can remain hidden in the body for years before causing any symptoms. That's why up to 85% of the estimated 3.9 million Americans infected with HCV don't even know that they have it…until decades later, by which time the virus has caused serious liver damage. As scar tissue replaces the liver's healthy tissue, a condition called cirrhosis, the organ can no longer function properly. HCV is the number-one reason for liver transplants…it also can cause liver cancer…and it leads to about 15,000 deaths in the US each year.

In about 20% of cases, the immune system fights off the virus on its own—but for the remaining 80% of people, HCV infection becomes a chronic and potentially deadly condition. And once infected, a person may transmit the virus to anyone who comes in contact with his or her blood.

A simple blood test that detects the presence of antibodies indicates whether a person has ever been infected with HCV, but the antibody test does not reveal whether the infection went away. For that, a second blood test is needed—the HCV RNA test (also called the HCV nucleic acid test), which detects the presence of the virus itself in the blood and indicates whether the infection is still active. If the HCV RNA test is positive, essential treatment can begin.

Worrisome recent study: Researchers at the Centers for Disease Control and Prevention (CDC) analyzed six years' worth of HCV data from eight different regions across the country, which identified more than 217,000 HCV patients. The shocker was that, of those patients, only 50.8% had undergone the HCV RNA test—there was no evidence that the other 49.2% had ever received that crucial RNA test after their antibody test came back positive! Without that second test, it's highly unlikely that those patients got the treatment that most of them undoubtedly needed.

The Boomer Connection

Baby boomers, meaning people born between 1945 and 1965, are particularly vulnerable to HCV.

A New Way to Fight Superbugs

In laboratory studies, high doses of vitamin B-3 dramatically increased the ability of immune cells to kill drug-resistant Staphylococcus aureus bacteria. This discovery may lead to a new option for treating staph infections that don't respond to antibiotics.

The Journal of Clinical Investigation

Reasons: Many were exposed to the virus before prevention programs (such as testing donated blood for the presence of the virus before using it for transfusions) were put in place...and many engaged in risky behaviors—meaning, multiple sex partners, illicit drug use—back in their youth. That's why the CDC and now the US Preventive Services Task Force, too, recommend that all boomers get the initial HCV antibody-screening test. Screening also is warranted for anyone who has a history of blood transfusion or organ transplant prior to 1992, when donors started getting screened for HCV...health-care workers who experience a needlestick injury... anyone with a history of sharing syringes... children born to HCV-positive mothers...and patients with HIV. (People born before 1945 are not considered to be at much risk because they were less likely to have been part of the IV drug scene and sexual revolution of the 1960s...and most likely would've developed symptoms of liver damage by now.)

Bottom line: If you've never had an HCV antibody test (or don't know whether you've had one), get one. Any doctor can order this blood test, which is simple and fairly inexpensive ($12 to $100, depending on your location and doctor) and may be covered by your insurance. If your HCV antibody test is positive, follow up with a hepatitis C RNA test to determine whether your infection is still active. Thanks to new therapies, the disease often can be cured—and the sooner you are diagnosed and treated, the more likely you are to recover.

This Vitamin Fights the Deadly Virus You Don't Know You Have

Gerardo Nardone, MD, is a professor in the department of clinical and experimental medicine of the gastroenterology unit at the University of Naples "Federico II" in Italy and coauthor of an article on hepatitis C published in *Gut*.

Unlike certain other types of viral hepatitis that can be prevented with vaccination, there is no vaccine for the hepatitis C (virus) HCV—and in about half of cases, the standard medications that have been used to treat HCV have failed to clear up the infection. As a result, about 70% of patients develop chronic hepatitis...and 30% of them progress to cirrhosis (scarring of the liver) and end-stage liver disease.

That's the bad news. The good news, according to a recent Italian study, is that adding vitamin B-12 to the standard regimen significantly improves the success rate for the treatment of this life-threatening disease.

How the study was done: HCV patients were randomly assigned to receive either the standard treatment of a twice-daily antiviral pill called *ribavirin* and a weekly injection of interferon...or these same medications plus monthly injections of 5,000 micrograms of vitamin B-12. Treatment continued for 24 to 48 weeks, and researchers checked periodically to see whether the virus was eliminated from the body.

Results: 12 weeks into the study, the response rate was already 21% higher among patients receiving vitamin B-12, compared with the standard treatment group...and six months after treatment ended, patients in the B-12 group were 34% more likely to be free of the virus. Interestingly, the beneficial effects of B-12 were especially pronounced among patients with a particularly difficult-to-treat type of HCV called genotype 1. Vitamin B-12 injections were not associated with any increased risk for side effects.

Update: The recent introduction of two antiviral drugs, *boceprevir* and *telaprevir,* now provides additional options for HCV patients. However, these medications can have serious side effects...they are very expensive...they raise concerns about the development of drug-resistant HCV strains...and, as with any new drug, their long-term risks are unknown. So until more is revealed about the new drugs, the study researchers say that the addition of vitamin B-12 represents a safe and inexpensive option for improving the effectiveness of the standard HCV treatment. In addition, it is possible that B-12 may even boost patients' response to these new drugs.

The Test Every Women Needs

Sexually active women over age 40 should get tested for the parasite Trichomonas vaginalis, a sexually transmitted disease (STD) that often has no symptoms.

Recent finding: 11% of women in their 40s and 13% of those over age 50 tested positive for Trichomonas vaginalis. Older women were more likely to test positive for the STD than younger women. If left untreated, trichomonas infection can cause pelvic inflammatory disease...inflammation of the vagina, urethra and cervix...and premature labor in pregnant women. Once detected, the STD can be easily treated with antibiotics.

Charlotte Gaydos, DrPH, professor in the division of infectious diseases, department of medicine, Johns Hopkins University School of Medicine, Baltimore, and leader of a study of 7,593 women, presented at the annual meeting of the International Society for STD Research.

Vampire Bacteria

A bacterial organism known as Micavibrio aeruginosavorus attaches to other bacteria and sucks out the nutrients. It targets only a few species, including one that causes serious lung infections.

Implication: With additional research, this bacteria could be developed into a type of "living antibiotic."

University of Virginia's College of Arts & Sciences

Better Cure for C. Diff Infection

Background: Clostridium difficile (C. diff), a dangerous bacterial infection that causes severe diarrhea, sometimes is difficult to treat with antibiotics and/or probiotics.

Recent study: When researchers implanted donated human stool from healthy family members into the intestines of 49 patients (average age 66) with C. diff, all of the patients recovered dramatically within four days, with no recurrence within the 100 days following treatment.

Theory: Healthy stool contains good bacteria that reestablish normal intestinal flora.

If you have C. diff that has not responded to antibiotics or probiotics: Ask your doctor about a fecal transplant.

Mayur Ramesh, MD, infectious diseases physician, Henry Ford Hospital, Detroit.

Killer Infection Has Mutated

Did you know that deaths from gastrointestinal infections more than doubled in the US, increasing from 7,000 a year in 1997 to more than 17,000 in 2007? Two-thirds of the deaths were caused by Clostridium difficile, a bacterium often contracted in hospitals and nursing homes that has become resistant to treatment.

Centers for Disease Control and Prevention, Atlanta. *www.CDC.gov*

When Strep Throat Moves to Your Toes (and Other Limbs)

William Schaffner, MD, professor and chair of the department of preventive medicine, Vanderbilt University School of Medicine, Nashville, and past president of the National Foundation for Infectious Diseases, Bethesda, Maryland.

There's a flesh-eating bacteria in the Southeast that's causing some concern. How, exactly, do you get this infection that can take your limbs or your life?

We put a call into William Schaffner, MD, past president of the National Foundation for Infectious Diseases and professor and chair of the department of preventive medicine at Vanderbilt University School of Medicine in Nashville.

He said that the technical name for this disease is necrotizing fasciitis and that it causes the bands of connective tissue that surround muscles, nerves and blood vessels to die.

The scariest part is that this contagious disease can move quickly throughout the body.

We asked him what we all can do to lower our odds of getting this type of infection. *This is what he had to say…*

How the Bacterium Infects You

Dr. Schaffner mentioned that though the disease has gotten a lot of press, it's still considered rare because it affects only about 500 to 800 people in the US each year. That said, if you're one of those 500 to 800 people, the disease can be devastating.

One reason that it's not more common is that coming into contact with the bacterium does not usually cause necrotizing fasciitis. In fact, many of us have the culprit, group A Streptococcus, in our throats and sometimes on our skin, without ever knowing it. A dangerous infection results only when the bacterium is able to find its way to a part of the body where it is not normally found—into muscle, fat or any tissue deep inside the body. The bacterium is able to get to those areas by taking advantage of vulnerabilities in our natural defenses, usually through wounds. Even then, our immune systems may be able to kill it off—but not always.

Symptoms to Look Out For

Dr. Schaffner said that when the infection occurs, it usually happens deep inside the body, so it may not be evident on the surface of your skin. Severe unrelenting pain that seems out of whack with your wound is frequently the first symptom. By the time the typical symptoms of infection (such as swelling, redness and fever) do appear, perhaps days later, they might not immediately be thought to be associated with the wound because of the time lag and because up until that point, it may have looked like your wound was healing well.

It's important to diagnose necrotizing fasciitis early because, as we mentioned before, it moves fast. So if you ever have pain that seems surprisingly severe for a particular injury or if you have a sore or wound that is becoming red and swollen instead of healing, get medical attention right away. Doctors suspecting necrotizing fasciitis will get a specimen from the wound to test for the bacterium and then will start treatment immediately.

Treat It and Beat It

Intravenous antibiotics are just part of the treatment. Surgery is almost always required to remove the infected tissue, and frequently, the surgeons need to go back several times to

Antibiotic Countdown

Because certain antibiotics may become less effective as bacteria develop resistance, infectious-disease specialists have called for the development of 10 new antibiotics by 2020.

Infectious Diseases Society of America

cut out more diseased tissue. Unfortunately, in some cases, the infection can be so overwhelming that the antibiotics and surgeons can't keep up. Sepsis (a blood infection), organ failure and even death can result, and, sadly, about 25% of people who get necrotizing fasciitis will die from it.

The best defense against necrotizing fasciitis is to avoid getting wounds altogether, but I know what you're thinking—that's impossible. So if and when you do get a wound, even a small one, don't take your safety for granted. Clean it and then keep it covered to reduce the chance of infection. Applying antibiotic ointment twice daily is a good idea, too, said Dr. Schaffner. And change the bandage daily, or more frequently if it gets soiled.

"It's especially important for people with chronic illnesses—such as people with cancer or diabetes or those taking steroids—to take good care of even small wounds," Dr. Schaffner said. "These people are more susceptible to getting flesh-eating bacteria infection because their immune systems are more vulnerable—and when they do get it, they have a poorer prognosis than a healthy person."

One more very important rule: Any wound beyond a superficial cut or scrape should be looked at by a health professional, who can ensure that it's cleaned properly. It's worth the time.

Skin Infections That Are Often Overlooked

Lawrence Eron, MD, associate professor of medicine at the John A. Burns School of Medicine at the University of Hawaii in Honolulu and infectious disease consultant at Kaiser Foundation Hospital, also in Honolulu.

The dangers associated with the highly drug-resistant, sometimes fatal "superbug" known as MRSA (methicillin-resistant Staphylococcus aureus) have been widely publicized.

MRSA, once a threat primarily in hospitals, long-term-care facilities and other health-care settings, is now appearing in a slightly mutated form in gyms, schools, military barracks and other settings where people may have skin-to-skin contact and/or share towels, linens or other items that can become contaminated. MRSA may turn life-threatening if the bacteria penetrate the skin, become blood-borne and reach other areas of the body, such as the heart or lungs.

What most people don't realize: The skin can harbor dozens of infectious organisms.

Example: The average handprint on a dinner plate might contain up to 35 species of bacteria, viruses or fungi.

Most of these organisms are harmless—and even those that are capable of causing disease are usually blocked from entering the body by the skin's protective barrier and/or destroyed by immune cells just beneath the skin's surface.

Danger: The skin typically has thousands of microscopic nicks or other openings that provide entry points for harmful germs—even if you don't have an obvious cut. To help prevent harmful bacteria from entering these tiny openings, wash your hands often with mild soap and warm water, and shave carefully. *Infections to avoid…**

Cellulitis

This skin infection, which can be mistaken for a scrape, bruise or spider bite, is caused by bacteria that enter the body through dry, flaky and/or cracked skin or other skin openings such as those caused by a cut, splinter or surgical wound.

Cellulitis typically occurs on the legs but can occur anywhere on the body—even on your hand. The infection usually originates in the upper layers (the dermis and

---

*To see examples of the many ways these infections can appear on the body, go to www.images.google.com and type in the name of each infection. Beware: Many of the images are graphic.

epidermis) of the skin but can also occur in deeper (subcutaneous) tissues, including the muscles and muscle linings. Infections in deeper tissues are more likely to cause serious symptoms and extensive tissue damage, such as severe swelling and pain, and formation of abscesses. Everyone is at risk for cellulitis, but those with weakened immunity (such as diabetes and dialysis patients) are at greatest risk.

What to look for: The affected area will be red, hot and tender. The redness spreads very quickly, and you may develop a fever (101°F or higher) and body aches. If the infection is severe, confusion or fecal incontinence also may occur. People with any of the severe symptoms described earlier should seek immediate medical care at a hospital emergency department.

Treatment: Oral antibiotics, such as *dicloxacillin* (Dycill) or *cephalexin* (Keflex). These are effective against Streptococcus and about half of the Staphylococcus organisms—common causes of cellulitis—and usually start to relieve symptoms within two days. Patients with more severe infections may require hospitalization and intravenous antibiotics.

To reduce your risk of developing cellulitis: Take a daily shower or bath. People who wash often and use plenty of mild soap are less likely to develop cellulitis or other skin infections.

Necrotizing Infections

The media often refer to these infections as "flesh-eating." This isn't entirely accurate. Several bacterial species can cause the necrosis (death) of infected tissue, but the bacteria don't eat the flesh, per se. Rather, they secrete toxins that break it down.

Necrotizing infections are rare—fewer than 1,000 cases occur each year in the US—but the fatality rate is quite high at 25% to 30%. These infections spread very rapidly—if you marked the edge of an infection with a pen, you might see the redness creep past the mark in as little as one hour.

Beware: Harmful Bacteria in Meat and Chicken

Antibiotic-resistant bacteria are in meat and poultry. Foodborne methicillin-resistant Staphylococcus aureus (MRSA) is less virulent than the strains that occur in hospital patients—but it still can cause illness.

Self-defense: Wash hands with soap and warm water before and after handling raw meat or poultry. Clean food-preparation surfaces with bleach or alcohol after use. Cook meat and poultry thoroughly.

Stuart B. Levy, MD, is director of Center for Adaptation Genetics and Drug Resistance, Tufts University School of Medicine, and president of Alliance for the Prudent Use of Antibiotics, both in Boston. He is author of *The Antibiotic Paradox* (HarperCollins).

What to look for: Skin redness and/or swelling that's warm to the touch. The initial infection, which can follow even a minor cut or puncture wound, resembles cellulitis. But a necrotizing infection is far more painful. As the infection progresses, you may develop very large, fluid-filled purple blisters (bullae), a high fever (104°F or higher), disorientation and a rapid heartbeat. If you develop any of these symptoms, seek immediate medical attention at a hospital emergency department.

Treatment: Intravenous antibiotics and surgery, sometimes requiring amputation, to remove infected tissue.

To reduce your risk of developing a necrotizing infection: Thoroughly clean even minor cuts and scrapes. Apply an over-the-counter antibiotic ointment, such as Neosporin or *bacitracin*, and keep the area covered with a clean dressing until the area is completely healed.

Folliculitis

This skin infection occurs at the root of a hair (follicle) and may produce a small pimple—or, less often, a larger, more painful pimple called a boil. Folliculitis tends to be more common in people with diabetes (which reduces resistance to infection) and those who live in hot, humid climates (excessive perspiration promotes growth of the bacterium that causes folliculitis).

What to look for: A small, white pimple at the base of a hair. Boils, also called abscesses, are larger than pimples (sometimes an inch or more in diameter), with a greater volume of pus. They tend to be warmer than the surrounding skin and can be intensely painful.

Treatment: The small pimples caused by folliculitis often disappear on their own within several days. Applying a topical antibiotic several times a day can prevent the infection from spreading. Apply a warm, moist compress (for 15 minutes four times daily for one to two days) to tender pimples or boils to help them drain.

Painful or unusually large boils should be lanced, drained and cleaned by a doctor. Do not "pop" them yourself. The risk for infection is high—and boils can be caused by MRSA. Antibiotics usually aren't necessary when boils are professionally drained and cleaned.

To reduce your risk of developing folliculitis: Wash your hands several times daily with soap…and take a daily shower or bath. If you have chronic, recurrent boils, use antibacterial soap.

What Your Cup of Joe Can Do

Coffee and tea drinkers are less likely to carry deadly bacteria. Researchers studied the health records of 5,555 people to examine links between consumption of coffee and tea and the likelihood of carrying methicillin-resistant Staphylococcus aureus (MRSA) in nasal passages.

Result: People who regularly drank hot coffee or hot tea were 50% less likely to carry MRSA in their noses.

Theory: Both coffee and tea contain chemicals with antimicrobial properties, which may rise up from the hot drinks in the form of vapor. However, frequent hand-washing is the best way to protect against MRSA.

Eric Matheson, MD, assistant professor of family medicine, Medical University of South Carolina, Charleston.

Nearly One in Four Teenage Girls Has a Sexually Transmitted Infection (STI)

Within one year of starting to have sex, 19.2% of girls ages 14 to 19 are infected with at least one of the five most common STIs—human papillomavirus (HPV), herpes simplex virus type 2, chlamydia, gonorrhea or trichomoniasis. The most common sexually transmitted infection is HPV, found in 18.3% of girls.

Sara E. Forhan, MD, MPH, researcher, National Center for HIV/AIDS Viral Hepatitis, STD and TB Prevention, Centers for Disease Control and Prevention, Atlanta, and leader of the analysis of STIs from National Health and Nutrition Survey (NHANES) 2003—2004 data from 838 teenage girls, published in *Pediatrics*.

Are Swollen Ankles a Serious Problem? It May Mean Cellulitis

Leo Galland, MD, director of the Foundation for Integrated Medicine in New York City…founder of Pilladvised.com, an online resource for learning about medications, supplements and food…and author of *Power Healing: Use the New Integrated Medicine to Cure Yourself* (Random House). *www.mdheal.org*

Dismissing ankle swelling as inconsequential can sometimes be a big mistake, according to Leo Galland, MD, a practicing physician, author and director

HPV May Return In Menopausal Women

In a recent study, the sexually transmitted human papillomavirus (HPV) was tracked in 843 women over two years.

Result: Among those over age 50 who were found to have an active HPV infection, researchers speculate that genital-tract changes due to aging or menopause-related hormone fluctuations may have been a factor in the recurrence of a dormant infection. This finding was true even among women who had been monogamous or abstinent for years. HPV can cause cervical cancer and other conditions.

Patti Gravitt, PhD, associate professor of epidemiology, Johns Hopkins Center for Global Health, Baltimore.

of the Foundation for Integrated Medicine in New York City. He explained, "In some cases, ankle swelling is a warning sign of a serious underlying medical condition that requires a doctor's attention or even emergency care." The bacterial infection cellulitis could be causing the problem. *Here are the warning signs to watch for...and what to do to protect yourself...*

Cellulitis usually affects the lower leg (but may occur elsewhere) and can spread quickly from the skin to the lymph nodes and bloodstream—with potentially life-threatening consequences.

Watch for swelling that...

- **Affects one ankle.**
- **Rapidly worsens.**

Accompanied by...

- **Redness, tenderness and heat in the affected area.**
- **Fever and/or chills.**

What to do: Immediately alert your doctor. You need antibiotics to keep the infection from spreading.

Reassuring: Most cases of ankle swelling are not caused by any hidden dire condition, but instead have a harmless or obvious cause, such as...

- **Fluid retention—brought on by an impending menstrual period, a recent high-salt meal or too many hours spent sitting still.** In this case, swelling affects both ankles, causes no discomfort, and goes away within a day or two.

Helpful: Sit down and elevate your legs, ideally higher than the level of your heart, for 30 minutes.

- **Varicose veins—which develop when tiny, one-way valves inside veins don't work well enough to keep blood circulating efficiently through the legs. One or both legs may be affected. Ask your doctor if you could benefit from wearing support stockings, which create a pressure gradient that helps prevent fluid from pooling in the legs.

Chapter 24

KEEP SAFE IN THE HOSPITAL AND OTHER HIGH-RISK LOCATIONS

Best Ways to Prevent Hospital Infections

We all know that infection is a very real risk during a hospital stay. And the numbers are staggering—at least 1.7 million Americans develop a hospital-acquired infection each year, and 99,000 people die from it. But aside from being vigilant about asking medical staff to wash their hands, is there really anything a patient can do to prevent infection? Absolutely! *There are several additional—and, in some cases, surprising—approaches…*

•**Start the conversation.** Many doctors never raise the subject of hospital-acquired infection unless the patient brings it up. So, bring it up! Ask your doctor what the overall infection rate is at the hospital where you are going to be treated. If he/she doesn't know, call the facility and ask for the infection control officer (required at every hospital). The infection rate should be below 6%. If it's above that, talk to your doctor about using a different hospital. But keep in mind that your overall medical status is an important factor. For example, people with diabetes are at higher risk for postsurgical infections, but

if presurgical blood glucose levels are well-controlled, infection rates drop. Cancer patients having surgical procedures have been found to have a higher risk of developing pneumonia after surgery. But getting a presurgical pneumonia vaccine or, in some cases, taking a presurgical antibiotic can lower that risk.

My advice: If you are being hospitalized for a specific health problem, be sure that your doctor is aware of any other medical conditions you may have.

•**Beware of certain procedures.** Research shows that certain procedures have relatively high risks for infection. For example, close to 10% of colorectal surgical patients develop surgical site infections (at the incision). Other procedures with high risks for infection include bladder catheterizations and the use of a breathing tube or intravenous (IV) line. But studies have found that, in some cases, wearing special surgical blankets and hats

Charles B. Inlander, consumer advocate and healthcare consultant based in Fogelsville, Pennsylvania. He was the founding president of the nonprofit People's Medical Society, a consumer advocacy organization credited with key improvements in the quality of US health care in the 1980s and 1990s, and is author of 20 books, including *Take This Book to the Hospital With You: A Consumer Guide to Surviving Your Hospital Stay* (St. Martin's).

before—and sometimes during—surgery can help your body fight infection.

My advice: Ask your doctor about steps that can be taken to keep you warm during surgery and/or when you are given IVs.

• **Check out the latest research.** Numerous medical studies have been published on just about all medical procedures. And most discuss infection risk.

My advice: Ask your doctor to discuss what the studies show are the infection risks associated with your procedure. Also ask about infection risks for other procedures that might be appropriate. For example, an open surgical gallbladder removal has a higher infection risk than laparoscopic gallbladder removal.

• **Be alert at home.** Many infections do not become apparent until after you get home. An infection may also be contracted when a nurse or other health-care provider administers care in your home.

My advice: Be watchful for signs of infection, including increasing tenderness, redness or pus at an incision site, unexplained fever or internal pain that was unexpected in the course of your healing. When in doubt, immediately call your doctor.

Protect Yourself from Killer Bacteria

Edward K. Chapnick, MD, director of the division of infectious diseases at Maimonides Medical Center in Brooklyn, New York, and associate professor of medicine at Mount Sinai School of Medicine in New York City. He has published more than 30 medical journal articles on infectious diseases.

Imagine entering a hospital for heart surgery, a joint replacement or some other procedure. The treatment is successful, but you contract an infection during your hospital stay.

Each year, this happens to two million Americans. The infection is usually minor—a simple rash and fever that can be cured with antibiotics. But about 10% of hospital-acquired infections are serious. Some bacteria are resistant to most—if not all—antibiotics, and harmful organisms can quickly invade the bloodstream and damage skin, organs, muscles and/or bones. Approximately 99,000 Americans die of these hospital-acquired infections annually.

While most hospitals have stepped up their efforts to prevent infections, only recently have many patients become aware that they must be more assertive in protecting themselves.

How to Avoid Bacteria

Bacteria can live for hours—sometimes even days—on almost any surface and then transfer easily to skin. From there, bacteria can enter the body through breaks in the skin or via touching the eyes, nose or mouth. Hand-washing is the most effective way to help prevent the spread of bacteria and other infection-causing organisms. Other ways to protect yourself—or a loved one…

• **Ask doctors and nurses to disinfect medical devices.** To prevent the spread of bacteria or other germs, stethoscopes, blood pressure cuffs and other such medical devices should be cleaned with a disinfectant alcohol wipe before they touch your skin.

• **Avoid touching surfaces touched by other people.** Some people do their best to avoid touching tabletops, chairs, elevator doors or any other surface. If this is impractical, use alcohol-based disinfectant gels and/or wipes. To prevent a possible infection, avoid rubbing bare skin from any part of your body against these surfaces. In a recent study, about three-quarters of hospital rooms tested were contaminated with bacteria.

• **Be aware that visitors can carry germs into your hospital room.** Ask visitors not to sit on your bed—they can transfer bacteria from their clothes to the sheets …or use the bathroom in your room—they can transfer germs to bathroom surfaces. Even doctors' neckties can carry bacteria or other germs, research shows.

Hospital patients typically are at greater risk of contracting an infectious disease due to their weakened immunity, but it's also wise for hospital visitors to follow hygienic practices to avoid getting sick.

Prep Yourself

Patients themselves often carry bacteria, such as Staphylococcus aureus (staph), on their bodies and/or clothes when they check into the hospital. These germs don't always cause symptoms—up to 30% of healthy adults carry staph on their skin. However, if your skin is colonized with bacteria when you go for surgery, it can enter your body at the surgical site. *To protect yourself…*

• **Wash your body.** Three to five days before surgery, start showering or bathing daily using a special 4% chlorhexidine soap. Chlorhexidine is a powerful antiseptic agent that will help remove bacteria from the skin's surface. Chlorhexidine soap (such as Hibiclens or Betasept) is available over the counter at most drugstores. If it is not in stock, ask the pharmacist to order it.

Caution: Because this soap can irritate the skin or cause an allergic reaction in some people, do not use the soap for more than five days…avoid the use of other skin products during that time…and be sure that your doctor gives his/her consent to use the soap.

• **Don't shave.** No matter how careful you are, shaving causes microscopic nicks in your skin. Any break in the skin can potentially create an entry point for bacteria. For 72 hours before surgery, do not shave the surgical site, even if the site is on your legs, underarms or face. If your surgery typically requires shaving, ask your doctor if clippers can be used instead of a razor by hospital personnel before your surgery.

• **Ask for a staph test.** A week to 10 days before surgery, ask your surgeon to test you for methicillin-resistant Staphylococcus aureus (MRSA) by taking a nasal swab. If this test shows that you are a carrier of the bacterium, specific infection-control procedures will be used in the hospital. A topical antibiotic also may be prescribed.

Helpful: Almost everyone will be given an oral antibiotic within 60 minutes of receiving surgery to help prevent an infection. However, it's common for busy hospital staff to forget this routine medication. Be sure to remind your doctor.

If you're scheduled for surgery: Call your state's health department and ask if hospitals in the state are required to report infection rates. If so, get the latest report for the hospital where you'll be treated. Discuss any findings with your doctor.

Catheters and IVs

Having a catheter or intravenous (IV) line increases your risk for infection because bacteria from your own body or a health-care worker's hands can enter at the insertion site. Catheters are tubes that are used to drain liquids, such as urine, from the body. IV lines deliver fluids, such as medication and nutrients, directly into a vein. *You may not have a choice whether or not a catheter or IV is inserted, but always ask…*

• **Why is the catheter and/or IV there?** Often, a catheter or IV is used when a patient enters the emergency room, but is then forgotten for a time after it is no longer needed. If you don't know why you have a catheter or IV, ask.

• **How many days will I need the catheter and/or IV?** The answer largely depends on your condition, but it's important to let your doctor know that you want a catheter and/or IV removed as soon as possible. With urinary catheters, the risk for an infection increases by at least 5% each day it remains in place. That means that it should come out as soon as medically possible.

Helpful: Every day, ask your nurse or doctor whether the catheter can come out…don't wait for medical staff to think of removing it.

With peripheral IVs (the kind that are inserted into a vein in your hand or arm), the risk for infection is relatively low until the third or fourth day. If an IV has been in place for four days, ask when you are scheduled to have it replaced with a new one. (Central venous lines, which are inserted in large veins of the neck or chest, don't have the same risk and can stay in place almost indefinitely.)

Infection Risk Alert for C-Sections

William H. Barth, Jr., MD, chair of the Committee on Obstetric Practice at the American College of Obstetricians and Gynecologists in Washington, DC.

If you or someone you love is pregnant, take note—postsurgical infections can occur in an estimated 10% to 40% of women who deliver babies by Cesarean section (compared with an infection rate of 1% to 3% in women who deliver vaginally). To minimize infection risk, a mother undergoing a C-section has traditionally been given a dose of antibiotics, but not until after her baby is delivered and the umbilical cord clamped. This practice has been rooted in concerns that antibiotics given before delivery could get into the unborn baby's bloodstream and mask any infection the infant might have…or cause the baby to become antibiotic-resistant.

New guideline: Based on analysis of several large and recent studies, the American College of Obstetricians and Gynecologists (ACOG) now recommends that all women having C-sections should receive a single dose of an antibiotic (such as cephalosporin) as a preventive within 60 minutes before surgery.

Reason: Predelivery antibiotics significantly reduced infection rates in mothers without presenting any increased risk to newborns.

Expectant moms: These are new suggestions from ACOG, so discuss presurgical antibiotic use with your obstetrician if you are planning to deliver by C-section.

Better Way to Prevent Postsurgical Infection

An analysis of the medical records of 1,137 gastrointestinal (GI) surgery patients (average age 59.5) discovered that 14% of those who tested positive for methicillin-resistant Staphylococcus aureus (MRSA), based on a nasal swab, developed surgical site infections, compared with 9% of patients who did not have MRSA. It's common for adults to carry MRSA without having symptoms.

Theory: A carrier of the MRSA pathogen is more likely to become infected after surgery. If you're having GI or other major surgery: Talk to your doctor about MRSA screening prior to the procedure.

Harry T. Papaconstantinou, MD, chief of colorectal surgery, Scott & White Memorial Hospital, Temple, Texas.

Infection Protection for Cardiac Implant Patients

Bruce Wilkoff, MD, director of Cardiac Pacing and Tachyarrhythmia Devices at the Cleveland Clinic and a professor of medicine at Cleveland Clinic Lerner College of Medicine at Case Western Reserve University in Ohio. He is also the president of the Heart Rhythm Society. *www.HRSonline.org*

If you or someone you love has a cardiac implantable electronic device (CIED), such as a pacemaker or cardio defibrillator, you should know about a potentially deadly problem that is becoming incresingly common—CIED-related infection.

Between 1993 and 2008, the number of CIEDs in use doubled while the number of infections associated with the devices more than tripled, reaching 2.41%, according to recent study in the *Journal of the American College of Cardiology.* Sadly, 18% of patients with CIED infections do not survive for a year. For those who live, treatment can be economically devastating, with an average cost of more than $146,000.

Bruce Wilkoff, MD, director of Cardiac Pacing and Tachyarrhythmia Devices at the Cleveland Clinic, explained that most CIED-related infections are caused by staphylococcus aureus or staphylococcus epidermidis bacteria. Infection can get started if, at the time of surgery, bacteria contaminate the surface of the device, the patient's skin or the area in the chest beneath the skin where the surgeon creates a "pocket" to hold the CIED. The surgeon's scrupulous attention to proper sterile techniques can greatly reduce but not completely eliminate this risk. Sometimes an infection develops soon after surgery, but in other cases it becomes apparent only after a year or more has passed.

Could staph also get into the pocket long after the surgery—for instance, by migrating from some other infected site in the body? Dr. Wilkoff said, "It is possible but very uncommon, particularly for these staph bacteria. But about 10% of the time, other bacteria are involved…and 1% to 2% of patients could have the infection occur through another mechanism."

Compared with the infection risk after an initial implantation, the risk is four to six times greater when a patient has another surgery to replace a device (for instance, because its battery is depleted, a component has stopped working or the patient requires a device with additional features).

Reason: Reopening the pocket where the device was placed may allow a colony of bacteria that the body had previously "walled off" to overwhelm the immune system's defenses, Dr. Wilkoff explained. Since a CIED typically lasts about four to eight years, a patient is quite likely to need such repeat surgery.

Warning signs: There is no one symptom that appears in all cases of infection, Dr. Wilkoff said. *But see your doctor quickly if any of the following occur…*

• **You run a fever of 101° or higher.**

• **There is swelling, redness or pain at the site where the device was implanted.**

• **The skin covering the device becomes dimpled or oozes.**

• **The device appears to be shifting position.**

Be especially vigilant about watching for such signs if you have diabetes or compromised kidney function. Either of these conditions can increase your susceptibility to CIED-related infection.

If you do get a CIED infection: Both the device and all of its leads (wires that deliver energy from the CIED to the heart muscle) need to be removed and replaced.

Reason: Staph bacteria can bind to a sticky substance called fibronectin that circulates in the blood and clings to the surface of implanted devices. Once this biofilm of persistent bacterial bugs takes hold, it is very antibiotic-resistant and almost impossible to get rid of without removing the device.

Before and after the surgery, for a period that can range from several days to several weeks, you receive antibiotics through an IV. You may be given a temporary pacemaker or an external defibrillator during this time. When the infection is gone, your doctor will schedule another surgery to implant a new CIED, often before you go home.

To reduce your risk for a subsequent infection: It is best to use an experienced cardiologist who does a high volume of device implantation and device change procedures. Dr. Wilkoff suggested asking the doctor and/or hospital whether they report the number of CIED procedures they do on a Web site or in a booklet—the larger the number, the better the outcomes tend to be. Also, he noted that women sometimes ask to have the CIED implanted underneath a muscle so that it's less visible. But since this makes it more difficult to remove if an infection does develop, it's important to discuss the pros and cons with your doctor before opting for such placement. And, of course, follow your doctor's advice on minimizing CIED infection risk after surgery.

How to Combat Germs at the Gym—Deadly Bacteria Is On the Rise

Steven Zinder, PhD, ATC, a certified athletic trainer and assistant professor of exercise and sports science at University of North Carolina, Chapel Hill. He is lead author of the National Athletic Trainers' Association position paper on the causes, prevention and treatment of skin diseases in athletes, published in *Journal of Athletic Training*.

Even the cleanest health club provides an ideal environment for a variety of skin diseases. That's unfortunate because an estimated one-third of American adults has some type of skin disease at any given time. And more than half of all infectious diseases among athletes are contracted cutaneously, or through the skin.

The problem with health clubs is that they provide plenty of heat and humidity, along with the secretions from hundreds of perspiring bodies.

Result: Fungi, bacteria and viruses survive and may even proliferate on floor mats, towels, hand weights, treadmills, weight machines and other equipment. Viruses and bacteria may survive for hours on metal and other gym surfaces—some fungi can survive for years. And the skin chafing that occurs during workouts makes it easy for these organisms to penetrate the body's defenses.

Main Risks

Most skin infections, such as athlete's foot and jock itch, are an annoyance and easy to treat. They're unpleasant but unlikely to pose a serious threat.

One dangerous exception is community-acquired methicillin-resistant Staphylococcus aureus (CA-MRSA). This is a potentially life-threatening antibiotic-resistant bacteria that's increasingly found in exercise settings.

A study published in *The New England Journal of Medicine* showed that 42% of nasal swabs from professional football players tested positive for MRSA, even if the players did not have active infections.

Fortunately, most MRSA and other gym-acquired skin infections can be prevented. *How to protect yourself…*

•**Wash gym clothes after every workout.** Many people keep their exercise clothes in a duffel bag or backpack. They change into them at the gym and then pack them up and take them home, but they wear them repeatedly before putting them in the wash.

Unwashed athletic clothing—even when you didn't break a sweat—acts as a reservoir for disease-causing microbes. Wearing these clothes repeatedly increases the risk that the organisms will colonize and/or penetrate the skin. And if you wear clothes repeatedly and don't change before you leave the gym, it spreads the organisms to other areas, such as the seat of your car, where you or someone else can get infected.

Solution: Don't wear your exercise clothes out of the gym. Take them off as soon as you're done with your workout, and wash them when you get home. A normal wash cycle with hot water and detergent will eliminate virtually all germs.

It's just as important to wash the bag that you use to carry your gym clothes. Put it in the washing machine if it's washable. The easiest thing to do is use a mesh bag that you can throw in the washer with your clothes. If your bag is not washable, you can swab the inside with a solution made from one part bleach and 10 parts water. Never stuff your gym clothes into your briefcase or purse.

Also, wash a reusable water bottle when you get home.

•**Shower after your workout.** The longer infectious organisms stay on the skin, the higher the risk for infection.

Solution: Shower after each gym workout—and when you work out at home. When you shower, wash every part of your body including the bottoms of the feet, between the toes, the groin area and the lower and upper legs. Also, wear shower shoes, such as flip-flops, in the shower and locker room—but be sure to still wash your feet.

•**Use an antimicrobial liquid soap.** Soap bars, even when they're antibacterial, can harbor germs long enough to spread them from one part of the body to another—or, when the soap is shared, from person to person.

•**Be sure the liquid soap is labeled antimicrobial, not just antibacterial.** Antimicrobial soap kills a broader spectrum of pathogens. An antibacterial soap kills only bacteria.

•**Wash your hands before and after.** Because MRSA can live indefinitely in nasal secretions, and we all touch our noses frequently, the organism is readily transferred from one person to another.

Solution: Wash your hands—vigorously, for about 30 seconds, using an antimicrobial soap—when you arrive at the gym (in case you're bringing in germs) and again when you're done with your workout.

•**Use alcohol wipes.** Many people who exercise at health clubs carry a hand towel as they work out. They use it to wipe down exercise bars, the seats on rowing machines, etc. This is not effective for preventing infection. It only removes sweat/moisture left by the previous user—it does not eliminate microbes and can, in fact, transfer them to other surfaces.

Solution: If your gym provides spray bottles of disinfectant and paper towels, use those to clean every piece of equipment—the handles, bars, seats, etc.—before you use it, or bring along a package of alcohol wipes. You can reuse the same wipe for multiple areas as long as it's still damp with alcohol. I also recommend bringing your own floor mat (if you use one) and wiping it down with disinfectant or an alcohol wipe after each use.

•**Stay dry.** Tinea pedis (athlete's foot) is among the most common gym-acquired infections. Others include tinea cruris (jock itch) and tinea capitis or tinea corporis (ringworm).

These fungi tend to thrive in the areas of the body that accumulate moisture, such as the feet or the groin.

Solution: Dry your feet and groin thoroughly after showering. Don't put on your clothes until your entire body is completely dry.

Helpful: After your feet are dry, dust them with a moisture-absorbing powder—regular baby powder works well.

•**Avoid "cosmetic" shaving.** Those who shave more than just the face, legs and armpits are more likely to get a skin infection than those who shave only these traditional areas. Studies have shown that people who shave their "tender" areas, such as the chest or pubic area, are up to six times more likely to get MRSA than those who don't. Even a smooth, comfortable shave can create micronicks in the skin that make you vulnerable to bacterial infections.

Solution: Ideally, shave only your face, legs and/or underarms. And be sure to wash your entire body with an antimicrobial soap immediately after workouts. Never use a shared razor—if you shave at the gym, bring your own shaving gear.

The Scary Truth About Manicures

Neal B. Schultz, MD, assistant clinical professor of dermatology at Mount Sinai School of Medicine and owner of Park Avenue Skin Care, both in New York City. He also is the founder of www.dermtv.com and author of It's Not Just About Wrinkles (Stewart, Tabori and Chang). www.nealschultzmd.com

When you go to get your nails done, the manicurist may want to trim your cuticles or at least push them back. Don't do it! Fiddling with cuticles sets the stage for paronychia, an infection of the skin around the nails.

We discussed the importance of cuticles with Neal B. Schultz, MD, an assistant clinical professor of dermatology at Mount Sinai School of Medicine. He said that while most people think of a cuticle as just dead skin, its function is to seal the nail to the skin. When you cut a cuticle, you effectively cut your skin (even though, as when a callus is removed, it does not bleed)…and when you push back a cuticle, you separate the skin from the nail. Either way, you leave an opening for various types of germs to enter.

Potential result: The lack of protection can allow a paronychial infection to occur. Symptoms of this type of infection include painful, red, swollen areas of skin around the nails that leave fingers looking far from lovely.

When caused by bacteria, a paronychial infection is acute and its symptoms, which usually include pus, arise within one to three days. This type of infection can be treated with an oral antibiotic suitable for staph or strep…and it will get better faster, Dr. Schultz noted, if your dermatologist or primary care doctor also drains any pus.

When caused by yeast (typically the same Candida yeast that causes vaginal infections), a paronychial infection is chronic and "smolders" for weeks to months, Dr. Schultz said, though it will not form pus.

Common error: If you mistake yeast for a bacterial infection and try to treat it yourself with over-the-counter antibacterial ointment, you only feed the yeast by trapping moisture in the nail bed. What is needed instead is a topical prescription anti-yeast medication, such as *nystatin*.

Though a yeast infection takes months to cure, you should see improvement within a few weeks. As an alternative, you can try nonprescription *clotrimazole* (Lotrimin)—but this may work more slowly than nystatin.

Day-to-day care of healthy cuticles: If a bit of skin is sticking up from a cuticle, there is no harm in trimming that, Dr. Schultz said. Or if one section of cuticle has grown over a larger than normal portion of nail, it is safe to trim that excess—but only if you leave at least one-sixteenth of an inch of cuticle next to the skin and take care not to destroy the seal between the skin and the nail.

The Infection You Could Get at a Nail Salon

David A. Johnson, MD, professor of medicine and chief of gastroenterology at Eastern Virginia Medical School, Norfolk, Virginia.

Thanks to nail salons on every other corner, getting a manicure is remarkably easy these days. But a recent report from the Virginia Department of Health has a warning about routine nail salon visits. The report cautions that hepatitis B and hepatitis C—serious, bloodborne viral infections that affect the liver—are being transmitted in some nail salons and barbershops through cuts caused by contaminated instruments such as scissors, clippers and razors.

Knowing how easy it is to get nicked at a salon or barbershop, this news can be unsettling. To find out more, we called David A. Johnson, MD, professor of medicine and chief of gastroenterology at Eastern Virginia Medical School in Norfolk, Virginia, who presented the health department's report at an annual meeting of the American College of Gastroenterology.

What Caused the Stir?

Prompted by news of a hepatitis C case in Virginia that resulted from a manicure/pedicure, the Virginia Department of Health performed a comprehensive search of published medical literature on the topic from all over the world. They found 18 published reports since 1995 that included nail salons and/or barbershops, with most of these reports coming from outside of the US. This obviously isn't a large number of cases, but that shouldn't lull us into assuming that US salons and barbershops are safe, said Dr. Johnson. *Here's what's causing concern…*

It's unlikely that most cases of hepatitis would ever be directly connected with a salon or barbershop, since hepatitis B or C symptoms typically don't appear for 10 to 20 years after initial infection, he said. Let's say that you do end up with hepatitis someday— what are the odds that you're going to think to link your disease to that time a manicurist nicked your index finger 15 years earlier?

Health regulations in salons and barbershops are weak to nonexistent, Dr. Johnson said. He said that each state's board of cosmetology determines the rules—not each state's health department, surprisingly. And when it comes to regulations for disinfecting tools, there is wide variation. Some states, such as Texas, require sterilization of all equipment, while others lack specific regulations for disinfection. But even when a state's rules are strict, there is often little to no enforcement or understanding by the salon employees performing the service, said Dr. Johnson—so the protection of customers is likely to vary widely from salon to salon.

So how likely are you to get infected with hepatitis at a salon or barbershop? "The true magnitude of risk in the US has yet to be defined," said Dr. Johnson. "It hasn't been thoroughly studied."

How Hepatitis Sneaks Into Your Body

The implements that are used repeatedly on many customers can—at any time—come into contact with a customer's blood. This could be from a minor nip during a manicure or shave or possibly from a customer's previous sore, scratch or insect bite. If this customer has hepatitis, the residue from even a tiny bit of blood will contaminate equipment. Without proper disinfection, hepatitis C may remain in an active state on a surface for two weeks or longer, and hepatitis B may remain on a dry surface for seven days. And then if that infected tool is used on another person and nicks him/her, too (or if the instrument merely touches an open sore), the virus may travel into his or her body.

Getting hepatitis B or C is particularly scary, because during its years undercover in your body, the virus damages the liver. Then one day your first symptom may suddenly be a severe health issue, such as liver failure.

Salon Safety—What to Look For

The first thing you should do when you go back to your salon or barbershop is ask the manager, "How do you disinfect your tools?" Dr. Johnson said to look for a two-step procedure. First, they should clean off the implements with a brush or in soap and warm water or through ultrasound. The second step is to place the implements in a disinfecting solution for several minutes. (In many salons, this is the familiar blue liquid.)

Caution: Those seemingly high-tech UV light cabinets that are found in many salons now do not necessarily kill all germs—particularly bloodborne pathogens, like the hepatitis B and C viruses.

If you ask your salon about its disinfection procedures and are satisfied with its answers—then OK. On the other hand, if you still don't like what you see, shop around for a different salon—with hygiene procedures being the first thing on your check list.

Another strategy: Buy your own implements and bring them with you to the salon. Many salons have "file bags" or drawers for regular customers to store implements that are used only on them. This may reduce your risk but won't eliminate it, since there is still a chance that inappropriate disinfecting procedures might cross-contaminate your implements with another customer's. So your safest bet is to bring your own tools back and forth with you and disinfect them yourself—or ask your salon if they have any disposable tools that they can use on you.

If you do get nicked with a tool at a salon, you should ask for first aid—or at least thoroughly wash the wound with soap—to kill as many germs as possible and ask your doctor immediately whether or not you should be checked for the hepatitis virus, said Dr. Johnson.

Dr. Johnson hopes that this analysis will trigger more research on the topic in the US—and also encourage state cosmetology boards to create and enforce stricter rules nationwide. Most importantly, he said, "I am hopeful that this analysis will make both health-care providers as well as the people who use these services aware of a significant potential risk for preventable infection." But in the meantime, instead of reading a magazine during your next salon visit, keep an eye on that disinfectant solution—and make sure that it isn't there just for show.

Bikini Wax Warning

Cherie A. LeFevre, MD, director of the Vulvar and Vaginal Disorders Specialty Center, St. Louis University School of Medicine.

Are there any health risks associated with the Brazilian bikini wax?

Yes. Pubic hair serves the purpose of protecting the very delicate tissues in the vaginal area. It traps moisture and allows for its quick evaporation and keeps bacteria away from the skin and vaginal opening. After a Brazilian bikini wax (that removes all hair in the pubic area), most women will experience swelling, redness and slight irritation for a few days.

In addition, a Brazilian bikini wax as well as a standard wax (that removes hair only at the bikini line) can lead to microabrasions of the skin, which allow bacteria access to the body and can lead to folliculitis (infection around the hair follicles), ingrown hairs or cellulitis (bacterial infection of the skin).

Cellulitis can be a serious infection that requires antibiotics to treat and can even lead to sepsis (a systemic blood infection) and hospitalization.

If you really believe that you need a bikini wax to feel comfortable wearing a swimsuit, make sure that the salon disinfects waxing tools and that the aesthetician wears gloves.

Women who are diabetic, have chronic kidney or liver disease or immune disorders have a greater risk for infection and should avoid waxing or shaving the pubic region.

Dangerous Spa Foot Baths

Skin infections from spa pedicures are becoming common.

Self-defense: Broken skin should not come in contact with foot-bath water. Don't shave, wax or use hair-removal cream on legs in the 24 hours before going to a foot spa. Don't go to the spa if you have skin damage, such as cuts or bug bites, on your feet or lower-leg area. Ask salon workers if foot spas are disinfected after each customer and again at night with a hospital disinfectant.

Recommendations from the US Environmental Protection Agency.

Surprising Places Where Germs Hide—Bacteria and Viruses Often Lurk in "Hot Spots" You'd Never Expect

Elizabeth Scott, PhD, assistant professor of biology and codirector of the Center for Hygiene & Health in Home & Community at Simmons College in Boston. *www.simmons.edu/hygieneandhealth.* A member of the scientific advisory board of the International Forum on Home Hygiene, she is coauthor of *How to Prevent Food Poisoning: A Practical Guide to Safe Cooking, Eating and Food Handling* (Wiley).

Seasonal flu viruses can often be found in places that many people would never suspect. This is also true of other harmful microbes, such as methicillin-resistant Staphylococcus aureus (MRSA) bacteria, and bacteria, including Escherichia coli and salmonella, that cause foodborne illness.

What you may not know: It's been estimated that about one in three Americans are carriers (and transmitters) of staph bacteria—usually in amounts so small that no infection occurs in the carrier.

Since it's impossible to completely avoid dangerous microbes, one of the best ways to stay healthy is to be aware of germ "hot spots"—including ones that often are over-looked, such as…

• **Telephone receivers (and cell phones), TV remote controls, computer keyboards and copying machines.** Most of us know to wash our hands after touching public door-knobs or handrails, but we may not consider the microbes on telephone receivers (and cell phones), TV remote controls and computer keyboards in public places, at work or even in our own homes.

Other areas to be wary of include the control buttons on office copying machines, handles of communal coffeepots, elevator buttons and shared books or tools.

It's best to assume that any inanimate sur-face—such as Formica, stainless steel or even paper—that could have been touched by an-other person may be infected with viruses or bacteria. If you touch your mouth, nose and/or eyes (the body's main entry points for infectious organisms) after touching the in-fected surface, you may be exposed to the germ.

Cold viruses and many bacterial infections are primarily transmitted by such surface contact. Flu viruses—including the H1N1 and seasonal flu—tend to be transmitted through the air (via coughs and sneezes) but also can be passed through surface contact.

What you may not know: Since bacteria and cold and flu viruses can survive for up to several days on inanimate surfaces, you can be exposed to germs long after the infected person has contaminated the area. Scientists have estimated that 80% of all human infec-tions are transmitted via hand-to-hand or surface contact.

Self-defense: After touching inanimate surfaces (such as those described earlier) in a public place—or at home, if someone in your household is sick—wash your hands thoroughly with plain soap for 20 seconds under running water. Then dry them thor-oughly with a paper towel or air dryer.

Or apply hand-sanitizing gel containing at least 62% alcohol, such as Purell Instant Hand Sanitizer or Germ-X, as soon as pos-sible after touching such surfaces.

If someone in your home or office is sick: Each day, clean surfaces that are touched by others with a cleansing wipe or other product (such as those made by Lysol or Clorox) that is registered with the Environmental Protec-tion Agency (EPA)—check the product label for an EPA registration number. This means the product can be used as a disinfectant. Or simply squirt alcohol-based hand sanitizer on a paper towel and wipe the surface.

Important: Use wipes and gels that kill bacteria and viruses. These broader-spec-trum cleansers are sometimes labeled "anti-microbial"—not "antibacterial."

• **Paper money.** A 2008 Swiss study found that some strains of flu virus can survive on paper money for up to three days—and for up to 17 days when mixed with mucus.

In addition, a University of California re-searcher cultured 68 $1 bills and found that all but four had colonies of dangerous bacte-ria, including the variety that cause staph in-fections and pneumonia. Coins tend to have lower levels of bacteria and viruses—perhaps because they contain trace metals that help inhibit such microbes.

Self-defense: To reduce your exposure to germs, use credit or debit cards in place of paper currency as often as possible dur-ing daily transactions, and wash your hands with soap or use a hand sanitizer after touch-ing paper money.

• **Doctors' waiting rooms.** Studies have found that germs are transmitted at a particu-larly high rate in the waiting areas of doctors' offices—especially by touching countertops, pens and even magazines.

Self-defense: As much as possible, avoid touching shared surfaces (such as those de-scribed above), and wash your hands imme-diately after your doctor visit.

If hand-washing is inconvenient, keep hand sanitizer in your pocket or purse and carry your own pen to sign papers at doctors' offices and stores.

• **Pets.** An increasing body of evidence shows that dogs—and cats, especially—car-ry MRSA bacteria. It's believed that these animals are exposed to the germs by human carriers and that the bacteria contaminate the animals' coats, skin and saliva, where it can then be transmitted to other animals and people. MRSA bacteria can, of course, infect humans, but it also can make cats and dogs sick.

Important finding: A random study conducted at the University of Guelph in Canada found that 2% to 3% of dogs carry MRSA bacteria. Meanwhile, in a study of 35 homes, researchers at Simmons College in Boston found that people who have cats in their homes are eight times more likely to have MRSA bacteria on household surfaces than those without household cats.

Self-defense: Wash your hands or use a hand sanitizer after touching your pet…make sure any cuts or abrasions you may have are covered with a bandage before touching an animal…do not let pets lick your face…wash pets' food and water bowls in a sink separate from the one used to prepare your own food…and wear gloves whenever touching an animal that has an open wound.

• **Microwave ovens, countertops and salt and pepper shakers.** Most of us know that we need to clean kitchen faucet handles and sinks, sponges and cutting boards to avoid exposure to foodborne microbes. However, some surfaces tend to be overlooked, such as microwave oven controls—which are touched frequently, often while users are handling raw food—and countertops, which are high-contact areas for raw food. Research shows that salt and pepper shakers also are likely to be contaminated.

Self-defense: Immediately after preparing any raw food—including fruit and vegetables as well as meat, fish or poultry—wipe down any surfaces you may touch (such as microwave controls, countertops and salt and pepper shakers) with antimicrobial cleanser, or use a mixture of one part household bleach diluted in 10 parts water. Apply the cleanser with paper towels or disposable rags. If you use sponges, put them in the dishwasher each time you run it—or rinse, then microwave them for one minute at high power several times a week. Do not place sponges that contain metal fibers in the microwave.

• **Bathroom sink handles.** In one survey of the homes of 30 adults with colds, bathroom sink handles were identified as the place most likely to harbor traces of cold virus.

Self-defense: If anyone in your family has a cold or flu—or any other respiratory, skin or gastrointestinal infection—clean bathroom sink handles (as well as other potentially contaminated objects, such as doorknobs and light switches) at least once daily with antimicrobial cleanser.

INDEX